This book is due for return on or before the last date shown below.

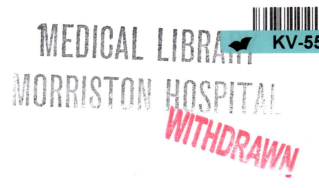
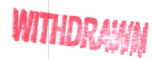

Radiofrequency Catheter Ablation of Cardiac Arrhythmias

Basic Concepts and Clinical Applications

Second Edition

Edited by

Shoei K. Stephen Huang, MD

Professor of Medicine
Associate Dean for International Affairs
Director, Laboratory Animal Center
National Taiwan University College of Medicine
Director, Cardiac Electrophysiology and Pacing Service
National Taiwan University Hospital
Taipei, Taiwan

and

David J. Wilber, MD

Professor of Medicine
Director, Clinical Electrophysiology
The University of Chicago
Chicago, Illinois

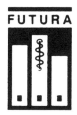

Futura Publishing
Company, Inc.
Armonk, New York

Library of Congress Cataloging-in-Publication Data

Radiofrequency catheter ablation of cardiac arrhythmias : basic concepts
   and clinical applications / edited by Shoei K. Stephen Huang and David
   Wilber. — 2nd ed.
      p. cm.
   Includes bibliographical references and index.
   ISBN 0-87993-438-7 (alk. paper)
   1. Catheter ablation.   2. Arrhythmia—Interventional radiology.
I. Huang, Shoei K. II. Wilber, David.
   [DNLM: 1. Tachycardia, Supraventricular—therapy. 2. Atrial
Fibrillation—therapy. 3. Catheter Ablation—methods. 4. Tachycardia,
Ventricular—therapy. WG 330 R129 1999]
RD598.35.C39R33   1999
617.4'12—dc21
DNLM/DLC
for Library of Congress   99-36034
                                                            CIP

Copyright © 2000

Published by
Futura Publishing Company, Inc.
135 Bedford Road
Armonk, New York 10504

LC #: 99-36034
ISBN #: 0-87993-438-7

Printed in the United States of America.

Printed in acid-free paper.

Dedication

To my children, Priscilla, Melvin, and Jessica

and

To my mother, Shing-Tzu Lin and late father, Yu-Shih Huang.

SKSH

To my colleagues and partners at the University of Chicago
whose skill, dedication and enthusiasm contributed greatly to this endeavor

and

To my wife, Sandy, and daughter, Jesse
Who provide the ultimate perspective.

DJW

Foreword

The past 20 years have witnessed a total revolution in the manner of treatment of patients with cardiac arrhythmias. Before the era of ablation, the treatment of arrhythmias was totally palliative, involving life-long dependence on drug therapy. Even if effective, the patient was exposed to potentially serious side effects and expenses associated with long-term drug treatment.

In 1982, we introduced the technique of catheter ablation involving direct-current shocks applied to the AV junction for control of drug resistant supraventricular arrhythmias. This technique had many pitfalls. While it obviated the need for drug therapy, the patients became pacemaker-dependent and those with atrial fibrillation still required anticoagulant therapy.

In 1987, the first reported clinical use of radiofreqeuncy (RF) energy for ablative procedures was reported; this energy form had many ideal features (Chapters 1–4) allowing for graded energy delivery to focal myocardial areas as opposed to the explosive discharge (associated with widespread damage) characteristic of high energy direct-current shocks.

Use of RF energy has resulted in developments where catheter ablation may now be offered as first line therapy for most supraventricular arrhythmias (Chapters 7–14, 20–28). In addition, catheter ablation can now be offered as first line therapy for patients with idiopathic forms of ventricular tachycardia (Chapters 29, 30) while great strides are continuing in improved mapping and ablation for patients with ventricular tachycardia associated with structural cardiac disease (Chapters 32, 33).

Of great import are the procedures that have been introduced for cure of atrial fibrillation. These procedures involve use of either linear ablation of atrial tissue (Chapters 18, 19) or ablation of foci which serve to trigger this arrhythmia (Chapter 17).

The text by Huang and Wilber is a remarkable effort to update both the electrophysiologist and specialist, as well as the general cardiac clinician in the realm of catheter ablation. In an era where rapid advances often make texts relatively obsolete by the time of publication, the editors and authors provide up to date, cutting edge information on all aspects of this burgeoning field. The work provides both the depth and breadth required by the specialist, but also provides excellent practical clinical information to allow the clinician greater knowledge and insight relative to the use of ablative therapy.

This second edition of the book contains virtually all the major therapeutic advances currently available, and the editors are to be congratulated for an excellent job. There will no doubt be further editions as our knowledge in this area expands. This is, in fact, the way cardiac electrophysiology has grown. A deeper understanding of arrhythmia mechanisms (particularly for atrial fibrillation) allows for introduction of newer modalities of therapy. We are indebted to the editors for providing us with the current platform, from which newer procedures and techniques will emerge.

Melvin Scheinman, M.D.
Professor of Medicine
University of California, San Francisco Medical Center

Preface

The initial clinical use of radiofrequency energy for the ablation of cardiac arrhythmias was reported in 1987. Over the past 12 years, the practice of radiofrequency catheter ablation has diffused from a small number of specialized centers to routine clinical use in a broad range of settings. The North American Society of Pacing and Electrophysiology maintained a voluntary registry between 1989 and 1993. During this time, the number of reported ablation procedures increased from 500 to nearly 15,000 annually in the United States. By 1998, estimates from industry and insurance databases indicate that between 80,000 and 100,000 ablation procedures were performed in the United States alone. The trajectory of growth worldwide has followed a similar path.

Since publication of the first edition of this book in 1994, not only the scope, but also the techniques and tools of radiofrequency ablation have evolved dramatically. Much of this new information has been made available only through subspecialty journals or national and international scientific presentations. The primary goal of the current edition is to provide a comprehensive and contemporary summary of the technical and clinical aspects of radiofrequency catheter ablation in a single volume. It is our hope that it will become a valued resource for reference, teaching, and daily decision-making. The primary audience for this book is trainees and established practitioners in clinical electrophysiology. However, it should prove useful for general cardiologists, nurses, technicians, and all who care for patients with cardiac arrhythmias. Fully two-thirds of the chapters are newly written for this edition, and the remaining chapters have been extensively revised and updated. We solicited the participation of a talented range of clinical scientists and leading practitioners. The majority of these contributors have made substantial independent contributions to the field in the areas covered by their individual chapters. Whatever the limitations of this multi-author approach, it is more than offset by an impressive breadth and depth of scientific and practical experience.

The book is divided into several sections. Part 1 is devoted to the fundamental principles of radiofrequency ablation, including biophysics, the pathophysiology and pathology of lesion formation, and the use and limitations of various monitoring techniques. A thorough grasp of this knowledge base is a fundamental prerequisite for the intelligent practice of catheter ablation. Parts 2–6 provide a systematic approach, including the most recent technical and strategic advances, to the ablation of specific cardiac arrhythmias: atrial tachycardia and flutter, atrial fibrillation, atrioventricular nodal reentrant tachycardia, tachycardias related to accessory atrioventricular connections, and ventricular tachycardia. Part 7 addresses issues of patient safety, complications, follow-up, and future perspectives.

A conceptual revolution in the field of cardiac ablation has been underway for several years. It is highlighted by an increasing appreciation for the role of specific anatomic structures and sites in genesis and maintenance of a broad range of cardiac arrhythmias. This knowledge has been translated into effective anatomically-based ablation strategies. As a corollary, anatomically based imaging has assumed greater importance. These issues are addressed in individual chapters where appropriate, but are covered more broadly in specific chapters on intracardiac echocardiography and electroanatomic imaging.

New catheter technology has always been an enabling feature of the field. Recently introduced tools, including the use of multipolar catheters for mapping and ablation, and electrode tip cooling during radiofrequency application, are discussed in individual chapters. Other new technical innovations are covered in chapters on specific arrhythmias. However, the pace of technological innovation invariably outstrips both publication times and the ability to provide an informed perspective of ultimate utility. It is probable that several new technologies and strategies currently in preliminary evaluation and planning stages will find their way into the chapters of future editions.

Finally, we sought to preserve and convey the fundamental excitement, energy and challenge of a maturing discipline. This book is published at a time of extraordinary recent advances and future opportunities to provide curative therapy and long-term relief for patients suffering with cardiac arrhythmias. They remain our ultimate teachers, and the focus of our collective efforts.

DJW
SKSH

Contributors

Boaz Avitall, M.D., Ph.D., F.A.C.C.
Associate Professor of Medicine, Director, Electrophysiology Services, Section of Cardiology, Department of Medicine, University of Illinois at Chicago, Chicago, Illinois

Helen Barold, M.D.
Clinical Cardiac Electrophysologist, JFK Medical Center, Atlantis, Florida

S. Serge Barold, M.D.
Director of Research, North Broward Hospital District Electrophysiology Institute, Broward General Hospital, Fort Lauderdale, Florida

Saroja Bharati, M.D., Ph.D.
Director, Maurice Lev Congenital Heart and Conduction System Center, The Heart Institute for Children, Christ Hospital and Medical Center, Oak Lawn, Illinois, Professor of Pathology, Rush Medical College, Rush-Presbyterian-St. Luke's Medical Center, Chicago, Illinois, Clinical Professor of Pathology, Finch University of Health Sciences/Chicago Medical School, North Chicago, Illinois

Ulrika Birgersdottir-Green, M.D.
Division of Cardiology, Department of Medicine, University of California San Diego School of Medicine, San Diego, California

Alfred E. Buxton, M.D.
Professor, Cardiology Section, Department of Medicine, Temple University School of Medicine and Temple University Hospital, Philadelphia, Pennsylvania

Hugh G. Calkins, M.D.
Director of the Arrhythmia Service and Cardiac Electrophysiology Laboratory, Johns Hopkins Hospital, Associate Professor of Medicine, Johns Hopkins University, Baltimore, Maryland

Riccardo Cappato, M.D.
St. Georg Hospital, Hamburg, Germany

Mau-Song Chang, M.D.
Professor of Medicine, National Yang-Ming University School of Medicine, and Director, Veterans General Hospital, Taipei, Taiwan

Shih-Ann Chen, M.D.
Professor and Director of Cardiac Electrophysiology, Division of Cardiology, Department of Medicine, National Yang-Ming University School of Medicine, and Veterans General Hospital, Taipei, Taiwan

Chern-En Chiang, M.D.
Associate Professor, Division of Cardiology, Department of Medicine, National Yang-Ming University, School of Medicine, and Veterans General Hospital, Taipei, Taiwan

Jacques Clémenty
Chef de service, Centre Hospitalier Universitaire de Bordeaux, Hôpital Cardiologie du Haut-Lévêque, Bordeaux, France

Philip A. Cooke, M.B.B.S.
Fellow in Cardiac Electrophysiology, University of Chicago, Chicago, Illinois

Robert F. Coyne, M.D.
Fellow in Cardiac Electrophysiology Allegheny University Hospitals, Philadelphia, Pennsylvania

N.A. Mark Estes III, M.D.
Director, Cardiac Arrhythmia Service, New England Medical Center, Boston, Massachusetts

Gregory K. Feld, M.D.
Director, Electrophysiology Program, Professor of Medicine, Division of Cardiology, Department of Medicine, University of Californi-San Diego School of Medicine, San Diego, California

Peter L. Friedman, M.D., Ph.D.
Cape Cod Cardiovascular Associates, Hyannis, Massachusetts

Gopal N. Gupta, B.S.
Section of Cardiology, Department of Medicine, University of Illinois at Chicago, Chicago, Illinois

David Haines, M.D.
Professor of Internal Medicine, Division of Cardiology, Department of Medicine, University of Virginia, Charlottesville, Virginia

Michel Haïssaguerre, M.D.
Professeur, Centre Hospitalier Universitaire de Bordeaux, Hôpital Cardiologie du Haut-Lévêque, Bordeaux, France

Ray W. Helms, B.S.E.
Section of Cardiology, Department of Medicine, University of Illinois at Chicago, Chicago, Illinois

Mélèze Hocini, M.D.
Centre Hospitalier Universitaire de Bordeaux, Hôpital Cardiologie du Haut-Lévêque, Bordeaux, France

Munther K. Homoud, M.D.
Co-director, Cardiac Electrophysiology and Pacemaker Lab, Cardiac Arrhythmia Service, New England Medical Center, Boston, Massachusetts

Henry H. Hsia, M.D.
Associate, Cardiology Section, Department of Medicine, Temple University School of Medicine and Temple University Hospital, Philadelphia, Pennsylvania

Shoei K. Stephen Huang, M.D.
Professor of Medicine, Associate Dean for International Affairs, Director, Laboratory Animal Center, National Taiwan University College of Medicine. Director, Cardiac Electrophysiology and Pacing Service, National Taiwan University Hospital, Taipei, Taiwan

Pierre Jaïs
Practicien Hospitalier, Centre Hospitalier Universitaire de Bordeaux, Hôpital Cardiologie du Haut-Lévêque, Bordeaux, France

John Kall, M.D.
Assistant Professor of Medicine, University of Chicago, Chicago, Illinois

Jonathan M. Kalman, M.B.B.S., Ph.D.
Section of Cardiac Electrophysiology, Department of Medicine and Cardiovascular, The Royal Melbourne Hospital, Parkville, Australia

Martin R. Karch, M.D.
Deutsches Herzzentrum Muenchen, Abteilung Fuer Kardiologie/Elektrophysiologie, Muenchen, Germany

G. Neal Kay, M.D.
Director, Clinical Electrophysiology Section, Division of Cardiovascular Disease, University of Alabama at Birmingham, Birmingham, Alabama

Dusan Kocovic, M.D.
Director, Electrophysiology Laboratory, Hospital of the University of Pennsylvania, Assistant Professor of Medicine, University of Pennsylvania School of Medicine, Philadelphia, Pennsylvania

Karl-Heinz Kuck, M.D.
St. Georg Hospital, Hamburg, Germany

Ling-Ping Lai, M.D.
Lecturer of Medicine, National Taiwan University College of Medicine, Attending Staff, Cardiac Arrhythmias and Electrophysiology, National Taiwan University Hospital, Taipei, Taiwan

Jonathan Langberg, M.D.
Professor, Emory University Hospital, Emory University School of Medicine, Division of Cardiology, Atlanta, Georgia

Thomas Lavergne, M.D.
Hôpital Broussais, Paris, France

Randall J. Lee, M.D., Ph.D.
Section of Cardiac Electrophysiology, Department of Medicine and Cardiovascular Research Institute, University of California-San Francisco, San Francisco, California

Shih-Huang Lee, M.D.
Associate Professor, Division of Cardiology, Department of Medicine, National Yang-Ming University, School of Medicine, and Director of Cardiac Electrophysiology, Shin-Kong Memorial Hospital, Taipei, Taiwan

Michael D. Lesh, S.M., M.D.
Associate Professor of Medicine, Director, UCSF Atrial Arrhythmia Center, Department of Medicine, University of California-San Francisco, San Francisco, California

Maurice Lev, M.D.
Professor of Pathology, Rush Medical College, Congenital Heart & Conduction System Center, The Heart Institute for Children, Palos Heights, Illinois

Albert Lin, M.D.
Assistant Professor of Medicine, University of Chicago, Chicago, Illinois

James C. Lin, Ph.D.
Professor, Department of Electrical Engineering and Computer Science and Department of Bioengineering, University of Illinois at Chicago, Chicago, Illinois

Jiunn-Lee Lin, M.D.
Associate Professor of Medicine, National Taiwan University College of Medicine, Director, Cardiac Electrophysiology Laboratory, National Taiwan University Hospital, Taipei, Taiwan

Mahadevappa Mahesh, M.D.
Chief Physicist, Johns Hopkins Hospital, Research Associate, Johns Hopkins University, Baltimore, Maryland

J. Michael Mangrum, M.D.
Division of Cardiology, Department of Medicine, University of Virginia, Charlottesville, Virginia

Frank Marchlinski, M.D.
Professor of Medicine, Director, Cardiac Electrophysiology, University of Pennsylvania Health System

Ali A. Mehdirad, M.D.
Cardiac Electrophysiologist, Mercy Cardiology Corporation, St. Louis, Missouri

Fernando Mera, M.D.
Fellow in Electrophysiology, Carlyle Fraser Heart Center, Emory University School of Medicine, Division of Cardiology, Atlanta, Georgia

William M. Miles, M.D.
Southwest Florida Heart Group, Fort Myers, Florida

John Miller, M.D.
Cardiology Section, Department of Medicine, Temple University School of Medicine and Temple University Hospital, Philadelphia, Pennsylvania

Michael M. Mollerus, M.D.
Division of Cardiology, Department of Medicine, University of California San Diego School of Medicine, San Diego, California

Larry Nair, M.D.
Fellow in Cardiac Electrophysiology, Duke University Medical Center

Sunil Nath, M.D.
Colorado Springs Cardiologists, Colorado Springs, Colorado

Jeffrey Olgin, M.D.
Assistant Professor of Medicine, Krannert Institute of Cardiology, Department of Medicine, Indiana University School of Medicine, Indianapolis, Indiana

Feifan Ouyang, M.D.
St. Georg Hospital, Hamburg, Germany

Franz X. Roithinger, M.D.
Universitaetsklinik Fuer Innere Medizin, Klinische Abteilung Fuer Kardiologie, Innsbruck, Austria

Lawrence Rosenthal, M.D
Assistant Professor of Medicine, Associate Director of the Electrophysiology Laboratory, University of Massachusetts Medical Center, Worcester, Massachusetts

Steven A. Rothman, M.D.
Associate, Cardiology Section, Department of Medicine, Temple University School of Medicine and Temple University Hospital, Philadelphia, Pennsylvania

Michael Schlüter, Ph.D.
St. Georg Hospital, Hamburg, Germany

Dipen C. Shah
Centre Hospitalier Universitaire de Bordeaux, Hôpital Cardiologie du Haut-Lévêque, Bordeaux, France

Hossein Shenasa, M.D.
Department of Medicine, Division of Cardiology, Duke University Medical Center, Durham, North Carolina

Jerold S. Shinbane, M.D.
Heart Place, Dallas, Texas

Grant Simons, M.D.
Department of Medicine, Division of Cardiology, Duke University Medical Center, Durham, North Carolina

William Stevenson, M.D.
Cardiology Department, Brigham and Women's Hospital, Boston, Massachusetts

S. Adam Strickberger, M.D.
Division of Cardiology, Department of Internal Medicine, University of Michigan Medical Center, Ann Arbor, Michigan

John F. Swartz, M.D.
Cardiology of Tulsa, Inc., Tulsa, Oklahoma

Ching-Tai Tai, M.D.
Associate Professor, Division of Cardiology, Department of Medicine, National Yang-Ming University, School of Medicine, and Veterans General Hospital, Taipei, Taiwan

Yasuhiro Taniguchi, M.D.
International Fellow in Electrophysiology, Gunma University School of Medicine, Gunma, Japan

Gregg W. Taylor, M.D.
University of Alabama at Birmingham, Birmingham, Alabama

Patrick Tchou, M.D.
Head, Section of Cardiac Electrophysiology and Pacing, Department of Cardiology, Cleveland Clinic Foundation, Cleveland, Ohio

George Van Hare, M.D.
Medical Director, Pediatric Arrhythmia Center, Pediatric Cardiology, Lucille Packard Children's Hospital, Stanford University, Palo Alto, California

Ismail Vergara, M.D.
Department of Medicine, Division of Cardiology, Duke University Medical Center, Durham, North Carolina

Alan B. Wagshal, M.D.
Department of Cardiology, Soroka Hospital, Beer-Sheva, Israel

Edward P. Walsh, M.D.
Chief, Electrophysiology Division, Department of Cardiology, Children's Hospital, Boston, Massachusetts

Paul J. Wang, M.D.
Associate Director, Cardiac Electrophysiology and Pacemaker Lab, Cardiac Arrhythmia Service, New England Medical Center, Boston, Massachusetts

Ming-Shien Wen, M.D.
Associate Professor of Medicine, Chang Gung Medical College, Attending Cardiologist, Chang Gung Memorial Hospital, Taipei, Taiwan

J. Marcus Wharton, M.D.
Department of Medicine, Division of Cardiology, Duke University Medical Center, Durham, North Carolina

David Wilber, M.D.
Professor of Medicine, Director of Clinical Electrophysiology, University of Chicago, Chicago, Illinois

Mark A. Wood, M.D.
Associate Professor of Medicine, Division of Cardiology, Medical College of Virginia, Richmond, Virginia

Delon Wu, M.D., F.A.C.C.
Professor of Medicine and Chancellor, Chang Gung Medical College, Attending Cardiologist, Chang Gung Memorial Hospital, Taipei, Taiwan

San-Jou Yeh, M.D.
Professor of Medicine, Chang Gung Medical College, Attending Cardiologist, Chang Gung Memorial Hospital, Taipei, Taiwan

Adam Zivin, M.D.
Division of Cardiology, Department of Internal Medicine, University of Michigan Medical Center, Ann Arbor, Michigan

Contents

Part I: Fundamental Aspects of Radiofrequency Energy Applications

Part II: Radiofrequency Ablation of Atrial Tachycardia and Flutter

Part III: Radiofrequency Catheter Ablation for Control of Atrial Fibrillation

Part VI: Radiofrequency Catheter Ablation of Ventricular Tachycardia

Part VII: Miscellaneous Topics

Part I

Fundamental Aspects of Radiofrequency Energy Applications

Chapter 1

Historical Aspects of Radiofrequency Energy Applications

Shoei K. Stephen Huang, M.D.,
Jiunn-Lee Lin, M.D.

Introduction

The introduction of radiofrequency (RF) current for catheter ablation of cardiac arrhythmias represented a significant stride and an important tool for catheter ablation procedures compared to direct current (DC) energy. However, RF current is not new to medicine, having been used in electrosurgery for over 60 years. It is worth mentioning that the history of destructive therapeutic techniques can be summed up by the statement that every new destructive technology that has been devised has been used in the human body for clinical purposes. Table 1 lists these technologies. Some of them are rational; others border on the diabolical. Cryogenic lesion making, chemical poisons, focal irradiation, and the laser have been used extensively. They all perhaps suffer from the same difficulties, namely, that the lesion is difficult to control and, in many cases, nonspecific. Throughout the years, the RF technique has apparently emerged as the most successful and effective energy source for clinical applications in many specialties.

The History of Radiofrequency Lesion Making

RF energy for lesion making has a very early historical root. In 1891, D'Arsonval applied the principle of using alternating current to avoid the undesir-

From Huang SKS, Wilber DJ (eds.): *Radiofrequency Catheter Ablation of Cardiac Arrhythmias: Basic Concepts and Clinical Applications,* 2nd ed. Armonk, NY: Futura Publishing Company, Inc. ©2000.

Table 1
Methods and Energy Sources for Lesion Generation

- Radiofrequency heating
- Direct current heating
- Cryogenics
- Focused ultrasound
- Microwave heating
- Laser heating
- Chemical destruction
- Induction heating
- Radiation
- Mechanical methods

able effect of neuromuscular stimulation during surgical procedures[1] and thus introduced the concept of RF current application. Subsequently, at the turn of the 20th century, ham radio operators first experienced the searing and cauterizing effects of RF current by inadvertently contacting the components of their transmitting and receiving radio sets. The first application of RF current for clinical use took place when the famous neurosurgeon Harvey Gushing, with his technician W.T. Bovie, carefully studied the use of high-frequency current for the purpose of electrocoagulation. This technique, which primarily used spark gap power amplifiers, has been in use since the 1920s for coagulation of blood vessels during surgery.[2] It was at that time that the first prototype electrosurgical generator became available. It is still as important today as it was when it was recognized by Dr. Gushing in the 1920s and 1930s. The first

Table 2
History of the Use of Radiofrequency Energy for Therapeutic Lesion Formation

Early 20th century: Ham radio operators experimenting with radio waves burned their fingers, thereby accidentally discovering potential for radio waves to generate localized heating.

1920s: Dr. Harvey Gusing and his technician, W.T. Bovie, used radiofrequency currents for electrocoagulation in neural tissue and introduced the first prototype electrosurgical generator.

1950s: Drs. W. Sweet and V. Mark showed that radiofrequency produced much more reproducible and controllable neural lesions than direct current energy.

Late 1950s: Drs. S. Aranow and B. Cosman developed first commercially available radiofrequency lesion generator for neurosurgery at Massachusetts General Hospital.

1960s–present: Growing applications of radiofrequency lesion generators, in conjunction with advances in technologies, have spread to neurosurgery, urology, dermatology, oncology, and cardiology.

Mid-1980s: Dr. S. Huang and coworkers introduced use of radiofrequency energy for cardiac lesion formation for control of cardiac arrhythmias.

Late 1980–2000: Widespread use of radiofrequency catheter ablation technique to successfully treat a variety of supraventricular and ventricular tachycardias in conjunction with the evolving designs of the new electrode catheter and mapping system.

commercially available lesion generators for the purpose of therapeutic controlled lesions in the brain were built by S. Aranow and B. Cosman after the pivotal suggestion made by Drs. W. Sweet and V. Mark, who demonstrated that high-frequency lesions made in the RF range were very reproducible and had sharp, well-defined borders.[3,4] These RF lesion generators were put into service at the Massachusetts General Hospital in the mid- to late 1950s. Since then, the field of RF lesion making has continued to grow and has paralleled the advances of solid-state devices and the methodology of modulating the waveform and controlling the output impedance and voltage by monitoring the probe tip temperature. These changes have enabled wide applications of RF current in many medical areas, particularly in the field of neurosurgery,[5–9] dermatological oncology,[10] and for the control of chronic pain syndrome.[11] The history of RF current application to therapeutic lesion formation is highlighted in Table 2.

The History of Applications of Radiofrequency Energy to Catheter Ablation Therapy for Cardiac Arrhythmias

Radiofrequency energy was first used as an alternative energy source in the experimental treatment of cardiac arrhythmias in a closed-chest canine model in February 1985 by Huang and coinvestigators, who found they were able to safely and effectively ablate the atrioventricular (AV) junction with a conventional 2-mm-tipped electrode catheter.[12,13] Before the introduction of RF catheter ablation technique, DC and laser energies were used to induce complete AV block in both animals and humans via a transvenous catheter.[14–18] Because of difficulties in controlling energy delivery and potential serious side effects of DC and laser ablation, Huang and his colleagues at the University of Arizona in Tucson began animal experiments using a 750 kHz microbipolar RF output from a SSE4 electrosurgical generator (Valleylab, Boulder, Colorado). Subsequently, Hoyt and Huang investigated several parameters that may influence RF lesion making.[19] The factors that were studied and shown to be significant on the bovine myocardial ablation in vitro included electrode size, electrode-tissue contact pressure, pulse power, and duration. Specific investigations of impedance rise and the accompanying coagulum formation at the electrode tip were later reported by Ring and Huang,[20] whereas special evaluations of the effects of temperature at the electrode-tissue interface on the lesion growth and the phenomenon of sudden impedance rise at the boiling point were well described by Haines (see Chapter 3).[21,22]

Since the initial introduction of RF catheter ablation, a wealth of studies of RF ablation of cardiac tissue in animal models, including the ventricles,[23–27] the coronary sinus,[28–30] the atrium,[31–34] and the tricuspid annulus,[31–35] have emerged. While RF current was safely and effectively applied in animals and humans[36–39] for complete AV junction ablation (see Chapter 15), interest was growing in modification of AV conduction to avoid implantation of a permanent pacemaker. The ability to induce partial AV block by titration of RF power output and duration was initially demonstrated in the animal experiments.[40–42] When applying this modification technique to humans in an attempt to treat 3 patients with refractory AV nodal reentrant tachycardia (AVNRT), it was incidentally found that the fast pathway of the dual AV nodal pathways was abolished with prolongation of antegrade AV conduction.[43] This technique, which was later regarded as the anterior approach method or fast-pathway ablation, has been substantiated in many other series[44–48] (see Chapter 21) and can be used as an alternative to slow-pathway ablation after the latter technique had failed (see Chapter 22). Selective ablation of the slow pathway of AV nodal reentry (the posterior approach method) was first described by Roman and Jackman et al[49] and has become an attractive approach and often the first choice to treat patients with AVNRT.[47,48,50,51] More importantly, production of the discrete lesion by RF ablation has enhanced our ability to understand the anatomy and the physiology of the AV nodal reentry at the critical AV junctional area (see Chapter 20).

Aside from successful clinical applications to ablate or to modify the AV junction, with the continuing improvement in catheter mapping technique and the understanding of the arrhythmogenic substrate, RF catheter ablation has become the standard therapeutic strategy in the treatment of: Wolff-Parkinson-White syndrome; AV reentrant tachycardia incorporating accessory pathways (see Chapters 23–28) [52–55]; atrial tachycardia (see Chapters 7–11)[56,57]; typical and atypical atrial flutter (see Chapters 12–14)[58,59]; and sustained ventricular tachycardia with (see Chapters 32 and 33) or without (see Chapters 29–31) structural heart disease.[60–63] Moreover, attention has been paid to increase the efficiency of RF ablation by the incorporation of a thermistor or a thermocouple in the distal ablation electrode,[64–66] use of the internal irrigation electrodes (see Chapter 35)[67] and the design of large-sized or other special types of ablation electrodes (see Chapter 39).[68–70] The temperature monitoring during RF catheter ablation improves the efficiency of energy delivery and reduces unnecessary impedance rise and coagulum formation. The very large ablation electrode, probably better equipped with a pair of separately-located thermistors,[70] could facilitate the creation of a long, linear lesion in the tissue with a critical reentry substrate. Ablation electrodes with intrinsic irrigation function can help cool down the catheter tip temperature and promote the deep-layer lesion formation, which is particularly attractive in the management of arrhythmogenic foci in the scar tissue or hypertrophied musculature.[66,67]

Recently, the success rate of RF catheter ablation technique for the treatment of cardiac arrhythmias has increased immensely by combining with the intracardiac echocardiography and the three-dimensional computerized mapping system. Intracardiac echocardiography using a 10 MHz rotating ultrasound transducer mounted on a 10F catheter has been used to directly visualize the detailed atrial anatomy and help identify the inferior vena cava-tricuspid annulus isthmus for RF ablation of atrial flutter,[71,72] and nicely aids in ablation of atrial tachycardia arising from the crista terminalis (see Chapter 14).[73] Lately, an ablation electrode incorporated with a magnetic field emitting device can easily rebuild the three-dimensional anatomy of the cardiac chambers by stepwise endocardial mapping and calculation of vector directions (see Chapter 36).[74,75] The revolutional integration of the computerized geometrical reconstruction not only enhances our understanding of the pathophysiology of cardiac arrhythmias but also creates a breakthrough in the arrhythmia therapy, especially for ablation of typical or atypical atrial flutter, incisional atrial tachycardia, or even atrial fibrillation.[76–78]

Summary

The RF lesion-making technique was established and has become solidified over the past several decades.[79,80] The lasting advantages and control of the RF lesion suggest that it is indeed the superior methodology in many areas of clinical practice, especially in the nervous system and catheter ablation of cardiac arrhythmogenic foci. Like the course of history in neurosurgery, it appears in the last few years that the use of RF current for cardiac ablation is showing the same or even better signs of success than it did in neurosurgery. There are many reasons the RF lesioning method has been so successful and why the paradigm from other clinical experience will also pertain in cardiology. The most important of these advantages can be succinctly summarized as follows:

1. RF currents (unmodulated sinusoidal waveforms at a relatively high frequency) do not cause any dangerous or unpleasant stimulation or sensory effect.
2. The RF lesion is well circumscribed and definable.
3. With temperature control, the RF lesion can be quantified from 1 patient to the next, and adverse effects, such as charring, boiling, and sticking, can be avoided.
4. The RF electrodes are amenable directly to various important targetry methods, such as impedance monitoring, stimulation, and recording during energy application.
5. The RF electrode is robust and can be made in a variety of configurations to suit a particular anatomical region or target.
6. RF energy output is easily controllable and can be simply delivered to electrodes that are used for routine diagnostic electrophysiologic study without a need for a special transmitter (such as a fiberoptic for laser, antenna for microwave, or transducer for ultrasound energy).

Thus, it is anticipated that a widespread application of RF current as an energy source to catheter ablation therapy of cardiac arrhythmias will continue and that RF catheter ablation will become a standard of care and the first line of treatment for symptomatic cardiac arrhythmias.

References

1. D'Arsonval M. Action physiologique des courants alternatifs. *Comp Rend Soc Biol* 1891;43:283–287.
2. McLean A. The Bovie electrosurgical current generator. *Arch Surg* 1929; 18:1863–1870.
3. Sweet WH, Mark VH. Unipolar anodal electrolyte lesions in the brain of

man and cat: report of 5 human cases with electrically produced bulbar or mesencephalic tractotomies. *Arch Neurol Psychiatry* 1953;70:224–234.

4. Cosman BJ, Cosman ER. *Guide to Radiofrequency Lesion Generation in Neurosurgery.* Burlington, MA: Radionics, Inc, 1974. Radionics Procedure Technique Series Monographs.

5. Brodkey JS, Miyazaki Y, Ervin FR, et al. Reversible heat lesions with radiofrequency current: a method of stereotactic localization. *J Neurosurg* 1964;21:49–53.

6. Fox JL. Experimental relationship of radiofrequency electrical current and lesion size for application to percutaneous cordotomy. *J Neurosurg* 1970; 33:415–421.

7. Alberts WW, Wright EW, Feinstein B, et al. Sensory responses elicited by subcortical high frequency electrical stimulation in man. *J Neurosurg* 1972;36: 80–82.

8. Organ LW. Electrophysiologic principles of radiofrequency lesion making. *Appl Neurophysiol* 1976;39:69–76.

9. Cosman ER, Nashold BS, Ovumann-Levitt J. Theoretical aspects of radiofrequency lesions in the dorsal root entry zone. *Neurosurgery* 1984,15: 945–950.

10. Dickson JA, Calderwood SK. Temperature range and selective sensitivity of tumors to hyperthermia: a critical review. *Ann N Y Acad Sci* 1980;335: 180–205.

11. Pawl PP. Percutaneous radiofrequency electrocoagulation in the control of chronic pain. *Surg Clin North Am* 1975;55:167–179.

12. Huang SK, Jordan N, Graham A, et al. Closed-chest catheter desiccation of atrioventricular junction using radiofrequency energy-a new method of catheter ablation [abstract]. *Circulation* 1985;72(suppl 3):III389.

13. Huang SK Bharati S, Graham AR et al. Closed-chest catheter desiccation of the atrioventricular junction using radiofrequency energy: a new method of catheter ablation. *J Am Coll Cardiol* 1987;9:349–358.

14. Gonzalez R, Scheinman MM, Margaretten W, et al. Closed-chest electrode-catheter technique for His bundle ablation in dogs. *Am J Physiol* 1981;241: H279–282.

15. Scheinman MM, Morady F, Hess DS, et al. Catheter-induced ablation of the atrioventricular junction to control refractory supraventricular arrhythmias. *JAMA* 1982;248:851–855.

16. Gallagher JJ, Svenson RM, Kasell JM, et al. Catheter technique for closed-chest ablation of the atrioventricular conduction system: a therapeutic alternative for the treatment of refractory supraventricular tachycardia. *N Engl J Med* 1982;306:194–200.

17. Narula OS, Bharati S, Chan MC, et al. Microtransection of the His bundle with laser radiation through a percutaneous catheter: correlations of hisologic and electrophysiologic data. *Am J Cardiol* 1984:54:186–192.

18. Narula OS, Boveja BK, Cohen DM, et al. Laser catheter-induced atrioventricular nodal delays and atrioventricular block in dogs: acute and chronic observations. *J Am Coll Cardiol* 1985;5:259–267.

19. Hoyt RH, Huang SK, Marcus FI, et al. Factors influencing transcatheter radiofrequency ablation of the myocardium. *J Appl Cardiol* 1986;1: 469–485.

20. Ring ME, Huang SKS, Graham AR, et al. Determinants of impedance rise during catheter ablation of bovine myocardium with radiofrequency energy. *PACE* 1989;12:1502–1513.

21. Haines DE, Watson DD. Tissue heating during radiofrequency catheter ablation: a thermodynamic model and observations in isolated perfused and superfused canine right ventricular free wall. *PACE* 1989;12:962–976.

22. Haines DE, Verow AF. Observations on electrode-tissue interface temperature and effect on electrical impedance during radiofrequency ablation of ventricular myocardium. *Circulation* 1990;82:1034–1038.

23. Huang SK, Graham AR, Hayt RM, et al. Transcatheter desiccation of the canine left ventricle using radiofrequency energy: a pilot study. *Am Heart J* 1987; 114:42–49.

24. Huang SKS, Graham AR, Wharton K. Radiofrequency catheter ablation of the left and right ventricles: anatomic and electrophysiologic observations. *PACE* 1988;11:449–459.

25. Ring ME, Huang SKS, Graham AR, et al. Catheter ablation of the ventricular septum with radiofrequency energy. *Am Heart J* 1989; 117:1233–1240.

26. Haverkamp W, Hindricks G, Gulker H, et al. Coagulation of ventricular myocardium using radiofrequency alternating current: biophysical aspects and experimental findings. *PACE* 1989;12:187–195.

27. Oeff M, Langberg JJ, Franklin JO, et al. Effects of multipolar electrode radiofrequency energy delivery on ventricular endocardium. *Am Heart J* 1990; 119:599–607.

28. Huang SKS, Graham AR, Bharati S, Lee MA, Gorman G, Lev M. Short- and long-term effects of transcatheter ablation of the coronary sinus by radiofrequency energy. *Circulation* 1988;78:416–427.

29. Jackman WM, Kuck K-H, Naccarelli GV, et al. Radiofrequency current directed across the mitral annulus with a bipolar epicardial-endocardial catheter electrode configuration in dogs. *Circulation* 1988;78:1288–1298.

30. Langberg JJ, Griffin JC, Herre JM, et al. Catheter ablation of accessory pathways using radiofrequency energy in the canine coronary sinus. *J Am Coll Cardiol* 1989;13:491–496.

31. Lee MA, Huang SK, Graham AR, et a1. Radiofrequency catheter ablation of the canine atrium and tricuspid annulus. *Circulation* 1987;76(suppl 4):IV-405.

32. Chauvin M, Wihelm J-M, Dumont P, et al. The ablation of canine atrial tissue by high-frequency currents: anatomical and hisological findings. *J Electrophysiol* 1988;2:407–414.

33. Lavergne T, Prunier L, Guize L, et al. Transcatheter radiofrequency ablation of atrial tissue using a suction catheter. *PACE* 1989;12:177–186.

34. Lee MA, Huang SK, Graham AR, et al. Transcatheter radiofrequency ablation in the canine right atrium. *J Interven Cardiol* 1991;4:125–133.

35. Jackman WM, Kuck K-H, Naccarelli GV, et al. Catheter ablation at the tricuspid annulus using radiofrequency current in canines [abstract] . *J Am Coll Cardiol* 1987;9:99A.

36. Lavergne T, Guize L, Le Heuzey JY, et al. Closed-chest atrioventricular junction ablation by high-frequency energy transcatheter desiccation. *Lancet* 1986;2:858–859.

37. Budde T. Breithardt G, Borggrefe M, et al. Initial experiences with high-frequency electric ablation of the AV conduction system in the human. *Z Kardiol* 1987:76:204–210.

38. Huang SKS, Lee MA, Razgan ID, et al. Radiofrequency catheter ablation of the atrioventricular junction for refractory supraventricular tachyarrhythmias [abstract]. *Circulation* 1988;78(suppl 2):II-156.

39. Langberg JJ, Chin MC, Rosenquist M, et al. Catheter ablation of the atrioventricular junction with radiofrequency energy. *Circulation* 1989;80:1527–1535.

40. Huang SKS, Bharati S, Graham AR, et al. Chronic incomplete atrioventricular block induced by radiofrequency catheter ablation. *Circulation* 1989;80:951–961.

41. Marcus FI, Blouin LT, Bharati S, et al. Production of chronic first degree atrioventricular block in dogs using closed-chest electrode catheter with radiofrequency energy. *J Electrophysiol* 1988;2:315–326.

42. Lopez Merino V, Sanchis J, Chorro FJ, et al. Induction of partial alterations in atrioventricular conduction in dogs by percutaneous emission of high-frequency currents. *Am Heart J* 1988:115:1214–1221.

43. Huang SKS, Chenarides J. Gasdia G. Abolition of the dual pathways and retrograde conduction in patients with atrioventricular nodal reentrant tachycardia by radiofrequency catheter ablation [abstract]. *Circulation* 1989;80(suppl 2):II-41.

44. Goy JJ, Fromer M, Schlaepfer J, et al. Clinical efficacy of radiofrequency current in the treatment of patients with atrioventricular node reentrant tachycardia. *J Am Coll Cardiol* 1990;16:418–423.

45. Lee MA, Morady F, Kadish A, et al. Catheter modification of the atrioventricular junction with radiofrequency energy for control of atrioventricular nodal reentry tachycardia. *Circulation* 1991;83:827–835.

46. Huang SKS. Advances in applications of radiofrequency current to catheter ablation therapy. *PACE* 1991;14:28–42.

47. Jazayeri MR, Hempe SL, Sra JS, et al. Selective transcatheter ablation of the fast and slow pathways using radiofrequency energy in patients with atrioventricular nodal reentrant tachycardia. *Circulation* 1992;85:1318–1328.

48. Langberg JJ, Leon A, Borganelli M, et al. A randomized prospective comparison of anterior and posterior approaches to radiofrequency catheter ablation of atrioventricular nodal reentry tachycardia. *Circulation* 1993;87:1551–1556.

49. Roman CA, Wang X, Friday KJ, et al. Catheter technique for selective ablation of slow pathway in AV nodal reentrant tachycardia [abstract]. *PACE* 1990;13:498.

50. Jackman WM, Beckman KJ, McClelland JH, et al. Treatment of supraventricular tachycardia due to atrioventricular nodal reentry by radiofrequency catheter ablation of slow-pathway conduction. *N Engl J Med* 1992;327:313–318.

51. Wu D, Yeh SJ, Wang CC, et al. A simple technique for selective radiofrequency ablation of the slow pathway in atrioventricular node reentrant tachycardia. *J Am Coll Cardiol* 1993;21:1612–1621.

52. Borggrefe M, Budde T, Podczeck A, et al. High frequency alternating current ablation of an accessory pathway in humans. *J Am Coll Cardiol* 1987;10:576–582.

53. Jackman WM, Wang X, Friday KJ, et al. Catheter ablation of accessory atrioventricular pathways (Wolff-Parkinson-White syndrome) by radiofrequency current. *N Engl J Med* 1991;324:1605–1611.

54. Calkins H, Sousa J, El-Atassi R, et al. Diagnosis and cure of the Wolff-Parkinson-White syndrome or paroxysmal supraventricular tachycardia during a single electrophysiologic test. *N Engl J Med* 1991;324:1612–1618.

55. Schlüter M, Ceiger M, Siebels J, et al. Catheter ablation using radiofrequency current to cure symptomatic patients with tachyarrhythmias related to an accessory atrioventricular pathway. *Circulation* 1991;84:1644–1661.

56. Walsh EP, Saul JP, Hulse JF, et al. Transcatheter ablation of ectopic atrial tachycardia in young patients using radiofrequency current. *Circulation* 1992;86:1138–1146.

57. Chen SA, Chiang CE, Yang CJ, et al. Radiofrequency catheter ablation of sustained intra-atrial reentrant tachycardia in adult patients: identification of electrophysiologic characteristics and endocardial mapping technique. *Circulation* 1993;88:578–587.

58. Feld GK, Fleck RP, Chen PS, et al. Radiofrequency catheter ablation for the treatment of human type I atrial flutter: identification of a critical zone in the reentrant circuit by endocardial mapping techniques. *Circulation* 1992;86:1233–1240.

59. Cosio FG, Lopez-Gil M, Goicolea A, et al. Radiofrequency ablation of the inferior vena cava-tricuspid valve isthmus in common atrial flutter. *Am J Cardiol* 1993;71:705–709.

60. Morady F, Harvey M, Kalbfleisch SJ, et al. Radiofrequency catheter ablation of ventricular tachycardia in patients with coronary artery disease. *Circulation* 1993; 87:363–372.

61. Stevenson WG, Khan H, Sager P, et al. Identification of reentry circuit sites during catheter mapping and radiofrequency ablation of ventricular tachycardia late after myocardial infarction. *Circulation* 1993;88:1647–1670.

62. Klein LS, Shih HT, Hackett FK, et al. Radiofrequency catheter ablation of ventricular tachycardia in patients without structural heart disease. *Circulation* 1992;85:1666–1674.

63. Nakagawa H, Beckman KJ, McClelland JM, et al. Radiofrequency catheter ablation of idiopathic left ventricular tachycardia guided by a Purkinje potential. *Circulation* 1993;88:2607–2617.

64. Langberg JJ, Calkins H, El-Atassi R, et al. Temperature monitoring during radiofrequency catheter ablation of accessory pathways. *Circulation* 1992; 86:1469–1474.

65. Gillette PC, Case CL, Calkins HG, and the Atakr Investigators Group. Closed loop temperature controlled radiofrequency catheter ablation [abstract]. *Circulation* 1993;88(suppl 1):I-165.

66. Kottkamp H, Hindricks G, Horst E, et al. Subendocardial and intramural temperature response during radiofrequency catheter ablation in chronic myocardial infarction and normal myocardium. *Circulation* 1997;95:2155–2161.

67. Nakagawa H, Yamanashi WS, Piths JV, et al. Comparison of in vivo tissue temperature profile and lesion geometry for radiofrequency ablation with a saline-irrigated electrode versus temperature control in a canine thigh muscle preparation. *Circulation* 1995;91:2264–2273.

68. Langberg JJ, Gallagher M, Strickberger SA, et al. Temperature-guided radiofrequency catheter ablation with very large distal electrodes. *Circulation* 1993;88:245–249.

69. Kuck KH, Schlüter M. The split-lip electrode catheter-improvement in accessory pathway potential recording [abstract]. *J Am Coll Cardiol* 1993; 21:173A.

70. McRury ID, Panescu D, Mitchell MA, et al. Nonuniform heating during radiofrequency catheter ablation with long electrodes: monitoring the edge effect. *Circulation* 1997;96:4057–4064.

71. Olgin J, Kalman J, Fitzpatrick A, et al. Role of right atrial structures as barriers to conduction during human type I atrial flutter: activation and entrainment mapping guided by intracardiac echocardiography. *Circulation* 1995;92:1839–1848.

72. Kalman J, Olgin JE, Saxon LA, et al. Activation and entrainment mapping defines the tricuspid annulus as the anterior barrier in typical atrial flutter. *Circulation* 1996;94:398–406.

73. Kalman JM, Olgin JE, Karch MR, et al. "Crista tachycardias": origin of right atrial tachycardias from the crista terminalis identified by intracardiac echocardiography. *J Am Coll Cardiol* 1998:31:451–459.

74. Shpun S, Gepstein L, Hayam G, et al. Guidance of radiofrequency endocardial ablation with real-time three-dimensional magnetic navigation system. *Circulation* 1997;96:2016–2021.

75. Kottkamp H, Hindricks G, Breithardt G, et al. Three-dimensional electromagnetic catheter technology: electroanatomical mapping of the right atrium and ablation of ectopic atrial tachycardia. *J Cardiovasc Electrophysiol* 1997;8:1332–1337.

76. Swartz J, Pellersels G, Silvers J, et al. A catheter-based curative approach to atrial fibrillation in humans [abstract]. *Circulation* 1994;90:I-335.

77. Haïssaguerre M, Gencel L, Fischer B, et al. Successful catheter ablation of atrial fibrillation. *J Cardiovasc Electrophysiol* 1994;5:1045–1052.

78. Haïssaguerre M, Jaïs P, Shah DC, et al. Right and left atrial radiofrequency catheter therapy of paroxysmal atrial fibrillation. *J Cardiovasc Electrophysiol*. 1996;7:1132–1144.

79. Kugler JD, Danford DA, Deal BJ, et al, for the Pediatric Electrophysiology Society. Radiofrequency catheter ablation for tachyarrhythmias in children and adolescents. *N Engl J Med* 1994; 330:1481–1487.

80. Zipes DP. Radiofrequency ablation: what is left? *Eur Heart J* 1995;16(suppl G):24–27.

Chapter 2

Physical Aspects of Radiofrequency Ablation

James C. Lin, Ph.D.

Introduction

Electromagnetic energy in the frequency region below 300 GHz is non-ionizing and has wavelengths in air longer than 1 millimeter. Energy with wavelengths longer than 10 meters (lower than 30 MHz) have propagation properties that differ greatly from those of wavelengths that approximate the human body's physical dimensions. Furthermore, at wavelengths closer to the millimeter limit of the spectrum, electromagnetic energy behaves as infrared radiation. It is customary for telecommunications use to divide the spectrum into bands with specific designations. Since its interaction with biological media differs according to the specific spectral band, these properties can give rise to different applications. The radiofrequency (RF) band of 300 kHz to 30,000 kHz (or 0.3 to 30 MHz with wavelengths from 1000 meters to 10 meters) is used in medicine for ablating, coagulating and cauterizing tissue. Although frequencies below 300 kHz can also be used for cardiac ablation, frequencies lower than 10 kHz are avoided to prevent stimulation of excitable muscular and cardiac tissues.

When RF energy is used, the applied voltage induces a current to flow between a small electrode inside or on the surface of the body to a large, grounded, dispersive electrode on the surface. In cauterizing tissue, a train of short RF pulses at high voltage is delivered through a pair of electrodes to create cutting and coagulation. For catheter ablation, RF energy is applied as a sinusoidal current through a small endocardial electrode to provide effective tissue heating.[1]

From Huang SKS, Wilber DJ (eds.): *Radiofrequency Catheter Ablation of Cardiac Arrhythmias: Basic Concepts and Clinical Applications,* 2nd ed. Armonk, NY: Futura Publishing Company, Inc. ©2000.

RF Energy Propagation in Tissue

A characteristic of RF frequency is that the associated wavelength is at least an order of magnitude longer than the dimensions of the human body. Its propagation behavior is therefore quasistatic and can be approximated using Laplace's formulation in electromagnetic field theory.[2,3]

The absorption of RF energy in tissues is governed by the electrical properties of tissue, specifically the dielectric permittivity and conductivity. Biological tissues are composed of macromolecules, cells, and other membrane-bound substances. At low frequencies, the behavior of dielectric permittivity is dominated by mobile ions associated with fixed charges on cell membranes and the resultant membrane capacitance. An applied electric field causes charges to accumulate at boundaries that separate different tissue regions such as intracellular and extracellular spaces.

At RF frequencies, insufficient time is allowed during each cycle to permit complete charging of the cell membranes. This behavior gives rise to a decrease in the value of dielectric permittivity through the RF frequency. Moreover, cell membranes become progressively short-circuited for frequencies above 1 kHz. This facilitates the participation of intracellular fluid in current conduction. It causes the conductivity to increase as the frequency increases. At the RF frequencies used for ablation, the conductive energy dissipation is considerably higher than dielectric energy dissipation. Accordingly, a reasonable approximation is obtained by neglecting dielectric permittivity and considering only the tissue conductivity such that Laplace's equation becomes

$$\nabla \cdot \sigma \nabla V = 0 \tag{1}$$

where σ is the tissue electrical conductivity and V is the electrical potential. The density of current (J) flowing at any point in the tissue is given from Ohm's law,

$$\mathbf{J} = -\sigma \nabla V. \tag{2}$$

The current flow is impeded by tissue resistance (which is related inversely to conductivity) and RF energy is extracted or transferred to the tissue. The transferred or absorbed energy is converted to heat in accordance with Joule's law which states

$$\mathbf{W} = \mathbf{J}^2/\sigma = \sigma (\nabla V)^2 \tag{3}$$

where **W** denotes the rate of energy absorption or the heating potential generated by RF energy as applied through the catheter electrode in a unit volume of tissue. The SI unit of **W** is watt per cubic meter.

A solution to equation (1) requires that V be specified at all points of the boundary throughout the region of interest. A pertinent set of boundary conditions is the voltage on the surface of the electrodes. In the case of unipolar ablation, RF energy is delivered from the electrode at the catheter tip inside the heart to a large, flat dispersive electrode on the skin surface. The voltage distribution between the active and dispersive electrodes in a homogeneous tissue is approximately given by

$$V(r) \sim V_o/r \tag{4}$$

where V_o is the voltage on the surface of the spherical unipolar electrode and r is the radial distance from the active electrode. The inverse proportion of voltage distribution to radial distance indicates a lower risk of cardiac stimulation or muscle contraction associated RF energy from cardiac ablation at 100 volts or less, which is the usual voltage used in RF ablation. The current density and time rate of heat generation are given, respectively, by

$$\mathbf{J} \sim -\sigma V_o/r^2 \tag{5}$$

$$\mathbf{W} \sim \sigma V_o^2/r^4 \tag{6}$$

Clearly, RF energy absorption decreases as the fourth power of distance from the active electrode. The rapid decrease suggests that applied RF energy diverges from the small electrode. Consequently, active tissue heating is localized to a very short distance from the electrode-tissue interface. For effective cardiac ablation, it is essential to maintain direct contact between the RF electrode and cardiac tissue. Slight pressure exerted on the myocardium by the catheter is useful. If the density of tissue (p) is known, $\mathbf{W}$ can also be expressed as a specific absorption rate (SAR) quantity in units of W/kg, such that

$$SAR = \mathbf{W}/\rho. \tag{7}$$

Note that SAR is a measure of the rate of RF energy deposition at points surrounding the catheter electrode. This distribution of SAR serves as the source of lesion formation in cardiac ablation following thermalization of absorbed RF energy. Figure 1 illustrates the SAR measured in a tissue-equivalent model for a catheter electrode operating at 500 kHz. It can be seen that the drop in SAR is about 7.5 dB/mm away from the electrode. At 3 millimeters the decrease is about 20 dB or 100 times.[4] The size of lesion produced would be the combined result of SAR, duration of RF application, and heat conduction in tissue.

RF heating would quickly become insignificant beyond a few millimeters from the active electrode. Heating would fall well below the thermal noise floor at the dispersive electrode on the body surface, provided that the dispersive electrode is large and in good contact everywhere. Increasing RF power delivery influences the magnitude of active heating (SAR) and its subsequent passive spread in lesion formation by RF ablation, but it has less influence on the region of active heat generation.

Desiccation and coagulation of tissue close to the electrode would decrease the tissue's electrical conductivity and raise the resistance to current flow. This, in turn, would further impede effective tissue heating and limit the size of RF-induced lesions. Lesions beyond the immediate vicinity of the electrode-tissue interface occur as a result of passive heat transfer from the shallow high temperature region. Indeed, studies have shown that RF-induced lesions increase rapidly in size during the initial period of power application. Subsequently, the rate of increase diminishes rapidly as the resistance rises at the electrode-tissue interface and the current flow falls.[5-7] This inevitable phenomenon of thermal lesion production may be assessed through changes in the impedance of the catheter electrode. It is noteworthy that measures to maintain good

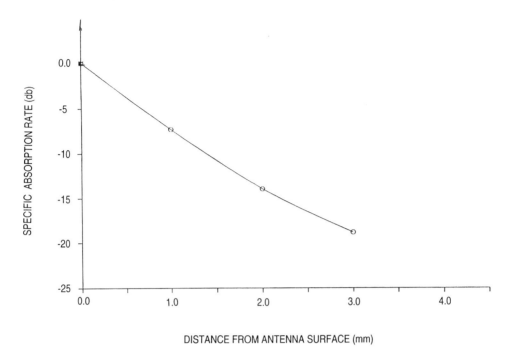

Figure 1. Measured SAR profile in a tissue-equivalent model for a RF catheter electrode operating at 500 kHz. Note that the drop in SAR is about 7.5 dB/mm away from the electrode. The decrease is about 20 dB or 100 times at 3 millimeters. (Adapted from [4].)

electrode-tissue contact such as increasing the contact pressure can enhance RF coupling to the tissue.[8]

The RF behavior of the electrode may be characterized by considering an equivalent circuit model of the electrode-tissue interface with a parallel combination of resistance, R, and capacitance, C. The effect of coagulative reaction of tissue on the input impedance of the catheter electrode during ablation is to introduce a resistance, R_o, in series with the R-C combination such that the impedance of the electrode becomes

$$Z = R_o + R/(1 + j2\pi f\, RC). \tag{8}$$

Biological tissue (muscle, for example) exhibits relatively large capacitance (on the order of microfarads/cm^2) and the resistance, R, is about 100 ohms at RF frequencies. Therefore, equation 8 can be approximated by

$$Z \sim R_o - j[1/(2\pi f\, C)]. \tag{9}$$

Thus, the electrode impedance is directly proportional to the series resistance arising from tissue reaction to ablation. Changes in electrode impedance provide a convenient way to monitor ablation effectiveness and to ascertain proper current flow during ablation procedures.[9,10] In particular, a rise in electrode impedance during ablation would indicate coagulative adhesion of tissue components at the electrode-tissue interface. This situation is demonstrated in Figure 2 where voltage, current, and electrode tip temperature were recorded simultaneously during an in vitro experiment.[11] The impedance, Z, is given by

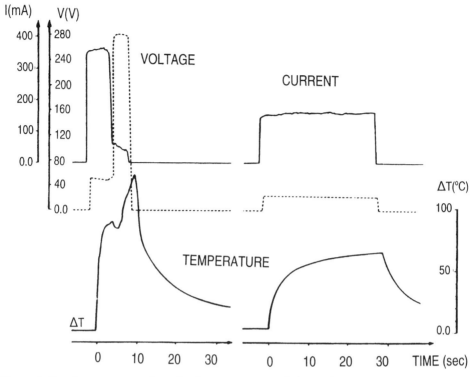

Figure 2. Simultaneous recording of voltage, current, and electrode tip temperature during an in vitro experiment illustrating the variation of impedance with temperature and tissue coagulation protein denaturation. The impedance, Z, is given by the ratio of voltage over current or V/I. (Adapted from [11].)

the ratio of voltage over current, or V/I. The graph on the right-hand side of the figure shows a typical rise in electrode tip temperature as a function of time following RF application. The maximum temperature reached is about 90°C. The accompanying impedance is stable and well-behaved. Similarly, the impedance remained relatively steady, and the electrode tip temperature initially rose smoothly, as shown on the graph to the left. As temperature continues to rise above 90°C, blood clots. The desiccated and coagulated tissue raises the resistance to current flow across the electrode-tissue interface. The impedance rises sharply (voltage jumps and current drops due to poor coupling between the electrode and adjacent tissue). The dramatic reduction in RF current flow is followed by a sharp decrease in temperature. This thwarts effective tissue heating and limits the size of RF-induced lesions.

Temperature Elevation in Tissue

In clinical practice the information of interest is temperature elevation and distribution in tissue. The dynamic temperature variation in tissue is a function of tissue composition, blood perfusion, thermal conductivity of tissue, and heat generation due to metabolic processes in addition to RF energy absorption.

The Pennes approximation to biological heat transfer via diffused conduction and blood convection in tissue can provide useful insights into RF ablation under the condition of uniform tissue perfusion by blood.[12] Specifically, the Pennes bio-heat transfer equation states that

$$d/dt \, (\rho cT) = \mathbf{W} + \eta \, \nabla^2 \, T - V_s \, (T - T_o) \tag{10}$$

where T is the temperature in tissue (°C), T_o is the temperature in blood and tissue (°C), ρ is the density of tissue (kg/m³), c is the specific heat of tissue (J/kg (°C)), $\mathbf{W}$ is the heating potential generated by RF power deposition (W/m³), θ is the coefficient of heat conduction of tissue (W/(°C m³)), and V_s is the product of flow rate and heat capacity of blood (W/(°C m³)). The numerical values of these parameters for muscle tissue are: ρ = 1000 (kg/m³), c = 3500 (J/kg °C), and η = 0.508 (W/(°C m³)). However, heat transfer by blood convection is considerably faster in well-perfused tissue, as is seen by a high V_s = 7.780 × 10⁶ (W/(°C m³)). Note that this equation neglects metabolic heat production since the usual period of RF application is 30 to 60 seconds, a period insufficient for significant metabolic heat contribution to tissue ablation.

The temperature distribution produced by RF ablation electrodes can be computed using the iterative technique of finite difference formulation of the bio-heat equation. The distribution of RF heating potential $\mathbf{W}$, calculated from Laplace's equation 1 and equation 6 serves as the driving source responsible for tissue temperature elevation. In addition, temperature distribution can also be measured using in vitro preparations and phantom models of cardiac tissue. However, it is only practical to measure the electrode tip temperature during the cardiac ablation procedure using currently available temperature probes.[13] Indeed, tip temperature-guided RF catheter ablation with large distal electrodes is used to improve lesion size.[14] It is important to recognize the distinctions among the electrode temperature, the temperature at the electrode-tissue interface, and the temperature in the tissue. The differences can be substantial if the temperature probe is far from the electrode-tissue interface.[15] Nevertheless, temperature monitoring and temperature control are valuable tools during RF ablation procedures because they provide important information regarding the adequacy of tissue heating. They also minimize the development of coagulum and maximize lesion size.[16]

The range of tissue temperatures used for RF catheter ablation is 50°C to 90°C with 60°C to 70°C as the target or optimal temperature for many temperature-controlled catheters.[14–18] Within this range, smooth desiccation of the tissue can be expected. If the temperature is lower than 50°C, no or only minimal tissue necrosis is expected. Figure 3 shows the time course of rising temperature produced by a 500 kHz endocardial RF electrode in a phantom model of muscle. It can be seen that the temperature in muscle near the electrode tip rose rapidly from 37°C to 52°C. A steady state temperature was reached in 5.0 seconds in this case. The actual rise in tissue temperature is controlled by the amount of power delivered and the duration of application.

The heat conduction term $\eta \, \nabla^2 \, T$ in equation 10 is a passive phenomenon that takes place slowly in muscle tissue. Therefore, with limited RF power deposition or heat generation at greater depths, the rate of temperature rise in cardiac muscle is only augmented weakly by heat conduction. Thus, prolonged

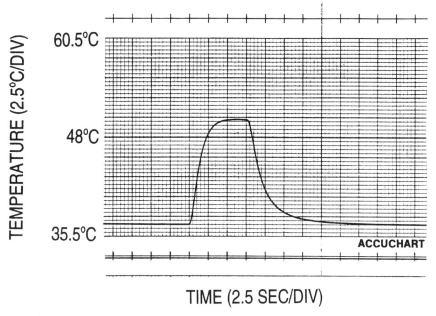

Figure 3. The time course of temperature rise produced by a 500 kHz endocardiac RF electrode in a phantom model of muscle. The temperature in phantom muscle near the electrode tip rose rapidly (by 15°C) in less than 5 seconds and reached steady-state in 5.0 seconds in this case.

RF power application (greater than 60 seconds) will not yield any significant increase in lesion size, since the half-time of thermal lesion growth is about 10 seconds.[5,6] Also, increasing the output power to heat deep lying tissues often results in excessive temperatures at the electrode-tissue interface without the desired enlargement of lesion size. However, with increased power delivery, the lesion size can be augmented somewhat by expanding the contact area between the endocardiac electrode and tissue at the interface. Viable approaches include extending the unipolar tip electrode length from 4 millimeters to 6 millimeters or longer[14] or connecting several electrodes of a quadripolar catheter in unipolar fashion for simultaneous delivery of RF energy.[19] Since temperature elevation and lesion formation rely on tissue resistance and current density, both approaches to increasing electrode size are limited by effective current density for ablation. Moreover, as the size of the endocardial electrode increases, the relative current density increases throughout the rest of the body, including the heart. It can be notably increased at the electrode-skin interface of the same dispersive electrode. Increasing the surface area of the dispersive electrode in contact with the skin can mitigate this phenomenon somewhat.

Note also that lesion formation is restrained by convective cooling from flowing blood. The convective heat exchange term, V_s $(T - T_o)$ in equation 10 serves to moderate temperature elevation in myocardial tissue because heat can be actively transported away from the generating site. Thus, sites with faster blood circulation, such as those near the mitral valve, require greater RF power delivery than those with slower blood circulation.

Mechanical Determinants of Lesion Size

Although RF catheter ablation has undergone explosive growth as the preferred treatment for a variety of arrhythmogenic substrates, the lesions induced by direct RF current heating are relatively small and shallow.[18,20,21] Several limiting factors with RF catheter ablation were mentioned above: small size of the electrode tip, divergent current flow, and coagulum formation around the catheter tip. RF techniques such as increasing power delivery, enlarged electrode tip or a serially connected quadripolar catheter, and monitoring and controlling the electrode temperature and impedance can overcome some of these limitations to enhance catheter ablation and produce larger and deeper lesions. However, all of these techniques are fundamentally frustrated by the effective current density needed for ablation through resistive heating.

Mechanical means of cooling or decreasing the electrode-tissue interface temperature can prevent excessive temperature buildup and subsequent coagulum formation at the interface during high power application. A lower temperature would minimize the incidence of electrode impedance rise stemming from tissue coagulation. However, at a given power level, a longer duration of RF energy application is required to allow accumulation of direct resistive RF heating to occur in deeper lying tissues.

One method of active cooling uses saline infusion through the catheter lumen and the ablation electrode during RF power application. It has been shown that saline irrigation during catheter ablation can produce significantly larger lesions.[22,23] Saline irrigation maintained a low electrode-tissue interface temperature at high power. It prevented any impedance rise and produced a higher temperature in deeper tissues than in the electrode-tissue interface. A technically less demanding but interesting approach in reducing the electrode-tissue interface temperature uses electrode tips made of gold.[24] Deeper lesions (7.2 versus 5.8 millimeters) were observed when RF energy was delivered to a gold rather than platinum tip electrode. It was proposed that since gold has nearly 4 times the thermal conductivity as platinum, the rate of heat removal by the circulating blood from the gold electrode-tissue interface is greater.

The coupling of RF energy to the endocardium is facilitated by maintaining a slight pressure from the electrode. In addition, the efficacy of RF catheter ablation depends on catheter-tissue orientation and the angle of electrode contact. With ablation catheters positioned parallel, perpendicular, or oblique to the myocardium, it was found that tissue temperature differed significantly with perpendicular or oblique placement as compared to the parallel electrode-tissue orientation.[25,26] The lesions were larger and deeper for an oblique electrode angle. As suggested in Figure 4, the difference would increase further with blood flow passing through the ablation site.[25,27]

Summary

RF ablation has become the preferred treatment modality for a variety of cardiac arrhythmias. RF energy delivered through a small endocardiac elec-

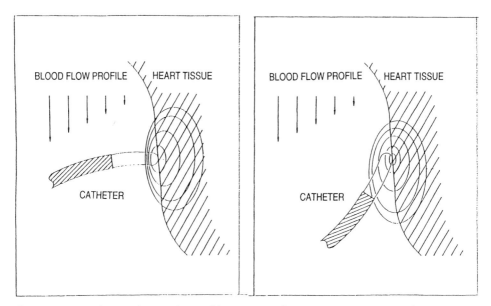

Figure 4. Dependence of RF catheter ablation on catheter-tissue orientation. The tissue temperature differs significantly with perpendicularity or obliqueness to the endocardium, as compared to the parallel electrode-tissue orientation. The difference would increase with blood flow passing through the ablation site. (Adapted from [27].)

trode is responsible for tissue modification and for producing the conduction block. An important precaution is that the dispersive electrode must be large (greater than 150 square meters) and in uniform contact with the skin to safely guard against high current density occurring at the edges. The biophysical aspects of RF cardiac ablation described in this chapter indicate that the dissipation or absorption of RF energy in the immediate vicinity of the electrode is the source of tissue temperature elevation and the subsequent lesion formation in RF ablation. The divergent nature of RF current flow from the catheter electrode and the rapid dissipation of RF energy by tissue resistance limit the depth and size of lesions produced. Several electronic and mechanical techniques can be invoked to enhance catheter ablation, produce larger and deeper lesions, and overcome some of the aforementioned limitations. However, all of these techniques are fundamentally baffled by the effective current density required for ablation through resistive heating. Treatment of certain subepicardial arrhythmogenic substrates remains a challenge for RF ablation.

Thermal microwave energy has been investigated for its potential in producing larger and deeper lesions. Unlike RF ablation, microwave energy is delivered through a radiating antenna mounted to the tip of a catheter. A dispersive electrode at the body surface is not needed. Tissue heating is produced exclusively by absorption of radiated microwave energy in the biological dielectric.[3] As compared to RF ablation, endocardial microwave antennas should increase the volume of direct heating since the lesion size is determined by the antenna radiation pattern, microwave power and duration of power delivery.

Comparison of phantom and in vivo results from RF and microwave ablation catheters showed that the volume of direct heating is indeed larger and that microwave energy is suitable for transcatheter ablation procedures.[4,28–32] Several microwave catheter antennas have been developed with efficient energy transfer into the myocardium.[30,33–35] Good dielectric and impedance matching and minimal power is reflected within the catheter transmission line or from the antenna.

References

1. Wagshal AB, Huang SKS. Application of radiofrequency energy as an energy source for ablation of cardiac arrhythmias. In: Lin JC, ed. *Advances in Electromagnetic Fields in Living Systems. Vol. 2.* New York, NY: Plenum Press, 1997. pp 205–254.
2. Michaelson SM, Lin JC. *Biological Effects and Health Implications of Radiofrequency Radiation.* New York, NY: Plenum Press, 1987.
3. Lin JC. Engineering and biophysical aspects of microwave and radiofrequency radiation. In: Watmough DJ, Ross WM, eds. *Hyperthermia.* Glasgow, Scotland: Blackie, 1986. pp 42–75.
4. Lin JC, Wang YJ, Hariman RJ. Comparison of power deposition patterns produced by microwave and radiofrequency cardiac ablation catheters. *Electronics Letter* 1994;30:922–923.
5. Blouin LT, Marcus FI. The effect of electrode design on the efficiency of delivery of RF energy to cardiac tissue in vitro. *PACE* 1989;12:136–143.
6. Wittkampf FHM, Hauer RNW, Robles de Medina EO. Control of RF lesion size by power regulation. *Circulation* 1989;80:962–968.
7. Nathan S, Dimarco JP, Haines DE. Basic aspects of radiofrequency ablation. *J Cardiovasc Electrophysiol* 1994;5:863–876.
8. Hoyt RH, Huang SKS, Marcus FI, Odell RS. Factors influencing transcatheter radiofrequency ablation of the myocardium. *J Appl Cardiol* 1986; 1:469–486.
9. Wagshal AB, Pires LA, Bonavita GJ, et al. Does the baseline impedance measurement during radiofrequency catheter ablation influence the likelihood of an impedance rise? *Cardiology* 1996;87:42–45.
10. Strickberger SA, Weiss R, Knight BP, et al. Randomized comparison of 2 techniques for titrating power during radiofrequency ablation of accessory pathways. *J Cardiovasc Electrophysiol* 1996;7:795–801.
11. Kottkamp H, Hindrick G, Haverkamp W, et al. Biophysical aspects of radiofrequency ablation: significance of sudden rises of impedance. *Z Kardiol* 1992;81:145–151
12. Pennes HH. Analysis of tissue and arterial blood temperatures in the resting human forearm. *J Appl Physiol* 1948;1:93–122.
13. Haines DE, Watson DD. Tissue heating during RF catheter ablation: a thermodynamic model and observations in isolated perfused and super perfused canine right ventricular free wall. *PACE* 1989;12:962–976.
14. Langberg JJ, Gallagher M, Strickberger AS, et al. Temperature-guided ra-

diofrequency catheter ablation with very large distal electrode. *Circulation* 1993;88:245–249.

15. McRury ID, Whayne JG, Haines DE. Temperature measurement as a determinant of tissue heating during radiofrequency catheter ablation: an examination of electrode thermistor positioning for measurement accuracy. *J Cardiovasc Electrophysiol* 1995;6:268–278.

16. Dinerman JL, Berger RD, Calkins H. Temperature monitoring during radiofrequency ablation. *J Cardiovasc Electrophysiol* 1996;7:163–173.

17. Pires LA, Huang SKS, Wagshal AB, et al. Temperature-guided radiofrequency catheter ablation of closed-chest ventricular myocardium with a noval thermistor-tipped catheter. *Am Heart J* 1994;127:1614–1618.

18. Wen ZC, Chen SA, Chiang CE, et al. Temperature and impedance monitoring during radiofrequency catheter ablation of slow AV node pathway in patients with atrioventricular nodal reentrant tachycardia. *Int J Cardiol* 1996;57:257–263.

19. Mackey S, Thornton L, He S, et al. Simultaneous multipolar radiofrequency ablation in the monopolar mode increases lesion size. *PACE* 1996; 19:1042–1048

20. Langberg JJ, Lee NA, Chin M, et al. Radiofrequency catheter ablation: the effect of electrode size on lesion volume in vivo. *PACE* 1990;13:1242–1248.

21. Nathan S, Dimarco JP, Haines DE. Basic aspects of radiofrequency ablation. *J Cardiovasc Electrophysiol* 1994;5:863–876.

22. Mittleman RS, Huang SKS, Deguzman WT, et al. Use of the saline infusion electrode catheter for improved energy delivery and increased lesion size in radiofrequency catheter ablation. *PACE* 1995;18:1022–1027.

23. Nakagawa H, Yamanashi WS, Pitha JV, et al. Comparison of in vivo tissue temperature profile and lesion geometry for radiofrequency ablation with a saline-irrigated electrode versus temperature control in a canine thigh muscle preparation. *Circulation* 1995;91:2264–2273.

24. Simmons WN, Mackey S, He DS, et al. Comparison of gold versus platinum electrodes on myocardial lesion size using radiofrequency energy. *PACE* 1996;19:398–402.

25. Kongsgaard E, Steen T, Jensen O, et al. Temperature guided radiofrequency catheter ablation of myocardium: comparison of catheter tip and tissue temperatures in vitro. *PACE* 1997;20:1252–1260

26. Panescu D, Whayne JG, Fleischman SD, et al. Three-dimensional finite element analysis of current density and temperature distributions during radiofrequency ablation. *IEEE Trans Biomed Eng* 1995;42:879–890.

27. Cosman ER, Rittman WJ. Physical aspects of radiofrequency energy applications. In: Huang SKS, ed. *Radiofrequency Catheter Ablation of Cardiac Arrhythmias*. Armonk, NY: Futura Publishing Co., 1995. pp 13–23.

28. Lin JC, Beckman KJ, Hariman RJ. Microwave ablation for tachycardia. *Proc IEEE/EMBS Int Conf* 1989;1141–1142.

29. Lin JC, Beckman KJ, Hariman RJ, et al. Microwave ablation of the atrioventricular junction in open heart dogs. *Bioelectromagnetics* 1995;16:97–105.

30. Lin JC, Hariman RJ, Wang YJ, et al. Microwave catheter ablation of the

atrioventricular junction in closed-chest dogs. *Med Biol Eng Comput* 1996;34:295–298.

31. Langberg JJ, Wonnell T, Chin MC, et al. Catheter ablation of the atrioventricular junction using a helical microwave antenna: a novel means of coupling energy to the endocardium. *PACE* 1991;14:2105–2113.

32. Whayne JG, Nath S, Haines DE. Microwave catheter ablation in myocardium in vitro. *Circulation* 1994;89:2390–2395.

33. Lin JC, Wang YJ. The cap-choke catheter antenna for microwave ablation treatment. *IEEE Trans Biomed Eng* 1996;43:657–660.

34. Lin JC, Wang YJ. A catheter antenna for percutaneous microwave therapy. *Microwav Opt Technol Lett* 1995;8:70–72.

35. Lin, JC. Catheter microwave ablation therapy for cardiac arrhythmias. *Bioelectromagnetics* 1999;20:120S–132S.

Chapter 3

Pathophysiology of Lesion Formation by Radiofrequency Catheter Ablation

Sunil Nath, M.D., David E. Haines, M.D.

Radiofrequency (RF) catheter ablation has emerged as the treatment of choice for reentrant supraventricular arrhythmias associated with accessory pathway conduction or the atrioventricular node.[1] The primary mechanism of tissue injury by RF ablation is likely to be thermally mediated.[2–5] Reversible loss of conduction can be demonstrated within seconds of initiating RF delivery, which may be caused by an acute electrotonic effect.[1,5] The accelerated beats frequently observed at the onset of RF delivery may be caused by thermally or electrotonically induced cellular automaticity or triggered activity.[5] Irreversible loss of electrophysiological function can usually be demonstrated immediately after a successful RF ablation; however, this finding may be delayed for up to several hours after the procedure. There may also be late recovery of electrophysiological function after an initially successful ablation. The underlying pathophysiological mechanisms that account for these early and late electrophysiological effects of RF ablation have not been fully elucidated. This chapter discusses the pathophysiological effects of RF catheter ablation with particular emphasis given to the cellular and tissue responses to hyperthermia and electrical field stimulation.

Thermal Injury

The mode of tissue heating by RF is resistive electrical heating, which means that only a thin rim of tissue in immediate contact with the RF electrode is directly heated. The remainder of tissue heating occurs as a result of heat

From Huang SKS, Wilber DJ (eds.): *Radiofrequency Catheter Ablation of Cardiac Arrhythmias: Basic Concepts and Clinical Applications,* 2nd ed. Armonk, NY: Futura Publishing Company, Inc. ©2000.

conduction from this rim to surrounding tissues. The temperature rise at the electrode-tissue interface is rapid ($t_{1/2}$, 7 to 10 seconds), and the steady-state temperature is usually maintained between 80°C and 90°C. However, because of the time required for heat conduction to deeper tissue sites, the rate of tissue temperature rise beyond the immediate vicinity of the RF electrode is much slower, resulting in a steep tissue temperature gradient,[3] but will continue to rise for several seconds after termination of energy delivery.[6] RF lesion size has been shown to be proportional to the electrode-tissue interface temperature, with higher temperatures resulting in larger lesions.[3] However, temperatures above 100°C are associated with coagulum formation on the RF ablation electrode and an electrical impedance rise, which potentially limits lesion size.[4]

Studies using mammalian cell culture lines have shown that cellular survival during hyperthermia is both time and temperature dependent.[7] Higher temperatures lead to both a more rapid and a greater degree of cell death (Figure 1). RF catheter ablation typically results in high temperatures (70°C to 90°C) for short durations of time (up to 60 seconds) at the electrode-tissue interface but significantly lower temperatures at deeper tissue sites. This leads to rapid tissue injury within the immediate vicinity of the RF electrode but relatively delayed myocardial injury with increasing distance from the RF electrode. Irreversible myocardial injury, as demonstrated by histochemical staining, has been reported to occur at an isotherm of 52°C to 55°C in an in vitro model of RF ablation using superperfused and perfused porcine right ventricular free wall.[8] In this model, RF power was adjusted to maintain an electrode-

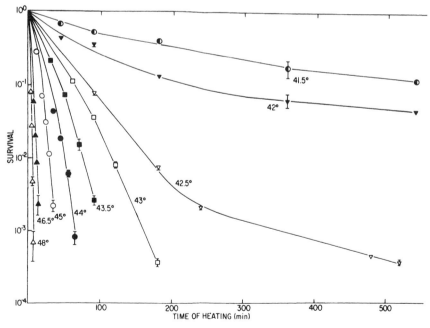

Figure 1. Survival of Chinese hamster ovary fibroblasts heated at various temperatures (T; 41.5° to 48°C) as a function of the heating time (minutes). As shown, cellular survival is both temperature- and time-dependent (Reprinted from Bauer and Henle[6] with permission.)

tissue interface temperature of 85°C for 60 seconds. Clinically, the mean electrode-tissue interface temperature (as measured by a thermistor-tipped ablation catheter) associated with permanent block of accessory pathway conduction was $62 \pm 15°C$.[9] Another clinical study examined the relationship of temperature to physiological effect using a power ramping protocol in patients undergoing atrioventricular (AV) junctional ablation. The mean temperature measured at the electrode-tissue interface was $51 \pm 4°C$ during hyperthermia-induced junctional automaticity, $58 \pm 6°C$ during reversible complete heart block, and $60 \pm 7°C$ during ablations that resulted in permanent complete heart block.[10] However, the values recorded by the catheter-mounted sensors may represent an underestimation of the critical temperature required for a physiological effect within the targeted arrhythmia substrate because of the sensors' remote location from the RF electrode and the falloff of tissue temperature with increasing distance from the electrode.

Although the cellular and tissue responses to hyperthermia have been described in detail[5,11,12] (see below), the exact pathophysiological mechanisms of heat-induced cellular and tissue injury are not fully understood.

Cellular Effects

Hyperthermia has profound effects on cellular electrophysiology, structure, and function. These include effects on the plasma membrane, the cytoskeleton, the nucleus, and cellular metabolism.

Electrophysiology

Hyperthermia exerts significant effects on many components of the sarcolemmal membrane and the intracellular structures such as the sarcoplasmic reticulum and mitochondria. It is anticipated that perturbation of these structures by hyperthermic exposure will result in impairment of cellular excitability and excitation-contraction coupling. Ge et al[13] tested the effects of RF catheter ablation on local action potentials in a model of superfused canine epicardial strips. They observed a loss of resting membrane potential, a decrease in dV/dt, and shortening of the action potential duration up to 6–8 mm from the lesion edge. However, severe abnormalities were only recorded within 2 mm of the pathological lesion.

The myocardial cellular electrophysiological effects of hyperthermia have been described in an in vitro model of isolated guinea pig right ventricular papillary muscle.[5] Hyperthermia was found to cause significant changes in myocardial cellular electrophysiological properties including: 1) marked depolarization of the resting membrane potential at temperatures $\geq 45°C$; 2) changes in the action potential characterized by a temperature-dependent increase in the maximal rate of rise and a temperature-dependent decrease in action potential amplitude and duration; 3) reversible loss of cellular excitability at a median temperature of 48.0°C (range 42.7°C to 51.3°C); 4) irreversible tissue injury only at temperatures ≥50°C; and 5) the development of abnormal automaticity at temperatures >45°C. These experimental observations have provided some insight into the temperatures that are required to produce reversible and irreversible myocardial injury during RF ablation. In addition, the finding of thermally-induced automaticity may explain the accelerated junctional beats frequently noted during RF ablation of the atrioventricular node or the "slow" atrioventricular nodal pathway.

Another in vitro study studied the effects of hyperthermia on myocardial conduction velocity in a model of superfused canine myocardium. Conduction was recorded from a multielectrode plaque during pacing at 600 milliseconds. At temperatures between 38.5°C and 45.4°C, conduction velocity was supranormal. In the intermediate hyperthermic range (45°C to 50°C), conduction was slowed. Transient conduction block and automaticity were observed with temperatures of 49.5°C to 51.5°C, and permanent block with temperatures ranging from 51.7°C to 54.4°C. Thus, the effects of brief hyperthermic exposure altered myocardial electrophysiology in vitro in a fashion similar to that seen in the clinical setting.[14]

Plasma Membrane

The plasma membrane is composed of a phospholipid bilayer and integral proteins that float within this bilayer. The hydrophobic, nonpolar hydrocarbon chains of the phospholipids face each other in the middle of the membrane, and the polar heads of the phospholipids are oriented to the aqueous phase inside and outside the cell. The degree of molecular motion of the hydrocarbon chains, which is primarily determined by the degree of saturation of the carbon-carbon bonds in the hydrocarbon chain, effects the fluidity of the membrane. Unsaturated hydrocarbon side chains allow more molecular motion and, hence, make the membrane more fluid. Pure phospholipid bilayers are thought to undergo phase transitions at different temperatures, resulting in different molecular orders. Below these transition temperatures, the phospholipids are in a solid-like state, while at temperatures above the phase transitions, the phospholipid bilayer becomes more fluid-like. Studies using cultured mammalian cells that have been heated to various temperatures have indicated 2 phase transitions. One transition occurs at 8°C, and the other between 23°C and 36°C.[15] No phase transition changes have been noted between 37°C and 45°C;[16] however, possible transition changes at temperatures above 45°C have not been investigated.

Membrane proteins serve as intracellular and extracellular receptors, transmembrane transporters, ion-specific channels, and ion-specific pumps. Hyperthermia is thought to cause protein conformational changes that result in protein inactivation. Studies using cultured mammalian cells have demonstrated that exposure of cells to temperatures of 39°C to 46°C results in inhibition of plasma membrane transport functions.[17] Intracellular ionic changes have also been observed after hyperthermic exposure. These changes depend on the cultured cell line used, as well as the magnitude and duration of the temperature change. Exposure of cultured Chinese hamster ovary cells to 42°C for

15 minutes resulted in an increase in intracellular K^+ uptake, which was inhibited by ouabain,[18] suggesting that this was due to an increased activity of the Na^+, K^+-ATPase pump. Other studies have reported a decrease in intracellular K^+ content when cultured mammalian cells were exposed to temperatures of 41°C to 43°C for 30 to 60 minutes, possibly because of an increased permeability of the plasma membrane to K^+ and consequent K^+ efflux from the cell.[19] Potassium efflux has not been a universal finding, since other studies have shown no change in intracellular K^+, Na^+, Cl^- or Mg^{2+} content after heating cultured cells to between 42°C and 45.5°C for 30 to 40 minutes.[20–22]

The precise mechanism of thermally induced myocardial injury is not defined at the present time. Preliminary experiments have been performed with an isolated guinea pig right ventricular papillary muscle model as described above. Papillary muscle tension was used as a surrogate marker for intracellular free calcium. It was observed that temperatures ≥45°C lead to increases in resting tension, and temperatures ≥50°C cause irreversible contracture of the myocardium.[23] Other studies using cultured mammalian cells, such as HT-29 human colon cancer cells and HA-1 Chinese hamster ovary fibroblasts, have reported increases in cytosolic calcium concentration during exposure to 44°C and 45°C, respectively.[24,25] In addition, an increase in calcium permeability of the plasma membrane at least partly mediated the heat-induced rise in cytosolic calcium concentration and was not prevented by calcium channel blockers.[25] One hypothesis of hyperthermia-induced myocardial injury that is consistent with these observations is that nonspecific injury to the sarcolemmal membrane occurs with temperatures ≥45°C. Extracellular sodium and calcium may then enter into the cell through the damaged plasma membrane resulting in depolarization and an increase in resting tension of the myocardium, respectively. The extracellular calcium influx into the cell may initially be buffered by calcium uptake into the sarcoplasmic reticulum and mitochondria, which may yield reversible myocardial injury at temperatures between 45°C and 50°C. However, in isolated sarcoplasmic vesicles from rabbit skeletal muscle, calcium accumulation rapidly declines at temperatures ≥50°C.[26] Additionally, sarcoplasmic reticulum ATPase activity is also inhibited at temperatures ≥50°C.[26] Therefore, it is hypothesized that irreversible injury to the myocardium occurring at temperatures ≥50°C is mediated by cytosolic calcium overload due to calcium influx across the sarcolemmal membrane and inhibition of the intracellular calcium buffering systems.

Cytoskeleton

Mammalian cells are composed of a cytoskeletal filamentous network composed of 3 types of filaments: microfilaments, microtubules, and intermediate filaments. In cultured cells, microfilaments, which are primarily composed of actin, form cytoplasmic bundles known as stress filaments. Stress filaments have also been shown to contain myosin, α-actinin, and tropomyosin in addition to actin. Stress filaments provide structural support to the plasma membrane and are responsible for maintaining cellular shape and morphology. Ex-

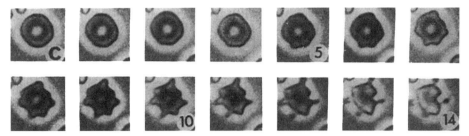

Figure 2. Alternate frames (50 frames/sec) of a human erythrocyte heated at a rate of 1°C/sec. Erythrocyte fragmentation occurs at a temperature of 50°C (Reprinted from Coakley and Deeley[27] with permission.)

posure of cultured Chinese hamster ovary cells to a temperature of 45°C was demonstrated to result in a rapid disruption of the stress filaments.[27] Heat-induced damage to the stress filaments may be caused by depolymerization of the actin-containing microfilaments, dissociation of the microfilament bundles, or a combination of both. Fragmentation of human erythrocytes has been shown to occur within 1 second at 50°C[28] and may be the result of heat-induced denaturation of the major erythrocyte cytoskeletal protein spectrin (Figure 2).[29] In cultured mammalian cells, hyperthermia causes blebbing of the plasma membrane, which has been correlated with the loss of cellular viability (Figure 3).[30] Blebbing of the plasma membrane also occurs after exposure of cultured cells to trypsin, local anesthetics, actinomycin D, and cytochalasin.[28] These agents are known to affect the cellular cytoskeleton. Thus, heat-induced blebbing of the plasma membrane and cell death observed in cultured cells may be caused by disruption of the cytoskeletal network.

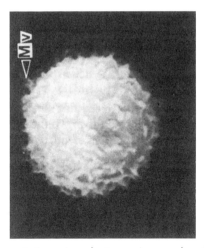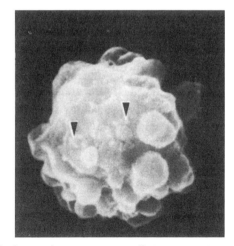

Figure 3. Scanning electron micrographs of Chinese hamster ovary cells in suspension. Left panel: Control cell at 37°C. The cell surface contains numerous microvilli (Mv). Right panel: After heating the cell at 45.5°C for 10 minutes, the cell surface contains numerous blebs. Small remnants of microvilli can still be observed (arrowheads.) (Reprinted from Borrelli et al[28] with permission.)

Nucleus

Hyperthermia causes a disruption of both nuclear structure and function. Morphological studies have shown vesiculation of the nuclear membrane, decreased heterochromatin content, and a prominent condensation of cytoplasmic material into the perinuclear region following thermal exposure.[31,32] One of the substructures within the nucleus is the nucleolus, which is the site of ribosomal RNA transcription and processing. The nucleolus appears to be a very heat-sensitive organelle in cultured mammalian cells. Changes in nucleolar structure and inhibition of nucleolar function have been observed at temperatures ranging from 41°C to 45°C.[33] Heating of cultured mammalian cells to 42°C to 45°C results in an inhibition of DNA synthesis as measured by a reduced incorporation of tritiated thymidine into cellular DNA.[34] Heat-induced inhibition of DNA synthesis appears to be caused by both a reduced initiation of DNA synthesis and depression of DNA chain elongation.[34,35] Whether heat is a direct cause of DNA damage is controversial.[36] Most studies indicate that hyperthermia alone does not cause DNA strand breaks. In some reports, DNA strand breaks have been observed, but in these cases they usually developed after the period of heating and were dependent on both the duration and temperature of the hyperthermic exposure.[34] The post-hyperthermic development of DNA strand breaks has been suggested to result primarily from cellular necrosis.[37]

A reproducible experimental finding is that hyperthermia results in an increase in nuclear protein content that appears to correlate with heat-induced cell killing (Figure 4).[11,38,39] Several studies have suggested that a significant

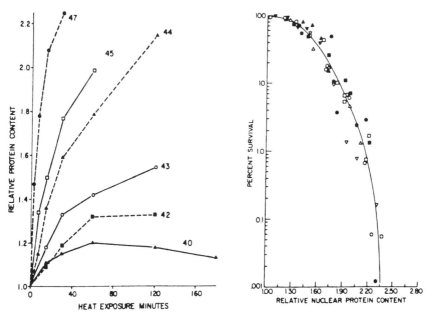

Figure 4. Panel (*left*): The effects of heating at various temperatures on the nuclear protein content of HeLa cells. Panel (*right*): Cellular survival as a function of protein content in HeLa cells immediately after heating to 45°C (Reprinted from Roti Roti and Laszlo[9] with permission.)

portion of the heat-induced excess nuclear protein is associated with the nuclear matrix.[32] The exact identity of this excess nuclear protein is not completely known, although one form has been identified as a heat shock protein known as HSP 70.[40] This protein is thought to translocate from the cytoplasm into the nucleus during cellular heat exposure. The exact pathophysiological role of HSP 70 is not known.

An alternative hypothesis for the increase in nuclear protein content is that hyperthermia causes disruption of the cell's cytoskeletal network, which leads to collapse of this structure toward the nucleus and absorption of cytoskeletal protein into the nuclear matrix.[41] The presence of this protein then results in disruption of nuclear function.[11]

Cellular Metabolism

Hyperthermia has been reported to cause alterations in cellular metabolism. Morphological changes including swelling, prominent cristae, and enlargement of the intracisternal spaces are observed in the mitochondria of cultured mammalian cells exposed to 42°C for several hours.[42] In addition, metabolic studies have revealed inhibition of both respiration and glycolysis (aerobic and anaerobic) in tumor tissue and cultured tumor cells exposed to temperatures of 42°C to 43°C.[43] The exact mechanisms involved in heat-induced inhibition of cellular energy metabolism and the association with structural changes of the mitochondria remain to be determined.

The effects of hyperthermia on myocardial cellular metabolism have not been reported. Our laboratory has investigated the effects of RF ablation on myocardial creatine kinase activity, an important enzyme in myocardial cellular metabolism.[44] Although clinical studies have shown no significant increases in serum creatine kinase activity after RF ablation, we postulated that this may be caused by thermal inactivation of the enzyme within the ablation zone. Serial RF ablations were performed on the epicardial surface of porcine left ventricle to test this hypothesis. Ten minutes after the ablation, a transmural tissue core 2 mm in diameter was taken from the center of the RF lesion. The sample was then rapidly frozen and sectioned longitudinally in 1-mm slices. The creatine kinase activity and total protein content were measured within each 1-mm slice of tissue and compared with controls. The creatine kinase activity within a typical RF lesion was calculated to be 29% of control. This study suggests that RF ablation results in loss of creatine kinase activity because of thermal inactivation of the enzyme.

Tissue Effects

Hyperthermia and Microvascular Blood Flow

Erythrocyte velocity and vessel luminal diameter have been measured within the microvasculature of rabbit granulation tissue exposed to temperatures of 40°C to 52°C for 60 minutes.[45] In this study, microvascular blood flow increased with temperature up to a critical value of 45.7°C but then rapidly declined at temperatures above this value. Histological studies using rat skeletal muscle exposed to temperatures of 43°C to 45°C for 20 minutes have demonstrated microvascular endothelial cell swelling and disruption, intravascular thrombosis, and neutrophil adherence to venular endothelium within 5 minutes of hyperthermic exposure. This was followed by an inflammatory cell infiltrate consisting of neutrophils and mononuclear macrophages which was most evident 6 to 48 hours after the hyperthermic insult (Figure 5).[46–48]

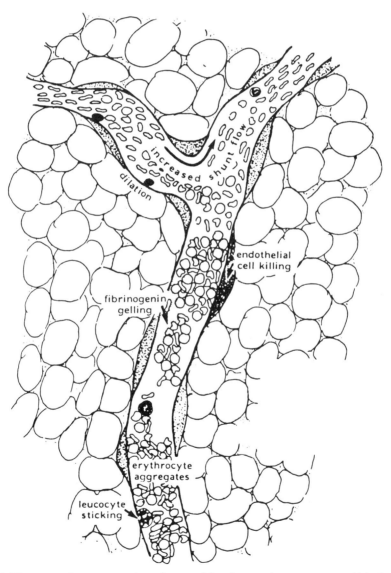

Figure 5. Diagrammatic representation of some of the changes that may occur within the microcirculation during hyperthermia (Adapted from Reinhold and van den Berg[44] with permission.)

Myocardial contrast echocardiography has been used to study the effects of RF ablation on myocardial microvascular blood flow in vivo using an open-chest canine model.[49] This study reported a marked reduction in microvascular blood flow within the acute pathological RF lesion. A significant reduction in microvascular blood flow extending beyond the edge of the acute pathological lesion was also demonstrated and was characterized by findings consistent with microvascular endothelial injury. The study concluded that the region of acute tissue injury produced by RF ablation was more extensive than the area of acute pathological injury, as demonstrated by histochemical staining.

The microvascular ultrastructure is dramatically altered in response to hyperthermia. Exposure of pial microvessels to 43°C resulted in platelet activation evidenced by degranulation, aggregation, and discoid platelets. The endothelial cells showed focal lucency, denudation vacuole formation, and membrane rupture.[50] Ultrastructural examination of the border zone region beyond the edge of an acute RF lesion in ventricular myocardium demonstrated marked endothelial changes. These included basement membrane disruption, plasma membrane dissolution, and erythrocyte stasis. These changes could be observed as far as 6 mm from the edge of the acute lesion. Thus, progression or resolution of the RF-induced tissue injury outside the acute pathological lesion may explain the late electrophysiological effects of RF ablation.[49]

Inflammatory Response

Acute and chronic histological studies of RF lesions in dogs after catheter ablation of the atrioventricular junction have been reported.[2,51] Light microscopic examination of RF lesions 4 to 5 days after the ablation has revealed well-circumscribed areas of coagulation necrosis surrounded by a peripheral zone of hemorrhage and inflammatory cells (consisting of mononuclear cells and neutrophils).[2] Chronic RF lesions examined 2 months after the ablation have shown fibrosis, granulation tissue, fat cell deposition, cartilage formation, and chronic inflammatory cell infiltration.[51] The contribution of the inflammatory response in the lesion border zone to lesion growth in the first 48 hours has not been determined.

Ultrastructure

Profound ultrastructural changes have been observed in ventricular myocytes in the border zone outside the region of acute coagulation necrosis of RF lesions (Figure 6). The general appearance of the near border zone (within 3 mm of the lesion's edge) was markedly disrupted with absent or severely distorted plasma membranes, missing basement membranes, and extravasation of erythrocytes. The mitochondria were swollen with discontinuous cristae membranes, and the T-tubules and sarcoplasmic reticulum were either absent or severely distorted. The sarcomeres were severely contracted or were extended with loss of myofilament structure. The far border zone (3–6 mm from lesion edge) showed similar but less severe ultrastructural changes. The

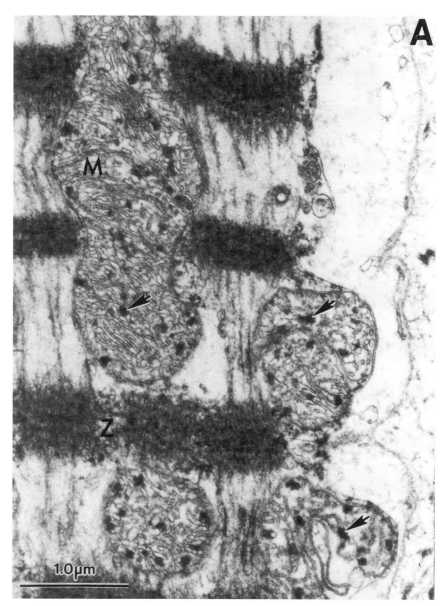

Figure 6. Electron micrographs at 33,000 × from 3 different regions outside of the edge of the acute pathological lesion created by RF ablation of ventricular myocardium. Panel A is a sample from the near border zone (within 3 mm of the lesion border), (*continued*)

plasma membranes were still severely damaged, but the mitochondria were less deranged, and the sarcomeres showed variability in their contractile state. Gap junctions were very distorted or absent in the near zone, but appeared normal in the far border zone. The intercalated discs showed only minimal structural distortion.[52] Immunochemical staining of the intercellular gap junction protein connexon 43 in a canine model of atrial fibrillation confirmed the observation that the density of gap junctions adjacent to regions of RF catheter ablation is markedly reduced.[53]

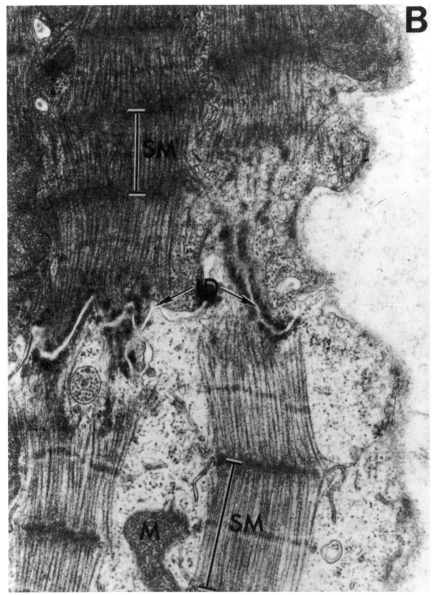

Figure 6. *(continued)* panel B is a sample from the far border zone (3–6 mm from the lesion border) and *(continued)*

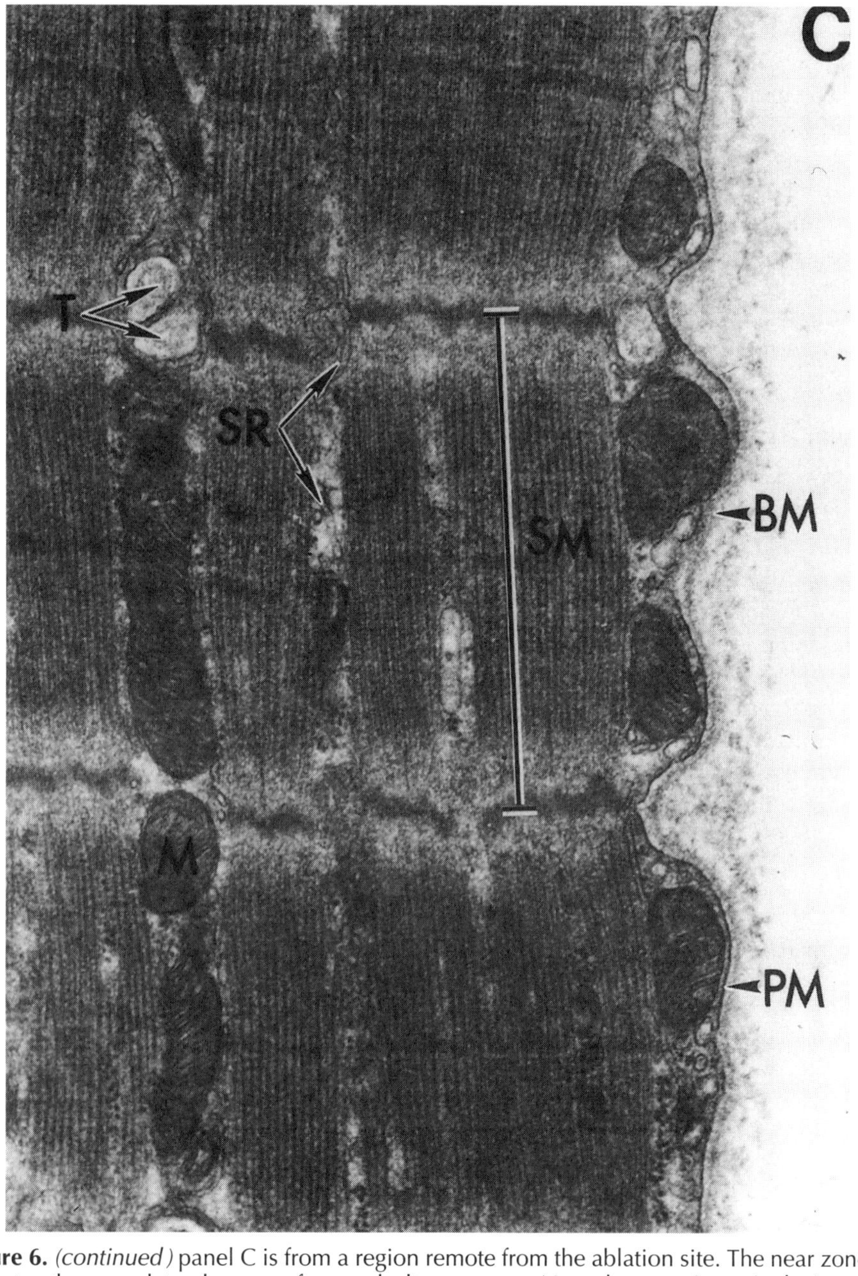

Figure 6. *(continued)* panel C is from a region remote from the ablation site. The near zone illustrates the complete absence of normal ultrasturcture. Note the prominent inclusions (arrowheads) in the remnants of mitochondria, thickened Z-lines, loss of myofilaments and absent plasma and basement membranes. From the far border zone, variation in sarcomere length among adjacent myocytes and disruption of the plasma and basement membranes are observed. The remote region demonstrates normal ultrastructural architecture of the myocytes. BM = basment membrane; ID = intercalated disc; M = mitochondrion; PM = plasma membrane; SM = sarcomere; SR = sarcoplasmic reticulum; Z = Z-line.[51]

Electrical Injury

Assessing the effects of radiofrequency current in the absence of tissue heating has been challenging, since significant heating invariably occurs within 1 or 2 seconds of onset of energy delivery. It has been observed clinically that an electrophysiological effect may be observed in the absence of significant temperature rise measured from catheter-mounted temperature sensors.[54] This could represent a direct electrical effect on myocardial conduction, or could alternatively reflect the inadequacy of surface temperature recording in representing the peak tissue temperature, particularly in high flow conditions.[55] Nonetheless, the contribution of direct electrical injury to the myocyte deserves further scrutiny.

Cellular Response to High-Intensity Electrical Fields

The response of cultured chick embryo myocardial cells to high-intensity electric field stimulation has been reported by Jones et al.[56] Stimuli of 60 to 200 V/cm resulted in cellular membrane depolarization and a progressive decrease in both action potential amplitude and duration. After intermediate levels of stimulation in the range of 60 to 80 V/cm, the cells exhibited an increase in automaticity. Further studies by the same investigators have demonstrated the incorporation of fluorescein labeled dextrans ranging in molecular mass from 4 to 20 kd into cultured chick embryo myocardial cells and indicated the presence of cellular blebbing following stimuli of 50 to 200 V/cm (Figure 7).[57] These data suggest that the cellular depolarization observed after high-intensity electric field stimulation may be caused by the formation of transient sarcolemmal microlesions that allow nonspecific ion exchanges across the plasma membrane.

Cellular Response to High-Intensity Radiofrequency Current

Cell biologists have used the technique of cell poration (i.e., reversible permeabilization of the cell membrane) to introduce genetic material into cells.[58] Cell poration has traditionally been induced by subjecting cells to a high-intensity direct-current electrical field. Although the response of myocardial cells to a RF field has not been investigated, the use of RF current to induce cell poration has been reported.[59] Cultured eukaryotic fibroblast cells were placed in a medium with DNA plasmids containing the cloramphenicol acetyltransferase gene. Using high-amplitude alternating-current fields (0.5 to 5 kV/cm) for brief durations (2 milliseconds), the study demonstrated intracellular incorporation of the plasmid DNA material. The most effective gene transfection (and, thus, the optimal electroporation) occurred when the field strength was between 1.8 to 2.1 kV/cm. Higher field strengths resulted in a marked decrease in cellular survival (Figure 8). A proposed mechanism for cell poration is that it is caused by a reversible dielectric breakdown of the cellular plasma membrane, resulting in the formation of membrane permeant pores. Comparable studies of the

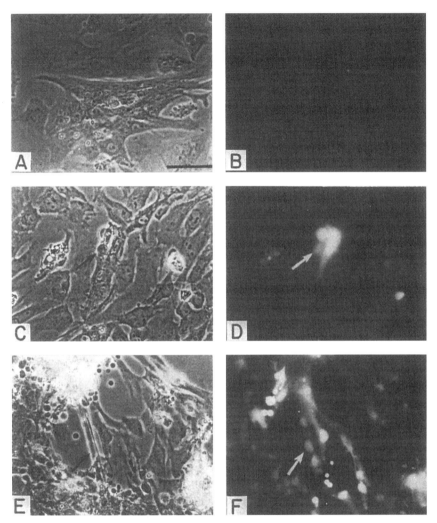

Figure 7. Panel A: Phase micrograph of myocardial cells 10 minutes after delivery of a "dummy shock." Cells were subjected to all treatment phases except that the shock was not delivered. Panel B: Fluorescence micrograph of same field showing lack of 10-kd dextran incorporation. Panel C: Phase micrograph of myocardial cells ≈ 10 minutes after 6 100-V/cm shocks (5-millisecond rectangular wave). A bleb is indicated by the arrow. Panel D: Fluorescence micrograph of same field showing incorporation of 10-kd dextrans. Circular fluorescent area corresponding to bleb in panel C is indicated by arrow. Panel E: Phase micrograph of myocardial cells ≈ 10 min after 6- to 200-V/cm shocks showing extensive damage including blebs (indicated by arrow). Panel F: Fluorescence micrograph of same field showing incorporation of 10-kd dextrans. Fluorescent area corresponding to bleb in panel E is indicated by arrow. All micrographs are same magnification; and bar represents 50 μm (Reprinted from Jones et al[50] with permission.)

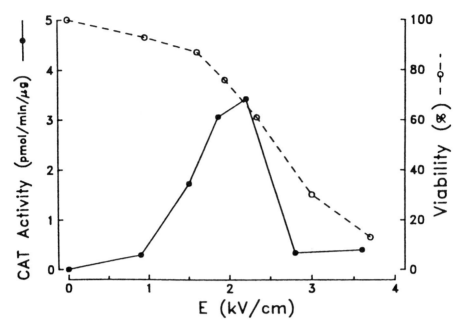

Figure 8. Cloramphenical acetyltransferase (CAT) activity and cellular survival as a function of the field strength (E) of the applied radiofrequency field. (See text for details.) (Reprinted from Chang[51] with permission.)

effects of lower energy alternating currents with a longer exposure duration on cell poration have not yet been reported.

Demonstration of the direct effect of electrical injury from RF current in the absence of heating has not been demonstrated in myocardial preparations using current amplitudes in the range that is used during clinical catheter ablation. Simmers et al[59] assessed the effects of radiofrequency energy and tissue heating on myocardial conduction in vitro. In this experiment, an isthmus was surgically created in a preparation of canine ventricular myocardium superfused at 37°C. They then heated this tissue with radiofrequency energy and measured the temperature at which conduction block through the isthmus was observed in response to pacing. Transient conduction block was observed at 50.7±3.0°C, and irreversible conduction block was observed at 58.0±3.4°C. The threshold temperatures for conduction block were similar to those observed in response to those seen after heating from a pure thermal source.[14] Therefore, the authors concluded that the dominant effect of physiological injury from radiofrequency heating was thermal. Further work must be performed to elucidate this question.

Conclusion

Although there are comparatively few studies on the pathophysiological effects of RF catheter ablation in vivo, a working framework can be established based on the biological effects of hyperthermia and electrical field stimulation which have been extensively reported in the literature (Table 1).

Table 1
Possible Biological Effects of RF Ablation

Thermal	
Cellular Effects	
Plasma membrane	
phospholipids	Possible changes in membrane fluidity[15]
proteins	Inhibition of membrane transport proteins[17]
	Kinetic and/or structural changes to ion channels and ion pumps[18–22]
Cytoskeleton	Disruption of stress filaments,[27] loss of plasma membrane support, and membrane blebbing[30]
Nucleus	Loss of nuclear structure and function[31–38,40]
Cellular metabolism	Inhibition of cellular metabolism[43]
	Denaturation of metabolic proteins[44]
Tissue Effects	
Microvasculature	Damage to microvasculature and reduced microvascular blood flow[45,47–50]
Inflammatory response	Secondary inflammatory response to initial thermal injury[2,47,51]
Electrical	
Plasma membrane	Formation of transient nonspecific ion-permeant pores in plasma membrane[56–58]

The initial, reversible loss of conduction observed immediately after the initiation of RF energy delivery may be caused by an electrotonic and/or heat-induced cellular depolarization. The speculated mechanisms responsible for depolarization include the transient formation of nonspecific ionic permanent pores in the plasma membrane by the RF electrical field and/or heat-induced effects on ion-channel/ion pump structure and kinetics. Cellular depolarization could result in spontaneous automaticity and may be the electrophysiological mechanism underlying the accelerated beats observed at the onset of RF ablation.[5] Irreversible loss of electrophysiological function immediately after a successful ablation is probably caused by thermal tissue injury, which results in a focal region of coagulation necrosis. The extent of tissue injury produced by RF ablation in vivo appears to be larger than the region of acute coagulation necrosis, which results in a border zone of acutely injured but viable myocardium. A secondary inflammatory response and/or ischemia as a consequence of microvascular damage may cause progression of tissue injury within the border zone. Progressive tissue injury may result in RF lesion extension over time and may be the pathophysiological mechanism for the late loss of electrophysiological function observed after RF ablation. Alternatively, resolution of the RF-induced tissue injury within the border zone may lead to late recovery of electrophysiological function, which has been reported to occur in approximately 5% to 10% of patients after an initially successful ablation.

References

1. Huang SKS. Advances in applications of radiofrequency current to catheter ablation therapy. *PACE* 1991;14:28–42.

2. Huang SK, Bharati S, Graham AR, et al. Closed chest catheter desiccation of the atrioventricular junction using radiofrequency energy-a new method of catheter ablation. *J Am Coll Cardiol* 1987;9:349–358.

3. Haines DE, Watson DD. Tissue heating during radiofrequency catheter ablation: a thermodynamic model and observations in isolated perfused and superfused canine right ventricular free wall. *PACE* 1989;12:962–976.

4. Haines DE, Verow AF. Observations on electrode-tissue interface temperature and effect on electrical impedance during radiofrequency ablation of ventricular myocardium. *Circulation* 1990;82:1034–1038.

5. Nath S, Lynch C III, Whayne JG, et al. Cellular electrophysiological effects of hyperthermia on isolated guinea pig papillary muscle: implications for catheter ablation. *Circulation* 1993;88:1826–1831.

6. Wittkampf FH, Nakagawa H, Yamanashi WS, et al. Thermal latency in radiofrequency ablation. *Circulation* 1996;93:1083–1086.

7. Bauer KD, Henle KJ. Arrhenius analysis of heat survival curves from normal and thermotolerant CHO cells. *Radiat Res* 1979;78:251–263.

8. Whayne JG, Nath S, Haines DE. Microwave catheter ablation of myocardium in vitro: assessment of the characteristics of tissue heating and injury. *Circulation* 1994;89:2390–2395.

9. Langberg JJ, Calkins H, El-Atassi R, et al. Temperature monitoring during radiofrequency catheter ablation of accessory pathways. *Circulation* 1992; 86:1469–1474.

10. Nath S, DiMarco JP, Mounsey JP, et al. Correlation of temperature and pathophysiological effect during radiofrequency catheter ablation of the AV junction. *Circulation* 1995;92:1188–1192.

11. Roti Roti JL, Laszlo A. The effects of hyperthermia on cellular macromolecules. In: Urano M, Double E, eds. *Hyperthermia and Oncology, Vol. 1: Thermal Effects on Cells and Tissues.* Utrecht, The Netherlands: VSP, 1988. pp 13–56.

12. Raaphorst GP. Fundamental aspects of hyperthermic biology. In: Field SB, Hand JW, eds. *An Introduction to the Practical Aspects of Clinical Hyperthermia.* London, England: Taylor and Francis; 1990. pp 10–54.

13. Ge YZ, Shao PZ, Goldberger J, et al. Cellular electrophysiological changes induced in vitro by radiofrequency current: comparison with electrical ablation. *PACE* 1995;18:323–333.

14. Simmers TA, de Bakker JMT, Wittkampf FHM, et al. Effects of heating on impulse propagation in superfused canine myocardium. *J Am Coll Cardiol* 1995 May;25(6):1457–1464

15. Lepock JR. Involvement of membrane in cellular responses to hyperthermia. *Radiat Res* 1982;92:433–438.

16. Mehdi SQ, Recktenwald DJ, Smith LM, et al. Effect of hyperthermia on murine cell surface histocompatibility antigens. *Cancer Res* 1984;44: 3394–3397.

17. Slusser H, Hopwood LE, Kapiszewska M. Inhibition of membrane transport by hyperthermia. *Natl Cancer Inst Monogr* 1982;61:85–87.

18. Stevenson AP, Galey WR, Tobey RA. Hyperthermia-induced increase in potassium transport in Chinese hamster cells. *J Cell Physiol* 1983;115:75–86.

19. Yi PN. Cellular ion content changes during and after hyperthermia. *Biochem Biophys Res Comm* 1979;91:177–182.
20. Vidair CA, Dewey WC. Evaluation of a role for intracellular Na^+, K^+, CA^{2+}, and Mg^{2+} in hyperthermic cell killing. *Radiat Res* 1986;105:187–200.
21. Boonstra J, Schamhart DHJ, DeLaat SW, et al. Analysis of K^+ and Na^+ transport and intracellular contents during and after heat shock and their role in protein synthesis in rat hepatoma cells. *Cancer Res* 1984;44:955–960.
22. Borrelli MJ, Carlini WG, Ransom BR, et al. Ion-sensitive microelectrode measurements of free intracellular chloride and potassium concentrations in hyperthermia-treated neuroblastoma cells. *J Cell Physiol* 1986;129:175–184.
23. Nath S, Lynch C III, Whayne JG, et al. Calcium overload: the mechanism for acute myocellular injury during radiofrequency catheter ablation? [abstract] *Circulation* 1993;88(suppl 1):I–399.
24. Stevenson MA, Calderwood SK, Hahn GM. Rapid increases in inositol triphosphate and intracellular Ca^{++} after heart shock. *Biochem Biophys Res Commun* 1986;137:826–833.
25. Mikkelsen RB, Reinlib L, Donowitz M, et al. Hyperthermia effects on cytosolic (Ca^{2+}): analysis at the single cell level by digitized imaging microscopy and cell survival. *Cancer Res* 1991;51:359–364.
26. Inesi G, Millman M, Eletr S. Temperature-induced transitions of function and structure in sarcoplasmic reticulum membranes. *J Mol Biol* 1973;81: 483–504.
27. Glass JR, DeWitt RG, Cress AE. Rapid loss of stress fibers in Chinese hamster ovary cells after hyperthermia. *Cancer Res* 1985;11:258–262.
28. Coakley WT. Hyperthermia effects on the cytoskeleton and on cell morphology. In: Bowler K, Fuller BJ, eds. *Temperature and Animal Cells.* Cambridge, England: Company of Biologists, 1987. pp 187–211.
29. Coakley WT, Deeley JOT. Effects of ionic strength, serum protein and surface changes on membrane movements and vesicle production in heated erythrocytes. *Biochim Biophys Acta* 1980;602:355–375.
30. Borrelli MJ, Wong RSL, Dewey WC. A direct correlation between hyperthermia-induced membrane blebbing and survival in synchronous G1 CHO cells. *J Cell Physiol* 1986;126:181–190.
31. Warters RL, Roti Roti JL. Hyperthermia and the cell nucleus. *Radiat Res* 1982;92:458–462.
32. Warters RL, Yasui LS, Sharma R, et al. Heat shock (45°C) results in an increase of nuclear matrix protein mass in HeLa cells. *Int J Radiat Biol* 1986;50:253–268.
33. Simard R, Bernhard W. Heat sensitive cellular function located in the nucleolus. *J Cell Biol* 1967;34:61–76.
34. Wong RSL, Dewey WC. Molecular studies on hyperthermic inhibition of DNA synthesis in Chinese hamster ovary cells. *Radiat Res* 1982;92:370–395.
35. Wong RSL, Dewey WC. Effect of hyperthermia on DNA synthesis. In: Anghileri LJ, Robert J, eds. *Hyperthermia in Cancer Treatment, Vol. 1.* Boca Raton, FL: CRC Press, 1986. pp 80–89.
36. Raaphorst GP, Feeley MM. Hyperthermic damage and its repair or fixation measured at the cellular level. In: Sugahara T, Saito M, eds. *Hyperthermic Oncology, Vol. 2.* Kyoto, Japan: Taylor and Francis, 1989 pp 181–182.

37. Warters RL, Henle KJ. DNA degradation in Chinese hamster ovary cells after exposure to hyperthermia. *Cancer Res* 1982;42:4427–4432.

38. Roti Roti JL, Henle KJ, Winward RT. The kinetics of increase in chromatin protein content in heated cells: a possible role in cell killing. *Radiat Res* 1979;78:522–531.

39. Roti Roti JL. Heat-induced cell death and radiosensitization: molecular mechanisms. *Natl Cancer Inst Monogr* 1982;61:3–10.

40. Welch WJ, Feramisco JR. Nuclear and nucleolar localization of the 72000-dalton heat shock protein in heat-shocked mammalian cells. *J Biol Chem* 1984;259:4501–4513.

41. Coss RA, Wachsberger PR. Role of cytoskeletal damage in heat killing of G1 populations of CHO cells. In: Fielden EM, Fowler JF, Hendry JH, Scott D, eds. *Proceedings of the Eighth International Congress on Radiation Research.* London, England: Taylor and Francis, 1987 pp 340.

42. Welch WJ, Suhan JP. Morphological study of the mammalian stress response: characterization of changes in cytoplasmic organelles, cytoskeleton and nucleoli, and appearance of intranuclear actin filaments in rat fibroblasts after heat-shock treatment. *J Cell Biol* 1985;101:1198–1211.

43. Dickson JA, Calderwood SK. Effects of hyperglycemia and hyperthermia on the pH, glycolysis, and respiration of the Yoshida sarcoma in vivo. *J Natl Cancer Inst* 1979;63:1371–1381.

44. Haines DE, Whayne JG, Walker J, et al. The effect of radiofrequency catheter ablation on myocardial creatine kinase activity. *J Cardiovasc Electrophysiol* 1995;6:79–88.

45. Dudar TE, Jain RK. Differential response of normal and tumor microcirculation to hyperthermia. *Cancer Res* 1984;44:605–612.

46. Reinhold HS, van den Berg AP. Effects of hyperthermia on blood flow and metabolism. In: Field SB, Hand JW, eds. *An Introduction to the Practical Aspects to Clinical Hyperthermia.* London, England: Taylor and Francis, 1990 pp 77–107.

47. Badylak SF, Babbs CF, Skojac TM, et al. Hyperthermia-induced vascular injury in normal and neoplastic tissue. *Cancer* 1985;56:991–1000.

48. Ferguson MK, Seifert FC, Replogle RL. Leukocyte adherence in venules of rat skeletal muscle following thermal injury. *Microvasc Res* 1982;24:34–41.

49. Nath S, Whayne JG, Kaul S, et al. Effects of radiofrequency catheter ablation on regional myocardial blood flow: Possible mechanism for late electrophysiological outcome. *Circulation* 1994;89:2667–2672.

50. Fahim MA, el Sabban F. Hyperthermia induces ultrastructural changes in mouse pial microvessels. *Anat Rec* 1995;242:77–82.

51. Huang SK, Bharati S, Lev M, et al. Electrophysiological and histologic observations of chronic atrioventricular block induced by closed-chest catheter desiccation with radiofrequency energy. *PACE* 1987;10:805–816.

52. Nath S, Redick JA, Whayne JG, et al. Ultrastructural observations in the myocardium beyond the region of acute coagulation necrosis following radiofrequency catheter ablation. *J Cardiovasc Electrophysiol* 1994;5:838–845.

53. Elvan A, Huang XD, Pressler ML, et al. Radiofrequency catheter ablation

of the atria eliminates pacing-induced sustained atrial fibrillation and re-duces connexon 43 in dogs. *Circulation* 1997;96:1675–1685.

54. Tracy CM, Moore HJ, Solomon AJ, et al. Thermistor guided radiofrequency ablation of atrial insertion sites in patients with accessory pathways. *PACE* 1995;18:2001–2007.

55. Nakagawa H, Yamanashi WS, Pitha JV, et al. Comparison of in vivo tissue temperature profile and lesion geometry for radiofrequency ablation with a saline-irrigated electrode versus temperature control in a canine thigh muscle preparation. *Circulation* 1995;91:2264–2273.

56. Jones JL, Lepeschkin E, Jones RE, et al. Response of cultured myocardial cells to countershock-type electric field stimulation. *Am J Physiol* 1978;235: H214–H222.

57. Jones JL, Jones RE, Balasky G. Microlesion formation in myocardial cells by high-intensity electric field stimulation. *Am J Physiol* 1987;253:H480–H486.

58. Chang DC. Cell poration and cell fusion using an oscillating electric field. *Biophys J* 1989;56:641–652.

59. Simmers TA, de Bakker JM, Wittkampf FH, et al. Effects of heating with radiofrequency power on myocardial impulse conduction: is radiofrequency ablation exclusively thermally mediated? *J Cardiovasc Electrophysiol* 1996;7:243–247.

Chapter 4

Determinants of Radiofrequency-Induced Lesion Size

Boaz Avitall, M.D., Ph.D., Ray Helms B.S.E.

Introduction

There are numerous factors involved in determining the size of lesions generated using radiofrequency (RF) energy. The degree of contact between the ablating electrode and the cardiac tissue is one of the most important determinants. Other factors include the magnitude and duration of power delivery, the characteristics of the ablating electrode, the orientation of the electrode in reference to the tissue, the RF energy delivery protocol (bipolar versus unipolar), and the tissue heat dissipation characteristics. Adjustments in any of these variables can have a significant impact on the dimensions of generated radiofrequency lesions. In this chapter, each of these subjects will be discussed in detail based on the current published data, including papers and abstracts.

Lesion Size Measurements

Lesion Dimensions

Experimental studies of lesion size have been performed using various methods of describing lesion dimensions. Some investigators summarize dimensions in the format of overall lesion volume, while others discuss lesion width and depth separately. Discussions of lesion volume can be difficult to compare because many different formulas have been used to calculate volume from width and depth measurements. These formulas are based on various as-

From Huang SKS, Wilber DJ (eds.): *Radiofrequency Catheter Ablation of Cardiac Arrhythmias: Basic Concepts and Clinical Applications,* 2nd ed. Armonk, NY: Futura Publishing Company, Inc. ©2000.

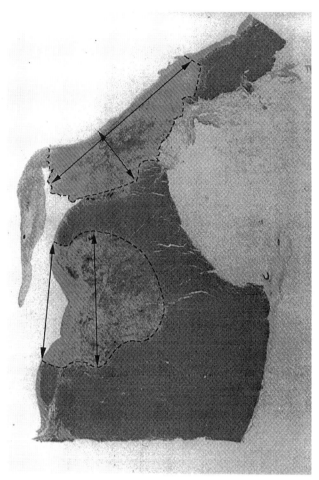

RF Lesion

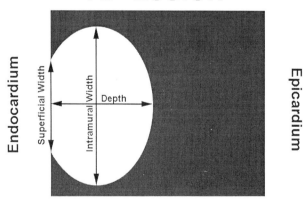

Figure 1. Lesion dimensions: the shape of a typical RF lesion is shown in the bottom panel. An example of a gross RF lesion in ventricular and atrial tissues is shown in the top panel. Note that the maximal ventricular lesion width is located intramurally, not at the electrode-tissue interface, whereas on the atrial lesion at the AV junction the endocardial lesion width closely approximates the lesion width.

sumptions about the three-dimensional shape of the lesion including a prolate spheroid,[1] a truncated hemisphere,[2] and a half ellipsoid.[3]

Separate discussions of width and depth are more informative than simply calculating an overall lesion volume. There is evidence that the growth of lesion depth and width follows different time courses. In a study of lesion dimensions, Avitall et al found that while endocardial lesion width matures within 20 seconds, lesion depth requires much more time (from 90–120 seconds) to reach a maximum level.[4]

Mature RF lesions within ventricular myocardium have a maximal lesion width located intramurally, not at the endocardial surface (Figure 1). Since the endocardial surface is cooled by intracavitary blood flow, the endocardial lesion width matures earlier than the intramural width and depth. The measurement of lesion width should be made after bisecting the lesion, so the true maximum width is documented.

Since some arrhythmogenic tissues may be located deep within the myocardium, adequate lesion depth is necessary for successful ablation. A large calculated volume may be due to a larger than average lesion width with a depth that is insufficient for successful therapy. A suboptimal amplitude or shortened duration of energy delivery, formation of coagulum on the electrode surface due to overheating, or poor electrode-tissue contact, may contribute to inadequate lesion depth maturation.

Estimation of Lesion Size via Intracardiac Echocardiography

Several studies have shown that lesion generation during RF ablation can be assessed using intracardiac echocardiography (ICE). In an in vivo canine study, Chan et al found that the dimensions measured via ICE were slightly overestimated, but were highly correlated with measurements made during post-procedural gross tissue observation.[5] In contrast to this study, Kalman et al found that in vitro ultrasound measurements tended to underestimate the lesion depth and width measured pathologically, with the width having a greater discrepancy.[6] The true utility of ICE in monitoring lesion maturation during RF ablation needs further clarification.

The Importance of Electrode-Tissue Contact and Orientation

The ablation of cardiac tissues with radiofrequency energy occurs via resistive heating. Therefore, maintaining adequate contact between the ablating electrode and the target cardiac tissue is a necessity for successful ablation. Without contact, no lesion may be created. The importance of good electrode-tissue contact has been the subject of discussion in multiple publications.[4,7–13]

Endocardial electrode-tissue contact is difficult to quantify in the intact heart. Therefore, numerous in vitro contact studies have been performed to determine the effects of different levels of contact on lesion generation parameters such as temperature, impedance, and power.

Hoyt et al demonstrated the significance of contact in generating RF lesions. Their in vitro study of epicardial lesions concluded that the force of contact is directly proportional to lesion diameter and depth in animals.[2] In this investigation contact pressure was set at 0, 5, 10, and 20 grams and 20 watts of power was applied for 5 seconds. In addition, the force of contact was shown by Haines and associates to be proportional to temperature and lesion volume in animals.[13]

The in vivo effects of varying electrode-tissue contact on lesion size, temperature, and impedance was investigated by Avitall et al.[4] This study suggested that close monitoring of the changes in temperature and impedance provides important information regarding the degree of contact between the catheter and the tissue. In this study the hearts of mongrel dogs were exposed, and the chest cavity was filled with heparinized blood, kept at a constant temperature of 37°C via a temperature-controlled bath. A catheter holder (Figure 2) was constructed so that a 4 mm temperature-monitoring ablation electrode could be positioned at different levels of contact (-5, 0, $+1$, $+3$ mm) with the epicardial surface. For investigative purposes, contact was defined as "good" when the electrode was pressed 3 mm ($+3$ contact) or 1 mm ($+1$ contact) into the epicardium. "Poor" contact was present when the electrode was either lightly pressed against the epicardium (0 contact) or retracted 5 mm (-5 contact) inside the holder so that the electrode did not make contact with the epicardium. During -5 contact the electrode was totally bathed in the circulating blood.

RF energy was applied for a maximum of 120 seconds to create a total of 12 lesions in the anterior free wall of the left ventricle at various contact and power levels (-5, 0, $+1$, and $+3$ contact at 10, 20, and 30 watts). When a rapid rise in impedance was noted, power application was terminated. The data collected included temperature and impedance values during energy application and lesion dimensions (width and depth).

Lesion Width

The lesion width appeared to mature within 30–40 seconds at each of the power and contact levels. As shown in Table 1, with 0 contact an increase in power from 10 to 30 watts resulted in an increase in lesion width from 5.2 ± 0.8 mm to 7.1 ± 1.0 mm ($P<0.05$). With $+3$ contact, the lesion width increased further to a maximum of 9.9 ± 1.3 mm at 30 watts ($P<0.05$ versus 0 contact, 30 watts) despite having an abbreviated RF power application time of only 35 ± 13 seconds.

Lesion Depth

Lesion depth required over 90 seconds to mature. With 0 contact the lesion depth increased from 4.6 ± 1.1 mm to 7.9 ± 0.7 mm ($P<0.01$) with RF power levels of 10 and 30 watts, respectively. As the power level increased to 30 watts,

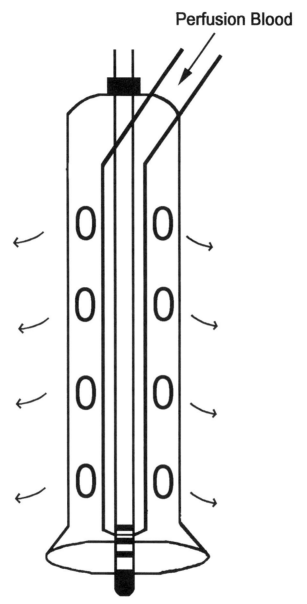

Perfusion Blood

Figure 2. Catheter holder used in contact study to place the electrode at various electrode/tissue contact levels (−5, 0, +1, +3) in isothermal circulating blood (37°C). A locking mechanism at the proximal end of the holder can be adjusted to maintain the appropriate contact level as the holder is placed on the epicardium with enough force to maintain stable positioning on the epicardium without compression. The stiff perfusion tube prevented the distal end of the catheter from shifting side-to-side.

Table 1
Lesion Width and Depth as a Function of Contact, Power, and Time (N=5)

Contact	Width (mm)			Depth (mm)		
	0	*+1*	*+3*	*0*	*+1*	*+3*
10 Watts	*5.2±0.8	*5.7±0.7	*5.8±0.4	*4.6±1.1	*6.2±1.6	+7.7±1
Time(s)	120±0	120±0	120±0	120±0	120±0	120±0
20 Watts	6±1.1	7.1±1.1	7.8±2.3	6.5±0.6	8.2±1.5	+9.2±1.2
Time(s)	120±0	86±32	99±32	120±0	86±32	99±32
30 Watts	7.1±1	7.7±1	+9.9±1.3	7.9±0.7	8.7±1.8	7.9±1.3
Time(s)	104±22	36±20	35±13	104±22	36±20	35±13

*$P<0.05$ vs. 30 watts
+$P<0.05$ vs. 0 mm

the RF application time decreased to 104±22 seconds due to tissue/electrode overheating and char formation that prevented further lesion growth. As shown in Table 1, the maximum lesion depth of 9.2±1.2 mm was achieved with 20 watts and +3 contact ($P<0.05$ versus +3 contact, 30 watts). Using this power and contact level, impedance rose in only 2 of 5 lesions with an average RF application time of 99±32 seconds. With 10 watts at the +3 contact level, power could be applied for the full 120 seconds and the lesion depth reached at 7.7±1.0 mm, but increasing the power to 30 watts frequently resulted in impedance rises and, therefore, shortened the RF application time to 35±13 seconds. This produced a lesion depth of 7.9±1.3 mm, which is not significantly different from the lesions generated with 10 watts and +3 mm contact. Thus, the avoidance of impedance rises can allow for longer power application and greater depth maturation.

Impedance and Temperature Monitoring Indicating Electrode-Tissue Contact and Lesion Formation

Both temperature and impedance can provide useful insights into the status of electrode-tissue contact[4] and lesion formation.[1,4–16] Though they cannot be directly measured in the clinical setting, electrode-tissue contact and lesion width and depth maturation can be indirectly estimated by tracking changes in temperature and impedance.

Initial Impedance Level

Both in vitro and in vivo studies have shown that increased electrode-tissue contact results in increased initial impedance levels. In a study of isolated pig myocardium using a specially designed catheter with 4 mm tip and ring electrodes, Remp et al found that impedance could be used to distinguish between contact with blood versus myocardium.[17] In addition, they concluded that increasing contact pressures were associated with increasing impedances and lesion volumes. Strickberger et al used two-watt pulses during ablations in humans with standard 4 mm tip ablating electrode catheters to determine whether the impedance might differ for poor versus firm contact.[18] With firm contact the average impedance level was $22\pm13\%$ higher versus poor contact ($139\pm24\ \Omega$ versus $113\pm16\ \Omega$).

Impedance Trend

Impedance trends for four different contact levels while applying 20 watts of RF power are shown in Figure 3.[4] With increasing electrode-tissue contact, the rate and level of impedance decrease is magnified. With poor electrode-tissue contact, the maximum impedance decreases with 20 and 30 watts were 6 ± 6 Ω and $9\pm5\ \Omega$, respectively, and the impedance plateaued after a few seconds of power application. With the electrode in good contact, the maximum impedance decreases with 20 and 30 watts were $25\pm2\ \Omega$ and $20\pm6\ \Omega$, respectively, and the rate of the impedance decrease required 40 seconds of power application to reach a plateau.

Several in vitro studies have investigated the relationship between impedance and electrode-tissue contact. Grogan et al studied impedance in an in vitro, saline perfused model.[19] Power levels of 3–20 watts were applied to saline-perfused left ventricle (LV) tissue or to saline alone. A 10% decrease in impedance was recorded during application to the tissue, whereas no decrease

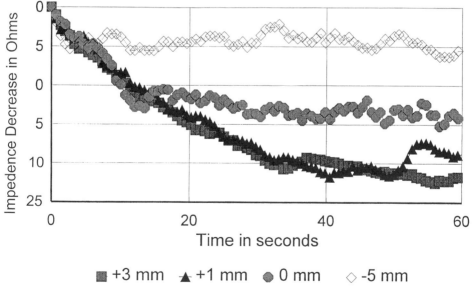

Figure 3. Impedance change from baseline versus time during the first 60 seconds using 20 watts of power with the electrode floating in blood (-5), lightly touching the epicardium (0), in good contact ($+1$), and in very good contact ($+3$).

was noted during the applications to saline alone. In perfused pig heart preparation, Dorwarth et al compared impedance trends for constant power (8, 12, 17 watts for 10–80 seconds) to temperature-controlled (70, 80, 90°C for 30–90 seconds) RF energy delivery.[20] During the constant power applications, an initial drop in impedance (82±8 Ω to 71±6 Ω was found to correlate with the induced lesion size. During the temperature-controlled ablations, there was no significant increase or decrease in the impedance.

In a clinical study of 24 patients, Harvey et al measured impedance during ablations to determine the usefulness of continuous impedance monitoring.[14] An initial drop in impedance of 10 Ω was found to be 78% sensitive and 88% specific for predicting evidence of tissue heating, as gauged by interruption of conduction or a rapid impedance rise due to coagulum formation. This same study concluded that initial values of voltage, current, or impedance were not predictive of effective versus ineffective applications. In an investigation of 24 patients, Strickberger et al found impedance monitoring to be an effective substitute for temperature monitoring during the ablation of accessory pathways.[18] The ablation procedure was successful in all 12 of the temperature monitoring procedures and unsuccessful in one of 12 patients in the impedance monitoring protocol. Otherwise, there was no significant difference in procedure duration, fluoroscopic time, or the number of applications that resulted in coagulum formation.

Temperature

In an in vitro investigation, Chan et al studied the power requirements needed to create lesions using temperature control set at a target temperature of 80°C for various contact pressures (0, 1, 20, 50, and 100 grams).[21] The power required to ablate the tissue at 80°C increased as the contact pressure decreased at each of 5 superfusate flow rates (0, 1, 2, 4, and 8 L/minute). This corroborates with the in vivo epicardial findings of Avitall and associates in their study which found that as the electrode-tissue contact increases, the amount of temperature rise also increases, as shown in Figure 4.[4] With the electrode floating in blood, the average maximum temperature increase with 20 and 30 watts was only 7±1°C and 11±2°C, respectively, and the temperature plateaued shortly after the initiation of power application. With good electrode-tissue contact, the temperature increase within the first 10 seconds was significantly greater than the temperature increase with poor contact and reached a maximum of 60±1°C after 60 seconds of power application.

Correlation of Width and Depth with Temperature and Impedance

In addition to providing insight into electrode-tissue contact, the impedance decrease and temperature increase also correlate well with both lesion width and depth according to Avitall and associates (Figure 5).[4] They found the best correlation between the lesion width and the maximum average temperature increase

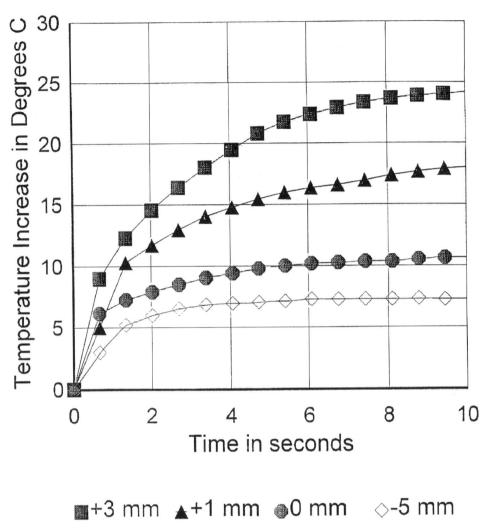

Figure 4. Average temperature increase above baseline versus time using 20 watts of RF power with the electrode floating in blood (−5), lightly touching the epicardium (0), in good contact (+1), and in very good contact (+3).

($R^2=0.9$). Lesion depth, however, correlated better with maximum average impedance decrease ($R^2=0.68$ for impedance versus $R^2=0.44$ for temperature).

Biobattery as an Indirect Measure of Temperature and Contact

In 2 studies—in vitro and in vivo—He et al evaluated the use of a "biobattery" galvanic current model to predict the temperature at the electrode-temperature interface.[22,23] In both investigations, catheters with 4 mm tip electrodes with thermocouples were used to ablate tissues with a generator capable of measuring galvanic current. In the in vitro study the correlation between

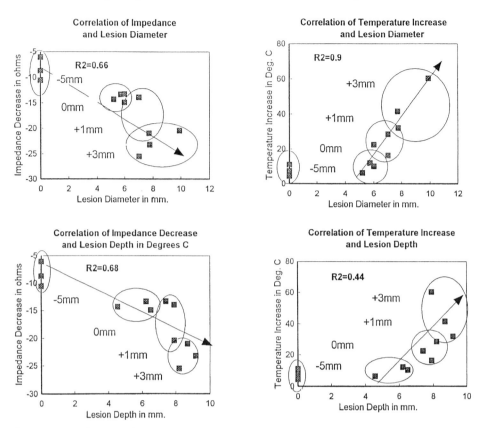

Figure 5. Impedance and temperature versus lesion width and depth using 20 watts of power with the electrode floating in blood (−5), lightly touching the epicardium (0), in good contact (+1), and in very good contact (+3). The correlation value (R^2) is shown on each panel.

the measured temperature and the galvanic current was 0.98 for temperatures between 36°C and 75°C. In the in vivo study, the correlation between temperature and galvanic current was 0.98 and 0.97 for 2 standard catheters from different manufacturers. Since temperature provides insight into electrode-tissue contact and lesion formation, this biobattery technique might be helpful in generating lesions using non-temperature-controlled catheters.

The Use of ICE to Aid in Evaluating Electrode-Tissue Contact and Orientation

Recent studies have described the use of intracardiac ultrasound to enhance maintenance of adequate electrode-tissue orientation and contact. Kalman et al reported that ICE can detect changes in tip location and stability and can therefore be used to help establish good electrode-tissue contact.[24] In another study, Kalman et al compared the use of ICE, fluoroscopy, and electrocardiograms (ECGs) to the use of only fluoroscopy and ECGs in evaluating contact prior to lesion generation.[25] They defined 3 levels of contact: poor, average, and good. In

27% of the RF applications with good contact as determined by fluoroscopy and ECG, ICE found that the contact conditions were actually poor. The size of the lesions generated with good contact were considerably larger than those generated with average or poor contact. The authors suggest that ICE can aid in obtaining good contact, and, therefore, lesion size can be maximized.

The orientation of the ablating electrode in reference to the tissue may have a significant effect on lesion size. Chan et al evaluated the difference in lesion maturation for perpendicular versus parallel orientations in canines.[26] They evaluated lesions created with 4, 6, 8, 10, and 12 mm electrodes and found that larger lesions were created with the electrodes oriented parallel to the tissue. This study concluded that ICE could be used to determine orientation and ensure proper contact to maximize lesion size.

Power and Energy

Numerous investigations have analyzed the relationship between lesion dimensions, the amplitude and duration of power delivery with both 2 mm and 4 mm electrodes. With 2 mm electrodes there is a higher probability that the electrode will be fully embedded within the tissue, with little or no exposure to the blood. If this is the case, all the power will be dissipated within the tissue. With larger electrodes much of the electrode may be bathed in fluid. Therefore, some of the power will be shunted through the blood rather than into the tissue. This contact scenario is probably common with 4 mm electrodes, especially when the catheter is not imbedded within ventricular trabeculations.

In Vitro Studies

2 mm Electrode

Hoyt and Hoffman both performed in vitro studies with short power durations using 2 mm electrodes.[2] Using excised bovine left ventricles, Hoyt et al concluded that pulse power and duration were the most significant variables influencing myocardial damage.[2] They created lesions with 1–50 watts of power applied for 2–20 seconds and found that diameter and depth both increased as power amplitude and duration increased (Figure 6). Hoffman et al studied the effects of power amplitude (17, 29, 32, 41, and 57 watts for 10 seconds) and duration (3, 6, and 9 seconds at 57 watts) on lesion generation in excised pig myocardium in a circulating blood bath.[27] For these relatively short application times, they concluded that the lesion depth was influenced more by the amplitude of the power, whereas the lesion area was affected more by the duration of power delivery. The short duration of power application in these 2 studies did not allow for full depth maturation, thus making depth a function of power. Haines et al applied RF power for a much longer duration and found that 35–45 seconds of power delivery were required to obtain maximal lesion size in an in vitro preparation using a 1.6 mm electrode.[13]

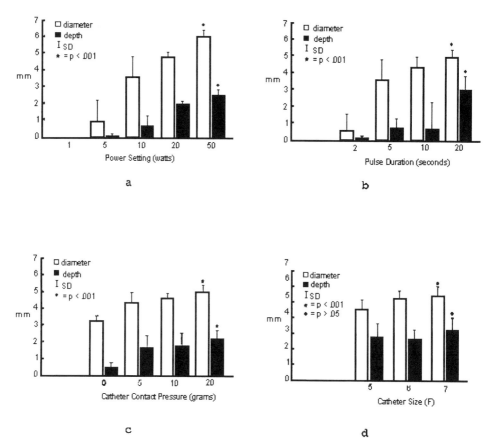

Figure 6. Lesion depth and diameter versus power, pulse duration, contact pressure, and catheter size. Lesions were created with 1–50 watts of power applied for 2–20 seconds in an in vitro preparation using 2 mm electrodes. (Image used by permission.[2])

In Vivo Studies

In the intact heart, the ability to control lesion dimensions by adjusting power delivery is limited due to the variable nature of the convective cooling effects of circulating blood. Furthermore, in contrast to in vitro studies in which contact or contact pressure may be carefully controlled, the electrode-tissue contact may vary significantly in in vivo studies.

2mm Electrodes

In an in vivo epicardial study, Bardy et al evaluated lesion volume while varying the duration (5, 10, 15, and 20 seconds) and amount (20, 40, and 60 volts) of RF voltage delivered.[28] They concluded that lesion volume rises as a function of time and power (Figure 7). At each voltage level, the lesion depth,

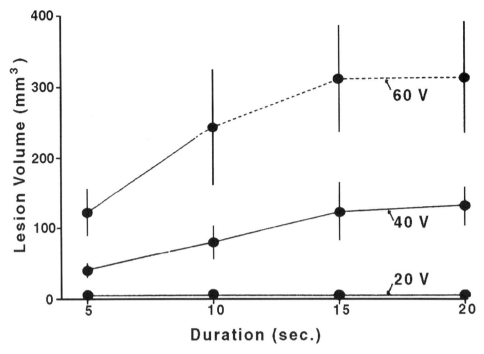

Figure 7. Lesion volume versus power and pulse duration. Lesions were created with 20, 40, and 60 volts applied for 5, 10, 15, and 20 seconds in an in vivo preparation using 2 mm electrodes. (Image used by permission.[28])

diameter, and volume increased as the duration increased from 5 to 15 seconds. Increasing the duration to 20 seconds at 40 volts did not result in increased lesion diameter. Furthermore, at 60 volts neither lesion depth nor diameter increased significantly when the duration was increased from 15 to 20 seconds. A study by Wittkampf et al used power levels of up to 9 watts and created lesions for 5, 10, 20, 30, and 60 seconds in canine ventricles using an endocardial approach. They concluded that lesion size (measured as a composite of length, width, and depth) matured within 20 seconds and increased in size with higher power for all exposure durations.[12]

Lesion Maturation with 4 mm Electrodes

Simmers et al evaluated the effects of pulse duration (5, 10, 20, 30, and 60 seconds) on lesion dimensions[29] with 4 mm electrodes at a fixed level of 25 watts. They concluded that 90% of maximum dimensions were reached within 20 seconds of the initiation of power delivery. Lesion depth was found to have matured within the first 10 seconds, while lesion diameter required more time, approximately 30 seconds.

These results stand in contrast to those described by Avitall et al[4] which noted that the lesion depth matures much more slowly than the width: the depth required 90 seconds to mature while the width required 30–40 seconds. It would be prudent for the user of this technology to apply RF power for 60–90 seconds if full lesion maturation is desired.

Cooled-tip Technology

With the development of cooled-tip technology, it is possible to deliver higher energy levels for longer periods of time while avoiding overheating leading to a rapid impedance rise and subsequent coagulum formation. This allows for the creation of much larger lesions than can be generated with standard technology.

Atrial Tissue

Recently, great energy has been focused on the development of technology for the ablation of atrial arrhythmias. Because the atrial walls are much thinner than the ventricles, the power requirements are different. The power required to create transmural lesions in the atria are much less than for ventricular tissues. Avitall and associates used fixed power levels of 1, 5, 10, 15, 20, and 30 watts for 30 seconds to create epicardial lesions with a standard 4 mm tip electrode.[30] The lesion diameter increased with increasing power. For power levels of 20 and 30 watts, all lesions were completely transmural.

Generator Frequency

Most standard RF generators produce signals in the range of 500–750 kHz. Some recent studies have investigated the lesion dimensions that can be produced using higher frequencies. Kovoor et al compared lesion dimensions for frequencies of 100, 600, 1200, and 2000 kHz.[31] Lesions were generated with a 1 mm long electrode (diameter = 0.8 mm) using temperature control at a setting of 90°C. They found that lesion width was not statistically different for the various frequencies, but the depth increased with higher frequency. Bru et al generated lesions to create AV block in sheep with a generator frequency of 27 MHz and an electrode of unknown size.[32] The power levels required for successful ablation were between 30 and 100 watts, and the generated lesions ranged from 3–45 mm in diameter and 1–15 mm in depth. The utility of RF generators with frequencies other than 500–750 kHz with standard catheter technology (4 mm electrodes) remains to be explored.

Unipolar versus Bipolar Energy Delivery

Most RF lesions are created by applying energy in a unipolar fashion between an ablating electrode touching the myocardium and a grounded reference patch electrode placed externally on the skin. The goal of cardiac tissue ablation is to eliminate arrhythmogenic foci with the least amount of tissue damage. The unipolar configuration is best suited to this goal because it creates a highly localized lesion, with the least amount of surface injury. Energy can also be applied in a bipolar mode between 2 endocardial electrodes. This method may prove to be useful in increasing the efficiency of creating long linear lesions for the ablation of atrial fibrillation. Haines et al compared the delivery of RF energy in unipolar and bipolar modes in the generation of lesions at the tricuspid/inferior vena cava isthmus using 2 3 mm electrodes spaced 3 mm apart.[33] Unipolar energy was found to generate lesions that were longer (14.9±1.6 mm versus 9.2±1.5 mm) and wider (8.1±1.8 versus 5.6±1.5) than bipolar energy. Anfinsen et al used a different electrode configuration to test the lesion dimensions created with unipolar versus bipolar RF energy delivery to the right atrial free wall in pigs.[34] Energy was applied via the distal 4 mm tip electrodes of 2 standard 7F catheters placed 6–8 mm apart on the endocardial surface. In contrast to the Haines study, the lesions generated via bipolar power delivery were longer and wider than those created via unipolar delivery, though the depth of the lesions did not differ between the 2 methods. In a similar but in vitro investigation by Anfinsen et al, bipolar energy delivery was found to provide a greater lesion length than unipolar delivery, but width and depth were not found to differ significantly between the 2 methods.[35]

Pulsed Power Application

By applying power in a pulsatile manner, the convective cooling blood currents may aid in avoiding overheating at the electrode-tissue interface and subsequent rapid impedance rises, therefore allowing the creation of larger lesions. An in vitro study by Nakagawa et al investigated the creation of lesions using pulsed power delivery with a saline-irrigated electrode.[36] A fixed level of 70 volts was applied via 3 techniques for 180 seconds or until a popping sound was heard. Power was applied in one of 3 ways: continuously, on for 5 seconds then off for 5 seconds, or on for 4 seconds then off for 5 seconds. The largest lesion diameter (16.5±1.7 mm) and depth (10.3±1.1 mm) were generated with the 5-on/5-off method of power delivery; the comparable dimensions with continuous power delivery were 13.1±1.8 and 6.5±1.0, respectively. With continuous power delivery 24 of 24 applications resulted in a popping sound while the popping frequency decreased to 5 of 36 and 0 of 13 for the 5-on/5-off and 4-on/5-off methods, respectively. The use of pulsed power delivery may allow for the creation of larger lesions because the power may be applied over a longer period of time allowing the lesion to mature more completely.

Reference Patch Electrode Location and Size

The standard method of ablating cardiac tissues involves applying RF power in a unipolar fashion from an electrode on a catheter to a reference patch placed on the patient's back. Tomassoni et al investigated lesion dimensions for standard and nonstandard locations of the reference electrode.[37] The reference electrode was either placed directly opposite the catheter tip on the thorax or placed in a simple anterior or posterior position. Placing the electrode patch opposite the catheter resulted in increased lesion surface area, depth, and volume. Otomo et al studied lesion dimensions for 2 different reference patch electrode sizes in a canine thigh muscle preparation.[38] They compared a 252 cm^2 patch (2 standard patches) to a 63 cm^2 patch (one-half a standard patch). Lesions were created with a 4 mm electrode with 20 watts of power for 60 seconds. In the preparation with the larger patch, the lesion depth and volume were significantly increased as opposed to the preparation with the smaller patch (depth = 7.4 ± 0.8 versus 5.1 ± 1.1 mm, volume = 368 ± 131 versus 152 ± 50 mm^3). These results suggest that the RF current path and skin reference electrode interface present significant impedance for the ablation current flow, therefore dissipating part of the power. Increasing the patch size and placing the reference patch at the path of least resistance for the ablation current provides for increased heating at the electrode-endocardial interface and thus increased ablation efficiency.

Heat Dissipation

Tissue Heating

The dimensions of a lesion created with radiofrequency power are determined by the amount of tissue heated above the critical temperature for producing irreversible myocardial damage, 50°C.[39] Because radiofrequency tissue damage is the result of resistive heating, good contact between the ablating electrode and the tissue is necessary for successful lesion generation. Appropriate contact between the electrode and the tissue to be ablated is usually evident via a rapid rise in temperature.[4,9,40,41] Upon the initiation of fixed level energy application, the temperature at the electrode-tissue interface rises monoexponentially to reach steady state within a few seconds (see Figure 4).[4,42] The rapid maturation of lesion width is related to the temperature increase at the electrode-tissue interface, which is a direct function of the current density. Deeper tissues are not heated as a direct result of the dissipation of electrical energy because tissue heating decreases as a function of $1/r^4$. Therefore, deep tissues are heated via conductive heating from the tissue near the electrode-tissue interface (Figure 8).[43,44] This conductive heating has been shown to require 1 to 2 minutes to equilibrate.[4,40,45]

Heating with Fixed Power Levels

Many studies have shown that monitoring electrode tip temperature can provide information about tissue heating and lesion maturation during application of fixed levels of radiofrequency power. Using 2 mm electrodes to deliver 3–25 watts of RF power for 10 seconds, Hindricks and associates found that the

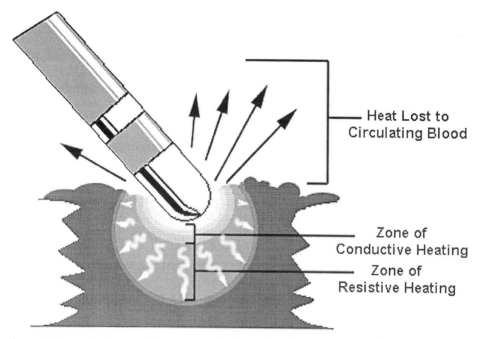

Figure 8. Tissue heating via RF power application. Superficial tissue near the electrode-tissue interface is ablated via resistive heating, while deeper myocardium is heated via conductive heating. The flow of blood near the electrode-tissue interface and in coronary vessels cools the myocardium via convection.

temperature integral had a higher correlation with lesion dimensions than with total applied energy or maximum temperature in in vitro and in vivo studies.[8] In similar studies using 2 mm electrodes to deliver 2.5–50 watts for 10 seconds, Haverkamp et al concluded that under in vivo conditions monitoring the temperature at the catheter tip improved the ability to predict lesion dimensions.[45] Extending the duration of power application to 90 seconds, Haines et al reported lesion size to be directly proportional to peak electrode-tissue interface temperature for constant power levels from 0.2–52 watts using a 2 mm electrode.[41] In a recent study using 4 mm electrodes and fixed power levels of 10 or 25 watts for 60 seconds, Wittkampf and associates documented the rise in temperature 3 mm deep to the electrode-tissue interface.[40] The temperature rise in the tissue was on average 2.4 times higher for the 25 watt versus the 10 watt ablations. Therefore, the authors concluded that the tissue temperature rise is proportional to power level. Langberg and associates performed RF ablations on 20 patients by delivering 20, 30, 40, and 50 watts for 20 seconds each or until an impedance rise occurred.[42] Though overall power output did not predict temperature, at any given site there was a clear-cut positive dose-response relationship between power and temperature. Each of these studies contributes to the conclusion that temperature monitoring is a useful means of guiding fixed power level RF ablations.

Closed-Loop Automatic Temperature Control

Maintaining the temperature at the electrode-tissue interface below 100°C results in significantly less coagulum formation on the ablation electrode and a decreased incidence of impedance rises and tissue tearing (Figure 9).[9,41,44] Monitoring the temperature at the electrode-tissue interface to prevent overheating can allow for longer power application and increased lesion dimensions.[44] Therefore, the application of RF power using closed-loop automatic temperature control has become a useful ablation technique. Haines et al applied RF power to maintain electrode tip temperature at 80°C for 120 seconds in an isolated right ventricle (RV) free wall preparation.[1] As shown in Figure 10, tip temperature was found to correlate closely with lesion depth (r = 0.92) and width (r = 0.88). In addition, tip temperature was a better predictor of lesion size than measurements of power, current, or energy. The temperature measured at the electrode-tissue interface does not necessarily reflect the temperature within the tissue itself. With increasing distance lateral to the electrode-tissue interface, the maximum temperature decreases rapidly (Figure 11).[1] Because circulating blood cools the tissue near the interface, the temperature measured by a thermistor or thermocouple at the electrode-tissue interface tends to be cooler than within the tissue directly below the electrode.[46–49] The tissue underneath the electrode may be 15°C to 20°C hotter than the measured temperature within the electrode. The orientation of the temperature-measuring element affects the degree of this difference.[48] Fleischman et al showed that the temperature measured from a sensor placed at the electrode tip provides a closer estimate of the actual tissue temperature than a centrally located sensor (Figure 12).[49] The measured temperature is affected by the sen-

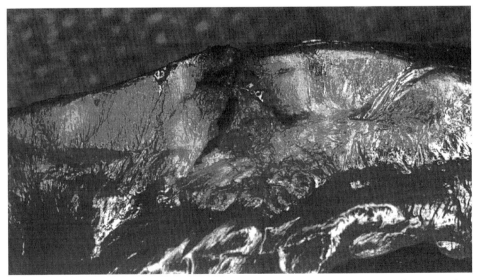

Figure 9. Intramural shredding of tissues resulting from explosions caused by gas formation during boiling with 30 watts applied via a 4 mm electrode pressed 3 mm into the epicardium.

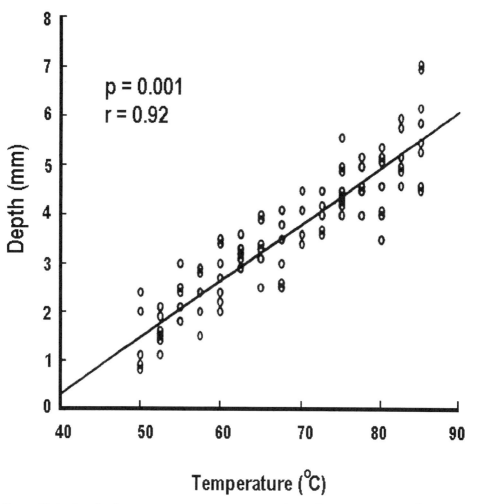

Figure 10. Lesion depth versus temperature: at a target electrode-tip temperature of 80°C, RF power was applied for 120 seconds to create 104 lesions. There is a strong linear relationship between lesion depth and temperature. (Image used by permission.[1])

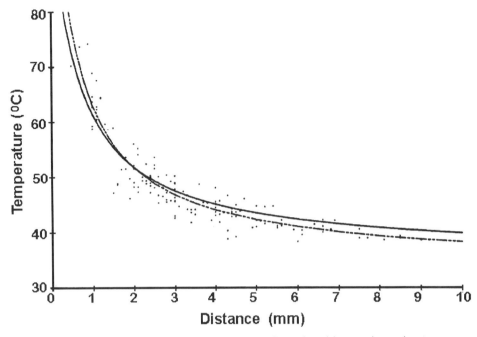

Figure 11. Maximum temperature versus distance from the ablating electrode. At a target electrode-tip temperature of 80°C, RF power was applied for 120 seconds to create 104 lesions. The temperature measured 2 mm below the epicardium decreased rapidly as a function of distance from the ablating electrode. (Image used by permission.[1])

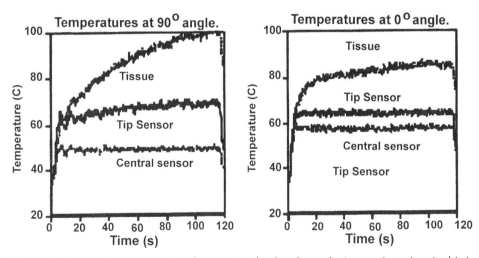

Figure 12. Temperature versus time for a perpendicular electrode-tissue orientation. In this in vitro preparation, power was adjusted to maintain a target temperature of 50°C at the central sensor. The temperature measured from a sensor placed at the electrode tip provides a closer estimate of the tissue temperature than a centrally located sensor, though neither closely estimates the actual tissue temperature. The tissue temperature was measured 1 mm below the electrode-tissue interface. (Image used by permission.[49])

sor's position, the electrode-tissue contact, and the degree of cooling by intra-cavitary blood flow. Thus, when using an automatic closed-loop temperature control system the target temperature should be set at 70°C to 80°C and maintained for 1 to 2 minutes to maximize lesion maturation while avoiding impedance rises and popping due to overheating at the electrode-tissue interface.

Electrode Radius and Length

If the RF power level were adjusted to maintain a constant current density, lesion width would increase proportionally to the electrode-tissue contact area. However, this assumes that the electrode-tissue contact, tissue heat dissipation, and blood flow are uniform throughout the electrode-tissue interface. As the electrode size increases, the likelihood that these assumptions are true diminishes due to variability in cardiac chamber trabeculations and curvature, tissue perfusion, and intracardiac blood flow, which will affect the heat dissipation and contact. These factors will result in unpredictable lesion size and uniformity for electrodes greater than 8 mm long. The character of lesions created with temperature control depends on the placement of the temperature sensor or sensors relative to the portion of the electrode that is in contact with the tissue. Thus, the orientation of the ablating electrode and its temperature sensors will determine the appropriate target temperature required to create maximal lesions while avoiding coagulum formation due to overheating at any location within the electrode-tissue interface.

Ventricular Lesion Generation via 2 to 12 mm Electrodes

Electrode Radius

In vitro studies have shown that lesion formation can be influenced by the size of the electrode-tissue interface.[2,50,51] Hoyt et al reported that increasing the electrode diameter (5F, 6F, 7F) results in a significant increase in lesion diameter, but not depth, in an in vitro study.[2] This study used power applications of 20 seconds only, so the lesions were not allowed to fully mature. Haines and associates evaluated the correlation between electrode radius and lesion transmural (depth) and transverse radii.[50] Lesions were created in a perfused RV free wall using temperature control at a setting of 60°C for 90 seconds. As shown in Figure 13, a strong correlation was noted between electrode radius and lesion transmural (r = 0.89) and transverse radii (r = 0.85).

Electrode Length

Theoretically, longer electrodes would be expected to create larger lesions if the power level was increased accordingly to maintain a constant current density. Langberg et al investigated the effects of distal electrode length (2, 3,

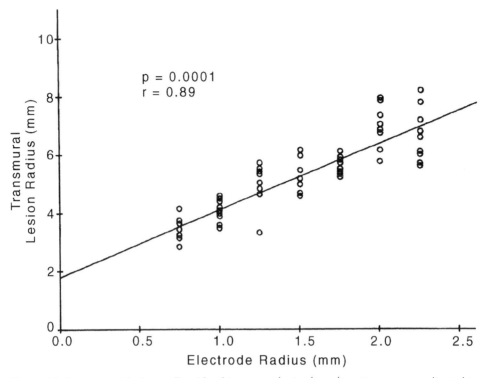

Figure 13. Transmural lesion radius (depth) versus electrode radius. Power was adjusted to maintain a target temperature of 60°C in this in vitro preparation. Electrodes with larger surface areas require higher powers to maintain the target temperature, and can create deeper lesions at a fixed target temperature. (Image used by permission.[50])

4, 6, 8, and 10 mm) on ventricular lesion volume in vivo.[51] Instead of attempting to maintain a constant current density, a constant power of approximately 13 watts was applied until a maximum of 500 joules of energy had been delivered or a rapid impedance rise occurred. For this power level, the optimum electrode length was 3–4 mm. Increasing the electrode length from 2 mm to 3 or 4 mm more than doubled the lesion volume (from 143 to 303 and 326 mm³, respectively), but increasing the length beyond 4 mm resulted in smaller lesions, presumably because of decreasing current density.

Studies using temperature control have shown that 8 mm electrodes optimize lesion dimensions in ventricular myocardium. Langberg et al compared the use of 8 mm and 12 mm electrodes versus standard 4 mm electrodes at a target temperature of 80°C for 60 seconds.[51,52] Lesions created with 8 mm electrodes were nearly twice as deep and four times as large as lesions made with 4 mm electrodes. The 12 mm electrodes produced lesions with depths and volumes that were smaller than with 8 mm electrodes and slightly larger than with 4 mm electrodes. In addition, the 12 mm electrodes were associated with charring and crater formation. McRury and associates evaluated 4, 8, and 10 mm electrodes delivering up to 150 watts with temperature controlled at 65, 80, and 90°C.[53,54] The lesion volume more than doubled when the size was increased from 4 mm to 8 mm for each of the target temperatures. The volume increase from 8 to 10 mm^3 at each target temperature was minimal.

In a canine thigh muscle preparation, Otomo and associates compared lesions created with 4 mm versus 8 mm tip electrodes with power delivered for 60 seconds under temperature control.[38] The target temperature was set at 60°C for a perpendicular electrode-tissue orientation and 90°C for a parallel orientation. The larger (8 mm) electrode produced significantly deeper lesions than the 4 mm electrode in both preparations (7.8±0.8 mm versus 6.6±0.5 mm at 60°C target; 8.3±0.7 mm versus 7.2±0.5 mm at 90°C target).

Atrial Lesion Generation via 4 mm to 12 mm Electrodes

Chan et al investigated the creation of atrial lesions with electrodes of various sizes (4, 6, 10, and 12 mm) with parallel versus perpendicular orientations.[26] The temperature at the electrode-tissue interface was maintained at 75°C for 60 seconds with up to 65 watts of power. Lesion area increased with increasing electrode length and was maximized at 10 mm for parallel orientation (55±78 mm versus 31±12 mm with a 4 mm electrode) and 12 mm for perpendicular orientation (70±40 mm versus 59±38 mm with a 4 mm electrode).

Segmented/Multiple Electrodes

Since ventricular tachycardia (VT) ablations may require large, deep lesions, several investigations have studied the application of RF energy to multiple electrodes to increase lesion dimensions.

Multiple Bipolar Power Applications with Four 2 mm Electrodes

In 2 investigations, Oeff and associates applied bipolar RF power (7–35 watts) between the proximal, middle, and distal pairs of electrodes on a catheter with four 2 mm electrodes.[54,55] The catheter was removed so that it could be cleaned and then the process was repeated 9 to 11 times at each target site. The surface area and volume of these lesions was much greater than that of lesions created with single applications. The average lesion volume was 0.84±0.38 versus 0.12±0.06 cm^3, and the average lesion surface area was 3.7±1.2 versus 0.29±0.15 cm^2.

Unipolar versus Bipolar Constant Voltage Application with 2 4 mm Electrodes

Chang et al placed 2 separate catheters with 4 mm tip electrodes next to one another horizontally to create lesions in isolated bovine myocardium.[56] They compared lesion generation at a fixed level of 30 volts in bipolar versus unipolar mode and with one versus both electrodes. Lesion volumes were calculated for interelectrode distances ranging from 2 to 7 mm. Lesions produced by simultaneous delivery to both electrodes were twice the size of lesions created with one electrode. Lesion volume and depth decreased with increasing interelectrode distance. In addition, for a given power level, bipolar delivery produced larger lesions than unipolar power application.

Unipolar Fixed Power Applications with 2 and 4 mm Electrodes

Two studies using unipolar RF power via multiple electrodes have been reported. Avitall and associates used a catheter with a distal 2 mm electrode and 3 additional 2 mm electrodes spaced 0.5 mm apart on its shaft to create lesions in the LV of 5 dogs.[57] Lesions were made by applying 10, then 20, then 30 watts of power for 60 seconds or until an impedance rise occurred. Lesion dimensions were compared for the use of electrodes 1 and 2 versus 1, 2, 3, and 4. While the depth was not significantly different, the length and width were greater for the 1-2-3-4 method versus the 1–2 method (length = 13±3.7 versus 9.3±2 mm, width = 8.7±2 versus 6.7±0.8 mm).

In a study using a quadripolar catheter, Mackey et al compared lesions created in vitro and in vivo with a distal 4 mm electrode versus simultaneous application via the distal 4 mm electrode and 3 2 mm electrodes placed 2 mm apart on the shaft.[58] The power was set at 12 watts for the distal tip ablations and 35 watts for the quadripolar applications. These power settings were defined based on preliminary studies documenting the highest power levels with impedance rise rates of less than 20%. In both the in vivo and in vitro studies, the lesions were twice as long with the 4 mm electrodes than with just the distal electrode. There was a trend toward increasing lesion depth with the quadripolar applications in both sets of experiments with a more substantial increase in the in vivo experiment.

Temperature Control with a 4 mm Electrode and a 3.5 mm Electrode

Baal and associates compared the use of a 4 mm distal tip electrode alone versus simultaneous ablation with the distal electrode and a 3.5 mm electrode on the catheter shaft using temperature control.[59] The target temperature was set at 80°C and maintained for 60 seconds. Using electrodes 1–2 versus 1 alone significantly increased the lesion depth (4.9±0.7 mm versus 4.5±0.5 mm) and volume (210±61 mm^3 versus 123±43 mm^3).

Coiled Electrodes

In attempting to create long lesions in the atria, several investigators have evaluated the use of coiled wire electrodes.[60–65] Long coiled electrodes are advantageous because they do not inhibit catheter flexibility as do the long ring electrodes. Experiments using multiple coils in the range of 4–12.5 mm at various interelectrode distances have concluded that these electrodes can create long atrial lesions, but they are limited in their ability to consistently create completely contiguous and transmural lesions.

Ablation with Saline Infusion

Active Fixation/Saline Electrode

Hoey and associates reported using a catheter with a tip that can be actively screwed into ventricular tissue from the endocardium.[65,66] After the tip is screwed into the tissue, saline is infused during RF energy application creating a "virtual electrode" that can be visualized via fluoroscopy. Lesions measuring $10 \times 10 \times 9$ mm were created using 50 watts of RF power for 2 minutes. With power applied for 4 minutes, the lesion size increased to $17 \times 15 \times 14$ mm. There was no evidence of thrombus formation, desiccation, or wall perforation.

Cooled-Tip

Numerous investigators have explored the use of saline to cool the electrode-tissue interface. There are 3 primary methods of cooling the electrode-tissue interface that have been investigated in animal models (Figure 14). Chilled saline can be circulated through the electrode via internal lumens in the body of the catheter. Fluid can be forced through the catheter lumen and out of pores in the electrode's distal tip. Finally, saline can be injected through a sheath placed around the catheter. There are advantages and disadvantages to each method, but all achieve the same general results. Larger lesions can be generated due to a reduction in overheating at the electrode-tissue interface and a decreased incidence of impedance rises which allows for higher levels of energy to be applied for longer durations.

Animal Studies

While there have been a great number of abstracts published regarding cooled-tip ablations, this discussion will focus on the results documented in 3 manuscripts, one utilizing a circulating saline catheter[67] and 2 using electrodes with pores.[68,69] In addition, an abstract comparing the 3 methods of tip cooling will be described.[70]

In an open-chest sheep study, Ruffy et al used a cooled-tip ablation catheter with a 4 mm tip electrode through which saline was circulated.[67] Lesions generated during endocardial LV ablations with this catheter were compared to lesions created with a standard temperature-control catheter with a 4 mm tip electrode used to maintain the temperature at the electrode-tissue

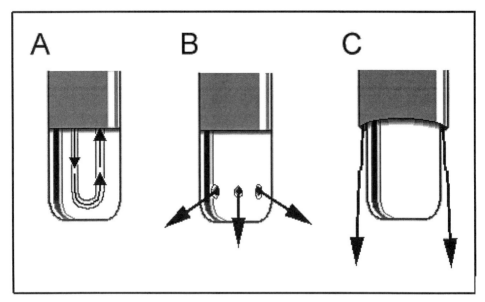

Figure 14. Three cooled-tip ablation methods. Chilled saline can be circulated through the electrode via internal lumens in the body of the catheter (A), fluid can be forced through the catheter lumen and out of pores in the electrode's distal tip (B), and saline can be injected through a sheath placed around the catheter (C). Larger lesions can be generated due to a reduction in overheating at the electrode-tissue interface and a decreased incidence of impedance rises which allows for higher levels of energy to be applied for longer durations.

interface just below 100°C. An average of 22 ± 4.5 watts of power was delivered using the cooled-tip catheter. Power was delivered for 43 ± 11 seconds with the temperature-controlled catheter and for 49 ± 7 seconds for the cooled-tip catheter. In 27 applications of power with the cooled-tip catheter, there were no impedance rises, but with the noncooled catheter 11 of the 28 ablations resulted in impedance rises. The cooled-tip catheter created lesions with significantly larger average maximum widths and depths. Average lesion volume was 1247 ± 521 mm^3 for the cooled-tip catheter and 436 ± 177 mm^3 for the temperature-controlled catheter.

In an investigation using catheters with 2 mm electrodes, Mittleman and associates compared a standard electrode to a custom-designed electrode with 2 side pores and one distal pore through which room-temperature saline could be infused.[69] Power was applied for 60 seconds at fixed levels of 10 and 20 watts to the endocardium of canine left ventricles. For both power levels, the length, width, and depth of the lesions created with the cooled-tip catheter were significantly larger than with the standard catheter (Figure 15).

In a canine thigh muscle preparation, Nakagawa et al used a catheter with a 5 mm distal electrode equipped with a centrally-located thermistor and 6 irrigation holes.[68] Power was delivered for 60 seconds or until an impedance rise occurred. Three separate protocols were used: a constant 66 volts, 20–66 volts adjusted to maintain the temperature measured at the thermistor between 80°C to 90°C, or a fixed level of 66 volts with saline irrigation. Impedance rises occurred during all 39 applications at a fixed level of 66 volts with no irrigation, but only 6 of 75 irrigated ablations. There were no impedance rises for the temperature-controlled ablation, but the average power level for these applications was only 38±6 volts. The lesions created with constant power and saline irrigation were significantly larger than those made with the other 2 methods (Table 2).

Demazumbder and associates compared all 3 methods of cooled-tip ablation using catheters with 5 mm tip electrodes.[70] Each electrode was irrigated with saline at a flow rate of 20 cc per minute. Constant RF power of 50 watts was applied for 60 seconds or until an impedance rise occurred. Lesion depth was greatest with the sheath infusion (8.2±0.4 mm) and the electrode with pores (7.6±0.8 mm). Due to impedance rises, the power application was abbreviated for the internal cooling catheter (32±16 seconds) resulting in shallower lesions (4.9±1.2 mm).

Human Investigations

Two studies have shown that cooled-tip catheters can be used to ablate VT in humans. Stevenson et al used a series of 41 RF applications to ablate 3 VTs in a 64-year-old man.[71] The temperatures recorded from the electrode tip

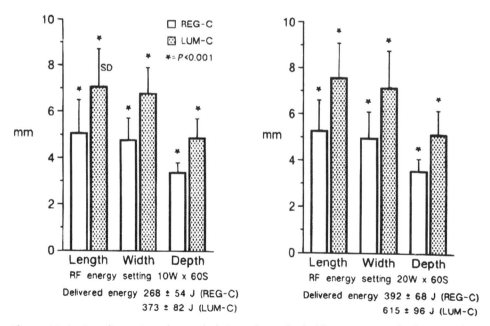

Figure 15. Lesion dimensions for cooled-tip and standard ablations. A standard 2 mm electrode was compared to a custom-designed 2 mm electrode with 2 side pores and one distal pore through which room-temperature saline could be infused. Power was applied for 60 seconds at fixed levels of 10 and 20 watts to the endocardium of canine left ventricles. For both power levels the length, width and depth of the lesions created with the cooled-tip catheter (LUM-C) were significantly larger than with the standard catheter (REG-C).

Table 2
Lesion dimensions for three power delivery protocols[68]

	66V	Temp-control	66V + saline
Depth (mm)	4.7±0.6	6.1±0.5	9.9±1.1
Diameter (mm)	9.8±0.8	11.3±0.9	14.3±1.5
Volume (mm³)	135±33	275±55	700±217

ranged from 31°C to 53°C. The patient received a transplant 18 days later and the lesions were evaluated. The investigators concluded that cooled RF ablation produces substantial lesions in regions of chronic infarction despite maintenance of electrode tip temperature below 55°C. Wilbur and associates used a cooled ablation system, which circulated saline through the tip electrode, to ablate VT in 37 patients.[72] They reported a 75% acute success rate and 77% of the patients had a 75% reduction in VT episodes in the 2 months post procedure versus 2 months before the ablation.

Material

Platinum electrodes have been the standard for most RF ablation catheters, but gold electrodes allow for greater power delivery without an impedance rise to create deeper lesions. Because gold has nearly four times the thermal conductivity of platinum, Simmons and associates investigated the use of gold versus platinum electrodes. This in vitro study utilized both 6F 2 mm and 7F 4 mm electrodes.[3] The power was initiated at 4 watts for the 2 mm studies and 12 watts for the 4 mm applications and increased in 2 watt increments until an impedance rise occurred. In both the 2 mm and 4 mm ablations, the maximum power that could be applied was higher for the electrodes made of gold versus platinum (2 mm: 8 watts versus 6 watts; 4 mm: 20 watts versus 14 watts). For the 2 mm electrodes, only the lesion depth was significantly increased for the gold versus platinum electrodes (6.7±0.7versus 4.7±0.5). In the 4 mm experiments, lesion depth, length, and volume were significantly increased for the gold electrodes (depth = 7.2±1.4 versus 5.8±0.7 mm; length = 8.0±0.9 versus 6.5±0.8 mm; volume = 195±69 versus 115±39 mm³).

Conclusions

The dimensions of a lesion created with radiofrequency power are determined by the amount of tissue heated above the critical temperature for producing irreversible myocardial damage, 50°C. Because radiofrequency tissue damage is the result of resistive heating, good contact between the ablating electrode and the tissue is necessary for successful lesion generation. Without contact, no lesion will be created. Appropriate contact between the electrode and the tissue to be ablated is usually evident via a rapid rise in temperature and a drop in the catheter to ventricular tissue impedance by greater than 10 Ω. With good contact, upon the initiation of fixed level energy application, the temperature at the electrode-tissue interface rises monoexponentially to greater than 15°C within 4 seconds using 20 watts of RF power.

The rapid maturation of lesion width is related to the temperature increase at the electrode-tissue interface, which is a direct function of the current density. Deeper tissues are not heated as a direct result of the dissipation of electrical energy because tissue heating decreases as a function of $1/r^4$. Therefore, deep tissues are heated via conductive heating from the tissue near the electrode-tissue interface. This conductive heating has been shown to require 1 to 2 minutes to equilibrate.

The character of lesions created with temperature control depends on the placement of the temperature sensor or sensors relative to the portion of the electrode that is in contact with the tissue. Thus, the orientation of the ablating electrode and its temperature sensors will determine the appropriate target temperature required to create maximal lesions while avoiding coagulum formation due to overheating at any location within the electrode-tissue interface. For most of the currently used catheters equipped with temperature sensors the target temperature should be set at 70°C to 80°C.

There are numerous factors involved in determining the size of lesions generated using RF energy. Following are the factors that could increase the lesion size and which have been summarized in this chapter:

1. Increased catheter to tissue contact.
2. Maximal RF power level, which does not result in tissue overheating.
3. RF power application time as long as 1–2 minutes.
4. Catheter ablating electrodes that are 8 mm long to ablate ventricular tissues which are adjusted to make full tissue contact by contacting the tissue side to side as well as in a perpendicular orientation; current density has to be maintained the same as with 4mm long ablation electrode. Longer flexible electrodes (12mm or longer) are used to create linear lesions within the atria.
5. Increasing the ablating electrode radius while adjusting the power to maintain the current density.
6. Catheter to tissue orientation and contact can be monitored by intracardiac ultrasound.
7. Active cooling of the ablating electrode with saline infusion allowing increased power and intramural heating. Ablating electrode temperature monitoring must be set at 50°C to 55°C to avoid intramural tissue overheating.
8. Gold ablating electrode.
9. Summation of multi-electrode to increase the ablation electrode contact area.
10. Unipolar configuration of power between the catheter and the reference electrode.
11. Large reference electrode which presents the least amount of impedance to the RF current flow.

The most useful monitoring factor used during ablation with nonirrigated ablation electrodes is the temperature by using a thermocouple or thermistor which is embedded at the tip of the ablation electrode. To avoid overheating the temperature should be maintained at 70°C to 80°C. However, the goal of RF arrhythmia ablation is to minimize the amount of tissue damage while eliminating the arrhythmogenic foci. Adjustments in any of these variables can have a significant impact on the dimensions of generated radiofrequency lesions.

References

1. Haines D, Watson D. Tissue heating during radiofrequency catheter ablation: a thermodynamic model and observations in isolated perfused and superperfused canine right ventricular free wall. *PACE* 1989;12:962–976.
2. Hoyt R, Huang S, Marcus F, et al. Factors influencing transcatheter radiofrequency ablation of the myocardium. *J Appl Cardiol* 1986;1:469–486.
3. Simmons W, Mackey S, He D, et al. Comparison of gold versus platinum electrodes on myocardial lesion size using radiofrequency energy. *PACE* 1996;19:398–402.
4. Avitall B, Mughal K, Hare J, et al. Radiofrequency lesion depth versus width maturation: 2 contrasting parameters. *J Am Coll Cardiol* 1995; 705–1:41A.
5. Chan R, Johnson S, Seward J, et al. Accuracy of intracardiac ultrasound assessment of RF ablation lesion dimensions in the intact canine atrium and ventricle. *Circulation* 1995;92(8):3820;I–794.
6. Kalman J, Jue J, Sudhir K, et al. In vitro quantification of radiofrequency ablation lesion size using intracardiac echocardiography in dogs. *Am J Cardiol* 1996;77(2):217–219.
7. Haines D. The biophysics of radiofrequency catheter ablation in the heart: the importance of temperature monitoring. *PACE* 1993;16:587–591.
8. Hindricks G, Haverkamp W, Gulker H, et al. Radiofrequency coagulation of ventricular myocardium: improved prediction of lesion size by monitoring catheter tip temperature. *Eur Heart J* 1989;10:972–984.
9. Hoffmann E, Mattke JS, Dorwarth U, et al. Temperature-controlled radiofrequency catheter ablation of AV conduction: first clinical experience. *Eur Heart J* 1993;14:57–64.
10. Ring M, Huang S, Gorman G, et al. Determinants of impedance rise during catheter ablation of bovine myocardium with radiofrequency energy. *PACE* 1989;12:1502–1513.
11. An H, Saksena S, Janssen M, et al. Radiofrequency ablation of ventricular myocardium using active fixation and passive contact catheter delivery systems. *Am Heart J* 1989;118:69–77.
12. Wittkampf F, Hauer R, de Medina R. Control of radiofrequency lesion size by power regulation. *Circulation* 1989;80(4):962–968.
13. Haines D. Determinants of lesion size during radiofrequency catheter ablation: the role of electrode-tissue contact pressure and duration of energy delivery. *J Cardiovasc Electrophysiol* 1991;2:509–515.

14. Harvey M, Kim Y, Sousa J, et al. Impedance monitoring during radiofrequency catheter ablation in humans. *PACE* 1992;15:22–27.
15. Hoffman E, Remp T, Gerth A, et al. Does impedance monitoring during radiofrequency catheter ablation reduce the risk of impedance rise? [abstract] *Circulation* 1993;88(suppl):I165.
16. Strickberger S, Hummel J, Vorperian V, et al. A randomized comparison of impedance and temperature monitoring during accessory pathway ablation. *Circulation* 1993;88(4):I–295.
17. Remp T, Hoffman E, Dorwarth U, et al. A new catheter design for validation of preablation impedance as a marker for contact. *J Am Coll Cardiol* 1997;29(2):1021–1068;333A.
18. Strickberger S, Vorperian V, Man K, et al. Relation between impedance and endocardial contact during radiofrequency catheter ablation. *Am Heart J* 1994;128(2):226–229.
19. Grogan EW, Nellis SH, Subramanian R. Impedance changes during catheter ablation by radiofrequency energy: a potential method for monitoring efficacy of lesion generation. *J Am Coll Cardiol* 1987;9:95A.
20. Dorwarth U, Mattke S, Muller D, et al. Impedance monitoring during constant power and temperature-controlled radiofrequency catheter ablation. *Circulation* 1993;88(4):0877;I–165.
21. Chan R, Johnson S, Packer D. The effect of ablation electrode length and catheter tip/endocardial orientation on radiofrequency lesion size in the canine right atrium. *PACE* 1994;17:225;797.
22. He D, Marcus F, Lampe L, et al. Temperature monitoring during RF energy application without the use of thermistors or thermocouples. *PACE* 1996;19 (244):626.
23. He D, Sharma P, Marcus F, et al. In vivo experiment of radiofrequency (RF) energy application using bio-battery induced temperature monitoring. *J Am Coll Cardiol* 1997;29(2):123;32A.
24. Kalman J, Fitzpatrick A, Chin M, et al. Efficiency of heating with radiofrequency energy is related to stability of tissue contact: evaluation by intracardiac echocardiography. *Circulation* 1994;90(4, part 2):1454;I–270.
25. Kalman J, Fitzpatrick A, Olgin J, et al. Biophysical characteristics of radiofrequency lesion formation in vivo: dynamics of catheter tip-tissue contact evaluated by intracardiac echocardiography. *Am Heart J* 1997;133(1): 8–18.
26. Chan R, Johnson S, Seward J, et al. Effect of ablation catheter tip/endocardial surface orientation on radiofrequency lesion size in the canine ventricle *J Am Coll Cardiol* 1997;29(2):727–726;76A.
27. Hoffman E, Haberl R, Pulter R, et al. Biophysical parameters of radiofrequency catheter ablation. *Int J Cardiol* 1992;13:213–222.
28. Bardy G, Sawyer P, Johnson G, et al. Radiofrequency ablation: effect of voltage and pulse duration on canine myocardium. *Am J Physiol* 1990;258: H1899-H1905.
29. Simmers T, Wittkampf F, Hauer R, et al. In vivo ventricular lesion growth in radiofrequency catheter ablation. *PACE* 1994;17(2):523–531.
30. Avitall B, Hare J, Silverstein E, et al. Radiofrequency ablation of atrial tissues: power requirements. *J Am Coll Cardiol* 1994;(suppl):276A.

31. Kovoor P, Eipper V, Dewsnap B, et al. The effect of differing frequencies on lesion size during radiofrequency ablation. *Circulation* 1996;94(8):3953; I677.

32. Bru P, Lauribe P, Rouane A, et al. Catheter ablation using very high frequency energy: a new method without limitation due to impedance rise. *Circulation* 1994:90(4, part 2):2608;I–485.

33. Haines D, McRury I, Whayne J, et al. Radiofrequency ablation at the tricuspid-inferior vena cava isthmus: unipolar versus bipolar delivery. *Circulation* 1994;90(4):3202;I–594.

34. Anfinsen O, Kongsgaard E, Foerster A, et al. Radiofrequency catheter ablation of pig right atrial free wall: larger lesions but similar incidence of lung injury and diaphragmal paresis with two-catheter bipolar compared to unipolar electrode configuration. *Circulation* 1996;92(4):3260;I–557.

35. Anfinsen O, Kongsgaard E, Aass H, et al. Radiofrequency current ablation of thin-walled structures: an in vitro study comparing unipolar and bipolar electrode configuration. *PACE* 1996;19:594;714.

36. Nakagawa H, Wittkampf F, Imai S, et al. Pulsed current delivery combined with saline irrigation produces deeper radiofrequency lesions without steam "pop." *J Am Coll Cardiol* 1997;29(2):786–3;374A.

37. Tomassoni G, Jain M, Dixon-Tulloch E, et al. Ground patch location significantly effects radiofrequency ablative lesion dimensions. *J Am Coll Cardiol* 1997;29(2):750–6;203A.

38. Otomo K, Arruda M, Tondo C, et al. Why does a large tip electrode make a deeper lesion? *Circulation* 1995;92(8):3814;I–793.

39. Nath S, Lynch C, Whayne J, et al. Cellular electrophysiological effects of hyperthermia on isolated guinea pig papillary muscle: implications for catheter ablation. *Circulation* 1993;88(part 1):1826–1831.

40. Wittkampf F, Simmers T, Hauer R, et al. Myocardial temperature response during radiofrequency catheter ablation. *PACE* 1995;18(2):307–317.

41. Haines D, Verow A. Observations on electrode-tissue interface temperature and effect on electrical impedance during radiofrequency ablation of ventricular myocardium. *Circulation* 1990;82:1034–1038.

42. Langberg J, Calkins H, El-Atassi R, et al. Temperature monitoring during radiofrequency catheter ablation of accessory pathways. *Circulation* 1992; 86:1469–1474.

43. Avitall B, Khan M, Krum D, et al. Physics and engineering of transcatheter cardiac tissue ablation. *J Am Coll Cardiol* 1993;22:3:921–932.

44. Haines D. The biophysics of radiofrequency catheter ablation in the heart: the importance of temperature monitoring. *PACE* 1993;16:586–591.

45. Haverkamp W, Hindricks G, Gulker H, et al. Coagulation of ventricular myocardium using radiofrequency alternating current:biophysical aspects and experimental findings. *PACE* 1989;12:187–195.

46. Blouin L, Marcus F, Lampe L. Assessment of effects of a radiofrequency energy field and thermistor location in an electrode catheter on the accuracy of temperature measurement. *PACE* 1991;14:807–813.

47. McRury I, Whayne J, Mitchell M, et al. Electrode size and temperature effects on lesion volume during temperature-controlled RF ablation in vivo. *J Am Coll Cardiol* 1997;29(2):928;123A.

48. Kongsgaard E, Steen T, Amlie J. temperature guided radiofrequency catheter ablation: catheter tip temperature underestimates tissue temperature. *Circulation* 1994:90(4, part 2):1457;I–271.

49. Fleischman S, Panescu D, Whayne J, et al. In vitro study of temperature sensor placement during temperature-controlled radiofrequency ablation. *PACE* 1995;18:293;869.

50. Haines D, Watson D, Verow A. Electrode radius predicts lesion radius during radiofrequency energy heating: validation of a proposed hemodynamic model. *Circ Res* 1990;67(1):124–129.

51. Langberg J, Lee M, Chin M, et al. Radiofrequency catheter ablation: the effect of electrode size on lesion volume in vivo. *PACE* 1990;13:1242–1248.

52. Langberg J, Gallagher M, Strickberger S, et al. Temperature-guided radiofrequency catheter ablation with very large distal electrodes. *Circulation* 1993;88:245–249.

53. McRury I, Whayne J, Haines D. Temperature measurement as a determinant of tissue heating during radiofrequency catheter ablation: an examination of electrode thermistor positioning for measurement accuracy. *J Cardiovasc Electrophysiol* 1995;6(4):268–278.

54. Oeff M, Langberg J, Chin M, et al. Ablation of ventricular tachycardia using multiple sequential transcatheter application of radiofrequency energy. *PACE* 1992;15(8):1167–1176.

55. Oeff M, Langberg J, Franklin J, et al. Effects of multipolar electrode radiofrequency energy delivery on ventricular endocardium. *Am Heart J* 1990;119(3, part 1):599–607.

56. Chang R, Stevenson W, Saxon L, et al. Increasing catheter ablation lesion size by simultaneous application of radiofrequency current to 2 adjacent sites. *Am Heart J* 1993;125:1276–1284.

57. Avitall B, Hare J, Mughal K, et al. Segmented ablation electrode: a system for flexible lesion size. *Circulation* 1994;90(4, part 2):671;I–126.

58. Mackey S, Thornton L, He D, et al. Simultaneous multipolar radiofrequency ablation in the monopolar mode increases lesion size. *PACE* 1996; 19:1042–1048.

59. Baal T, Chen X, Kottkamp H, et al. Radiofrequency catheter ablation: improving lesion size achieved with conventional catheters. *Circulation* 1994; 90(4, part 2):1463;I–272.

60. Strickberger S, Davis J, Maguire M. Radiofrequency ablation of the atrium using sequential coil electrodes. *J Am Coll Cardiol* 1996;27(2):1037–1033;400A.

61. Mitchell M, McRury I, Haines D. Results of linear right atrial radiofrequency ablation with a temperature controlled, multiple coil electrode catheter. *J Am Coll Cardiol* 1996; 27(2):1037–1033;400A.

62. Fleischman S, Thompson R, Panescu D, et al. Flexible electrodes for long atrial lesions. *Circulation* 1996;94(8):3952;I–676.

63. Panescu D, Haines D, Fleischman S, et al. Atrial lesions by temperature-controlled radiofrequency ablation. *Circulation* 1996;94(8):2891;I–493.

64. Whayne J, Haines D, Panescu D, et al. Ring and coil electrodes for ablation of atrial fibrillation. *Circulation* 1996;94(8):2891;I–493.

65. Hoey M, Mulier P, Shake J. Pre-test mapping with cold Ringer's solution

via screw-tip catheter before radiofrequency ablation. *Circulation* 1995; 92(8):3813;I–793.

66. Hoey M, Mulier P, Shake J. Intramural ablations using screw-tip catheter and saline electrode produces predictable lesion sizes. *Circulation* 1995; 92(8):3818;I–794.

67. Ruffy R, Imran M, Santel D, et al. Radiofrequency delivery through a cooled catheter tip allows the creation of larger endomyocardial lesions in the ovine heart. *J Cardiovasc Electrophysiol* 1995;6:1089–1096.

68. Nakagawa H, Yamanashi W, Pitha J, et al. Comparison of in vivo tissue temperature profile and lesion geometry for radiofrequency ablation with a saline-irrigated electrode versus temperature in a canine thigh muscle preparation. *Circulation* 1995;91(8):2264–2273.

69. Mittleman R, Huang S, de Guzman, et al. Use of saline infusion electrode catheter for improved energy delivery and increased lesion size in radiofrequency catheter ablation. *PACE* 1995;18(5, part 1):1022–1027.

70. Demazumbder D, Kallash H, Schwartzman D. Comparison of different electrodes for radiofrequency ablation of myocardium using saline irrigation. *PACE* 1997;20(106):1076.

71. Stevenson W, Mitchell R, Friedman P, et al. Radiofrequency ablation lesions produced by a cool tip catheter in human infarction. *Circulation* 1996;94(8):124;I–22.

72. Wilbur D, Epstein A, Kay G, et al. Prospective randomized multicenter study with a new cooled radiofrequency ablation system for the treatment of ventricular tachycardia. *PACE* 1997;20:293;1123.

Chapter 5

Pathological Aspects of Radiofrequency Catheter Ablation of Cardiac Tissue

Saroja Bharati, MD and Maurice Lev, MD

A method of closed-chest catheter ablation of the atrioventricular (AV) junction using radiofrequency (RF) energy was introduced in detail by Huang and colleagues in 1987.[1] They demonstrated that catheter ablation of the AV junction with RF energy can produce acute or chronic AV block. This was documented with electrophysiological and histological correlations.[1,2] They showed that RF energy is a safe procedure with no serious complications such as perforations or hemorrhage. In addition, pathologically, the ablated areas were discrete and relatively well defined. These findings suggested a distinct advantage over catheter ablation of the AV junction with direct current shock or laser energy.

Later, Marcus and colleagues[3] and Huang and associates[4] demonstrated that ablation with RF energy has the potential application of creating incomplete AV block and modifying AV nodal conduction. Huang et al[5] and Langberg et al[6] showed that RF ablation of the coronary sinus area was feasible and has the potential to ablate the right- or left-sided accessory pathways. Ring et al[7] and Lee et al[8] also produced ablation in the ventricular septum and the right atrium, thereby suggesting that this method may be used to ablate arrhythmic foci originating from the ventricular septum and an atrial arrhythmic focus in cases of intractable right atrial tachycardia. Finally, Marcus and colleagues[9] have demonstrated in short- and long-term experiments that dissociation of AV conduction and refractoriness after application of RF energy to the canine AV node can be produced.

It is important that we understand the pathological findings of the ablated areas and the surrounding structures. Because the long-term outcome of these

From Huang SKS, Wilber DJ (eds.): *Radiofrequency Catheter Ablation of Cardiac Arrhythmias: Basic Concepts and Clinical Applications,* 2nd ed. Armonk, NY: Futura Publishing Company, Inc. ©2000.

patients is unknown today, it is important to understand the pathological changes following the use of RF energy. In this chapter, we will discuss our pathological findings of the conduction system and the entire heart following RF catheter ablation of the AV junction, the coronary sinus, the atria, the tricuspid annulus, and the ventricles. The experiments were conducted in canine models by various investigators. In addition, the AV junction of one human explanted heart where RF catheter ablation eliminated the slow pathway of AV nodal reentrant tachycardia is discussed.

Method of Study of the Conduction System

The ablated area including the entire AV junction was studied microscopically in all hearts in the following manner:

Blocks containing the AV node and its approaches, the AV bundle (the penetrating, the branching, and bifurcating portions), and the bundle branches up to the region of the moderator band were serially sectioned and every 20th section was retained. All sections were alternatively stained with hematoxylin and eosin and Weigert-van Gieson stains. In this manner, a mean of 500 sections was examined from each heart. The method of study of the conduction system has previously been reported.[24]

Closed-Chest Catheter Ablation of the AV Junction Using RF Energy: Electrophysiological and Histologic Observations of Acute AV Block

Huang and associates[1] produced complete AV block by means of RF catheter ablation in 11 dogs and second-degree AV block in 2. Complete AV block persisted in 9 of the dogs during 4- to 7-day follow-up. One had persistent 2:1 AV block and the other had persistent first-degree AV block. One of the 2 dogs with initial second-degree AV block developed complete AV block, and the other resumed normal conduction.

Pathology

At a gross level, well-delineated brownish round or oblong scar areas were present adjacent to the septal leaflet of the tricuspid valve (Figure 1). There were no hemorrhages, perforations, or thrombi.

Conduction System

Acute AV Block Created by RF Energy Using Bipolar Electrodes

In the acute experiments using bipolar electrode catheters, 2 dogs developed complete AV block, 1 with wide QRS and the other with narrow QRS com-

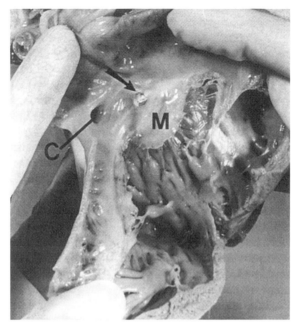

Figure 1. Complete AV block with narrow QRS complex created by RF ablation through a unipolar electrode catheter. Right atrial and right ventricular view demonstrates a discrete localized lesion at the AV junction. Note that the lesion is distinctly smaller than the previous one. M indicates medial leaflet of the tricuspid valve; C, coronary sinus. Arrow points to lesion created by ablation. Note the well-delineated margins. (From Huang et al[1]).

plex escape rhythm. The dog with wide QRS complex in the electrocardiogram showed extensive mononuclear cell and neutrophil infiltration and marked hemorrhage in the approaches to the AV node. There was well-delineated coagulation necrosis at the approaches to the AV node as well as in the AV node itself. The penetrating bundle showed increased eosinophilia. The cells of the beginning of the left bundle branch also showed coagulation necrosis, and there was vacuolization of the spongiosa of the aortic and tricuspid valves.

In the dog with narrow QRS escape rhythm, there was extensive infiltration of mononuclear cells, hemorrhage, and dissolution and well-delineated necrosis of the approaches to the AV node and the AV node up to the beginning of the AV bundle. In addition, the nerves were inflamed. The summit of the ventricular septum on the right side showed chronic inflammation. There was increased vacuolization of the basal spongiosa with hemorrhage and inflammation in the tricuspid valve.

Acute Block Created by RF Energy Using Unipolar Electrode Catheter

The conduction system of 1 dog that developed complete AV block and narrow QRS complex following RF energy produced by a unipolar electrode catheter showed that the AV node and its approaches (very close by), the prox-

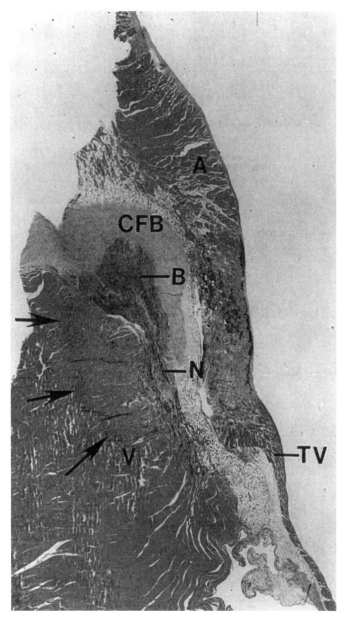

Figure 2. Microscopic examination of the ablated area from Figure 1. A low-power view of the end of the AV node and the penetrating bundle. The end of the node and the beginning of the penetrating bundle are replaced by hemorrhage, with area of coagulation necrosis extending to the adjacent atrial and ventricular myocardium. CFB indicates central fibrous body; A, atrial myocardium; TV, tricuspid valve; V, ventricular septum; B, the end of the node and beginning of the penetrating bundle; N, AV node. Arrows demarcate the discrete area of necrosis that extended to the summit of the ventricular septum, especially on the right side. (Hematoxylin and eosin stain. Magnification ×16.) (From Huang et al.[1])

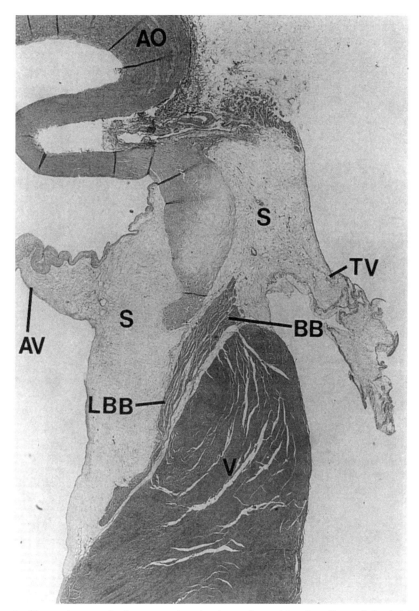

Figure 3. Photomicrograph demonstrating the intact branching bundle and the left bundle branch from Figures 1 and 2. AO indicates aorta; S, spongiosa; AV, aortic valve; TV, tricuspid valve; BB, branching bundle; V, summit of the ventricular septum; and LBB, left bundle branch. Note the marked increase in and vacuolization of the spongiosa of the aortic and tricuspid valves. (Hematoxylin and eosin stain. Magnification ×16.) (From Huang et al.[1])

imal part and the end point of the AV node, and the beginning of the AV bundle demonstrated hemorrhage, coagulation necrosis, and chronic inflammation (Figure 2). The necrotic area was well defined. The remainder of the penetrating bundle was intact (Figure 3) but showed coagulation necrosis and chronic inflammation. There was an increase in spongiosa of the aortic and tricuspid valves and vacuolization of central fibrous body. These lesions were less severe (less extensive) than those seen in bipolar experiments.

In summary, in the acute experiments, a well-delineated coagulation necrosis of the approaches to the AV node and the AV node, and in part the penetrating bundle, was created by RF ablation of the AV junction with clinically documented complete AV block. The lesion created by unipolar configurations appears to be better than that created by bipolar configurations.

Chronic AV Block Induced by Closed-Chest Catheter Desiccation with RF Energy: Electrophysiological and Histologic Observations

Complex AV block was achieved in 4 dogs immediately after ablation with a bipolar RF electrode catheter delivered at the AV junction. During 2 months of follow-up, 3 dogs had persistent complete AV block and a stable escape rhythm, and the other had persistent 2:1 AV block. At the end of 2 months of follow-up, repeat His bundle recordings revealed supra-His AV block in 2; in the other 2, His bundle potentials could not be recorded.[2]

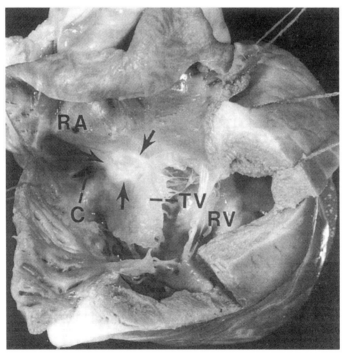

Figure 4. Chronic complete AV block produced by RF energy. Right atrial and right ventricular view showing the chronic changes in the AV nodal area. Note that there are no perforations in the tricuspid valve, right atrium, or right ventricle. Arrows point to the thickened whitish plaque area between the coronary sinus and the medial leaflet of the tricuspid valve. RA indicates right atrium; RV, right ventricle; C, coronary sinus; and TV, thickened tricuspid valve. (From Huang et al[2].)

Gross Pathology

A localized lesion was found between the septal leaflet of the tricuspid valve and the coronary sinus (Figure 4). There were no hemorrhages, edema, perforations, or thrombus formation. All the valves were normal.

Conduction System

In 1 dog the proximal portion of the node was fibrosed with tenuous connection with surrounding atrial myocardium Figure 5. The AV node and its ap-

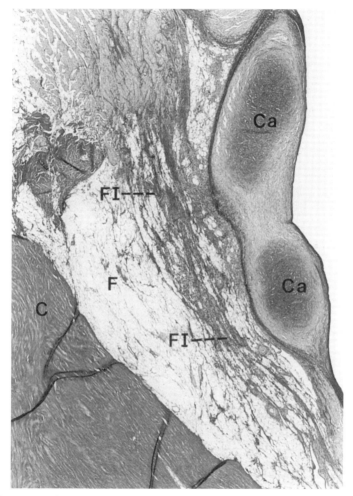

Figure 5. The approaches to the AV node and the beginning of the node (from Figure 4) are replaced by fibrosis, fat, and cartilage formation in the subendocardium of the right atrium. The AV node has tenuous connection with the atrium. C indicates central fibrous body; Ca, cartilaginous formation of the subendocardium of the right atrium pressing on the approaches to the node; F, fatty infiltration of the approaches to the atrioventricular node; and Fl fibrosis to the node and the beginning of the atrioventricular node. (Weigert-van Gieson stain. Magnification ×30.) (From Huang et al.[2])

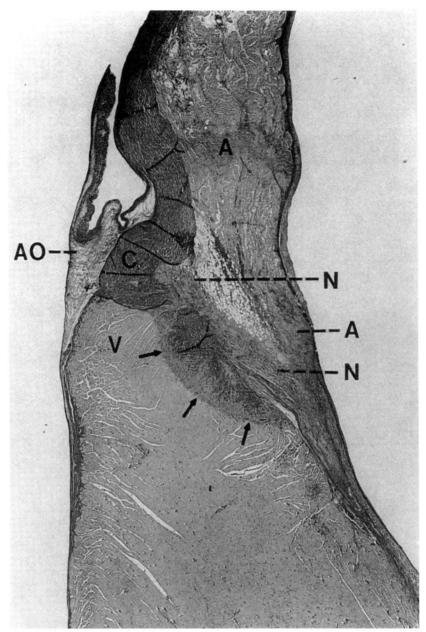

Figure 6. Chronic complete AV block produced by RF energy. The AV node is entering the central fibrous body. Note the AV node and the immediate approaches and the right side of the summit of the ventricular septum are replaced by granulation tissue. Arrows point to the localized well delineated area of the summit of the ventricular septum immediately beneath the atrioventricular node. Note also the fatty infiltration separating the superior approaches from the AV node. A indicates atrial approaches; AO, aortic valve; C, central fibrous body; N, AV node; and V, summit of the ventricular septum. (Weigert-van Gieson stain. Magnification ×17.25.) (From Huang et al.[2])

proaches were replaced by granulomatous tissue in 2 (Figure 6) and in 1 by fibrosis and cartilage. Thus, in all 4 dogs, the approaches to the AV node revealed varying amount of chronic inflammatory cells, fibrosis, fatty metamorphosis, and, in one, cartilage formation. The maximum damage occurred in the AV node in all dogs. See Figure 6. In addition, there was a varying degree of injury to the penetrating portion of the AV bundle. The dog with the wide QRS escape rhythm also had mild to moderate injury to the branching portion of the bundle, associated with absence of His bundle potential on the His bundle electrogram. The right side of the summit of the ventricular septum showed varying amount of granulation tissue with a well demarcated zone.

Our study therefore suggests that RF energy delivered at the AV junction can produce complete AV block both acutely and chronically, with maximum damage in the AV node and its approaches and varying amount of damage to the AV bundle, the tricuspid and aortic valves, and the summit of the ventricular septum. The lesions produced by this energy are quite discrete and well delineated when seen acutely as well as chronically, in contrast to the use of direct current energy where the ablated area is not well defined.

Chronic Incomplete AV Block Induced by RF Catheter Ablation

Huang and colleagues[4] induced chronic (first- and second-degree) AV block in 13 of 20 dogs. One dog progressed to complete AV block. Seven dogs remained in complete AV block. The conduction system was studied in 5 dogs, 2 with first-degree, two with 2:1 AV block, and one with complete AV block. The dogs were killed 8 to 12 weeks after the ablative procedure.

Pathology

There was no damage in the ablated and adjoining area, except for a well demarcated localized whitish scar between the septal leaflet of the tricuspid valve and the coronary sinus (Figure 7).

Conduction System

The basic pathology produced by the experimental procedure was found in the distal part of the atrial septum, the approaches to the AV node, and the AV node. The AV bundle and the bundle branches were minimally involved. There was fibrosis of the approaches to the AV node, extending from the endocardium on the right side of the septum, with chronic inflammatory cells, fatty metamorphosis, and cartilage formation. The AV node presented chronic inflammatory change and fibrosis. There were mild to moderate fibrotic changes in the bundle and bundle branches. In the 2 dogs with first-degree AV block there was less severe damage in the approaches to the AV node and the AV

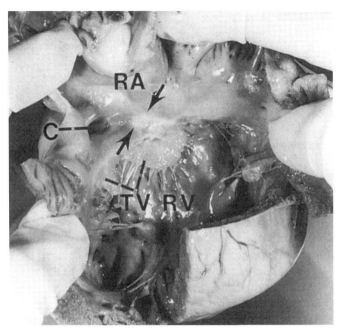

Figure 7. Chronic incomplete AV block. Right atrial and right ventricular view showing the effects of RF catheter ablation of the AV nodal area which produced chronic incomplete AV block. RA indicates right atrium; RV, right ventricle; TV, tricuspid valve; and C, coronary sinus. Arrows point to the atrioventricular nodal area that is thickened and whitened. (From Huang et al.[4])

node (Figure 8) when compared in dogs with 2:1 or third-degree AV block. The AV bundle was also distinctly less damaged in first-degree AV block compared with that seen in dogs with complex AV block.

In conclusion, RF catheter ablation of the AV junction may be achieved with production of chronic incomplete AV block. The modification of AV conduction is obtained by creating lesions in the approaches to the AV node and the AV node. These studies suggest that modification of AV nodal conduction can be accomplished in humans and may be found useful in managing intractable supraventricular arrhythmias.

Transcatheter Ablation of Coronary Sinus for Ablating Accessory Pathways with RF Energy

Huang et al[5] demonstrated in 1988 that RF catheter ablation of the coronary sinus can be accomplished with feasibility for potential interruption of left-sided accessory pathways in Wolff-Parkinson-White syndrome.

These investigators demonstrated no significant changes in the AV nodal refractoriness and conduction after catheter ablation of the coronary sinus in 20 dogs by means of RF energy. There was neither rupture of the coronary sinus nor occlusion of the coronary arteries (Figure 9). The chronic lesions were characterized by granulation tissue and fibrosis. Two dogs showed damage to

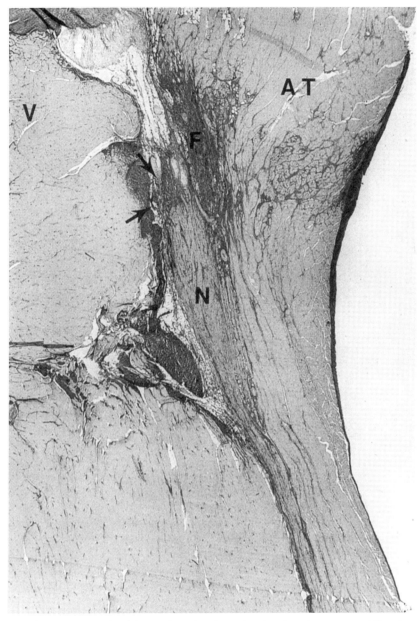

Figure 8. Photomicrograph of the AV junction from the dog that demonstrated first-degree AV block 12 weeks after the ablative procedure. Note the mild to moderate fibrosis of the approaches to the AV node and part of the distal end of the node. Nevertheless, the node maintains its continuity with its approaches and most of the nodal fibers are intact. AT indicates atrial approaches; F, fibrosis of the atrial septum; N, AV node; and V, ventricular septum. Arrows point to fibrosis present mostly in the distal part of the node. (Weigert-van Gieson stain. Magnification ×15.18.) (From Huang et al.[4])

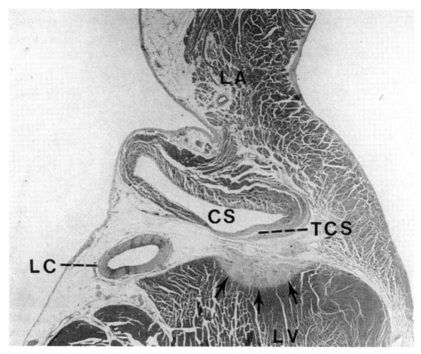

Figure 9. Photomicrograph of the coronary sinus showing the effect of RF ablation. Note the discrete area of fibrosis of the left ventricle produced by RF catheter ablation of the coronary sinus. CS, coronary sinus; LA, left atrium; LV, left ventricle; LC, left circumflex coronary artery; and TCS, fibrosis of part of the wall of the coronary sinus. Arrows point to the discrete scar on the left ventricle. (Hematoxylin and eosin stain. Magnification ×7.5) (From Huang et al.[5])

the branches of the underlying coronary artery, with necrotizing arteritis and arteriosclerosis.

Conduction System Findings

Four, 6, 8, and 12 weeks after the procedure 4 dogs were studied. There were very minimal chronic inflammatory changes with or without fibrosis in the conduction system. Discrete lesions were present in the coronary sinus similar to those previously seen.

It was therefore concluded that RF energy was relatively safe when ablation was attempted at the coronary sinus. This suggests that this technique has the potential for interruption of the left free wall and posteroseptal accessory pathways.

Catheter Ablation of Accessory Pathways with RF Energy in Canine Coronary Sinus

Langberg and colleagues[6] performed catheter ablations of accessory pathways by RF energy in 16 dogs in 1989. There were no arrhythmias after the procedure.

Gross Findings of the Coronary Sinus

A microscopic lesion was seen in 14 of the 16 dogs. The mean diameter of the lesions was approximately 11.6 × 4.3 × 2.8 millimeters in greatest dimension. The endocardium and mitral valvular apparatus were not involved in any of the dogs (Figure 10).

Findings of the Coronary Sinus Area

There was coagulation necrosis and hemorrhage of fat in the AV sulcus. The necrosis involved the entire thickness of the coronary sinus with a localized disruption of the elastic lamina (Figure 11). The left atrium and left ventricle were intact, as was the mitral valvular apparatus. In 1, the lesion extended to and affected the adventitia of the circumflex coronary artery with no changes in the media and intima.

Pathology of the AV Sulcus

Pathological changes in the AV groove were found in 11 of the 13 dogs in the form of internal proliferation and degeneration of the elastic lamina. In 3 dogs a chronic thrombus in the lumen of the coronary sinus was observed.

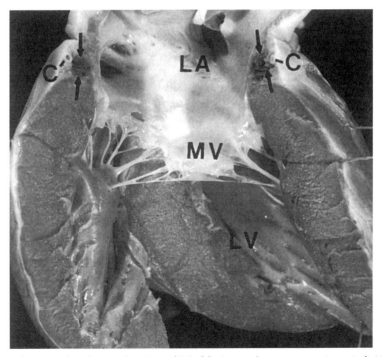

Figure 10. Three weeks after application of RF ablation to the coronary sinus. Left AV sulcus. C indicates circumflex coronary artery; LA, left atrium; LV, left ventricle; and MV, mitral valve. Arrows denote the extent of injury. (From Langberg et al.[6])

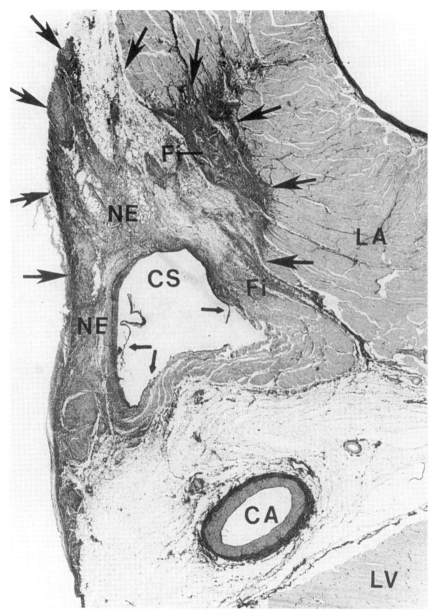

Figure 11. Lower power photomicrograph of the coronary sinus 1 hour after the ablative procedure. Large arrows delineate the extent of fibrosis and hemorrhage, and small arrows point to the intimal disruption in the coronary sinus. LA indicates left atrium; LV, left ventricle; CS, coronary sinus; CA, left circumflex coronary artery; NE, necrosis; FI, fibrosis. (Weigert-van Gieson stain. Magnification ×10.) (From Langberg et al.[6])

There was dense fibrosis and chronic inflammatory cells in the fat of the AV groove surrounding the coronary sinus. In 2, in addition, there was cartilage formation. The demarcation between the fibrotic and healthy myocardial tissue was quite sharp, especially in the areas of the lesion extending into the epicardial surface of the atrium and the ventricle.

The work of Langberg and Huang suggests that RF energy can be safely applied to the coronary sinus and may be useful in interrupting left-sided accessory pathways in the human.

Catheter Ablation of Ventricular Septum with RF Energy

In 1989 Huang and colleagues (Ring et al[7]) ablated the ventricular septum in 10 dogs with RF energy with no significant acute or late arrhythmias. Histologic examination of the ablated areas demonstrated well-delineated round or oval lesions with microscopic thrombi overlying 2 of the lesions.

Conduction System Studies

The conduction system was examined in 2 dogs, one 14 days and the other 7 days after the experimental procedure. There were minimal chronic inflammatory cells in the approaches to the AV node and in the AV node. The AV bundle and remainder of the conduction system were within normal limits.

In conclusion, catheter ablation of the ventricular septum with RF energy is feasible, appears to be safe, and produces discrete scar areas in the ventricular septum. This may provide an alternative to direct current energy for catheter ablation of ventricular tachycardias originating from the ventricular septum.

Transcatheter Radiofrequency Ablation in the Canine Right Atrium

In 1991 Huang and colleagues (Lee et al[8]) ablated the right atrium in 11 closed-chest dogs by means of transcatheter RF energy with no significant arrhythmias or complications. The animals were killed 0 to 29 days after the procedure. For a total of 47 attempted ablations, there were 36 well-delineated coagulative lesions in the atrium. The lesions at a gross level measured approximately 5×3 millimeters and 2.5 millimeters in depth. In 17% there was transmural necrosis without perforation, and a thin layer of mural thrombus was present in 14%.

In conclusion, transcatheter RF ablation in the canine right atrium can be accomplished and appears to be relatively safe for right atrial ablations in a short-term follow-up. The potential application of this method to ablate right atrial tachycardia foci may be entertained in selected cases of intractable arrhythmias of atrial etiology. However, it is emphasized that the approaches to the AV node, and the AV bundle may be involved unintentionally during the procedure, and the AV nodal conduction time may not be altered in the immediate future. However, in the long run, chronic scar tissue formation of the affected area of the distal conduction system may produce abnormalities in AV conduction and/or arrhythmias.

Transcatheter Ablation of Tricuspid Valve Annulus

When the ablation was performed at the tricuspid valve annulus close to the AV bundle, complete AV block occurred.[8] In one dog, where the ablative area extended from the tricuspid valve annulus to the ventricular septum, there was extensive hemorrhage and necrosis in the distal penetrating and beginning of branching portions of the AV bundle, bifurcating bundle, and the beginning of the bundle branches.

Dissociation of AV Conduction and Refractoriness After Application of RF Energy to the Canine AV Node: Acute and Chronic Observations

Marcus et al[9] recently demonstrated dissociation of AV conduction and refractoriness in 5 dogs that received RF ablation (5 others received a sham procedure). These dogs had an AH prolongation greater than 100% from baseline values, which persisted throughout the 2-month follow-up study. The AV nodal functional refractory period was prolonged only acutely. These findings indicate a dissociation between the effects on AV nodal conduction and refractoriness that was produced by this procedure. The 5 sham-treated controls showed no electrophysiological changes either acutely or chronically.

Pathology

In 4 hearts in which the conduction system was examined, thickened whitish plaque formation was seen involving the annulus of the septal leaflet of the tricuspid valve and extending close to the mouth of the coronary sinus to a varying degree (Figure 12). There were no perforations or hemorrhages.

Conduction System

The approaches to the AV node revealed minimum to moderate pathological change in the form of fibrosis, dissolution of tissue, chronic inflammatory cells, and fatty metamorphosis. In addition, there was cartilage formation in 3 dogs. The AV node maintained its continuity with the surrounding atrial myocardium to a varying degree. The penetrating portion of the bundle in general

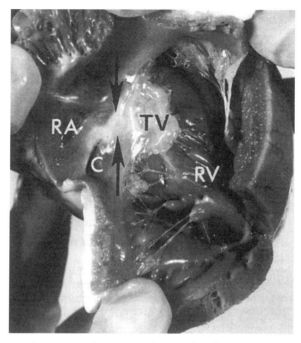

Figure 12. Chronic prolongation of AH interval 2 months after RF ablation of the AV junction. Right atrial and right ventricular view showing scar in the AV nodal area. RA indicates right atrium; RV, right ventricle; TV, septal leaflet of the tricuspid valve; and C, coronary sinus. Arrows point to the thickened whitened area at the region of the approaches to the atrioventricular node and the node itself. (From Marcus et al.[9])

revealed moderate fatty metamorphosis. The branching portion of the bundle showed very minimal fibrosis. The bifurcating AV bundle revealed mild to moderate fibrosis with acute degenerative changes. The beginning of the right and left bundle branches showed mild to moderate fibrosis and some acute degenerative changes. In summary, the changes in the approaches to the AV node and the AV node were distinctly less than that seen in previous studies in dogs where complete AV block was created by RF ablation.

It is concluded that chronic modification of the AV nodal conduction without concomitant change in refractoriness can be produced by RF energy delivered in the proximal portion of the AV node. Because the AV node itself shows at least a moderate amount of fibrotic change, it is conceivable that some of the cases might progress with time to late development of complete heart block after this procedure.

Histopathological Findings After RF Ablation of the Slow Pathway in a Patient With AV Nodal Reentrant Tachycardia

Although RF ablation appears to be the method of choice in the management of intractable arrhythmias in the human, there are practically no pathological studies documenting the effects after the ablative procedure. We studied one such case.

A 47-year-old man was diagnosed with nonischemic cardiomyopathy with severe congestive heart failure. His condition was complicated by recurrent episodes of supraventricular tachycardia of a narrow QRS morphology at a rate of 145 beats per minute. The episodes of tachycardia were associated with hypotension and exaggerated the symptoms of heart failure. An electrophysiological study demonstrated dual AV nodal pathways, and AV nodal reentrant tachycardia was reproducibly induced. RF ablation was applied at the site of presumed "slow-pathway" potentials close to the annulus of the tricuspid valve. AV nodal reentry could not be induced at the conclusion of the procedure and 1 week after ablation. A week after RF ablation he underwent orthotopic cardiac transplantation.

Gross Findings

Only a piece of the heart containing the AV junction was sent to us for evaluation. There was a recently ablated area very close to the annulus of the septal leaflet of the tricuspid valve, reddish brown in color, that measured 5 × 4 millimeters in an oblong shape (Figure 13).

Pathology of the Ablated Area

Histologically, the effects of RF energy were present in the approaches to the AV node extending from the tricuspid valve annulus, the surrounding atrial septum, and the adjoining right ventricular septum in the form of hemorrhage, edema, chronic inflammatory cells, and necrosis. This area measured approximately 0.5 centimeters in length, width, and depth (Figure 14). The RF energy did not affect the AV node.

Conduction System

The AV node revealed mild inflammatory changes with moderate to marked fatty metamorphosis and fibrosis. The node, in part, was somewhat flattened and was present in the central fibrous body. The small blood vessels were thickened and narrowed. The penetrating bundle likewise showed moderate to marked fatty metamorphosis and chronic inflammatory changes. The branching bundle was on the left ventricular side and was somewhat compressed by the right ventricular septal muscle. This likewise showed chronic inflammation and acute necrosis and fibrosis. The left bundle branch also revealed chronic mild inflammation, disruption at the middle, and replacement by fibrous tissue and linear formation. The bifurcating AV bundle showed moderate to marked fatty metamorphosis, and the bifurcation was intramyocardial

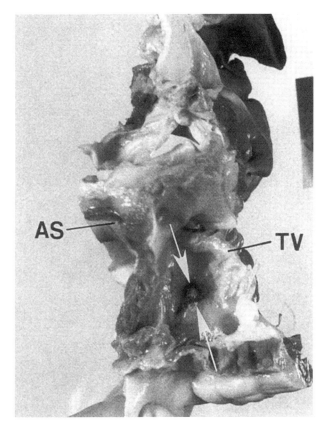

Figure 13. AV junction of the explanted heart showing the RF ablation in the posterior approaches to the AV node. AS indicates atrial septum; TV, septal leaflet of the tricuspid valve. The 2 white arrows point to the ablated area. Note an oblong dark area with a white central zone produced by RF energy.

on the left side. The entire course of the right bundle branch was intramyocardial, and this revealed considerable fatty metamorphosis in the beginning. The ventricular septum revealed focal fibrosis and arteriosclerosis.

Because the slow conduction was completely eliminated in this patient, we may conclude that the approaches to the AV node close to the annulus of the septal leaflet of the tricuspid valve and the tail end (proximal) of the AV node were probably responsible for the slow AV nodal pathway. The chronic inflammatory changes in the conduction system suggest that it is the secondary reaction of the ablative procedure.

The marked fatty infiltration of the approaches to the AV node, the AV node, and the AV bundle up to its bifurcating portion raises the issue of what role it might have played in the production of dual AV nodal pathways. The focal fibrosis of the ventricles probably represents the effects of previous repetitive tachycardia. This study demonstrates that selective ablation of the approaches to the AV node without involvement of the AV conduction system can indeed be accomplished in the human by RF energy.

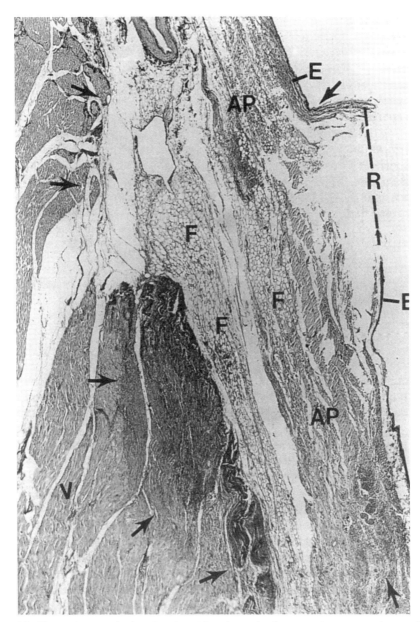

Figure 14. Photomicrograph showing the ablated area in the posterior approaches to the AV node. AP indicates posterior approaches to the AV node; F, fat in the approaches; E, right atrial endocardium; V, right side of the ventricular septum; and R, rupture of the right atrial endocardium as a result of ablation. Arrows demarcate the ablated area. (Hematoxylin and eosin stain. Magnification ×30.)

Summary

Today RF ablation is used successfully in humans to treat refractory cardiac arrhythmias. It is emphasized that long-term follow-up of the ablated patients is required before any definitive statements can be made as to the efficacy of this procedure and its long-term prognosis. Although it has been shown that RF ablation can be accomplished by catheter ablation of the AV junction from the left ventricular approach,[11] as well as in ablating atrial[12] and ventricular tachycardia foci, aortic valve perforation has occurred during ablation of a left-sided accessory pathway in a 15-year-old girl.[13] Recently, a 30% increase in incidence of mitral and aortic valve insufficiency was found during ablation of left-sided accessory connections. The long-range effect on the summit of the ventricular septum (right or left side) and the tricuspid, mitral, and aortic valves is not known today. Because the procedures are done with the help of fluoroscopy and His bundle catheters only, inadvertent damage to the vital part of the conduction system adjacent to the targeted area may result in complete AV block. Furthermore, the long-term effects of the residual scar tissue and/or its extension into the vital parts of the conduction system from the adjacent ablated area with the possibility of late development of arrhythmias or complete AV block still unknown. The cartilage formation in the ablated areas in the chronic canine experiments may be related to the type of tissue reaction, which may be different from that of humans. Likewise, the risk of fatal malignancy at a later date because of significant radiation exposure to both the patient and the physician during fluoroscopic imaging is stated to be 0.1%, and a risk of a genetic abnormality is 20 per million births.[14] These risks, however, are considered relatively negligible when compared with other alternatives available for managing these patients with intractable arrhythmias, such as surgery, pharmacological methods, or no treatment.

The relatively acute histopathological findings of the AV junction in the explanted human heart suggest that selective ablation of the posterior approaches to the AV node can be achieved without damaging the AV node during abolishment of the slow pathway in intractable AV nodal reentrant tachycardia. However, it is recommended that histopathology from *all* hearts (if possible) following RF ablation be examined carefully from the standpoint of the conduction system, the myocardium, and the valves when patients die, irrespective of the time and circumstances. This is because however selective the ablative procedure might be, the right ventricular side of the ventricular system adjacent to the approaches to the AV node is almost always affected. This may result in focal scar areas that might form a milieu for an arrhythmic event during an altered physiological state at a later date.

References

1. Huang SK, Bharati S, Graham AR, et al. Closed chest catheter desiccation of the atrioventricular junction using radiofrequency energy—a new method of catheter ablation. *J Am Coll Cardiol* 1987;9:349–358.

2. Huang SK, Bharati S, Lev M, et al. Electrophysiologic and histologic observations of chronic atrioventricular block induced by closed-chest catheter desiccation with radiofrequency energy. *PACE* 1987;10:805:816.

3. Marcus FI, Blouin LT, Bharati S, et al. Production of chronic first degree atrioventricular block in dogs, using closed-chest electrode catheter with radiofrequency energy. *J Electrophysiol* 1988;2:315–326.

4. Huang SK, Bharati S, Graham AR, et al. Chronic incomplete atrioventricular block induced by radiofrequency catheter ablation. *Circulation* 1989;80:951–961.

5. Huang SK, Graham AR, Bharati S, et al. Short- and long-term effects of transcatheter ablation of the coronary sinus by radiofrequency energy. *Circulation* 1988;78:416–427.

6. Langberg J, Griffin JC, Herre JM, et al. Catheter ablation of accessory pathways using radiofrequency energy in the canine coronary sinus. *J Am Coll Cardiol* 1989;13:491–496.

7. Ring ME, Huang SK, Graham AR, Gorman G, Bharati S, Lev M. Catheter ablation of the ventricular septum with radiofrequency energy. *Am Heart J.* 1989;117:1233–1240.

8. Lee MA, Huang SKS, Graham AR, Gorman G, Bharati S, Lev M. Transcatheter radiofrequency ablation in the canine right atrium. *J Interven Cardiol.* 1991;4:125–133.

9. Marcus FI, Blouin LT, Bharati S, Lev M, Hahn E. Dissociation of atrioventricular conduction and refractoriness following application of radiofrequency energy to the canine atrioventricular node: acute and chronic observations. *PACE* 1992;15(11):1702–1710.

10. Lev M, Bharati S. Lesions of the conduction system and their functional significance. In: *Pathology Annual 1974,* New York, NY: Appleton-Century Crofts, 1974 pp 157–208.

11. Sousa J, El-Atassi R, Rosenheck S, et al. Radiofrequency catheter ablation of the atrioventricular junction from the left ventricle. *Circulation* 1991;84:567–571.

12. Seifert MJ, Morady F, Calkins HG, et al. Aortic leaflet perforation during radiofrequency ablation. *PACE* 1991;14:1582–1585.

13. Minich LL, Snider AR, Dick M II. Doppler detection of valvular regurgitation after radiofrequency ablation of accessory connections. *Am J Cardiol* 1992;70:116–117.

14. Calkins H, Niklason L, Sousa J, et al. Radiation exposure during radiofrequency catheter ablation of accessory atrioventricular connections. *Circulation* 1991;84:2376–2382.

Chapter 6

Temperature Monitoring versus Impedance Monitoring during RF Catheter Ablation

Adam Zivin, M.D., S. Adam Strickberger, M.D.

Introduction

F (RF) catheter ablation has become a standard therapy for paroxysmal supraventricular tachycardias as well as other arrhythmias.[1-4] Cure of an arrhythmia with RF energy depends on heat-induced necrosis of tissue within a critical portion of the tachycardia substrate. Unsuccessful RF applications are due to either imprecise mapping or inadequate tissue heating. For this reason, an accurate assessment of heating at the electrode-tissue interface during ablation is useful and can usually be achieved with monitoring of either temperature or impedance. In general, the goal of ablation is to achieve a temperature of approximately 60°C at the electrode-tissue interface. This temperature goal, without excessive heating, can be achieved by titrating power to achieve a 5–10 Ω decrease in the measured impedance, or by titrating power to the desired temperature. The purpose of this chapter is to review impedance and temperature monitoring, and to discuss the value of these techniques to verify adequate, but not excessive, tissue heating during applications of RF energy.

Experimental Basis for Temperature Monitoring

Application of RF energy to myocardial tissue results in tissue destruction, primarily by generation of heat within the tissue. Tissue heating occurs by 2 primary mechanisms. The first mechanism is the Joule effect, or "resistive

From Huang SKS, Wilber DJ (eds.): *Radiofrequency Catheter Ablation of Cardiac Arrhythmias: Basic Concepts and Clinical Applications,* 2nd ed. Armonk, NY: Futura Publishing Company, Inc. ©2000.

heating," a consequence of direct RF-induced agitation of ions within the muscle. The magnitude of this resistive heating is dependent on the local strength of the electromagnetic field generated by the catheter and is proportional to the power density, which is, in turn, proportional to the square of the current density. Approximating the catheter tip as a sphere, the electromagnetic field and current decrease with the square of the distance from the catheter tip. This dictates that the magnitude of resistive heating will be inversely proportional to the fourth power of the distance from the electrode tip. Thus, resistive heating is responsible only for a thin lesion, less than 1 mm deep.[5] The second, and primary mechanism of tissue heating is thermal energy generated by the resistively heated tissue, and conducted into the deeper tissue.[6,7] The subendocardium reaches steady state temperature within 20 seconds, while tissue deeper than 5 mm heats more slowly and may take more than 60 seconds to reach the temperature required for tissue necrosis.[6,8]

In isolated guinea pig papillary muscles, abnormal automaticity has been demonstrated at tissue temperatures over 45°C, while reversible loss of electrical excitability to pacing stimuli occurs at 48°C, and irreversible loss of excitability at 50.5°C.[9] Other in vitro experiments have demonstrated irreversible tissue destruction at 54.6°C.[10] This is consistent with a target temperature of 55°C to 60°C that is usually required clinically.[11]

Experimental Basis for Impedance Monitoring

Biological tissues have electrically as well as thermally conductive properties. The electrical properties of tissues can be modeled as a resistor-capacitor network to account for the dielectric properties of lipid membranes and the conductive properties of cytoplasm and interstitial fluid.[12] The impedance, or opposition to current flow through a substance, is measured in ohms. Impedance is a sum of frequency-independent resistance and a frequency-dependent reactance that is primarily due to the capacitance of cell membranes. At lower frequencies, membrane capacitance exerts a comparatively large effect. However, at the higher frequencies used in RF ablation, the capacitive component becomes negligible, and the tissue impedance can be modeled as a simple resistor. The in vitro tissue resistivity of canine myocardium to RF energy at 300 kHz is 180–240 Ω per centimeter.[13] As tissue is heated, tissue ion mobility increases and the local tissue resistivity falls by approximately 2% per degrees centigrade.[13] This decrease in tissue impedance within the nascent lesion is the basis for impedance monitoring used during RF ablation. The impedance falls 5–10 Ω in clinically successful applications of RF energy, while larger decrements are noted when a coagulum formation is imminent.[14]

General Principles of Temperature and Impedance Monitoring

The clinical efficacy of a given RF application depends on both precise target site mapping and adequate lesion formation.[7,15,16] Both in vitro and in vivo there is a dose-response relationship between applied power and temperature if endocardial contact remains constant. In vivo, however, the efficiency of tissue heating (that is, tissue temperature per watt of applied power) is less predictable because it is affected by variations in catheter stability, contact pressure, orientation relative to the endocardium, effective electrode contact area, convective heat loss into the blood pool, and target location.[16,17] Thus, applied energy, power, and current are poor indicators of the extent of lesion formation, and actual electrode-tissue interface temperature remains the only predictor of actual lesion volume.[18,19] The purpose of temperature and impedance monitoring is to ensure adequate, but not excessive, heating at the electrode-tissue interface with a monitoring technique that is relatively insensitive to the uncertainties associated with catheter positioning in clinical application.

For a given power, temperatures tend to be higher at target sites associated with improved catheter stability and tissue contact, such as the ventricular side of the mitral annulus.[7,15,16] Targets on the atrial side of the tricuspid and mitral annuli, where catheter stability is more difficult to maintain and convective heat loss to intracavitary blood flow is greater, are associated with a lower efficiency of heating.[7,15,16]

The magnitude of the current delivered by a RF generator used in cardiac ablation is largely determined by the impedance between the ablation catheter and the ground electrode. In addition to intrinsic tissue properties, impedance is affected by such factors as catheter contact pressure, catheter electrode size, the presence of coagulum at the catheter tip, body surface area, and transthoracic diameter.[20] With firm catheter contact, the impedance at the onset of a RF application before tissue heating has occurred is typically 90–120 Ω. Due to the lower resistivity of blood, if contact is poor, the initial impedance is approximately 20–25% less.[21] Larger electrodes have a larger contact area at the endocardial surface, and also result in a lower impedance.[22] Similarly, the impedance decreases by roughly 10% if the surface area of the grounding electrode is doubled.[23] Impedance provides a useful qualitative assessment of tissue heating; like applied power and current, however, it does not correlate with lesion volume.[24]

Assessment of tissue heating at the electrode-tissue interface is not only to ensure adequate heating, but to prevent excessive heating which results in coagulum formation. Coagulum is an accumulation of fibrin, platelets, and other blood and tissue components at the ablation electrode which results from the boiling of blood and tissue serum. In vitro, coagulum formation is seen with catheter temperatures over 100°C, and despite being composed largely of blood constituents, it is not prevented by heparin administration.[25,26] Clinically, it is usually accompanied by an abrupt rise in impedance to greater than 250 Ω, and is associated with catheter temperatures over roughly 95°C. Because coagulum is an electrical insulator, its accumulation at the catheter tip prevents additional RF current delivery into the tissue. Preventing coagulum formation during applications of RF energy is therefore desirable, and can be achieved with either monitoring technique.

In summary, tissue necrosis occurs at a temperature of approximately 55°C, and is accompanied by a predictable fall in impedance. Figure 1 illustrates the time course of these variables for a typical RF application. In prac-

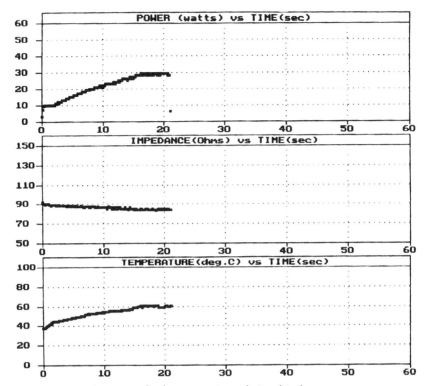

Figure 1. Representative example demonstrating relationship between temperature and impedance during an application of RF energy. Top panel has power (watts) on Y axis, while middle and bottom panels have impedance (Ω) and temperature (°C) respectively on Y axis. Temperature increases from 37°C to 61°C, and a corresponding decrease in impedance from 91 Ω to 84 Ω is observed. Note that power was titrated upwards to achieve this result. (Reproduced with permission).

tice, an application of RF energy associated with adequate heating can be verified with either impedance or temperature monitoring.

Impedance Measurement and Temperature Sensors

Measurement of impedance does not require any specific catheter-based sensor circuitry, and therefore can be performed with any catheter designed for RF ablation. However, not all RF generators are ideal for impedance monitoring. The RF generator must display consistent impedance determinations without large, rapid, measurement fluctuations.

Temperature monitoring requires a dedicated sensor within the catheter, and also requires associated circuitry. Two types of sensors are available for temperature monitoring with RF catheter ablation. A thermistor is a semiconductor, the intrinsic resistance of which changes in a predictable fashion with temperature. Thermistors are typically incorporated into the catheter tip and are thermally isolated from the surrounding electrode with an insulating sleeve. As currently used, accurate assessment of temperature requires that a thermistor be thermally isolated from the surrounding electrode and perpendicular to the electrode-tissue interface.[27] This last characteristic makes this technology difficult to employ in multiple electrode catheters. A thermocouple is composed of 2 metals that, when in contact with one another, generate a small current proportional to the ambient temperature. Measurement of this current allows quantification of the temperature. Thermocouples are usually placed within the catheter tip in contact with the distal electrode, and thus are less sensitive to catheter orientation than an embedded thermistor. This design, however, does not measure the temperature at the electrode-tissue interface per se, but rather reflects the average temperature of the electrode. This may underestimate true tissue heating due to convective cooling of the electrode and temperature averaging throughout the electrode body.[16]

The inherent accuracy of each type of sensor is similar but requires additional complexity and cost. Either sensor type can be used as part of a temperature monitoring, closed-loop feedback system whereby the RF generator automatically adjusts the power output to maintain a user-programmed temperature.

Practical Application of Temperature and Impedance Monitoring

To titrate RF energy using impedance monitoring alone, an initial generator output power of 20–30 watts is selected. The power is gradually increased to obtain a 5–10 Ω decrement in measured impedance. This change in impedance correlates with a tissue temperature of approximately 55°C to 60°C, which is the temperature needed for tissue necrosis.[7,14] When the target impedance is reached, the output should be adjusted as needed to maintain the impedance in the target range. An impedance change of 5–10 Ω is rarely associated with coagulum formation, but larger impedance decrements are associated with coagulum formation in at least 10% of energy applications and should therefore be avoided.[28] Manual power titration is frequently required throughout the RF energy application to maintain the impedance within the target range.

Temperature monitoring can be performed with manual power titration, but is usually done as part of a closed-loop temperature monitoring system that automatically adjusts the power to achieve the target temperature. When manual power titration is directed by temperature monitoring, the power is gradually increased beginning at 20–30 watts until the target temperature is achieved. The target temperature varies according to the arrhythmia substrate, but is approximately 50°C to 53°C for the slow pathway approach to ablation of atrioventricular nodal reentrant tachycardia (AVNRT), and 60°C for accessory pathway, AV junction, and ventricular tachycardia ablation.[4,7,11,29] With closed-loop temperature monitoring, the target temperature is selected, and the RF generator automatically adjusts the power to achieve the target temperature. With both manual and automatic power titration, change in power output is frequently required throughout the RF application to maintain the target temperature.

With or without a closed-loop system, the application of RF energy is continued if the desired clinical effect is observed within 5–10 seconds after the target temperature or impedance is achieved. If the desired end point—for example, loss of accessory pathway conduction—does not occur within this time, the failed application is probably due to inadequate mapping. Because subendocardial steady state tissue temperature is achieved within 20 seconds, if the target impedance or temperature is not achieved with maximum generator output within this time frame, the energy application can be terminated.[30] The inability to reach the target temperature or impedance suggests that endocardial contact is inadequate for tissue heating.

Impedance and Temperature Monitoring During Arrhythmia Ablation

For the slow pathway approach to ablation of AVNRT with a fixed power output of 32 watts, success was achieved at a mean temperature of 48.5°C and a maximum temperature of 54°C at the electrode-tissue interface.[29] The impedance decrease associated with successful energy applications was 2.4 Ω. This small change in measured impedance associated with successful applications precludes the clinical usefulness of impedance monitoring during ablation of AVNRT. The mean temperature associated with junctional ectopy was 47°C. Additionally, even during fixed power applications with 32 watts, coagulum formation was uncommon and not well predicted by either temperature or impedance measurements. Preliminary results of a randomized study comparing fixed power at 32 watts, to temperature monitoring to achieve a target temperature of 60°C, shows both strategies to be equally effective.[31] In clinical practice, because the efficiency of heating is so poor in this anatomic region, temperatures greater than 55°C are rarely achieved.[29,31] Practically speaking, the easiest technique for applying RF energy during ablation of AVNRT using the slow pathway approach is to use closed-loop temperature monitoring. We favor a target temperature of approximately 53°C. This approach is highly successful, and is rarely associated with coagulum formation, heart block, or tachycardia recurrence.[29,31]

Transient loss of accessory pathway function is observed at roughly 50°C, while permanent interruption of accessory pathway function is observed at approximately 60°C, though temperatures as low as 53°C may also result in permanent loss of accessory pathway function.[7] In a randomized comparison of impedance and temperature monitoring for ablation of accessory pathways using a target impedance decrement of 5–10 Ω and a target temperature of 60°C, a similar success rate was noted with no difference in fluoroscopy time, procedure duration, number of RF applications, or incidence of coagulum formation.[32]

For ablation of the AV junction using a thermistor-equipped catheter, successful ablation was routinely achieved at a temperature of 60°C. Temperatures of less than 60°C were associated with junctional ectopy, but not complete heart block.[11] Impedance monitoring has not been studied in this setting.

A recent study used temperature monitoring with closed-loop control for ablation of typical atrial flutter. Continuous applications of RF were used to produce linear lesions across the isthmus between the inferior vena cava and tricuspid annulus. Significant fluctuations in impedance and electrode-tissue interface temperature were noted throughout the application as catheter contact varied. A mean temperature of 61°C was associated with successful ablation.[33]

Limited impedance and temperature data are available for ablation of ventricular tachycardia. Most studies have used power outputs of 30–45 watts and targeted an impedance change of 5–10 Ω, or a temperature of 60°C to 70°C.[4,34-36] Furthermore, a recent experimental study suggests that similar heating patterns are observed in normal and infarcted ventricular myocardium during application of RF energy.[8] Therefore, based on in vivo and in vitro data, these impedance and temperature end points are reasonable, although studies to determine optimal values have not been published.

Clinical studies have used a wide range of available RF generators with equal success. No catheter or thermometry technology has been demonstrated to be superior in clinical use; however, closed-loop control of power output is easier to use than manual power titration. A formula for calculating tissue temperature from impedance measurements has been developed, and could be used for implementing an impedance based closed-loop feedback system.[37] At present, closed-loop power control for RF generators is only available using temperature monitoring.

Saline Cooled Catheters

Saline irrigated catheters cause peak tissue heating several millimeters from the electrode-tissue interface.[38] Because maximum tissue heating does not occur at the electrode-tissue interface, the value of temperature and impedance monitoring is limited with this type of catheter. The inability to assess tissue heating, and hence to titrate power to an objective end point, prevents the operator from determining if unsuccessful applications are due to inadequate mapping or inadequate heating. When using saline-irrigated catheters, RF energy is usually delivered with fixed power applications, or with slow, empiric, power titration.

Conclusion

Both temperature monitoring and impedance monitoring are helpful in assessing efficacy of RF energy delivery. A temperature of 60°C or a fall in impedance of 5–10 Ω during an energy application is indicative of adequate tissue heating for lesion formation. A temperature greater than 85°C or an impedance decrement of more than 10 Ω is predictive of eventual coagulum formation and should be avoided. Manual power titration using either technique is equally effective, although closed-loop power control is preferable and is currently only available utilizing thermometry. Catheters equipped for thermometry are more expensive, and are difficult to implement in multi-electrode ablation catheters. Impedance monitoring, although used infrequently now that closed-loop thermometry systems are available, may prove increasingly valuable when longer electrodes or multi-electrode catheters are available for clinical use.

References

1. Calkins H, Souza J, El-Atassi R, et al. Diagnosis and cure of the Wolff-Parkinson-White syndrome or paroxysmal supraventricular tachycardias during a single electrophysiologic test. *N Engl J Med* 1991;324:1612–1618.
2. Jackman WM, Beckman KJ, McClelland JH, et al. Treatment of supraventricular tachycardia due to atrioventricular nodal reentry by RF catheter ablation of slow-pathway conduction. *N Engl J Med* 1992;327:313–318.
3. Langberg JJ, Chin MC, Rosenqvist M, et al. Catheter ablation of the atrioventricular junction with RF energy. *Circulation* 1989;80:1527–1535.
4. Morady F, Harvey M, Kalbfleisch SJ, et al. RF catheter ablation of ventricular tachycardia in patients with coronary artery disease. *Circulation* 1993;87:363–372.
5. Haines DE, Watson DD, Verow AF. Electrode radius predicts lesion radius during RF energy heating: validation of a proposed thermodynamic model. *Circ Res* 1990;67:124–129.
6. Haines DE, Watson DD. Tissue heating during RF catheter ablation: a thermodynamic model and observations in isolated perfused and superfused canine right ventricular free wall. *PACE* 1989;12:962–976.
7. Langberg JJ, Calkins H, El-Atassi R, et al. Temperature monitoring during RF catheter ablation of accessory pathways. *Circulation* 1992;86:1469–1474.
8. Kottkamp H, Hindricks G, Horst E, et al. Subendocardial and intramural temperature response during RF catheter ablation in chronic myocardial infarction and normal myocardium. *Circulation* 1997;95:2155–2161.
9. Nath S, Lynch C, Whayne JG, et al. Cellular electrophysiological effects of hyperthermia on isolated guinea pig papillary muscle: implications for catheter ablation. *Circulation* 1993; 88(part I):1826–1831.
10. Whayne JG, Nath S, Haines DE. Microwave catheter ablation of myocardium in vitro: assessment of the characteristics of tissue heating and injury. *Circulation* 1994;89:2390–2395.
11. Nath S, DiMarco JP, Mounsey JP, et al. Correlation of temperature and pathophysiological effect during RF catheter ablation of the AV junction. *Circulation* 1995;92:1188–1192.
12. Ackman JJ, Seitz MA. Methods of complex impedance measurements in biologic tissue. *Crit Rev Biomed Eng* 1986;11(4):281–311.
13. Schwan HP, Foster KR. RF-field interactions with biological systems: electrical properties and biophysical mechanisms. *Proc IEEE* 1980;68(1):104–113.
14. Harvey M, Kim Y-N, Sousa J, et al. Impedance monitoring during RF catheter ablation in humans. *PACE* 1992;15:22–27.
15. Strickberger SA, Hummel J, Gallagher M, et al. Effect of accessory pathway location on the efficiency of heating during RF catheter ablation. *Am Heart J* 1995;129:54–58.
16. Calkins H, Prystowsky E, Carlson M, et al. Temperature monitoring during RF ablation procedures using closed loop control. *Circulation* 1994;90:1279–1286.
17. Panescu D, Whayne JG, Fleischman SD, et al. Three-dimensional finite el-

ement analysis of current density and temperature distributions during radio-frequency ablation. *IEEE Trans Biomed Eng* 1995;42:879–888.

18. Hindricks G, Haverkamp W, Gulker H, et al. RF coagulation of ventricular myocardium: improved prediction of lesion size by monitoring catheter tip temperature. *Eur Heart J* 1989;10:972–984.

19. Haines DE. Determinants of lesion size during RF catheter ablation: the role of electrode-tissue contact pressure and duration of energy delivery. *J Cardiovasc Electrophysiol* 1991;2:509–515.

20. Borganelli M, El-Atassi R, Leon A, et al. Determinants of impedance during RF catheter ablation in humans. *Am J Cardiol* 1992;69:1095–1097.

21. Strickberger SA, Vorperian VR, Man KC, et al. Relation between impedance and endocardial contact during RF catheter ablation. *Am Heart J* 1994;128:226–229.

22. Langberg JJ, Gallagher M, Strickberger SA, et al. Temperature-guided RF catheter ablation with very large distal electrodes. *Circulation* 1993;88: 245–249.

23. Nath S, DiMarco JP, Gallop RG, et al. Effects of dispersive electrode position and surface area on electrical parameters and temperature during RF catheter ablation. *Am J Cardiol* 1996;77:765–767.

24. Haverkamp W, Hindricks G, Gulker H, et al. Coagulation of ventricular myocardium using RF alternating current: biophysical aspects and experimental findings. *PACE* 1989;12(part II):187–194.

25. Haines DE, Verow AF. Observations on electrode-tissue interface temperature and effect of electrical impedance during RF ablation of ventricular myocardium. *Circulation* 1990;82:1034–1038.

26. Ring ME, Huang SKS, Gorman G, et al. Determinants of impedance rise during catheter ablation of bovine myocardium with RF energy. *PACE* 1989;12:1502–1513.

27. Blouin LT, Marcus FI, Lampe L. Assessment of effects of a RF energy field and thermistor location in an electrode catheter on the accuracy of temperature measurement. *PACE* 1991;14(part I):807–814.

28. Strickberger SA, Ravi S, Daoud E, et al. Relation between impedance and temperature during RF ablation of accessory pathways. *Am Heart J* 1995;130:1026–1030.

29. Strickberger SA, Zivin A, Daoud EG, et al. Temperature and impedance monitoring during slow pathway ablation in patients with AV nodal reentrant tachycardia. *J Cardiovasc Electrophysiol* 1996;7:295–300.

30. Wittkampf FHM, Hauer RNW, Robles de Medina EO. Control of RF lesion size by power regulation. *Circulation* 1989;80:962–968.

31. Strickberger SA, Daoud EG, Bogun F, et al. A randomized comparison of RF ablation of atrial ventricular nodal reentrant tachycardia with fixed power versus temperature monitoring. *PACE* 1996;19(part II):666A.

32. Strickberger SA, Weiss R, Knight BP, et al. Randomized comparison of two techniques for titrating power during RF ablation of accessory pathways. *J Cardiovasc Electrophysiol* 1996;7:795–801.

33. Wen Z, Chen S, Tai C, et al. Temperature monitoring in RF catheter ablation of atrial flutter using the linear ablation technique. *J Cardiovasc Electrophysiol* 1996;7:1050–1057.

34. Schwartzman D, Jadonath RL, Callans DJ, et al. RF catheter ablation for control of frequent ventricular tachycardia with healed myocardial infarction. *Am J Cardiol* 1995;75:297–299.
35. Wen M, Yeh S, Wang C, et al. RF ablation therapy in idiopathic left ventricular tachycardia with no obvious structural heart disease. *Circulation* 1994;89:1690–1696.
36. Kottkamp H, Hindricks G, Chen X, et al. RF catheter ablation of sustained ventricular tachycardia in idiopathic dilated cardiomyopathy. *Circulation* 1995;92:1159–1168.
37. Hartung WM, Burton ME, Deam AG, et al. Estimation of temperature during RF catheter ablation using impedance measurements. *PACE* 1995;18:2017–2021.
38. Nakagawa H, Yamanashi WS, Pitha JV, et al. Comparison of in vivo tissue temperature profile and lesion geometry for RF ablation with a saline-irrigated electrode versus temperature control in a canine thigh muscle preparation. *Circulation* 1995;91:2264–2273.

Part II

Radiofrequency Ablation of Atrial Tachycardia and Flutter

Chapter 7

Ablation of Ectopic Atrial Tachycardia in Children

Edward P. Walsh, MD

Introduction

Ectopic atrial tachycardia (EAT) is an uncommon rhythm disorder that involves inappropriately rapid impulse generation from a single atrial focus outside the sinoatrial node. This form of tachycardia can be incessant or present throughout large portions of the day, causing some patients to develop a secondary cardiomyopathy from the chronically elevated heart rates. Historically, the results of antiarrhythmic drug therapy, and even cardiac surgery, were suboptimal in this condition, but since chronic tachycardias such as EAT are among the few reversible causes of cardiomyopathy, alternate treatment options were explored aggressively. Radiofrequency (RF) ablation was thus adopted rather quickly as a potential management strategy for this condition,[1-7] and during the past decade has proven itself to be a highly effective intervention.

This chapter is intended as a brief review of the basic pathophysiology of EAT, with primary emphasis on the technique and results for RF ablation of the abnormal atrial focus. Although the number of patients undergoing EAT ablation is still small compared to the clinical experience with accessory pathway ablation, the results are no less remarkable when one considers that many of these patients benefited from prompt reversal of symptomatic ventricular dysfunction when EAT was successfully eliminated.

From Huang SKS, Wilber DJ (eds.): *Radiofrequency Catheter Ablation of Cardiac Arrhythmias: Basic Concepts and Clinical Applications,* 2nd ed. Armonk, NY: Futura Publishing Company, Inc. ©2000.

Background

Electrophysiology

The precise cellular mechanism of EAT is still incompletely understood. Beyond the fact that it is a primary atrial arrhythmia, our current understanding of EAT electrophysiology is still largely conjectural and is based upon gross inspection of the P wave on electrocardiogram, limited information from atrial stimulation in the clinical electrophysiology laboratory,[8] and a single microelectrode study of a surgically excised focus.[9] Most data would suggest that EAT is a disorder of automaticity.[10] Clinical observations which support this notion include:

1) Nearly incessant tachycardia with wide fluctuation of atrial rate in a pattern which parallels autonomic state (Figure 1).
2) Gradual "warm-up" in rate at time of EAT initiation, and "cool-down" or exit block at termination (Figure 2).
3) General inability to initiate or terminate EAT with programmed stimulation techniques.
4) Initiation or acceleration of EAT with administration of isoproterenol.
5) Reset behavior of the EAT focus to premature extrastimuli or prolonged rapid pacing similar to the sinoatrial node (Figure 3).
6) Inability to terminate EAT with external direct current (DC) cardioversion.

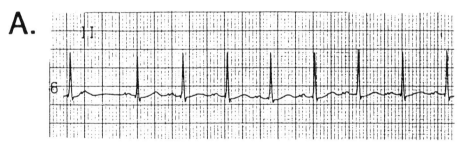

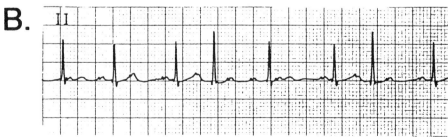

Figure 1. Surface electrocardiograms from a patient with incessant EAT before (A) and after (B) mild exercise, slowing variation in both atrial rate and AV conduction with changing autonomic state.

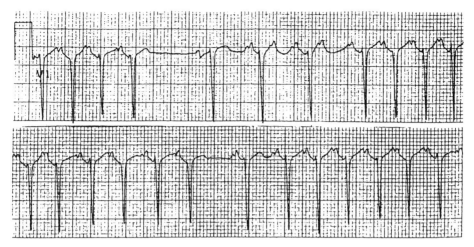

Figure 2. Surface electrocardiogram from a patient with episodic EAT, showing "warm up" of atrial rate at initiation and "cool down" at termination.

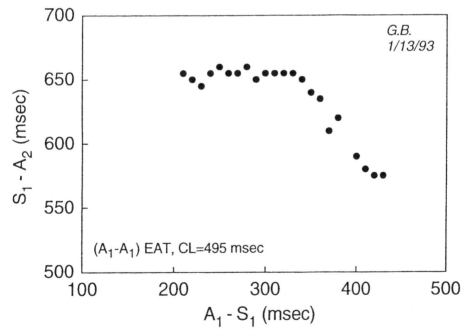

Figure 3. Effect of single atrial premature stimuli (S_1) on the timing of EAT focus discharge (A_1 and A_2). The curve is similar to data generated from measurement of sinoatrial conduction time, and demonstrates a clear reset zone.

The above features would seem to exclude classic reentry as a causative mechanism, but fail to distinguish between an abnormal automatic pacemaker site and triggered activity. However, microelectrode data from atrial tissue obtained during surgical EAT excision are available from a single case report[9] which demonstrated spontaneous diastolic phase 4 depolarization suggestive of abnormal automaticity. While the bulk of current evidence seems to support the notion that EAT is caused by focal automaticity, triggered activity still cannot be completely excluded, and it is possible that either mechanism could be operative in a given patient to cause a similar clinical picture.

The etiology of EAT is likewise poorly understood. Although this arrhythmia is sometimes observed as an acute (and usually transient) disorder after cardiac surgery, most cases involve an otherwise normal heart. Some small series have examined histology of cardiac and skeletal muscle biopsy specimens,[11] or resected atrial tissue from the region of the abnormal focus at time of arrhythmia surgery,[12] but the occasional pathological findings have been restricted to nonspecific fibrosis, cellular hypertrophy, and patchy fatty infiltrates. These features may simply reflect the generalized myopathy induced by chronic tachycardia as much as the pathophysiology of the arrhythmia. Very often, the tissue examined is completely normal.

Clinical Diagnosis

Despite uncertainty regarding etiology and cellular electrophysiology, the clinical picture of EAT is well described.[13] It is primarily a disorder of children and teenagers, but still accounts for about 5% of supraventricular tachycardia in the adult age group. Patients may be asymptomatic for many years with incessant EAT until ventricular dysfunction eventually leads to low cardiac output and pulmonary edema. In this setting, EAT may sometimes be mistaken for sinus tachycardia related to a primary myopathy. Patients may also present with relatively minor complaints of palpitations, dizziness, or exercise intolerance, at a time when ventricular function is still well preserved. Of the population (primarily pediatric) to be discussed in this chapter, the average age at first presentation was 12 years, and the presenting complaints related to cardiomyopathy in a significant percentage. Ventricular dysfunction appears to be less common in the older adult population who first present with EAT.[5]

The diagnosis can usually be made on the basis of surface electrocardiogram, which reveals a single abnormal P wave axis and/or morphology, with atrial rates that are inappropriately rapid for age and physiological state. Although EAT may arise from any site in the right or left atrium, the majority of EAT foci in young patients tend to cluster near either the right atrial appendage area or the region of the pulmonary veins.[3,12] There are thus two general P wave patterns to recognize. Right-sided foci in the appendage tend to produce a normal frontal plane P wave axis, but the vector of atrial depolarization in the horizontal plane is directed from anterior to posterior such that the P wave in leads $V_4R–V_2$ is predominately negative (Figure 4). Left-sided foci are usually more obvious in the frontal plane, where the P wave axis is typically measured in the range of $+90$ to $+180$ degrees (Figure 5).

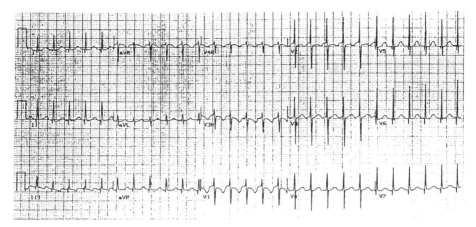

Figure 4. A twelve-lead electrocardiogram from a patient with EAT which was mapped to the region of the right atrial appendage.

The atrial rates during EAT are highly variable, ranging from minimum values of about 90 per minute, to as fast as 300 per minute, with average daily rates of about 140–170 per minute. In many young patients, the atrial tachycardia is incessant, with atrioventricular conduction ratios that are often 1:1 in the absence of medications. In the remainder, activity from the atrial focus is episodic, but may still account for more than 50% of the atrial rhythm over a 24-hour period. First degree and second degree (Mobitz type I) atrioventricular (AV) block are commonly seen while the patient is resting or asleep.

Electrophysiological testing is occasionally needed to confirm the diagnosis of EAT. While most left atrial foci are usually easy to diagnose based on P wave axis, right atrial foci and some right pulmonary vein foci are sometimes quite difficult to distinguish from sinus tachycardia on ECG. Activation sequence mapping may be required in such cases to determine the true site of ori-

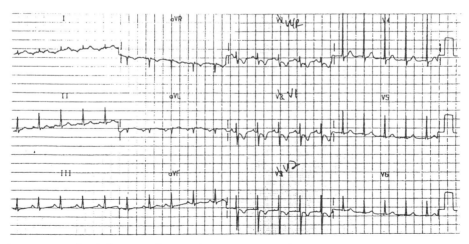

Figure 5. A 12-lead electrocardiogram from a patient with EAT which was mapped to the region of the left upper pulmonary vein.

gin of atrial rhythm. EAT can also be confused with atypical atrial flutter in rare cases where the degree of atrial rate variation is subtle. The inability to terminate an atrial tachycardia with pacing maneuvers and external cardioversion should make one suspicious of EAT.

EAT and Cardiomyopathy

The cardiomyopathy associated with chronic tachycardia (e.g., EAT, PJRT, and some forms of incessant ventricular tachycardia) is a peculiar one. The most notable feature of this syndrome is a prompt reversal of ventricular dysfunction when tachycardia is eliminated.[14] In animal models, dilated cardiomyopathy can be induced within 30 days when the atrium is paced chronically at rates that are approximately 3 times normal, and recovery occurs in about 2 weeks when pacing is terminated.[15] It is now known that this ventricular dysfunction is truly related to depressed contractile performance of individual myocytes, and is not simply a phenomenon of excess preload or high afterload. Multiple factors have been implicated as the cause of tachycardia-induced myopathy,[16] including: 1) alterations in cellular calcium homeostasis; 2) changes in cell ultrastructure involving decreased myofibril content; 3) alteration in Na^+,K^+-ATPase system; and 4) changes in beta-receptor function. The central biochemical derangement which induces these changes has not yet been identified.

In general, about one-half of young patients who are diagnosed with EAT will have some degree of depressed ventricular function at first presentation.[3] However, most clinical series also describe patients who tolerate tachycardia without ventricular failure for many years. There appears to be a reasonable correlation between the ventricular rate during EAT and left ventricular function on echocardiogram. In published pediatric series, mean heart rates of about 150–176 per minute were seen in patients with depressed function, compared to about 90–136 per minute for those with well preserved ventricular performance.[6,12,14]

The typical pattern for the myopathy seen with EAT involves a combination of reduced systolic function and ventricular dilation.[14] Either or both features may be evident at time of initial presentation. Immature or developing myocardium may be more susceptible to the effects of chronic atrial tachycardia than mature myocardium, perhaps because the rate of AV conduction tends to be quite brisk through a younger patient's AV node, although the exact explanation for this age-related difference is uncertain.[17]

Pharmacological Therapy for EAT

Although spontaneous resolution of EAT has been reported,[18] many patients have a chronic tachycardia that will require treatment, particularly if ventricular function is depressed. Drug therapy for this condition has been far from perfect. No single antiarrhythmic agent has been broadly effective, and potential negative inotropic and proarrhythmic side effects often limit their use.

The highest success rates have been observed with class Ic and class III drugs, with occasional successes reported for phenytoin and class II agents.[12,19,20] In a series of 45 young patients treated for EAT, Garson et al[12] found an effective drug in only 50%.

Verapamil and digoxin have minimal effect on the EAT focus, although they can be used acutely to slow the ventricular response rate, and may be useful diagnostically to establish the atrial origin of the disorder. Likewise, adenosine can be used to induce transient AV block for purposes of diagnosis. It may be of interest to note that we have observed several patients in whom adenosine clearly produced direct slowing or termination of EAT which persisted for several seconds after administration.

With the development of RF catheter ablation as definitive therapy for EAT, aggressive pharmacological trials are performed much less frequently for this disorder. At most centers, chronic drug therapy is used only for patients with mild symptoms and good ventricular function, using relatively benign agents such as β-blockers. The cases of patients with compromised ventricular performance, or those who fail to respond to β-blockers, are now often managed with catheter ablation as an early intervention.

Surgical Therapy for EAT

Arrhythmia surgery has been attempted for both right and left atrial EAT. Two approaches have been used. The first involved epicardial cryosurgery without cardiopulmonary bypass, but it was largely abandoned when it became evident that the lesions made in this manner were not always transmural due to endocardial warming by circulating atrial blood. Transient EAT suppression with early recurrence was not uncommon with the epicardial cryosurgical technique.[12] A more effective surgical method involved transmural incisions during cardiopulmonary bypass, with either direct removal of the EAT focus and a cuff of surrounding tissue, or isolation of a broad atrial region that contains the tachycardia site.[21–25] This technique was nearly 100% effective for EAT arising from the left atrium; however, the result for right atrial EAT surgery was less encouraging. It had been suggested that some patients with a right atrial EAT focus had more diffuse electrical pathology involving multiple arrhythmogenic foci, and that excision of one area simply allowed emergence of tachycardia from a new region of the right atrium.[12] This problem could be largely overcome with more generous excision of right atrial tissue, but the technique was still not as effective as surgery in the left atrium.

Another frustration with surgical intervention for EAT was the difficulty in maintaining active tachycardia while the patient was under anesthesia.[26] Sedative medications and surgical manipulation of the heart would sometimes suppress the EAT focus, even in patients who had demonstrated incessant tachycardia until the time of operation. This same problem may be encountered during transcatheter ablation for EAT, but is certainly of less consequence compared to a situation where the arrhythmia becomes quiescent after the chest is open. Although the surgical experience helped pave the way for catheter ablation of EAT, it is quite rare nowadays to perform surgery for this condition.

Development of Transcatheter Therapy for EAT

In light of the imperfect results with pharmacological and surgical therapy, several catheter approaches evolved to address EAT. The earliest method involved DC ablation of the normal AV conducting system, which permitted the atrial tachyarrhythmia to persist, but could control the ventricular response rate.[27] This intervention was generally effective for reversing cardiomyopathy due to EAT, and was well tolerated despite the loss of AV synchrony. The resultant need for a ventricular pacemaker was often the lesser of two evils, but it was obviously much more desirable to eliminate EAT directly and preserve normal AV conduction. Direct ablation of the EAT focus was first reported by Silka et al in 1984 using DC energy.[28] The procedure was successful in 2 of 4 patients with right atrial foci, and was not associated with acute complications, but DC ablation did not gain wide acceptance for treatment of EAT due primarily to the risk of perforation from barotrauma in the relatively thin walled atrium.

The introduction of RF current as an ablation energy source prompted a resurgence of interest in catheter therapy for EAT. Studies by Lee et al[29] and other investigators[30,31] in animal models demonstrated the transmural nature of RF lesions at the atrial level, which healed with well organized fibrous scars and did not result in acute or late perforation. The technique was quickly applied to both adult[1] and pediatric patients[2] with EAT beginning in 1990, with published results now suggesting an acute success rate of better than 90%, and a complication rate not dissimilar to accessory pathway ablation.

Technique for RF Ablation of EAT

The methodology and results for EAT ablation will be discussed in the context of the clinical experience at Boston Children's Hospital since 1990, involving 64 children and young adults. Admittedly, there may be subtle aspects of both the arrhythmia and the procedure in older patients that cannot be addressed by this review. Indeed, early descriptions of EAT ablation in an older population by Kay et al[4] and Tracy et al[5] reported some features that differed slightly from our institutional experience in younger subjects, including a higher percentage of EAT foci in the right atrium of adults, and a lower incidence of cardiomyopathy at initial presentation. Nevertheless, the basic principles of focus localization and ablation are similar, and it is likely that the experience with a pediatric population can be broadly applied to all age groups.

Patient Preparation

The key to a successful mapping and ablation session is the maintenance of high-level activity from the EAT focus, which permits rapid mapping and accurate evaluation of RF lesion efficacy. Frequently, EAT foci may become inactive in the laboratory environment due to sedative medications, possible autonomic influences of prolonged supine posture, patient anxiety, deviation from normal diet (e.g. caffeine intake), or other changes in daily activities that may have an impact on circadian variation of EAT activity. For all these reasons, antiarrhythmic drugs must be stopped far in advance of the study, and patients should be managed with the smallest effective doses of sedation throughout the procedure. When dealing with a pediatric population, it is still sometimes necessary to use deep intravenous sedation or even general anesthesia, but for older children and young adults we attempt to use only low doses of midazolam and narcotic for EAT procedures. Ultimately, despite these measures, mapping and ablation was impossible in 5 of our 64 patients (8%) owing to our inability to recreate or maintain the tachycardia in the electrophysiology laboratory despite prolonged efforts. In three of these patients, the EAT was episodic and relatively slow in rate to begin with, but we also experienced difficulty starting EAT in two others who had nearly incessant tachycardia until the time of the ablation procedure. Unlike reentry tachycardias, there are clearly features peculiar to EAT and other "automatic" tachycardias which occasionally defy our ability to replicate the disorder under controlled conditions.

When EAT is absent or very intermittent during the ablation procedure, we have used provocative pharmacological maneuvers in an effort to excite the abnormal focus, including isoproterenol, epinephrine, atropine, and aminophylline. Programmed atrial stimulation is performed after each pharmacological intervention if the EAT focus does not exhibit spontaneous activity. In general, we found isoproterenol alone to be the most effective stimulus for initiating EAT when the focus is inactive or only intermittently active during the ablation session. It was administered to nearly half of our patients in either episodic bolus form, or as a continuous infusion of 0.01–0.04 µg/kg/min, and had the desired effect in all but the 5 cases mentioned above. Atrial stimulation involving prolonged rapid bursts seemed to be a reliable trigger for inducing EAT in only two of our patients (both adults) in whom it was tested.

Whenever a patient with documented EAT happens to be in stable sinus rhythm upon arrival to the laboratory, we have adopted a policy of waiting until some EAT activity is observed before giving any sedation or inserting a full complement of catheters. We initially monitor the surface ECG carefully and begin isoproterenol through a peripheral intravenous line. If the EAT still remains quiescent, we then insert a single transvenous electrode catheter (using local anesthesia) for aggressive atrial stimulation, and eventually add atropine and aminophylline if necessary. It is certainly possible in our experience to perform successful EAT ablation even if only single ectopic atrial beats are seen, as long as they remain frequent and have a P wave morphology identical to the clinical tachycardia. However, if the ectopic focus is completely inactive despite the above measures, we abort the procedure, and consider retrying at a future date.

Mapping Techniques

Our institutional technique for EAT focus localization has emphasized analysis of bipolar signals from standard catheters with 2 mm electrode spacing, filtered in the range of 30–500 Hz. This technique has been supplemented in recent years with unipolar signals from the ablation tip electrode. The overall goal of mapping is to identify the electrical epicenter of atrial activation, which requires both a compulsive search for ideal electrograms, as well as clear knowledge of the atrial anatomy.

Prior to the procedure, it is quite helpful to examine gross atrial anatomy by standard echocardiography, particularly in any patient with ventricular dysfunction where the atria might be enlarged and distorted. During the procedure itself, we have also found it beneficial to perform biplane atrial angiograms (using RAO/LAO projections for right atrial foci, and AP/LAT projections for left atrial foci) to outline anatomic landmarks in difficult cases (Figure 6). Additional high-resolution anatomic information can be obtained during ablation using transesophageal echocardiography. Not only do these imaging techniques clarify atrial structure (including fine details of pulmonary veins and the appendages) along with ablation catheter tip position, but they also help display atrial septal anatomy to either confirm the presence of a patent foramen ovale, or to simplify Brockenbrough transseptal puncture[32,33] whenever the left atrium must be entered for mapping and ablation. We have not had experience with intracardiac echocardiography during EAT cases at our institution, nor have we felt it essential to pursue this technology for EAT patients given the

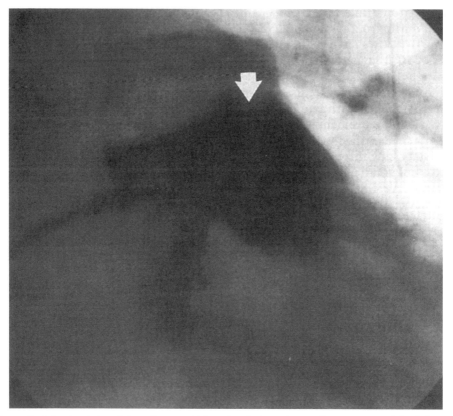

Figure 6. Selective left atrial angiogram (AP projection) outlining the anatomy of the left atrial appendage in a 10-year-old patient with left-sided EAT focus. The site of successful ablation was found along the roof of the appendage (arrow).

resolution possible with the more conventional tools, although we acknowledge its potential value in experienced hands.

The number of transvenous electrode catheters used for mapping can vary from 1 to 4 depending on patient size and the EAT focus location. In our youngest EAT patient (age 2 months), a successful procedure was possible with a single 5F bipolar ablation catheter and an esophageal electrode.[3] More typically, 3 or 4 multielectrode catheters are inserted for recording of the His bundle electrogram, the region of the SA node at the SVC-RA junction, and at least one other right atrial site. The right atrial activation sequence during EAT is first quickly examined for the region of earliest depolarization based on the bipolar recordings. In those cases where the EAT focus seems clearly localized near the right atrial appendage area, direct catheter entry into the left atrium for additional mapping is not performed. Instead, left atrial activation can be evaluated adequately with recordings from a coronary sinus electrode or a transesophageal electrode. However, in our experience, when EAT arises from any region other than the right atrial appendage, it is usually insufficient to rely on a coronary sinus electrode as the sole reflection of left atrial activation, and direct mapping within the left atrium will ultimately be mandatory at some point in the case. This is particularly true for left atrial foci localized near the right pulmonary veins which generate a misleading picture of early activation times along the posterior right atrium and late activation along the entire length of the coronary sinus.

With catheters in position, standard electrophysiological data should be collected to confirm the diagnosis of EAT[8] and to rule out concealed accessory pathways or AV nodal reentry as possible causes of the tachycardia. In addition, programmed atrial stimulation can be performed to test the reset response of the EAT focus to single premature beats and prolonged pacing. With only one exception in our 64 patients, EAT was never terminated with pacing maneuvers, and the reset behavior was in agreement with the pattern previously described for an automatic focus tachycardia.[10]

After the diagnosis is confirmed, preliminary mapping of the EAT focus is performed by moving the mapping/ablation catheter throughout multiple sites in the right atrium (and left atrium if necessary) under biplane fluoroscopic guidance (Figure 7). The local atrial activation times (measured as the earliest high-frequency and high-amplitude signal on a bipolar recording) can be indexed against the onset of the P wave on surface ECG to identify the likely site of EAT origin. Efforts should be made to select ECG leads with the most distinct P wave onset, but at times the P wave may be low in amplitude or obscured by a superimposed QRS or T wave, in which case a stable intracardiac reference (such as the low septal right atrial signal on the His bundle electrode) can be used for initial mapping. We have also found it useful at times to administer an AV node blocking drug such as verapamil or adenosine during mapping to uncover an obscured P wave onset. Local activation times in the general vicinity of an EAT focus should usually precede the onset of the P wave on ECG by a minimum of 20 milliseconds. Although some investigators have reported "fractionated" atrial electrograms from an EAT focus[34] this has not been our general experience. For the most part, the signals ultimately recorded from the site of successful ablation in our patients involved sharp and "normal-appearing"

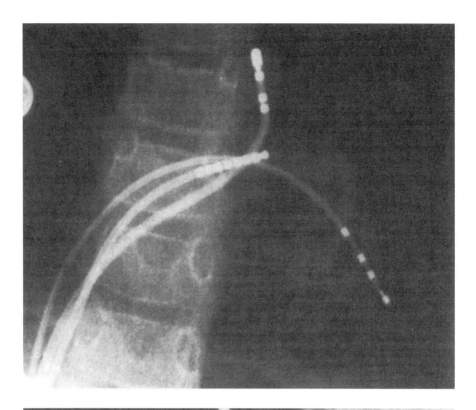

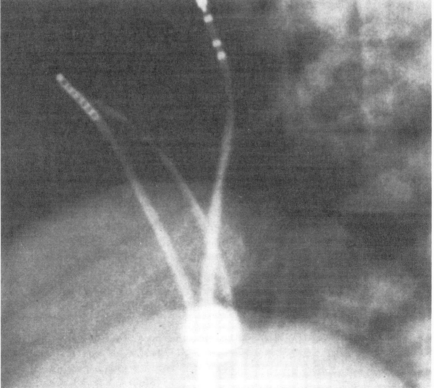

Figure 7. Fluoroscopic views (AP, top panel, and lateral projection, bottom panel) of electrode catheters in position for mapping of a left-sided EAT focus in a 6-year-old patient. The mapping/ablation catheter (MAP) has been positioned in the left atrium via transseptal puncture.

atrial electrical activity which was unique only in its early timing relative to the P wave (Figure 8). Occasionally, the electrogram was "complex" in the sense that it contained multiple rapid components (Figure 9), but similar signals can also be found during routine mapping in the normal atrium during sinus rhythm, particularly in the appendages and along the atrial septum, or at sites of prior unsuccessful RF applications. We have yet to identify a reliable and distinctive electrogram feature apart from activation time which correctly predicts a suitable site for effective EAT ablation.

Following preliminary localization, more precise mapping of the EAT focus can be accomplished with one of several techniques. The most basic exercise involves small movements of the catheter tip in the general target region until the site is identified with the earliest possible atrial activation relative to the P wave.[3] Using this method, we have identified sharp electrical activity on bipolar recordings at the site of successful ablation which preceded the P wave onset by 10–80 milliseconds (mean = 38 milliseconds). An alternate technique for precision mapping has been described by Tracy et al[5] involving a modification of "pace mapping." Intracardiac electrograms are recorded from several stable atrial electrodes during spontaneous EAT and during pacing from the tip of the mapping/ablation catheter. When the paced activation sequence map matched the spontaneous EAT map on all electrodes, RF applications were made with excellent results. Activation pace mapping would appear to be particularly well suited to patients in whom a clear P wave onset is difficult to identify on surface recordings, or those in whom the EAT is very sporadic. A third method for precision mapping involves the use of two mapping catheters which can be moved independently in a region of interest to "triangulate" the focus. This technique is easily used for right atrial foci, but is of limited use in the left atrium since it may necessitate multiple transseptal punctures. Finally, unipolar recordings from the ablation tip electrode during EAT mapping can be used to supplement conventional bipolar mapping. At sites of successful ablation we

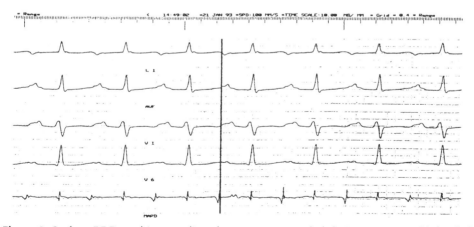

Figure 8. Surface ECGs and intracardiac electrograms recorded during mapping of left-sided EAT focus. The mapping/ablation catheter (MAP) is located at the site of successful ablation. The electrogram in this case contained no distinctive features, apart from early activation time relative to the onset of the surface P wave.

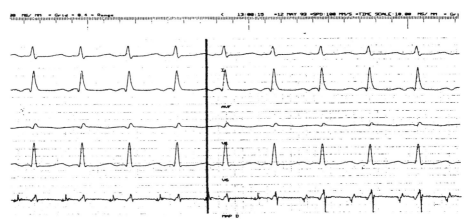

Figure 9. Surface ECGs and intracardiac electrograms recorded during mapping of a right-sided EAT focus. The mapping/ablation catheter (MAP) is located at the site of successful ablation. The electrogram in this case contained several rapid components, but was most notable for its early activation time. Similar "complex" signals can be found during mapping of normal atrial tissue. We did not observe true "fractionation" of atrial electrograms at the EAT focus in our patients.

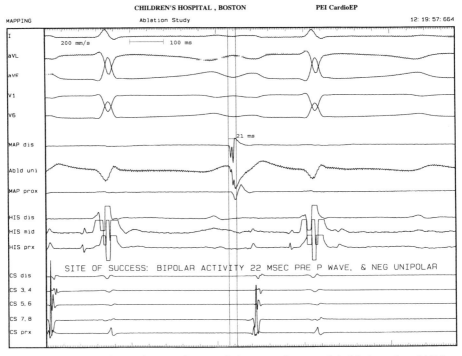

Figure 10. Bipolar and unipolar signals recorded at site of successful ablation of an EAT focus near the right upper pulmonary vein in a 16-year-old boy. Note the early activity from the distal mapping catheter which precedes the surface P wave onset by 21 milliseconds, and the simultaneous onset of a pure negative signal on the unipolar recording. Note also that the activation times on a coronary sinus catheter are late despite the left atrial location of the focus. Coronary sinus signals can be misleading in this disorder, and direct left atrial mapping is usually necessary.

have typically observed a purely negative unipolar signal, with an onset that coincides exactly with the rapid deflection of the bipolar signal (Figure 10).

In 6 of our patients, we noted the fortuitous occurrence of abrupt EAT termination related to simple mechanical pressure of the catheter tip over the target site, which correctly predicted the site of successful ablation.[3] This sign is not sufficiently common to be recommended as a routine mapping tool, but can be useful in the occasional patient where it is a reproducible phenomenon. We have observed that relaxation of catheter pressure on the focus allows EAT to resume promptly (usually within a few seconds, but occasionally requiring several minutes until recovery). When this finding was verified on 2 or more occasions at a site of early local activation in our patients, ablation was performed with consistently good results.

New technology for three-dimensional "nonfluoroscopic" mapping[35] will likely play an important role in EAT mapping in the future, since it combines the two critical components of activation times and atrial anatomy. Such equipment has recently been added to our laboratory and we have not yet had occasion to use it for EAT, although preliminary experience from elsewhere has been encouraging. We have had some experience with right atrial mapping of EAT using an investigational "basket" catheter[36] but were largely disappointed with the results. Since the "basket" did not record directly from the complex nooks and folds of the atrial chamber, the best it could provide was a general sense of the direction for EAT origin that did not seem superior to conventional linear catheter mapping.

Technique for RF Ablation

Once the focus is localized with the above maneuvers, RF applications can be delivered in a unipolar fashion from the distal electrode of the mapping/ablation catheter to an adhesive patch electrode positioned on the patient's leg or trunk. Prior to the availability of temperature monitoring technology, we would begin EAT ablation with an initial generator power of 20–25 watts. If the tachycardia was not affected within 10 seconds, the RF application was terminated and the catheter was repositioned slightly for a repeat attempt. If EAT stopped or changed rate noticeably during the 10-second "test application", the application was continued at the site for 30–60 seconds with the power increased to 35–45 watts. With modern temperature-control generators, we now use set temperatures of 70°C with "test applications" of less than 10 seconds, and 60-second applications at a site of success.

The response of the EAT focus to a successful RF application should be rapid, similar to that seen with a correctly positioned catheter in patients undergoing ablation for accessory pathways. Termination, or dramatic rate change, has typically been observed within 1–5 seconds of beginning the successful lesion in our patients. The most common response of the EAT focus has been abrupt termination (Figure 11), a pattern observed in the majority of our successful procedures. In about one-third of patients, there was transient acceleration of the EAT just preceding termination (Figure 12), and in two unusual cases we observed gradual slowing of EAT rate prior to termination (Fig-

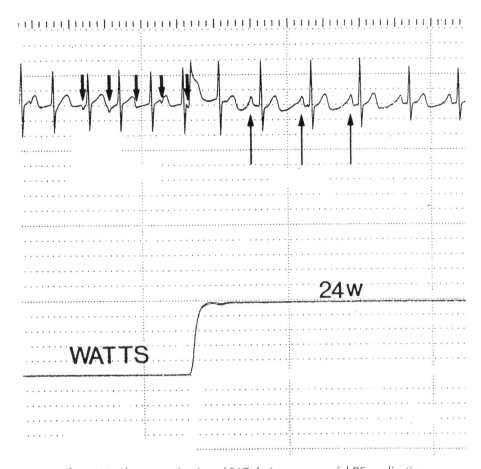

Figure 11. Abrupt termination of EAT during a successful RF application.

ure 13). The total time until EAT termination in our group ranged from 0.2–18.0 seconds (mean = 3.7 seconds). Prolonged RF applications beyond 10 seconds without accompanying change in EAT rate have almost always been nonproductive. However, in some patients we have observed that applications which were just slightly off target can cause acceleration of EAT without terminating the arrhythmia. In these cases, the EAT rate would remain elevated as long as RF discharge was in progress, but would return immediately to baseline rate when the application was discontinued. Such a finding probably suggests that the catheter is close to, but not exactly at, the proper target area. Continued RF application at a site which produces only acceleration (but not termination) after 15 seconds invites the possibility of transient injury to the EAT focus, which prohibits further mapping, and could well result in later EAT recurrence.

Following a successful RF lesion, we observe our patients in the laboratory with catheters in place for periods of 30 to 60 minutes. All are challenged with an infusion of isoproterenol, and if no EAT activity is observed, the study is terminated. A postprocedure echocardiogram is usually done to rule out pericar-

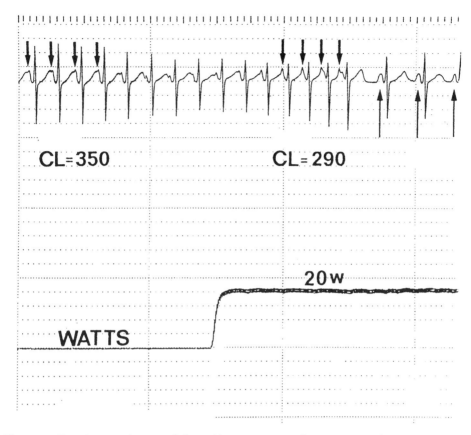

Figure 12. Transient acceleration, followed by termination, during a successful RF application.

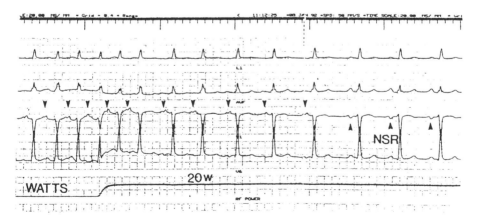

Figure 13. Transient slowing, followed by termination, during a successful RF application.

dial effusion in very young patients, or in patients regardless of age when RF applications are made very distally in the atrial appendages.

Institutional Results for EAT Ablation

Patient Characteristics

Since 1990 at Boston Children's Hospital, RF ablation has been attempted for 64 patients with EAT ranging in age from 2 months to 60 years (median 12.6 years), representing 6% of our total RF ablation volume. Excluded from this review are 9 additional patients who underwent ablation for a clinical picture of EAT but were found to have more than one automatic atrial focus during mapping, which possibly represents a different disease entity.

The majority of our EAT patients (67%) had some degree of impaired left ventricular systolic performance by echocardiographic criteria due to chronic tachycardia, including 12 cases with severe dysfunction (echocardiographic shortening fraction of less than 20%). Congenital heart defects were present in 6 patients; one had hypertrophic cardiomyopathy; one had idiopathic fibrous dysplasia of the anterior right atrium; and one older man had significant coronary artery disease. Apart from ventricular dysfunction, there was no demonstrable structural pathology in the remainder.

In 7 patients (11%), there were other documented supraventricular tachycardia mechanisms in addition to EAT. This involved atrial fibrillation or flutter in 5, classic AV nodal reentry in 1, and 1 patient had a concealed accessory pathway. In at least 3 of the 5 patients with atrial fibrillation or flutter, it seemed clear that the EAT served as the primary trigger for the atrial muscle reentry, since successful ablation of EAT alone resulted in elimination of both disorders.

Focus Location

Mapping of the EAT focus was possible for the 59 patients in whom EAT was spontaneously active or inducible in the laboratory. The focus was localized to the left atrium in 37 patients, and to the right atrium in 22 (Table 1). Left atrial foci clearly tended to cluster toward the orifice of various pulmonary veins or the left atrial appendage. The distribution pattern for right atrial foci involved clustering toward the appendage, with a fair number along the upper crista terminalis, not far distant from the area of the SA node. Normal SA node function was preserved after successful ablation along the upper crista in 6 of 7 patients, and the one exception had recovery of physiological sinus rates after 72 hours. It seemed likely to us that these upper crista sites represented true abnormal foci rather than inappropriate sinus tachycardia.

There were certainly exceptions to these general patterns, and it must be recognized that EAT can arise from nearly any region in the atria. About the only area which seems unlikely to be a potential site of EAT origin in our ex-

Table 1
Location of Mapped EAT Foci (n=59)

LEFT ATRIAL	n=36
Pulmonary veins	17
Left appendage	11
Along mitral valve ring	5
Other	3
RIGHT ATRIAL	n=22
Right appendage	9
Upper crista	7
Lower crista	4
Other	2

perience is the sinus venosus portion of the right atrium, located posterior to the crista terminalis. Whenever we have mapped relatively early activation times along the posterior portions of the right atrium, we invariably found that the EAT focus was actually arising from a right pulmonary vein or the left side of the atrial septum rather than the back wall of the right atrium. Our intra-cardiac mapping observations are in close agreement with the data previously reported for surgical therapy of EAT in a young population,[12] and except for the relative predominance of left atrial sites in our series, are also similar to re-ports of EAT ablation in an adult population.

Ablation Results

Radiofrequency ablation was attempted for the 59 patients in whom map-ping was possible, and was acutely successful in 56 (95%), all of whom left the hospital in normal sinus rhythm after an average hospital stay of 24 hours (Table 2). This required a mean of 4.3 "test lesions" of less than 10 seconds duration per patient, and a mean of 2.5 "therapeutic" applications of 30–60 seconds duration per patient. In 19 cases, EAT was permanently eliminated on the initial RF ap-plication. One of the 3 failures occurred in a patient who had an area of diffuse fi-brous dysplasia of unknown etiology involving the anterior right atrium.[3] Abla-tion was attempted at a site of early activation, but despite excellent signal quality, EAT would only accelerate and degenerate into atrial fibrillation. This patient was ultimately taken to surgery soon thereafter, and did well following resection of a large fibrotic region of right atrial muscle and an associated aneurysm. The 2 other failures involved patients with relatively minor symptoms in whom we elected to terminate the procedure after mapping and preliminary ablation attempts, out of concern that aggressive lesion creation would result in complications. Both patients had their foci in the right upper pulmonary vein. In one, atrial pacing at the site of the focus resulted in clear diaphragm twitch from phrenic nerve stimulation, and we feared the nerve would be damaged if we per-sisted with RF applications. In the other, the focus was mapped far more distally into the pulmonary vein than we were accustomed to seeing, and we were con-cerned that vein stenosis might occur if aggressive RF applications were made.

Table 2
Results for EAT (single focus) Mapping and Ablation:
Boston Children's Hospital, 1990–1998

TOTAL PATIENTS STUDIED	n=64
No EAT in laboratory	5 (8%)
EAT active or induced	59
ABLATION ATTEMPTED	n=59
Acute success	56 (95%)
Complications	1 (2%)
Recurrence	5 (9%)
2nd procedure success	3 of 3

Of the 57 patients in whom we eliminated EAT acutely, a total of 5 (9%) were noted to have EAT recurrence 1 week to 3 months after the procedure. Three underwent successful second ablation procedures, and one elected to resume medical therapy. Of interest, one other patient had a transient recurrence documented 10 days after ablation, but has subsequently been arrhythmia-free during 14 months of careful follow-up without treatment, and may be an example of a "late cure."

There was only one direct complication of RF ablation in this patient group, involving transient sinus node dysfunction in a 10-month-old child who had incessant EAT at rates in excess of 200 per minute, and severe mitral regurgitation related to left ventricular dilation. The EAT focus was mapped quite close to the sinus node, and was successfully ablated, although the initial recovery rhythm was sinus bradycardia and junctional escape beats. Within 72 hours sinus rhythm returned at physiological rates. No other complications were encountered.

The benefit of EAT elimination for the patients with ventricular dysfunction was dramatic. Of the 43 with depressed function prior to ablation, 39 have follow-up echocardiograms available that demonstrate normal ventricular function. The improvement usually occurred within 2 months of the ablation, although a rare patient required 9–12 months to normalize.

Future Directions

Ectopic atrial tachycardia can be managed by RF catheter ablation with a high rate of success, a reasonably low rate of recurrence, and acceptable risk. There are clearly technical aspects of EAT ablation that still require improvement, including the unpredictable nature of the focus activity which can become quiescent during a procedure and frustrate mapping efforts. A reliable maneuver which can reproducibly activate the focus under controlled conditions is still elusive, and is very likely to remain so until the exact cellular mechanism (or mechanisms) of EAT is better understood.

The use of combined data from bipolar and unipolar electrograms seems to allow very accurate focus localization, but ablation can still be technically challenging due to the complexities of atrial anatomy, particularly the regions of the pulmonary veins and appendages. Echocardiographic visualization, and the availability of three-dimensional electroanatomic mapping[35] equipment, will likely simplify these procedures in the future.

The risk of perforation at the ablation site (even in thin-walled structures like the appendages) appears to be negligible from both animal studies and accumulated human experience, but it is still unclear whether the scar could expand with time or become an arrhythmogenic focus in itself. The former concern is probably most relevant to the pediatric population, and is founded on the laboratory observation that atrial RF lesions created in young lambs tend to enlarge as the animal matures.[37] The long term significance of this finding is uncertain, but it does support a more conservative approach to very young patients with EAT unless medical therapy has clearly proven unsuccessful. The possibility of new arrhythmias from the ablation scar has been monitored carefully in all clinical series, and thus far there appear to be very few untoward electrophysiological effects. However, longer follow-up will be needed until this concern can be dismissed completely. In addition, there is now growing evidence from the experience with atrial fibrillation ablation in adults[38] that aggressive RF lesions made around the pulmonary veins can result in symptomatic vein stenosis. We have not encountered this so far in our population undergoing EAT ablation in or near the pulmonary veins, although we have not looked aggressively for the problem. Echocardiographic evaluation of pulmonary vein flow velocity has now been incorporated into the follow-up testing of all our patients who undergo ablation in this area.

Radiofrequency ablation is a highly-effective tool for dealing with the often difficult disorder of EAT. Indications are still being developed for deciding who and when to ablate, and until longer follow-up is available, reasonable caution must be exercised with patient selection. Finally, in our enthusiasm to perform a definitive procedure against this disease, it must be remembered that the etiology and cellular electrophysiology of EAT is still undetermined. Equal efforts must be directed toward a basic understanding of mechanism, if progress is to continue against this form of tachycardia.

References

1. Margolis PD, Roman CA, Moulton KP, et al. Radiofrequency catheter ablation of left and right ectopic atrial tachycardia [abstract]. *Circulation* 1990;82(suppl 3):III–718.
2. Walsh EP, Saul JP, Hulse JE, et al. Successful transcatheter ablation of ectopic atrial tachycardia using radiofrequency energy [abstract]. *PACE* 1991;14(suppl 2):II–656.
3. Walsh EP, Saul JP, Hulse JE, et al. Transcatheter ablation of ectopic atrial tachycardia in young patients using radiofrequency current. *Circulation* 1992;86:1138–1146.
4. Kay GN, Chong F, Epstein AE, et al. Radiofrequency ablation for treatment of primary atrial tachycardias. *J Am Coll Cardiol* 1993;21:901–909.
5. Tracy CM, Swartz JE, Fletcher RD, et al. Radiofrequency catheter ablation of ectopic atrial tachycardia using paced activation sequence mapping. *J Am Coll Cardiol* 1993;21:910–917.

6. Walsh EP. Ablation of ectopic atrial tachycardia in children. In: Huang SKS, ed. *Radiofrequency Catheter Ablation of Cardiac Arrhythmias.* Armonk, NY: Futura Publishing Co., 1995. pp 421–443.

7. Chen SA, Chiang CE, Chang MS. Ablation of atrial tachycardia in adults. In: Huang SKS, ed. *Radiofrequency Catheter Ablation of Cardiac Arrhythmias.* Armonk, NY: Futura Publishing Co., 1995. pp 445–458.

8. Gillette PC, Garson A. Electrophysiologic and pharmacologic characteristics of automatic ectopic atrial tachycardia. *Circulation* 1977;56:571–575.

9. de Bakker JM, Hauer RN, Bakker PF, et al. Abnormal automaticity as mechanism of atrial tachycardia in the human heart—Electrophysiologic and histologic correlation: a case report. *J Cardiovasc Electrophysiol* 1994;5:335–344.

10. Gillette PC, Crawford FC, Zeigler VL. Mechanisms of atrial tachycardia. In: Zipes DP, Jalife J, eds. *Cardiac Electrophysiology: From Cell to Bedside* Philadelphia: WB Saunders, 1990. pp 559–563.

11. Dunnigan A, Pierpont ME, Smith SA, et al. Cardiac and skeletal myopathy associated with cardiac dysrhythmias. *Am J Cardiol* 1984;53:731–737.

12. Garson A, Smith RT, Moak JP, et al. Atrial automatic tachycardia in children. In: Touboul P, Waldo AL, eds. *Atrial Arrhythmias: Current Concepts and Management.* St. Louis, MO: Mosby-Year Book, 1990. pp 282–287.

13. Keane JF, Plauth WH, Nadas AS. Chronic ectopic tachycardia of infancy and childhood. *Am Heart J* 1972;84:748–757.

14. Fishberger SB, Colan SD, Saul JP, et al. Myocardial mechanics before and after ablation of chronic tachycardia. *PACE* 1996;19:42–49.

15. Ogilvie RI, Zborowska-Sluis D. Effect of chronic rapid ventricular pacing on total vascular capacitance. *Circulation* 1992;85:1524–1530.

16. Spinale FG, Fulbright BM, Mukherjee R, et al. Relation between ventricular and myocyte function with tachycardia-induced cardiomyopathy. *Circ Res* 1992;71:174–187.

17. Tanake R, Spinale FG, Crawford FA, et al. Effect of chronic supraventricular tachycardia on left ventricular function and structure in newborn pigs. *J Am Coll Cardiol* 1992;20:1650–1660.

18. Mehta AV, Sanchez GR, Sacks EJ, et al. Ectopic automatic atrial tachycardia in children: clinical characteristics, management, and follow-up. *J Am Coll Cardiol* 1986;11:379–385.

19. Kunze KP, Kuck KH, Schluter M, et al. Effect of encainide and flecainide on chronic ectopic atrial tachycardia. *J Am Coll Cardiol* 1986;7:1121–1126.

20. Evans VL, Garson A, Smith RT, et al. Ethmozine: a promising drug for "automatic" atrial ectopic tachycardia. *Am J Cardiol* 1987;60:83f–86f.

21. Gillette PC, Wampler DG, Garson A, et al. Treatment of atrial automatic tachycardia by ablation procedures. *J Am Coll Cardiol* 1985;6:405–409.

22. Gillette PC, Garson A, Hesslein PS, et al. Successful surgical treatment of atrial, junctional, and ventricular tachycardia unassociated with accessory connections in infants and children. *Am Heart J* 1981;102:984–991.

23. Ott DA, Gillette PC, Garson A, et al. Surgical management of refractory supraventricular tachycardia in infants and children. *J Am Coll Cardiol* 1985;5:124–129.

24. Garson A, Moak JP, Friedman RA, et al. Surgical treatment of arrhythmias in children. *Cardiol Clin* 1985;7:319–329.
25. Seals AA, Lawrie GM, Magro S, et al. Surgical treatment of right atrial focal tachycardia in adults. *J Am Coll Cardiol* 1988;11:1111–1117.
26. Olssen SB, Blomstrom P, Sabel KG, et al. Incessant ectopic atrial tachycardia: successful surgical treatment with regression of dilated cardiomyopathy picture. *Am J Cardiol* 1984;53:1465–1466.
27. Langberg JJ, Chin MC, Rosenquist M, et al. Catheter ablation of the atrioventricular junction with radiofrequency energy. *Circulation* 1989;80: 1527–1535.
28. Silka MJ, Gillette PC, Garson A, et al. Transvenous catheter ablation of a right atrial automatic ectopic tachycardia. *J Am Coll Cardiol* 1985;5: 999–1001.
29. Lee MA, Huang SKS, Graham AR, et al. Radiofrequency catheter ablation of the canine atrium and tricuspid annulus [abstract]. *Circulation* 1987; 76(suppl 4):IV-405.
30. Huang SKS. Advances in applications of radiofrequency current to catheter ablation therapy. *PACE* 1991;14:28–42.
31. Lavergne T, Prunier L, Cuize L, et al. Transcatheter radiofrequency ablation of atrial tissue using a suction catheter. *PACE* 1989;12:177–186.
32. Brockenbrough EC, Braunwald E. A new technique for left ventricular angiocardiography and transseptal cardiac catheterization. *Am J Cardiol* 1966;6:1062–1064.
33. Keane JF, Lock JE. Manual techniques of cardiac catheterization: vessel entry and catheter manipulation. In: Lock JE, Keane JF, Fellows KE, eds. *Diagnostic and Interventional Catheterization in Congenital Heart Disease.* Boston, MA: Martinus Nijhoff, 1987. pp 29–30.
34. Lesh MD, Van Hare GF, Kwasman MA, et al. Curative radiofrequency (RF) catheter ablation of atrial tachycardia and flutter [abstract]. *J Am Coll Cardiol* 1993;21(2):374A.
35. Smeets JL, Ben-Haim SA, Rodriguez LM, et al. New method for nonfluoroscopic endocardial mapping in humans: accuracy assessment and first clinical results. *Circulation* 1998;97:2426–2432.
36. Triedman JK, Jenkins KJ, Colan SD, et al. Multipolar endocardial mapping of the right atrium using a basket catheter: acute and chronic animal studies. *PACE* 1997;20:51–59.
37. Saul JP, Hulse JE, Walsh EP. Late enlargemant of radiofrequency lesions in infant lambs: implications for ablation procedures in small children. *Circulation* 1994;90:492–499.
38. Robbins IM, Colvin EV, Doyle TP, et al. Pulmonary vein stenosis after catheter ablation of atrial fibrillation. *Circulation* 1998;98:1769–1775.

Chapter 8

Ablation of Atrial Tachycardia in Adults

Marcus Wharton, M.D., Hossein Shenasa, M.D., Helen Barold, M.D., Grant Simons, M.D., Ismael Vergara, M.D.

Introduction

Atrial tachycardias are defined as supraventricular tachycardias (SVTs) that arise solely within atrial tissues and are independent of atrioventricular (AV) nodal conduction, excluding AV nodal reentrant or AV reciprocating tachycardias. Traditionally defined, the electrocardiogram reveals a tachycardia with P waves separated by an isoelectric baseline and fixed or variable relationship to the QRS complexes depending on AV conduction.[1] If the site of origin is outside of the sinus nodal region, then the tachycardia is "ectopic"; whereas inducible atrial tachycardias arising from the sinus nodal region have typically been defined as sinus nodal reentrant tachycardia.[2–4] Electrocardiographically, atrial tachycardias are distinguished from atrial flutters by the slower atrial rate (typically <250 beats per minute) and the presence of an isoelectric baseline between P waves (i.e., the absence of "flutter waves").[1] Clinically, this helps distinguish relatively focal atrial tachycardias from large macroreentrant circuits, such as isthmus-dependent or independent atrial flutters. These distinctions arose from the different electrocardiographic characteristics of these arrhythmias and have been shown to have some clinical utility. However, as we shall see, this electrocardiographic nosology has definite limitations in the era of more detailed electrophysiological understanding of the focal atrial tachycardias in which focal tachycardias may electrocardiographically mimic atrial flutter and even atrial fibrillation[5–7] and macroreentrant atrial flutters with long

From Huang SKS, Wilber DJ (eds.): *Radiofrequency Catheter Ablation of Cardiac Arrhythmias: Basic Concepts and Clinical Applications,* 2nd ed. Armonk, NY: Futura Publishing Company, Inc. ©2000.

cycle lengths may mimic atrial tachycardias. Whether such electrocardiographic distinctions are useful in the era of electrophysiological definitions and ablation is questionable.[8] For purposes of this chapter, an atrial tachycardia is defined as a tachycardia of any rate and P wave pattern that is due to a relatively focal mechanism, be it reentrant, triggered, or automatic. Relatively focal implies that the sites of origin cannot be mapped spatially beyond a single point or few adjacent points with the resolution of a standard 4–5 mm tip catheter. If the arrhythmia can be mapped across a defined space (e.g., macro-reentrant atrial flutters, typical atrial fibrillation, or sinus tachycardia), it will not be considered an atrial tachycardia. Focal atrial tachycardias electrocardiographically simulating atrial fibrillation and flutter will be discussed at the end of this chapter.

Prevalence

Atrial tachycardias, by conventional definition, are the third most common form of SVT referred for ablation. In older studies, atrial tachycardias accounted for approximately 7–15% of all SVTs studied.[9–12] As a broader range of patients are referred in the era of ablation, the incidence of atrial tachycardia appears to be somewhat larger. In the ablation registry at Duke University Medical Center, atrial tachycardias (inclusive of sinus nodal reentrant tachycardia) account for approximately 13% of cases referred for ablation. The rate of referral of atrial tachycardias for ablation has been steadily increasing. In 1993, atrial tachycardia accounted for only 4% of SVT referred, compared to 18% in 1998. This still probably underestimates the actual frequency of atrial tachycardias in the overall population of SVTs, particularly as the understanding of focal mechanisms of atrial fibrillation expands the type of atrial tachycardia which are ablated.

Baseline Predictors

Several clinical features suggest that a patient may have an atrial tachycardia. Age is one predictor. The prevalence of atrial tachycardia in pediatric populations ranges from 11–34%.[12–14] Ko et al[12] showed that atrial tachycardia is the second most common mechanism of SVT in very young patients, comprising 16% of SVT in age groups less than 1 year of age and only exceeded by AV reciprocating tachycardia. After one year of age, AT is consistently the least common mechanism as the prevalence of AV nodal reentrant tachycardia (AVNRT) increases. Data from our laboratory have shown that the relative prevalence of atrial tachycardia in the adult ablation population steadily increases with age (Figure 1). As shown in the figure, atrial tachycardia comprises approximately less than 10% of SVT in age groups less than 40 years, but is greater than 20% in patients aged 60 years or more. Thus, the prevalence of atrial tachycardia appears to demonstrate a bimodal distribution, with higher frequency in the very young and older populations.

The history of cardiac disease or prior cardiac surgery also increases the

Type of SVT Ablation as Function of Age

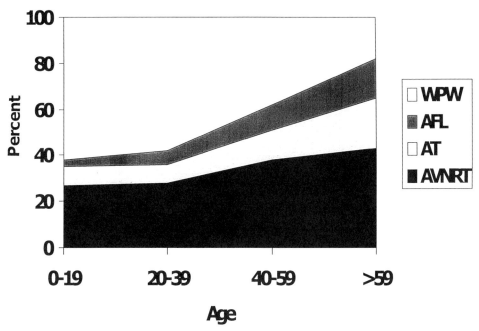

Figure 1. Graph of relative percentages of specific diagnoses of SVT referred for ablation at Duke University Medical Center between 1991–1998 compared to the age at the time of ablation. The Wolff-Parkinson-White (WPW) syndrome accounts for approximately 60% of ablations in patients <40 years of age and then progressively decreases with increasing age, whereas the relative percentages of AVNRT and atrial flutter (AFL) gradually increase with age. Atrial tachycardia (AT) is constant at 8% at ages <40 years, but increases to 22% for patients >59 years old.

suspicion of atrial tachycardia in patients with SVT. Although most patients with atrial tachycardia had cardiac disease in early studies,[11,14,15] more recent studies of patients with atrial tachycardia undergoing ablation have had a much lower prevalence of definable cardiac disease, with generally more than 70% of patients with atrial tachycardia not having definable cardiac disease.[9,16–27] In our experience, the prevalence of cardiac disease in the adult population is similar to that seen with AVNRT, probably reflecting the similar ages of the patients afflicted.

Electrocardiographic Evaluation

Electrocardiography can be helpful in the noninvasive determination of atrial tachycardia and in roughly approximating the site of origin. The electrocardiogram classically reveals abnormal P wave morphology and a long RP relationship during tachycardia. If the P waves are "retrograde" in appearance (inverted in the inferior limb leads), then a left or right posteroseptal tachycardia may be present, most commonly in the coronary sinus ostial region. However, the differential diagnosis includes AV reciprocating tachycardia using an accessory pathway which conducts slowly, or fast-slow or slow-slow variants of AVNRT.[28] Development of AV block during tachycardia strongly suggests atrial tachycardia, but does not totally exclude an atypical variant of AVNRT. P waves during tachycardia with other anomalous morphologies other than a retrograde morphology indicate atrial tachycardia. Identification of the P wave during tachycardia is thus helpful in suggesting a diagnosis. However, the P wave during atrial tachycardia cannot always be discerned, particular if there is 1:1 AV conduction and the P wave is buried in the preceding T wave or QRS complex. These cases may be mistaken for AV nodal dependent tachycardias unless transient AV block occurs or the tachycardia rate changes to allow identification of the P waves with an inconstant RP relationship (Figure 2). Atrial tachycardias arising from the high right atrium or the high posteromedial left atrium (e.g., right superior pulmonary vein) may generate P waves that

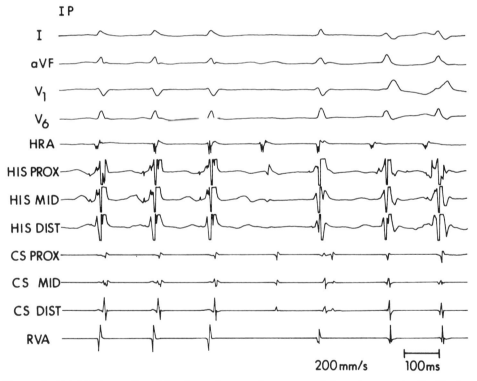

Figure 2. Atrial tachycardia arising from the superior aspect of the crista terminalis. During most episodes of the tachycardia, atrial activation occurs simultaneously with the preceding QRS complex, electrographically resembling typical AVNRT. However, spontaneous development of second degree AV block exposes the P wave and reveals earliest atrial activation in the high right atrium (HRA) rather than His bundle region (HIS) or coronary sinus (CS). Atrial-ventricular independence is further demonstrated by the inconstant relationship between the atrial and ventricular event in the last three complexes. Shown are surface electrocardiographic leads I, aVF, V$_1$ and V$_6$ and electrographic recordings from the HRA, HIS, CS and right ventricular apex (RVA). Other abbreviations: PROX = proximal; MID = middle; DIST = distal.

are similar to those in sinus rhythm. Unless an abrupt onset and/or termination are demonstrated, these rhythms may be difficult to distinguish from appropriate or inappropriate sinus tachycardia (Figure 3).

The ECG can also be useful for determining prior to ablation which patients may have a left atrial focus for their tachycardia and allow anticipation of the need for transseptal catheterization.[29,30] A predominantly negative or isoelectric P wave in leads I or aVL suggests a left atrial focus. However, P waves generated by posteromedial left atrial sites, such as the right superior pulmonary vein, may generate P waves which are upright in the left limb leads.[30] Although this seems unlikely for a left atrial source, closer scrutiny of atrial anatomy reveals that the posteromedial left atrium is posterior, rather than leftward, of the right atrium. The right superior pulmonary vein, which is a very common site of origin for left atrial tachycardias, is only a few centimeters from the head of the sinus node. Activation rapidly crosses the septum via Bachman's bundle to activate the right atrium in a fashion similar to sinus rhythm, explaining the similarities of P wave morphologies. However, lead V_1 may help distinguish left superior pulmonary veins sites from high right atrial sites, since posterior left atrial sites generate upright P waves in lead V_1, whereas high lateral right atrial sites generate negative or biphasic P waves in

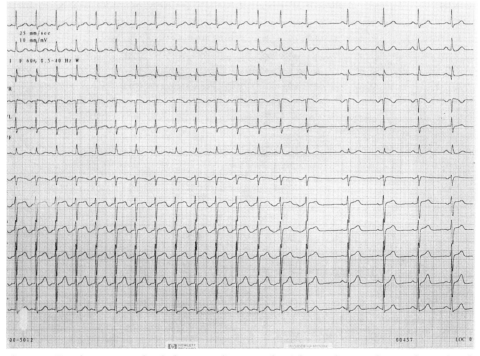

Figure 3. Simultaneous 12-lead electrocardiogram of a right atrial appendage tachycardia after an intravenous bolus of 6 milligrams of adenosine, which terminated the tachycardia without causing AV block. Note the similarity between the P wave during atrial tachycardia and sinus rhythm, suggesting relatively close proximity between the 2 sites. Specifically, note that the P wave during tachycardia is upright in lead I and negative in V_1, suggesting a right and anterior location.

V_1.[30] Negative P waves in the anterior precordial leads suggest an anterior right or left atrial freewall location. Clearly, such electrocardiographic patterns are only rough indicators of the site of origin of an atrial tachycardia; nonetheless, they provide an initial basis to guide mapping strategies. Preliminary work has suggested that body surface mapping to obtain P wave integral maps may provide a more effective means of localizing atrial tachycardias.[31]

Adenosine

Adenosine may be a useful tool for causing transient AV block to permit discernment of the P waves and allow noninvasive determination of the diagnosis of atrial tachycardia. Early studies suggested that adenosine caused transient AV block in almost all patients and rarely, if ever, terminated atrial tachycardia.[32,33] However, as referral population of patients with atrial tachycardia have changed in the ablation era, it has become obvious that most atrial tachycardias are actually terminated with adenosine, typically prior to the onset of AV block (see Figure 3). Studies have shown that the rate of termination of atrial tachycardia with adenosine range from 50–80%,[34–36] with less than 20% of atrial tachycardias terminated with adenosine demonstrating AV block prior to termination. Thus, demonstration of AV block with or without termination of SVT confirms the diagnosis of atrial tachycardia. However, the converse is not true. If AV block does not occur and the tachycardia terminates, atrial tachycardia is still a possible etiology for the SVT. Adenosine may also be helpful in establishing a mechanistic diagnosis, but, as will be seen, limitations may exist in its ability to distinguish triggered automaticity from microreentry.[22]

Mechanism of Atrial Tachycardia

Atrial tachycardias can be further classified by the presumed mechanism of the tachycardia, i.e., reentrant, triggered, or automatic. Delineation of the mechanism of tachycardia can be difficult, and means of distinguishing atrial tachycardia mechanism are fraught with exceptions.[8,37] Furthermore, it is not clear that making such mechanistic distinctions carries any clinical significance at the present time, although it is possible that such information could be useful in guiding pharmacological therapy. It is unlikely that this hypothesis will be tested in the present era of ablation.

Electrophysiological characteristics for each mechanism are shown in Table 1. The initial step in determining the mechanism of atrial tachycardia is to establish whether the arrhythmia can be initiated and terminated with premature atrial extrastimulation and/or burst pacing. Initiation and termination with pacing techniques are characteristics consistent with reentry or triggered automaticity.[22,37] Atrial tachycardias that cannot be initiated or terminated with pacing techniques are most likely due to an automatic mechanism, although it is possible that a reentrant or triggered focus cannot be activated with sufficient prematurity or rapidity due to entrance block or that initiation of

Table 1
Electrophysiological and pharamacological properties of different mechanisms of AT.*

	Reentry (N=27)	Triggered (N=7)	Automatic (N=9)
Electrophysiological Findings			
Inducible by pacing	100%	100%	0%
Terminated by pacing	100%	100%	0%
Resetting	100%	100%	0%
Entrainment	100%	0%	0%
DAD on MAP†	0%	100%	0%
Pharmacological Termination			
Adenosine	87%	100%	0%
Verapamil	96%	100%	0%
Propranolol	68%	100%	100%
Vagal manuever	7%	100%	0%

*Adapted from Chen S-A, et al. Electrophysiological mechanisms in successful radiofrequency catheter modification of atrioventricular junction for patients with medically refractory paroxysmal atrial fibrillation. *Circulation* 1994;90:1262–1278.
†Delayed afterdepolarization on monophasic action potential catheter.

reentry is dependent upon the site of stimulation. In response to rapid pacing, automatic tachycardias will demonstrate transient overdrive suppression, but will subsequently resume, typically with a gradual increase in the rate.[22,38]

The best means to distinguish reentrant from triggered atrial tachycardia is to demonstrate entrainment with concealed fusion (see Table 1).[22,39] Pacing 10–20 milliseconds faster than the atrial tachycardia at a site with presystolic activity or a discrete mid-diastolic potential can entrain a reentrant tachycardia to the pacing rate without changing the morphology of the P wave or the intracardiac electrogram sequence (Figure 4). The interval between the atrial electrogram at the site of entrainment and the onset of the P wave and the interval between the stimulus during entrainment and the onset of the P wave should be similar (less than 25 milliseconds).[39] To exclude pacing in a dead-end alley, the postpacing interval at the termination of concealed entrainment should be similar to the atrial tachycardia cycle length. Since entrainment is only seen with reentry, it confirms the mechanism. Although simple in principle, demonstration of concealed entrainment is frequently difficult clinically, even in atrial tachycardias that are presumed reentrant, because spatial separation of diastolic zones and exit sites are similar (focal by relative mapping terms) so that distinction of entrainment from simply pacing at the exit site of a focal tachycardia can be difficult. In our experience, demonstration of concealed entrainment is particularly important for the successful ablation of atrial tachycardias using small macroreentrant circuits such as occur in atrial scar from atrial infarcts, aneurysms or surgical cicatrix.

Reentrant and triggered atrial tachycardias can also show the property of resetting during premature stimulation during which a premature extrastimulus alters the return cycle of the next beat of atrial tachycardia (see Table 1). Several patterns of resetting exist.[22] A flat pattern exists when the return cycle is noncompensatory and remains the same value with decreasing coupling in-

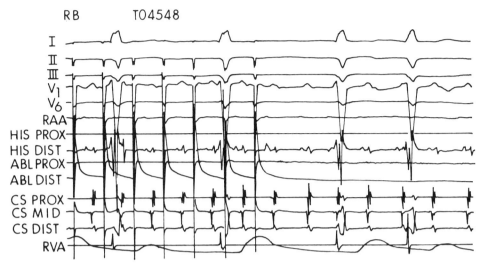

Figure 4. Concealed entrainment of a right atrial tachycardia at the border of a large area of atrial scar that recorded a minute mid-diastolic potential. The tachycardia is accelerated to the rate of a pacing on the ablation catheter and the P wave morphology and intracardiac activation sequence during pacing and tachycardia are the same. The postpacing interval cannot be determined in this example because the proximal ablation electrode is over scar and records no electrogram. The interval between the mid-diastolic potential and onset of P wave (not shown) is the same as the interval between the pacing stimulus and onset of P wave.

tervals. An increasing pattern exists when decreasing the coupling interval of the extrastimulus results in a gradual increase in the return cycle. This is classically felt to be due to reentry, since the increasingly premature extrastimulus causes increasing conduction delay in the zone of slow conduction of the reentrant circuit. A flat and then increasing (mixed) pattern commonly is seen with atrial tachycardias.[22] Again, this pattern is felt classically to be consistent with reentry. A fourth and rarely seen pattern of a decreasing return cycle with increasing prematurity of the extrastimulus is felt to be consistent with triggered automaticity since triggered arrhythmias have shown increasing amplitude of the delayed afterpotential (and consequently earlier triggered depolarization) with earlier extrastimuli. In practice, resetting patterns have not been shown to reliably distinguish between the reentry and triggered automaticity.[22]

Monophasic action potential (MAP) catheters have been suggested by some as being useful for distinguishing triggered automaticity from reentry (see Table 1). Chen et al[22] were able to demonstrate possible delayed afterdepolarizations on MAP recordings in patients with presumed triggered atrial tachycardia (Figure 5), but not in those with presumed reentry. However, a number of technical problems limit the applicability of this approach, most notably the production of "late potentials" due to mechanical artifacts. Furthermore, prospective validation that "late potentials" seen on MAP catheters placed near the site of origin of an atrial tachycardia are in any way related to the tachycardia mechanisms is not possible.

Pharmacological probes have also been used in attempts to distinguish mechanisms of atrial tachycardias (see Table 1). For ventricular arrhythmias,

VERAPAMIL

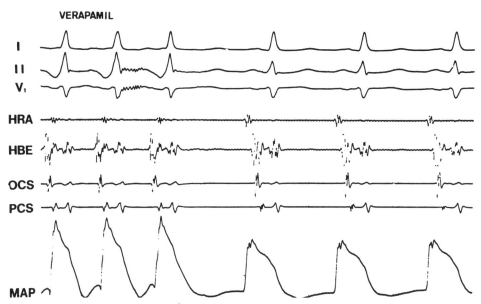

Figure 5. Example of delayed afterdepolarizations detected on a monophasic action potential (MAP) catheter during a presumed triggered atrial tachycardia (first 3 complexes), which are not present during sinus rhythm after termination with intravenous verapamil (last 3 complexes). Abbreviations as before; also, HBE = His bundle electrogram; OCS = orifice of coronary sinus; PCS = proximal coronary sinus. (Reproduced with permission from Chen SA, et al.[22])

adenosine has been shown to be mechanistically specific, terminating triggered but not reentrant or automatic ventricular tachycardias.[40] However, in the atrium, the effects of adenosine are more complex. Besides its antiadrenergic effect (which theoretically is the reason it terminates triggered ventricular tachycardia), adenosine also activates the $Ik_{ACh/Ado}$ channel which decreases action potential duration and decreases resting membrane potential.[38] Either of these effects, as well as the antiadrenergic effect, could be responsible for termination of atrial tachycardias due to microreentry,[22] and, in rare cases, macroreentry. Adenosine's frequent termination of atrial tachycardias due to reentry and triggered automaticity has been confirmed by Chen et al,[22] although others have suggested that adenosine should only terminate triggered atrial tachycardias or sinus nodal reentrant tachycardia.[8] Adenosine is useful for identifying automatic atrial tachycardias, which are transiently slowed, then terminated, with gradual resumption of atrial tachycardia without initiating premature atrial contractions.[8] Other pharmacological probes (e.g., β-adrenergic blockers and verapamil) have been tried, but again there is too much overlap with these probes to be useful in distinguishing reentrant and triggered mechanisms (see Table 1).

Sinus Nodal Reentrant Tachycardia

Paroxysmal atrial tachycardias arising from the high right atrium near the region of the sinus node that can be induced and terminated with atrial pacing techniques have been defined as sinus nodal reentrant tachycardia.[2–4] The hallmark diagnostically for these tachycardias is that the P wave during tachycardia and intracardiac atrial activation sequence is identical, or almost identical, to that during sinus rhythm. Slight variations can exist given the relatively long length of the sinus node just posterior to the crista terminalis along the upper half of the lateral right atrium. Detailed mapping studies in animals have suggested reentry within the sinoatrial (SA) nodal or perinodal tissues.[41] Clinically, it is not possible to tell if reentry is occurring in perinodal tissues, or simply in close proximity to perinodal tissues. Given the length of the sinus node along the upper half of the crista terminalis and the frequency of origin of atrial tachycardias along the full length of the crista terminalis,[42,43] it is difficult to proposed when sinus nodal reentry ends and cristal tachycardias begin. Furthermore, although consistent termination with adenosine, verapamil, and vagomimetic maneuvers has been used as indirect evidence that these tachycardias utilized SA nodal tissue, frequent termination of atrial tachycardias remote from the sinus node with these interventions raises serious questions regarding the specificity of these maneuvers.[22,34,35] Given the difficulty truly distinguishing SA nodal reentry from triggered or reentrant tachycardias arising from closely adjacent regions, no attempt is made in this review to distinguish SA nodal reentry from other atrial tachycardias.

Anteroseptal Atrial Tachycardias

Atrial tachycardias arising from the anteroseptal space in the region of the compact AV node and His bundle present a number of dilemmas.[44,45] First, they are commonly mistaken for atypical or even typical variants of AVNRT. However, ablation of the posterior AV nodal approaches will have no effect on these tachycardias. Although rarely seen with AV nodal reentry, demonstration of AV nodal block during a tachycardia with earliest atrial activation anteroseptally should suggest an atrial tachycardia. Unfortunately, adenosine usually terminates anteroseptal atrial tachycardias before the development of AV nodal block, but rapid ventricular pacing can be used to induce AV nodal block with continuation of the atrial tachycardia (Figure 6). In addition, the use of critically timed premature extrastimulation to result in concealed retrograde penetration of the AV node to prolong the AH interval, or shortening of the postpause AH, without altering the encompassing AA interval during tachycardia, also strongly supports the diagnosis of atrial tachycardia (see Figure 6), since AH alterations should alter the cycle length of AV nodal reentry in a parallel fashion, except in the unlikely circumstance that all of the AH delay is below the lower turnaround point. Man et al[46] demonstrated that the difference in the AH interval during tachycardia and during right atrial pacing at a similar cycle length was more than 40 milliseconds in most patients with atypical AV nodal reentry, but was less than or equal to 20 milliseconds in most patients with atrial tachycardia or AV reciprocating tachycardia using a slowly conducting accessory pathway, since the AV conduction pathway is the same in the latter two conditions but potentially dissimilar in atypical AVNRT. This observation may be used to distinguish anteroseptal atrial tachycardia from atypical, but not typical, variants of AVNRT.

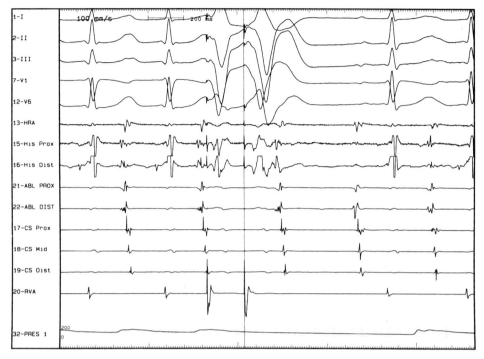

Figure 6. Use of 2 closely coupled ventricular extrastimuli to dissociate atrial activity from ventricular activity and fully expose the P wave during an atrial tachycardia arising from the anterior limbus of the foramen ovale. AV dissociation is clearly demonstrated between the third and fourth atrial complexes, completely excluding AV reciprocating tachycardia and very unlikely with atypical AVNRT. Note that the AA interval is not altered by the ventricular extrastimuli despite block of AV nodal conduction. Exposure of the P wave allows better timing of intracardiac events to the true P wave onset, which is hard to ascertain within the T wave during 1:1 AV conduction and which has isoelectric initial components in several leads (e.g., leads I and V_1). Earliest intracardiac activation is on the His bundle electrogram; the ablation (ABL) catheter is in the high posteromedial right atrium. The flat activation sequence across left, right, and septal atrial recording sites suggests a septal or near septal site of origin. PRES 1 = right femoral artery pressure recording.

Location of Site of Origin of Atrial Tachycardia

Review of almost all large series of patients with atrial tachycardia in which detailed mapping of the site of origin was performed reveals that the majority of atrial tachycardias, traditionally definied, arise from the right atrium.[17–27,47] As shown in Table 2, which is derived from recent studies of radiofrequency ablation of atrial tachycardia, all but one study showed that right atrial origins predominated. From the pooled data, 83% of atrial tachycardias arise from the right side. Studies revealing larger percentages of left atrial tachycardias have incorporated only pediatric patients,[16] suggesting that atrial tachycardia distribution may be different in pediatric and adult populations. The mechanism of tachycardia does not appear to alter this relationship.[22,23,25] As already alluded to, recent studies have suggested that the predominance of right atrial sites occur along the length of crista terminalis from the sinus nodal region to the coronary sinus and AV nodal complex.[42,43] The

Table 2
Results and complications in published studies of ablation of atrial tachycardia.

Study	N	R/L	Mech.	Success	Complic.	Recur.
Walsh et al (1992)	12	5/7	AAT	11 (92%)	1 (8%)	0
Chen et al (1993)	7	9/1	IART	7 (100%)	0	0
Kay et al (1993)	15	14/1	AAT (11) SANRT (4)	15 (100%)	1 (7%)	3 (19%)
Tracy et al (1993)	10	>8/2	NA	7 (88%)	0	2 (20%)
Goldberger et al (1993)	15	15/0	AAT (11) IART (4)	12 (80%)	0	2 (17%)
Shenasa et al (1993)	16	19/0	NA	16 (100%)	1 (6%)	0
Sanders et al (1994)	10	10/0	SANRT (10)	10 (100%)	0	0
Chen et al (1994)	34	34/7	AAT (6) IART (27) TAT (8)	32 (94%)	0	2 (6%)
Lesh et al (1994)	17	17/5	AAT (12) IART (8) SANRT (3)	16 (94%)	0	2 (11%)
Wang et al. (1995)	13	10/5	AAT (12) RAT (1) SANRT (2)	9 (69%)	1 (8%)	1 (8%)
Poty et al (1996)	36	33/3	AAT (16) RAT (15) SANRT (3) Unknown (2)	31 (86%)	0	4 (12%)
Pappone et al (1996)	45	36/9	NA	42 (93%)	3 (7%)	3 (7%)
Weiss et al (1998)	48	40/12	NA	44 (92%)	0	5 (10%)
TOTAL	278	253/52	—	252 (91%)	7 (3%)	24 (9%)

clustering of atrial tachycardias along this relatively narrow ridge of tissue has been likened to an atrial "ring of fire"[42] and have been termed "cristal" tachycardias.[43] Given this predominance of right atrial tachycardias along the crista terminalis, the crista terminalis should be used as the initial point of mapping, starting superiorly along the crista if the P wave frontal plane axis is normal and inferiorly along the crista if the P wave axis is superiorly directed. Preliminary studies have suggested that the presence of structural heart disease may increase the probability of right atrial location, but from sites other than the crista terminalis.[48]

Other sites of atrial tachycardia clustering include the pulmonary venous ostia, coronary sinus ostia, and perhaps the mitral and tricuspid valve rings. Marchlinski and colleagues[49,50] noted a second ring of fire around the mitral annulus, although this has not been a common site in our experience. Atrial tachycardias associated with venous structures, such as the coronary sinus or pulmonary veins, may arise from sites several centimeters away from the atrial freewall,[6,7,51] representing the fact that atrial myocardium wraps around these structures for some distance from their insertions into the heart.[52] As will be seen at the end of this chapter, left atrial and particularly pulmonary venous tachycardias may be even more common than suspected when consideration is given to focal atrial fibrillation and flutter.[5-7]

Mapping of Atrial Tachycardia

Mapping of focal mechanisms of atrial tachycardia can be a relatively simple task. Traditionally, mapping entails localizing the site of earliest presystolic activity relative to the onset of the P wave during tachycardia. Clearly, determining the onset of the P wave may be impossible if the preceding T wave or QRS complex is superimposed. In complicated cases, confusion can arise regarding the prematurity of a mapping site if the onset of the P wave has not been adequately defined in multiple electrocardiographic leads. This is particularly the case if there is an isoelectric early portion of the P wave resulting in mapping data that appears premature when in fact it is relatively late (see Figure 6). P waves during tachycardia should be assessed using multiple electrocardiographic leads and choosing the P wave with the earliest onset. To facilitate this, delivering premature ventricular extrastimuli to advance ventricular activation and repolarization to permit careful distinction of the onset of the P wave during tachycardia is extremely helpful. After determining the P wave onset, a surrogate marker, such as the high right atrium or a coronary sinus electrogram, can be used rather than the P wave onset.

Another useful means of mapping focal atrial tachycardias is to use one mapping catheter placed at a site of early presystolic activity and the second ablation catheter can then be manipulated around the reference mapping catheter to find even earlier sites of activation. The reference catheter allows a more obvious timing marker than the P wave to facilitate mapping. An extension of this approach is to use one ablation catheter as a reference, find an earlier site with a second ablation catheter, then move the first catheter to an even earlier site. The process is reiterated until the earliest definable site is established. This "dancing catheter technique" or "*pas de deux*" can be very useful in complicated cases in the right atrium, but obviously cannot easily be applied to left atrial tachycardias at the present time. However, the coronary sinus catheter may serve as an excellent reference catheter, especially in cases of left atrial tachycardias arising close to the mitral valve annulus. Importantly, the sequence of activation along the length of the coronary sinus catheter can frequently be misleading in tachycardias arising from the superior left atrium. Atrial activation times may be similar ("flat") along the length of the coronary sinus with right and sometimes left superior pulmonary vein tachycardias (Figure 7). The more inferiorly in the atrium the tachycardia arises, the more the coronary sinus electrodes will point to the appropriate location.

Left atrial mapping is best performed via the transseptal approach. Although the retrograde aortic and mitral approach can be performed, the circuitous route of the catheter with this approach greatly complicates fine movement of the catheter and catheter whip makes establishment of stable catheter contact difficult at best. Knowledge of the approximate location of the left atrial tachycardia is helpful in sheath selection for transseptal approaches. Although straight sheaths can be used in all cases, the approach to pulmonary venous tachycardias is greatly facilitated by the use of sheaths that are angled posteriorly.

Special consideration needs to be given to tachycardias that map to the midseptum, particularly if presystolic activity is not particularly premature

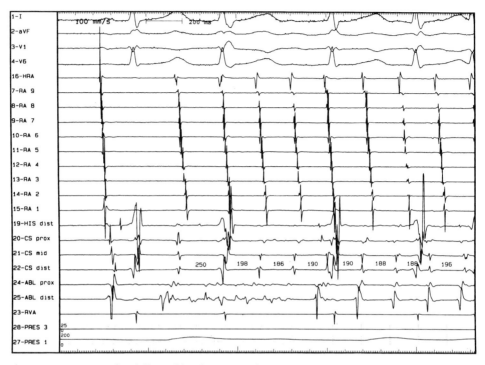

Figure 7. Sinus complex followed by the onset of a very rapid focal atrial tachycardia arising from the left superior pulmonary vein (focal atrial fibrillation). The ablation catheter is located at the ostium of left superior pulmonary vein and reveals an early, fractionated electrogram at the distal electrogram at the site of successful ablation. However, despite its origin from the left superior pulmonary vein ostium, note that the sequence of atrial activation in the coronary sinus is flat (first complex of tachycardia) and sometimes slightly eccentric (complexes 2–4). Also note in the first complex that the coronary sinus activation times are similar to those at the His bundle and high right atrium. Such a rapid activation is presumptively due to activation along Bachman's bundle of both the right and left atria. Abbreviations as before; RA 1–9 represents consecutive bipolar recordings along a duodecapolar catheter positioned along the crista terminalis, with RA 1 being along the inferior aspect. An isthmus ablation for atrial flutter had been previously performed causing activation along the crista terminalis catheter to run from high to low lateral right atrium.

(i.e., less than 30 milliseconds), signals are not fractionated, and multiple sites have similar activation times. Great care must be given in these cases to exclude a left atrial tachycardia using transseptal access to the left atrium. For tachycardias arising from the pulmonary veins, coronary sinus activation times may not clearly point to a left atrial site (see Figure 7). Again, with atrial tachycardias that map to the right anteroseptal space (His bundle region), great care needs to be given to the anteromedial left atrial septum or freewall since sites in these regions breakthrough early to the right anteroseptal region and ablation at the latter site may result in heart block. Unfortunately, it is not uncommon for atrial tachycardias to arise within the region of the anteroseptal space, but careful mapping and the use of low powers of radiofrequency (RF) can result in successful ablation without heart block in most cases.

Pace mapping has also been proposed as a useful means of localizing atrial tachycardias for ablation.[19,26,27] However, difficulties in precisely comparing P wave morphologies and intracardiac activation sequences limit its applicability. The spatial resolution of atrial pace mapping has been shown to be a couple of centimeters, which is much too imprecise to facilitate mapping of atrial tachycardia. Man et al[53] demonstrated that P waves with identical or near-identical morphology could be generated by pacing at sites as far apart as 1.7 centimeters in the right atrium and 3.2 centimeters in the left atrium. Despite these limitations, pace mapping may still occasionally be useful in trying to ablate nonsustained and difficult-to-induce atrial tachycardias. Pappone et al[26] reported that concordance of P wave morphology during tachycardia and pace mapping had a sensitivity of 86% and specificity of 37% for prediction of the successful ablation site. However, in our experience atrial pace mapping has rarely been required for atrial tachycardia ablation. Transient catheter-induced interruption of atrial tachycardia by the pressure of the catheter may also suggest an appropriate site for ablation.[26]

Newer mapping techniques are also evolving. Multielectrode expandable basket catheters have been developed and can be used to map the right atrium more rapidly.[54,55] Basket approaches are limited by several features, including that the electrode arrays do not expand to provide adequate contact with all of the atrium, do not permit immediate correlation of activation times to precise anatomic sites, and still require that a second ablation catheter be manipulated to the site identified. In addition, left atrial application of basket mapping arrays may be limited by the large diameter of the sheath required to allow passage to the left atrium. Electromagnetic three-dimensional mapping uses a single roving mapping catheter attached to a system that can precisely localize the catheter tip in three-dimensional space and store activation times on a three-dimensional anatomic reconstruction. Although traditional single-catheter mapping of the region of interest is still required, the ability to use the catheter localization system to steer precisely back to previously obtained sites of earliest activation greatly facilitates the ablation process.[56,57] Marchlinski et al[56] successfully ablated atrial tachycardia in 7 of 8 patients attempted and Kottkamp et al[57] successfully ablated 4 patients with only 1–2 RF applications using an electroanatomic mapping system. Noncontact mapping systems are also under development and may be useful for mapping atrial tachycardias.[58] Whether any of the above new technologies will allow more rapid ablation than traditional approaches has not been systematically studied.

Electrographic Criteria

Electrograms at the site of successful ablation are typically fractionated and demonstrate moderate to marked presystolic timing (Figure 8). Activation times are generally measured from the onset or first rapid deflection of the atrial electrogram to the onset of the P wave or surrogate marker during tachycardia. We prefer the onset of the local electrogram since it is easier to determine reproducibly when measuring heavily fractionated, low amplitude atrial electrograms. Average presystolic intervals at sites of successful ablation are generally greater than 30 milliseconds.[4,16–27] However, the key to successful

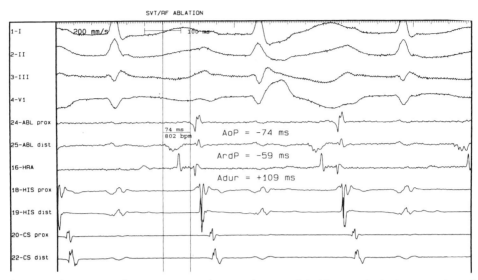

Figure 8. Electrogram characteristics at the site of successful ablation of a high posterolateral right atrial tachycardia occurring along the crista terminalis. Note that the local electrogram is markedly presystolic with an interval from the onset of the atrial electrogram to the onset of the P wave (the AoP interval) of −74 milliseconds and from the rapid deflection of the local electrogram (ArdP interval) of −59 milliseconds. In addition, the local electrogram is markedly fractionated, making distinction of the first rapid deflection arbitrary, and the duration of the local electrogram (Adur) is prolonged to 109 milliseconds.

mapping is finding the earliest site, since there is great variability in the presystolic interval that will be obtained at successful ablation sites. Presystolic activation times of more than 50 milliseconds are common, and presystolic activation greater than 100 milliseconds and mid-diastolic potentials can be seen occasionally. In addition, activation times of less than 30 milliseconds at sites of successful ablation can be seen, especially in children or patients with automatic atrial tachycardias.[16] Poty et al[25] have used unipolar mapping to localize the site of origin of atrial tachycardia and have shown that a QS atrial electrogram with a rapid initial deflection was highly predictive of the successful site of ablation. Given the high success rates with bipolar mapping of atrial tachycardia, it is unlikely that unipolar mapping will improve upon this, and it is unknown whether unipolar mapping will decrease procedure time compared to bipolar mapping.

Ablation Results

Multiple studies of RF ablation of atrial tachycardia have now been published and these are summarized in Table 2. Overall results are excellent, with acute success rates ranging from 69% to 100% with complication rates between 0 and 8% and recurrence rates between 0 and 20%.[4,16–27] In the pooled data of 278 patients (see Table 2), the averaged success rate was 91%, with a complication rate of 3% and recurrence rate of 9%. Acute success rates continue to increase as further experience is accumulated. Most studies have shown low rates of recurrence in follow-up, although a few studies have had late recurrences or development of new tachycardias in 10–20%.[18–20,23,25] The issue of development of previously undiagnosed atrial tachycardias suggests that, at least in some patients, there is the possibility that underlying atrial disease will progress to generate new foci. How commonly this occurs awaits long-term follow-up in a large group of successfully ablated patients. In addition, most studies have only attempted ablation in patients with relatively few atrial tachycardias. Less is known about the long-term results in patients with multiple tachycardias. Although long-term results in patients with multiple tachycardias are probably lower than patients with only 1–2 tachycardias,[25] long-term cures in patients with up to 5 atrial tachycardias have been accomplished (unpublished observation).

Special Problems with Atrial Tachycardia Ablation

Although atrial tachycardia ablation is generally relatively simple, special problems can be encountered which make mapping and/or ablation difficult. These problems include occurrence of atrial tachycardia at epicardial loci which are sufficiently removed from endocardial approaches to make conventional RF ablation difficult or impossible. Examples of such remote atrial tachycardia include those occurring in the epicardium or mid-myocardium of thick atrial structures, such as an enlarged crista terminalis, thickened pectinate muscles, lipomatous atrial septal hypertrophy,[59] or the mitral valve annulus,[27] or removed from the accessible endocardium, such as behind the purse-string suture closure of the cannulation site in the right atrial appendage created during cardiopulmonary bypass, within a small necked atrial diverticulum, or underneath atrial scar. Fortunately, these specific problems occur infrequently. Of note, epicardial atrial tachycardias along the mitral valve annulus can occasionally be successfully ablated from within the coronary sinus.[27,50] Atrial tachycardias arising from behind purse-string suture lines or small-necked atrial aneurysms can be isolated by circumferential ablation along the suture line or aneurysmal neck. Cooled RF ablation may also be useful for ablation of atrial tachycardia foci which are sufficiently removed from the accessible atrial endocardium as to be unablatable using conventional RF techniques.[60]

Complications of Ablation

As mentioned above, the rate of complications with atrial tachycardia ablation is approximately 3%.[4,16–27] There are few complications specific to ablation of atrial tachycardias. Despite the generally thin wall of the atria, cardiac perforation is uncommon and probably no more frequent than with ablation of other SVTs. However, the thin atria frequently do not limit lesion growth beyond the myocardium, so damage to noncardiac structures may occur, most notably damage to the right or left phrenic nerve with ablation of right or left lateral atrial freewall, superior vena cava, and left pulmonary vein tachycardias.

When ablating at these sites, the ability to pace the phrenic nerve should suggest attempting to find a slightly different site, or, if this is not possible, then applying RF current at very low powers and/or for short duration. In addition, and even if phrenic nerve pacing is not demonstrable, intermittent fluoroscopic visualization of the ipsilateral diaphragm movement should be performed during RF current application at high risk sites and RF ablation terminated if diaphragmatic excursion decreases. We have been able to safely ablate atrial tachycardias at sites demonstrating diaphragmatic pacing using the above safety guidelines. Other ablation site specific risks included the risk of sinus node dysfunction after ablation of atrial tachycardia arising from the sinus nodal region and complete heart block after ablation of atrial tachycardias occurring in the anteroseptal region. With regard to the risk of sinus node dysfunction after ablation of sinus nodal reentrant or other high cristal tachycardias, the risk is low[4] except with a few exceptions, notably older patients, especially if there is a history of preexisting sinus node dysfunction. Ablation of anteroseptal atrial tachycardias carries a high risk of complete heart block, given that these tachycardias may arise from sites associated with detectable His bundle potentials. Detailed mapping of both the right and left anteroseptal regions is required, since atrial tachycardias occurring along the anterior and anteroseptal left atrium will frequently have earliest right atrial activation at the His bundle region with a normal activation pattern along the posterior left atrium as recorded in the coronary sinus electrodes (Figure 6). For true anteroseptal atrial tachycardias, we and others[44] have been able to successfully ablate these tachycardias using detailed mapping to limit the total number of RF applications, low powers of RF current, and short RF application times. Nonetheless, the risk of complete heart block is still high and should be discussed with the patient before attempting ablation. Increasingly, atrial tachycardias arising within the pulmonary veins, coronary sinus, and superior vena cava are being identified. Recent data suggest that, at least with the pulmonary vein tachycardias, circumferential ablation may result in pulmonary vein stenosis and occlusion.[61] Given this concern, effort should be made to limit the number and power of RF applications applied to the pulmonary and other venous structures. In children, the size of an atrial lesion produced by RF ablation may increase with age. Saul et al[62] demonstrated in infant lambs that atrial lesion width increased 164% within one month of atrial myocardium ablation, but did not increase further out to approximately 6 months. Whether this lesion expansion creates clinical problems is unknown.

Focal Atrial Tachycardias Simulating Atrial Fibrillation

One of the most interesting recent developments regarding atrial tachycardias has been the demonstration that focal atrial tachycardias with very rapid, and frequently irregular, rates may simulate atrial fibrillation or atypical atrial flutters electrocardiographically (Figure 9). Such rapid atrial tachycardias simulating atrial fibrillation were first described by Scherf in work with aconitine-induced atrial fibrillation.[63] However, subsequent work by Moe,[64] Allessie,[65] and others[66] have suggested that most atrial fibrillation is probably

2:57pm **Atr-Flutter/Sinus**   93 BPM Size=x1

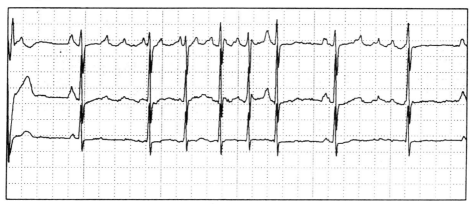

8:28pm **Atrial Flutter**   124 BPM Size=x1

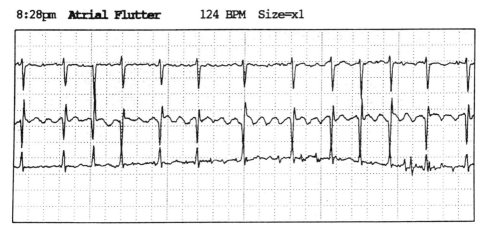

Figure 9. The upper panel (labelled "Atr-Flutter/Sinus") shows an electrocardiographic recording from a patient with focal atrial fibrillation. After the first sinus complex, there is a run of a
rapid atrial tachycardia with a cycle length varying from 180 to 240 milliseconds simulating
an atypical atrial flutter. After generating 5 QRS complexes, the atrial tachycardia terminates,
there is a single sinus complex, and then there is another burst of the nonsustained atrial tachycardia. Leads shown are modified V_2, V_5, and II from top to bottom, respectively. The lower
panel (labeled "Atrial Flutter") reveals a period of sustained, coarse atrial fibrillation in the same
patient. Because of the relative organization (coarseness) of the atrial fibrillation, the computer
labeled the arrhythmia at "atrial flutter," although the polymorphic and changing nature of the
fibrillatory waves is clearly seen. The patient was successfully ablated in the left superior pulmonary vein.

due to nonfocal reentrant mechanisms, such as multiple wandering wavelets.
Until recently, focal mechanisms of atrial fibrillation were not thought to be
clinically relevant. However, Haïssaguerre and colleagues[5–7] have recently
demonstrated in humans that atrial fibrillation can be due to, or initiated by,
rapidly firing atrial tachycardias (see Figure 7). If the atrial tachycardia activates very rapidly, conduction away from the focus may no longer be uniformly
centrifugal, and such nonuniformity results in a fibrillatory pattern of activation of the atria (what has been termed "fibrillatory conduction" in distinction

from true fibrillation).[65] It is also possible that these rapid atrial tachycardias induce typical atrial fibrillation and thus serve as a focal initiator of atrial fibrillation.[7]

Clinically, the syndrome of focal atrial fibrillation has been shown to occur predominantly in young patients with no or minimal heart disease,[5–7] although this observation may be heavily skewed by selection bias. Patients with heart disease can also have focal atrial fibrillation syndromes. Patients defined to date have had repetitive runs of nonsustained atrial tachycardia or atrial fibrillation, sustained atrial fibrillation, atypical morphologies of atrial flutter, typical atrial flutter and/or frequent atrial ectopy. The presence of frequently and spontaneously occurring atrial ectopy or arrhythmia is necessary, since mapping is aimed at localizing the onset of these arrhythmias and these arrhythmias do not appear to be inducible during electrophysiological study. Stimulation with β-adrenergic agonists may enhance the rate of spontaneous occurrence of atrial ectopy to allow mapping and ablation. Mapping is directed towards identifying the earliest site of atrial activation during the onset of these spontaneously occurring atrial extrasystoles,[7] or less commonly during sustained atypical atrial flutter-like rhythms. Electrograms at the site of successful ablation typically, but not always, have long presystolic intervals and marked fractionation (see Figure 7). Haïssaguerre et al[7] described a peculiar split potential on the atrial electrogram in sinus rhythm at the successful ablation site from the pulmonary veins, with the late component preceding all beats of tachycardia. Conduction into and out of the pulmonary veins has been shown to be very complex and slow,[67,68] potentially explaining the complexities of electrogram patterns seen in this region.

For reasons that are not known, these tachycardias most commonly occur from the ostia or within the pulmonary veins, but may also occur at other sites such as the sinus nodal region, superior vena cava, coronary sinus, or right or left atrial freewall locations.[6,7] Pertinent to mapping, these sites are frequently well within the pulmonary veins or other venous structures, not uncommonly 2–3 centimeters from the atrial freewall. The pulmonary veins are true venous structures, with an endothelial tunica intima and a thin smooth muscle tunica media. However, between the medial and adventitial venous layers there is a myocardial muscle sleeve consisting of two muscular layers, an inner circumferentially wrapped layer and an outer, longitudinally directed layer.[69] These myocardial layers are composed of working atrial myocardium in continuity with the atrial freewall. Microscopically, the pulmonary venous myocardium is identical to adjacent left atrial freewall myocardium.[69] Indeed, these myocardial sleeves have contractile function, and the myocardial sleeves of the pulmonary veins are proposed to function as a means to decrease pulmonary venous pressure under conditions of left atrial volume overload.[70]

The reason for the frequent occurrence of rapid atrial tachycardias from the pulmonary venous myocardium, and, to a lesser extent, from other venous myocardial sleeves, is not known. It is possible that the peculiarities of the fiber arrangement predispose to slow conduction and local reentry, explaining the split potential commonly seen at sites of ablation of these tachycardias. However, it is also possible that cells in the region of the venous structures have peculiar electrophysiological properties which predisposed them to have triggered or abnormal automaticity. Further studies will hopefully elucidate the mechanism(s) underlying these rapid focal atrial tachyarrhythmias. In addition, further information is needed about the frequency of focal atrial fibrillation in patients with atrial fibrillation and structurally normal hearts and the role that these focal atrial tachycardia play in initiating atrial fibrillation in patients with heart disease.

References

1. Chou T-C. *Electrocardiography in Clinical Practice.* Philadelphia, PA: WB Saunders Co., 1991.
2. Narula OS. Sinus node re-entry: a mechanism for supraventricular tachycardia. *Circulation* 1974;50:1114–1128.
3. Gomes JA, Hariman RJ, Kang PS, et al. Sustained symptomatic sinus node reentrant tachycardia: incidence, clinical significance, electrophysiological observations and the effects of antiarrhythmic agents. *J Am Coll Cardiol* 1985;5:45–57.
4. Sanders WE Jr, Sorrentino RA, Greenfield RA, et al. Catheter ablation of sinoatrial reentrant tachycardia. *J Am Coll Cardiol* 1994;23:926–934.
5. Haïssaguerre M, Marcus FI, Fischer B, et al. Radiofrequency catheter ablation in unusual mechanisms of atrial fibrillation: report of three cases. *J Cardiovasc Electrophysiol* 1994;5:743–751.
6. Jaïs P, Haïssaguerre M, Shah DC, et al. A focal source of atrial fibrillation treated by discrete radiofrequency ablation. *Circulation* 1997;95:572–276.
7. Haïssaguerre M, Jaïs P, Shah DC, et al. Spontaneous initiation of atrial fibrillation by ectopic beats originating in the pulmonary veins. *N Engl J Med* 1998;339:659–666.
8. Lesh MD, Kalman JM. To fumble flutter and tackle "tach"? Toward updated classifiers for atrial tachyarrhythmias. *J Cardiovasc Electrophysiol* 1996;7: 460–466.
9. Ganz LI, Friedman PL. Supraventricular tachycardia. *N Engl J Med* 1995;332:162–173.
10. Wellens HJJ. Atrial tachycardia: how important is the mechanism? *Circulation* 1994;90:1576–1577.
11. Wu D, Denes P, Amat-Y-Leon F, et al. Clinical, electrocardiographic and electrophysiological observations in patients with paroxysmal supraventricular tachycardia. *Am J Cardiol* 1978;41:1045–1051.
12. Ko JK, Deal BJ, Strasburger JF, et al. Supraventricular tachycardia mechanisms and their age distribution in pediatric patients. *Am J Cardiol* 1992;69:1028–1032.
13. Gillette PC. The mechanism of supraventricular tachycardia in children. *Circulation* 1976;54:133–139.
14. Garson A Jr, Gillette PC. Electrophysiological studies of supraventricular tachycardia in children, 1: clinical-electrophysiologic correlations. *Am Heart J* 1981;102:233–250.

15. Haines DE, DiMarco JP. Sustained intraatrial reentrant tachycardia: clinical, electrocardiographic and electrophysiological characteristics and long-term follow-up. *J Am Coll Cardiol* 1990;15:1345–1354.

16. Walsh EP, Saul JP, Hulse JE, et al. Transcatheter ablation of ectopic atrial tachycardia in young patients using radiofrequency current. *Circulation* 1992;86:1138–1146.

17. Chen S-A, Chiang C-E, Yang C-J, et al. Radiofrequency catheter ablation of sustained intra-atrial reentrant tachycardia in adult patients: identification of electrophysiological characteristics and endocardial mapping techniques. *Circulation* 1993;88:578–587.

18. Kay GN, Chong F, Epstein AE, et al. Radiofrequency ablation for treatment of primary atrial tachycardias. *J Am Coll Cardiol* 1993;21:901–909.

19. Tracy CM, Swartz JF, Fletcher RD, et al. Radiofrequency catheter ablation of ectopic atrial tachycardia using paced activation sequence mapping. *J Am Coll Cardiol* 1993;21:910–917.

20. Goldberger J, Kall J, Ehlert F, et al. Effectiveness of radiofrquency catheter ablation for treatment of atrial tachycardia. *Am J Cardiol* 1993;72:787–793.

21. Shenasa H, Sanders W Jr, Pressley J, et al. Safety and efficacy of radiofrequency catheter ablation of ectopic atrial tachycardia [abstract] *PACE* 1993;16:850.

22. Chen S-A, Chiang C-E, Yang C-J, et al. Sustained atrial tachycardia in adult patients: electrophysiological characteristics, pharmacological response, possible mechanisms, and effects of readiofrequency ablation. *Circulation* 1994;90:1262–1278.

23. Lesh MD, Van Hare GF, Epstein LM, et al. Radiofrequency catheter ablation of atrial arrhythmias: results and mechanisms. *Circulation* 1994;89:1074–1089.

24. Wang L, Weerasooriyq HR, Davis MJE. Radiofrequency catheter ablation of atrial tachycardia. *Aust NZ J Med* 1995;25:127–132.

25. Poty H, Saoudi N, Haïssaguerre M, et al. Radiofrequency catheter ablation of atrial tachycardias. *Am Heart J* 1996;131:481–489.

26. Pappone C, Stabile G, De Simone A, et al. Role of catheter-induced mechanical trauma in localization of target sites of radiofrequency ablation of automatic atrial tachycardia. *J Am Coll Cardiol* 1996;27:1090–1097.

27. Weiss C, Willems S, Cappato R, et al. High frequency current ablation of ectopic atrial tachycardia. Different mapping strategies for localization of right- and left-sided origin. *Herz* 1998;23:269–279.

28. Guarnieri T, German LD, Gallagher JJ. The long 'R-P' tachycardias. *PACE* 1987;10:103–117.

29. Zimerman LI, Shenasa H, Sorrentino RA, et al. Utility of P wave morphology on predicting site of origin of atrial tachycardia [abstract]. *PACE* 1995;18(II):861.

30. Tang CW, Scheinman MM, Van Hare GF, et al. Use of P wave configuration during atrial tachycardia to predict site of origin. *J Am Coll Cardiol* 1995;26:1315–1324.

31. Sippens-Groenewegen A, Roithinger FX, Scholtz DB, et al. Body surface mapping during left atrial pace mapping: evaluation of spatial differences in P-wave configuration. *J Am Coll Cardiol* 1998;31(suppl A):46A.

32. DiMarco JP, Sellers TD, Lerman BB, et al. Diagnostic and therapeutic use of adenosine in patients with supraventricular tachycardia. *J Am Coll Cardiol* 1985;6:417–425.

33. Camm AJ, Garratt CJ. Adenosine and supraventricular tachycardia. *N Engl J Med* 1991;325:1621–1629.

34. Shenasa H, Kanter RJ, Hamer ME, et al. Reappraisal of the efficacy of adenosine for the termination of ectopic atrial tachycardia [abstract]. *J Am Coll Cardiol* 1992;21:425A.

35. Hsieh I-C, Yeh S-J, Wen M-S, et al. Effects of adenosine on paroxysmal atrial tachycardia. *Am J Cardiol* 1994;74:279–281.

36. Crosson JE, Etheridge SP, Milstein S, et al. Therapeutic and diagnostic utility of adenosine during tachycardia evaluation in children. *Am J Cardiol* 1994;74:155–160.

37. Brugada P, Wellens HJJ. The role of triggered activity in clinical ventricular arrhythmias. *PACE* 1984;7:260–271.

38. Engelstein ED, Lippman N, Stein KM, et al. Mechanism-specific effects of adenosine on atrial tachycardia. *Circulation* 1994;89:2645–2654.

39. Stevenson WG, Sager PT, Friedman PL. Entrainment techniques for mapping atrial and ventricular tachycardias. *J Cardiovasc Electrophysiol* 1995;6:201–216.

40. Lerman BB. Response of nonreentrant catecholamine-mediated ventricular tachycardia to endogenous adenosine and acetylcholine. Evidence for myocardial receptor-mediated effects. *Circulation* 1993;87:382–390.

41. Allessie MA, Bonke FIM. Direct demonstration of sinus node reentry in the rabbit heart. *Circ Res* 1979;44:557–568.

42. Shenasa H, Merrill JJ, Hamer ME, et al. Distribution of ectopic atrial tachycardias along the crista terminalis: an atrial ring of fire? [abstract] *Circulation* 1993;88(II):I-29.

43. Kalman JM, Olgin JE, Karch MR, et al. "Cristal tachycardias": Origin of right atrial tachycardias from the crista terminalis identified by intracardiac echocardiography. *J Am Coll Cardiol* 1998;31:451–459.

44. Lai LP, Lin JL, Chen TF, et al. Clinical, electrophysiological characteristics, and radiofrequency ablation of atrial tachycardia near the apex of Koch's triangle. *PACE* 1998;21:367–374.

45. Katz A, Evans JJ, Fogel RI, et al. Septal atrial tachycardia: electrophysiological characteristics and radiofrequency ablation results [abstract]. *Circulation* 1996;94(Suppl 1);I-446.

46. Man KC, Niebauer M, Daoud E, et al. Comparison of atrial-His intervals during tachycardia and atrial pacing in patients with long RP tachycardia. *J Cardiovasc Electrophysiol* 1995;6:700–710.

47. Wharton JM. Atrial tachycardia: advances in diagnosis and treatment. *Cardiol Rev* 1995;3:332–342.

48. Verdino RJ, Burke MC, Kopp DE, et al. Differences in location and electrophysiological properties of atrial tachycardias in structurally normal and abnormal hearts [abstract]. *J Am Coll Cardiol* 1998;31(Supp A):292A.

49. Mallavarupu C, Schwartzman D, Callans DJ, et al. Radiofrequency catheter ablation of atrial tachycardia with unusual left atrial sites of origin: report of two cases. *PACE* 1996;19:988–992.

50. Marchlinski F, Schwartzman D, Saligan J, et al. Periannular left atrium—a second ring of fire? [abstract] *PACE* 1996;19(Part 2):593.

51. Hatala R, Weiss C, Koschyk DH, et al. Radiofrequency catheter ablation of left atrial tachycardia originating within the pulmonary vein in a patient with dextrocardia. *PACE* 1996;19:999–1002.

52. Nathan H, Eliakim M. The junction between the left atrium and the pulmonary veins: an anatomic study of human hearts. *Circulation* 1966;34:412–422.

53. Man KC, Chan KK, Kovack P, et al. Spatial resolution of atrial pace mapping as determined by unipolar atrial pacing at adjacent sites. *Circulation* 1996;94:1357–1363.

54. Triedman JK, Jenkins KJ, Colan SD, et al. Intra-atrial reentrant tachycardia after palliation of congenital heart disease: characterization of multiple macroreentrant circuits using fluoroscopically based three-dimensional endocardial mapping. *J Cardiovasc Electrophysiol* 1997;8:259–270.

55. Zrenner B, Hofmann F, Schneider MAE, et al. Three-dimensional computer-assisted animation of atrial tachyarrhythmias recorded with a 64-polar basket catheter. *J Am Coll Cardiol* 1998;31(Suppl A):511A.

56. Marchlinski F, Callans D, Gottlieb C, et al. Magnetic electroanatomic mapping for ablation of focal atrial tachycardias. *PACE* 1998;21:1621–1635.

57. Kottkamp H, Hindricks G, Breithardt G, et al. Three diminsional electromagnetic catheter technology: electroanatomical mapping of the right atrium and ablation of ectopic atrial tachycardia. *J Cardiovasc Electrophysiol* 1997;8:1332–1337.

58. Liu ZW, Jia P, Biblo LA, et al. Endocardial potential mapping from a noncontact nonexpandable catheter: A feasibility study. *Ann Biomed Eng* 1998;26:994–1009.

59. Shirani J, Roberts WC. Clinical, electrocardiographic and morphologic features of massive fatty deposits ("lipomatous hypertrophy") in the atrial septum. *J Am Coll Cardiol* 1993;22:226–238.

60. Jaïs P, Haïssaguerre M, Shah DC, et al. Successful irrigated-tip catheter ablation of atrial flutter resistent to conventional radiofrequency ablation. *Circulation* 1998;98:835–838.

61. Robbins IM, Colvin EV, Doyle TP, et al. Pulmonary vein stenosis after catheter ablation of atrial fibrillation. *Circulation* 1998;98:1769–1775.

62. Saul JP, Hulse JE, Papagiannis J, et al. Late enlargement of radiofrequency lesions in infant lambs. Implications for ablation procedures in small children. *Circulation* 1994;90:492–499.

63. Sherf D. Studies on auricular tachycardia caused by aconitine administration. *Proc Soc Exp Biol Med* 1947;64:233–239.

64. Moe GK, Abildskov JA. Atrial fibrillation as a self-sustaining arrhythmia independent of focal discharge. *Am Heart J* 1959;58:59–70.

65. Allessie MA, Rensma PL, Brugada J, et al. Pathophysiology of atrial fibrillation. In: Zipes DP, Jalife J, eds. *Cardiac Electrophysiology: From Cell to Bedside*. Philadelphia, PA: WB Saunders Co., 1990. pp 548–558.

66. Cox JL, Canavan TE, Schuessler RB, et al. The surgical treatment of atrial fibrillation: II. Intraoperative electrophysiological mapping and description

of the electrophysiological basis of atrial flutter and atrial fibrillation. *J Thorac Cardiovasc Surg* 1991;101:406–426.

67. Ludatscher RM. Fine structure of the muscular wall of the rat pulmonary veins. *J Anat* 1968;103:345–357.

68. Braun K. Pumping action of pulmonary veins. *Am Heart J* 1966;71:286–287.

69. Spach MS, Barr RC, Jewett PH. Spread of excitation from the atrium into the thoracic veins in human beings and dogs. *Am J Cardiol* 1972;30:844–854.

70. Zipes DP, Knope RF. Electrical properties of the thoracic veins. *Am J Cardiol* 1972;29:372–376.

Chapter 9

Ablation of Inappropriate Sinus Tachycardia

Michael D. Lesh, S.M., M.D., Martin R. Karch, M.D.,
Jonathan M. Kalman, M.B.B.S., Ph.D.,
Franz X. Roithinger, M.D., Randall J. Lee, M.D.,
Jerold S. Shinbane, M.D.

Introduction

The syndrome of inappropriate sinus tachycardia (IST) is an uncommon and perplexing disorder characterized by an increased resting heart rate (>100 bpm) or an exaggerated heart rate response to minimal exertion or change in body posture associated with markedly distressing symptoms of palpitations, fatigue, shortness of breath, and anxiety.[1-3] The P wave axis and morphology during tachycardia is similar or identical to that during sinus rhythm. Secondary causes of sinus tachycardia should be carefully excluded before establishing the diagnosis.

The recognition that the sinus node region is a distributed complex exhibiting rate-dependent site differentiation[4] allows for targeted ablation to eliminate the fastest sinus rates while maintaining some degree of sinus node function. In this chapter, we will review our approach to the electrophysiological management of these patients, including the use of intracardiac ultrasound guidance to position mapping and ablation catheters directly along the superior crista terminalis (CT).

From Huang SKS, Wilber DJ (eds.): *Radiofrequency Catheter Ablation of Cardiac Arrhythmias: Basic Concepts and Clinical Applications,* 2nd ed. Armonk, NY: Futura Publishing Company, Inc. ©2000.

Electrophysiology and Pathophysiology

The underlying mechanism for IST is still poorly understood. It may well be that the clinical syndrome of inappropriate sinus tachycardia in fact consists of several different disorders with multiple pathophysiologic mechanisms. In some patients, there may be a psychological component of hypersensitivity to somatic input. The anatomy of the sinus node complex has been well studied, as has its rich innervation with autonomic fibers.[5–8] The sinus node complex responds to changes in autonomic balance with changes in the rate of firing of the sinus complex. A reasonable hypothesis, therefore, is that IST represents a disorder of autonomic responsiveness of the sinus node. Indeed, studies have demonstrated a β-adrenergic hypersensitivity of the sinus node complex as well as a hyposensitivity to parasympathetic influences in patients with this disorder.[3] However, there may also be a primary abnormality of the sinus node function, as evidenced by a higher intrinsic heart rate (after total autonomic blockade) than that found in age-matched normal controls.[2,3]

From an epidemiological standpoint, there is the curious observation that almost all patients afflicted with IST are women, and many are health care workers such as cardiac nurses or physical therapists. The explanation for these findings is lacking. One possibility is that there is a presently unidentified occupational exposure. Or perhaps IST is actually more common in the population at large, but it is only those with access to sophisticated monitoring technology and who request, insist upon, and ultimately receive, referral to trained subspecialists such as cardiologists and electrophysiologists and who then undergo extensive evaluation and treatment. Surreptitious drug use including thyroid hormone, diuretics and stimulants must be considered in the differential diagnosis of any medical sophisticate with sinus tachycardia.

There may in some patients be an overlap between IST and disorders such as chronic fatigue syndrome and neurocardiogenic (vasovagal) syncope. One possibility is that IST may represent an autonomic neuritis or part of a spectrum of a more general autonomic neuropathy. Clearly, further research into the etiology of IST is required. Unfortunately, there is no "gold standard" to make a definitive diagnosis of IST. As discussed below, the diagnosis remains a clinical one after exclusion of other causes of symptomatic tachycardia. Thus, while ablation directed at the "end organ" of IST can be effective in some patients, it is hoped that more definitive treatment will emerge when the true etiology of this troubling and enigmatic disorder is more fully elucidated.

Diagnosis of IST

It should be emphasized that the diagnosis of IST must be made based on the complete clinical picture, not merely on the basis of invasive electrophysiological study. In other words, the sole purpose of the diagnostic electrophysiology study must be for the exclusion of other arrhythmias in a patient who has already had clear documentation of excessive heart rates with concomitant symptoms.

Patients with IST may have a variety of complaints such as palpitations, chest pain, shortness of breath, pre-syncope, etc. However, the importance of documenting as thoroughly as possible a close correlation of symptoms with electrocardiographic sinus tachycardia, and absence of symptoms with normal rates, cannot be overemphasized. A patient who experiences significant fatigue and palpitations when her rate is 80 or 90, as well as at a rate of 130 or 150, will not be likely to have symptomatic relief if the fastest rates are eliminated by ablative modification of sinus node function. This documentation may require multiple ambulatory monitors with a carefully completed patient diary, trans-telephonic event recorders, and exercise stress tests. Patients should not undergo invasive evaluation until this step is complete.

Once the diagnosis of IST is suspected on clinical grounds, an electrophysiology study is performed. The purpose of the electrophysiology study, as noted above, is to exclude other tachycardias that may mimic sinus tachycardia, such as atrial tachycardia arising near the superior aspect of the CT or right upper pulmonary vein, and to assure that tachycardia occurring spontaneously or, more likely with catecholamine infusion, acts in a manner consistent with an exaggeration of normal sinus node physiology. For example, the site of earliest atrial activation along the CT was demonstrated to change in response to autonomic activation.[9] Sympathetic stimulation causes an increase in heart rate with a cranial shift of the earliest atrial activation to the superior aspect of the CT; in contrast, vagal stimulation results in slowing of the heart rate with a more inferior focus.

Recalling that the sinus node pacemaker complex is anatomically situated within the sulcus terminalis on the epicardial surface and that the analogous endocardial structure is the CT, it is helpful to map atrial activation directly from the CT. However, the CT is not directly visible using standard fluoroscopy.

To overcome the limitations imposed by fluoroscopic imaging on the identification of endocardial landmarks, and the spatial relationship of electrode catheters to such structures, our laboratory has explored the use of intracardiac echocardiography (ICE) to identify endocardial structures[2,9–12] such as the CT, and in particular to guide mapping and ablation of sinus node tissue along the crista. A typical ICE image is shown in Figure 1. During ICE imaging the CT can be clearly identified in all our patients as a prominent ridge crossing in front of the superior vena cava from its septal insertion site to the lateral right atrial wall. The crista courses down the lateral right atrial wall and terminates in the posteroinferior right atrium as the eustachian ridge.

For activation sequence mapping along the CT, we typically place a 20 pole catheter (1mm interelectrode and 5 mm interbipole distance) along the crista with catheter positioning along the CT guided by continuous ICE imaging. The catheter is positioned on the CT from the superomedial aspect originating at the junction of the superior vena cava and right atrial appendage inferolaterally with continuation along the CT towards the junction of the inferior vena cava and right atrium. The second bipolar pair is positioned as a reference point at the junction of the superior vena cava and right atrium with the first bipolar pair extending to the superomedial aspect of the sinus node complex. Achieving adequate contact along the length of the CT is sometimes enhanced by deploying the 20 pole catheter through a long vascular sheath. Use of ICE to place a multipolar catheter on the CT is demonstrated in Figure 2.

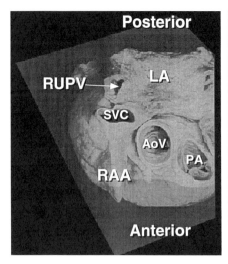
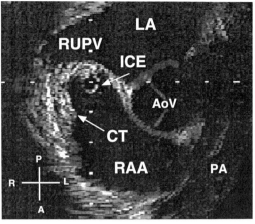

Intracardiac Echo

Figure 1. Example of transcatheter intracardiac ultrasound imaging. On the left is an anatomic specimen of the heart viewed from above. The right panel is the intracardiac echo image, a two-dimensional transaxial plane perpendicular to the shaft of the imaging catheter (ICE), which runs along the intercaval axis in this case. Structures seen at this level include the right upper pulmonary vein (RUPV) entering the left atrium (LA), the right atrial appendage (RAA) separated from the posterior smooth walled right atrium by the crista terminalis (CT) noted as a prominent ridge extending from the endocardial surface, the aortic valve (AoV) and pulmonary artery (PA). In most patients, the CT can be seen along the length of the right atrium, from superomedial to inferolateral, allowing placement of mapping catheters directly on or near the crista for assessment of its electrophysiological properties. SVC = 5 superior vena cava.

With the 20 pole catheter in place on the CT, as well as the usual catheters positioned for a complete electrophysiological evaluation (coronary sinus, His bundle region, and so on), attempts are made to induce tachycardia using programmed stimulation before and after catecholamine infusion. An intravenous infusion of isoproterenol is administered starting at 0.5 to 1 mcg per minute and titrated every 3 to 5 minutes to a maximum of 6 mcg per minute of isoproterenol with serial assessment of sinus cycle length and earliest activation site on the CT catheter. Atropine (1 mg) is also administered to assess maximum sinus cycle length.

The electrophysiological diagnosis for sinus tachycardia includes:

1. Failure to induce a clinical atrial or other supraventricular tachycardia using programmed stimulation; care must be taken in interpreting the relevance of such electrophysiological phenomenon as dual atrioventricular nodal physiology or AV nodal echo beats in patients in whom the only documented symptomatic tachycardia appears to have a sinus mechanism;

2. Despite autonomic manipulation (atropine or isoproterenol) earliest atrial activation always occurs along the CT as confirmed by the multipolar catheter placed using ICE directly on the CT;

3. There is generally a craniocaudal activation pattern along the CT during tachycardia, with the site of earliest atrial activation shifting up the CT at faster rates, and down the CT at slower rates; in distinction, while

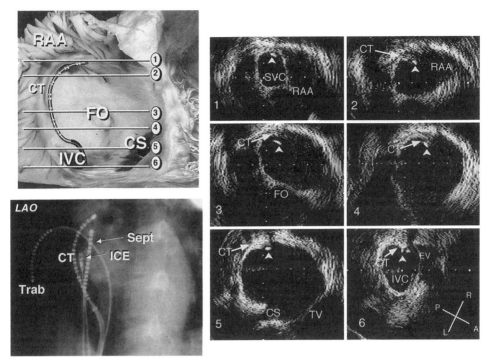

Figure 2. Anatomic view of the right atrium (with kind permission of Anderson and Becker; top left) showing sequential imaging planes (1 through 6) which correspond to intracardiac echo (ICE) images on the right. Note the presence of the CT (arrow) and a multipolar catheter overlying it (short arrow head) seen at each ICE level from superior (1) to inferior (6). On the bottom left is a radiograph in the left anterior oblique projection (LAO) showing catheters in place in the right atrium. In addition to a catheter on the CT, multipolar catheters are also present in this case on the septum (Sept) and trabeculated (Trab) right atrium. The ICE catheter itself is also seen. RAA = right atrial appendage; CS = coronary sinus; FO = fossa ovalis; TV = tricuspid valve; EV = eustachian valve.

focal atrial tachycardias may exhibit a change in the rate of firing in response to changes in autonomic stimulation, the site of earliest activation should remain nearly fixed;

4. There is a gradual increase and decrease in heart rate (compared to patients with focal automatic atrial tachycardia) with changes in autonomic tone or at the "initiation" and "termination" of the tachycardia.

Sinus Node Modification

After making a clinical diagnosis of IST and excluding other causes at electrophysiological testing, attempts can be made to modify sinus node function. Note that this is a clinical decision which must be made prior to the invasive procedure itself, since there is a wide overlap in the range of sinus rates in response to catecholamine infusion in those with and without the clinical syndrome of inappropriate sinus tachycardia.

The principle of sinus node modification is based in the concept of site-dependent rate differentiation. The importance of the anatomic distribution of impulse generation with changes in sinus rate is the hypothesis that sinus node function can be modified—the most rapid rates can be eliminated—by an ablative approach that creates a set of lesions along the superior aspect of the CT. Several studies using a variety of energy modalities have shown that sinus node function can be abolished.[13-15] The feasibility of modification of sinus pacemaker function using a catheter-based application of radiofrequency (RF) energy was recently demonstrated in dogs by Kalman and co-workers.[16] Since ICE allows clear visualization of the CT, it is logical to expect that ICE could be used to guide endocardial catheter ablation of the sinus node. The goal is to apply initial ablative lesions to the most superior aspect of the CT, with subsequent lesions progressing in a caudal direction down the CT to achieve an approximately 30% decline in maximal heart rate during infused isoproterenol and atropine. This often requires ablating 3 or 4 cm along the length of the CT, with a number of RF applications using standard ablation catheter technology. ICE is used to identify the CT, place the tip of the ablation catheter with firm contact on the CT, and in some cases to assess the lesion formed as a result (Figure 3). Power should be adjusted to achieve a tip temperate of 55° to 70°C. Speeding of the sinus heart rate followed by a marked subsequent heart rate reduction or the appearance of a junctional rhythm during ablation are indicators for successful ablation sites and therefore delivery of ablation energy should be continued for at least 60–90 seconds.

Through the use of ICE, lesions can be confined to the CT, or just anterior

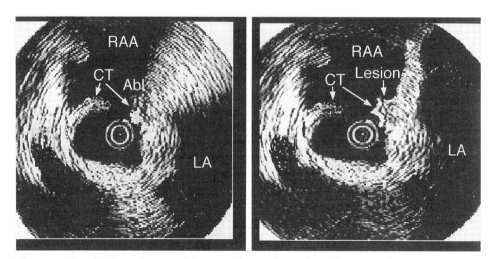

Figure 3. Use of ICE to place an ablation catheter electrode (Abl) against the crista terminalis (CT). Images have been obtained just below the SVC/RA junction with the right atrial appendage (RAA) seen. The CT is seen both on the lateral wall (CT) as well as on the septal surface as it has coursed in front of the SVC. On the left, the characteristic fan shaped artefact is seen shadowing the lateral aspect of the CT with firm and stable catheter tip contact to the tissue. On the right, the lesion created as a result of RF application. The clear circle in the center of each image is the ICE catheter itself. RUPV = right upper pulmonary vein; LA = left atrium; Ant = anterior; Post = posterior.

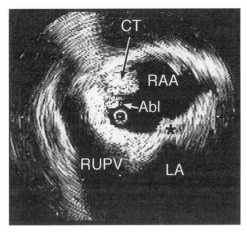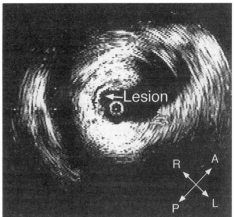

Figure 4. For a complete sinus node modification, the septal aspect of the CT must also be ablated. On the left, the ablation catheter is seen juxtaposed to the septal, or medial, aspect of the CT. On the right, the lesion is seen on the CT. The lateral aspect of the CT has an almost finger-like prominence. RUPV = right upper pulmonary vein. LA = left atrium. Ant = anterior. Post = posterior.

to it, in which case phrenic nerve damage will generally not be an issue since it is a posterior structure. However, if there is any question as to the course of the phrenic nerve in a given patient, pacing with a high output of 10 mA should be performed before delivery of RF energy.

Recall that there is a medial portion of the CT as it courses in front of the SVC. In our experience, this medial portion of the CT is the site of earliest activation for the fastest sinus rates, and ablation must be directed here for sinus node modification to be successful (Figure 4). In cases of failed sinus node modification, this most medial aspect of the CT is the site most often missed during the initial ablative attempt.

Complications and Follow-up Results

When performed with ICE, sinus node modification is generally a safe procedure. Just as in any interventional procedure, complications related to vascular access can occur. Cardiac perforation leading to tamponade has been rarely observed. This has most likely been due to penetration of a right ventricular electrophysiology catheter in a thin female patient with rapid and vigorous heart action due to high-dose catecholamine infusion. Therefore, when all attention is focused on activity in the atrium, it is important to take care that ventricular catheters do not migrate during the procedure. The use of a very flexible 5F pacing catheter is to be considered.

Early in our experience before the routine use of ICE, one patient developed a transient SVC syndrome that was likely related to extensive lesion creation at the SVC/right atrial junction. With a more targeted approach using ICE, this complication can be avoided. Further, risk of damage to the phrenic nerve should be minimized if ablative lesions are confined to the CT itself, or are placed just anterior to it.

Shinbane recently reported on the long-term follow-up of 25 consecutive patients (all female with an average age of 33 ± 8 years) who underwent sinus node modification using ICE to guide placement of a 20 pole CT catheter and RF energy applications to the superior aspect of the CT.[17] Acutely, a mean increase in maximal sinus cycle length of $21\pm24\%$ was achieved. At follow-up of 9 months or more, 37% have had sustained improvement of tachycardia symptoms, with 7 patients requiring additional procedures. Complete sinus node ablation with implantation of permanent pacemakers has been required in 3 patients, whose symptoms improved as a result. It should be noted that ablation of the atrioventricular junction with implantation of a dual chamber pacemaker is, by itself, inadequate therapy for these patients as they will continue to either track their sinus tachycardia or exhibit symptoms during mode switching or high-rate block. In our experience, it is difficult to program the pacemaker to avoid symptoms, and a primary sinus node ablation, rather than ablation of the AV node, is the ablative approach of choice. Given the relatively low rate of long-term success in relieving symptoms despite electrophysiological modification of sinus node function, further studies are needed to identify the optimal extent of ablation and the cohort of patients most likely to benefit from such a procedure.

Summary

IST is an usual but highly symptomatic arrhythmia seen almost exclusively in young women. Its exact etiology is unknown, and it may well be a heterogeneous disorder. The unusual high baseline heart rate and/or the inappropriate increase in heart rate during minimal activity can be debilitating. A tight correlation between symptoms and tachycardia, exclusion of secondary causes of sinus tachycardia and other arrhythmia mechanisms such as atrial tachycardia, and failure of pharmacological therapy are indications for considering sinus node modification. This procedure can be safely done but should be guided by intracardiac echocardiography for visualizing the underlying substrate, to shorten fluoroscopy time and decrease the number of RF energy applications. In cases of recurrent symptoms in the most refractory of cases after an initial attempt to modify the sinus node, a more aggressive ablation attempt can be performed with the goal being total ablation of the sinus node with subsequent dual chamber pacemaker implantation.

References

1. Bauernfeind RA, Amat-Y-Leon F, Dhingra RC, et al. Chronic nonparoxysmal sinus tachycardia in otherwise healthy persons. *Ann Intern Med* 1979;91:702–710.
2. Lee RJ, Kalman JM, Fitzpatrick AP, et al. Radiofrequency catheter modifi-

cation of the sinus node for "inappropriate" sinus tachycardia. *Circulation* 1995;92(10):2919–2928.

3. Morillo C, Klein G, Thakur R, et al. Mechanism of "inappropriate" sinus tachycardia: role of sympathovagal balance. *Circulation* 1994;90:873–877.

4. Boineau JP, Canavan TE, Schuessler RB, et al. Demonstration of a widely distributed atrial pacemaker complex in the human heart. *Circulation* 1988;77(6):1221–1237.

5. Anderson KR, Ho SY, Anderson RH. Location and vascular supply of sinus node in human heart. *Br Heart J* 1979;41:28–32.

6. James TN. Anatomy of the human sinus node. *Anat Rec* 1961;141:109–116.

7. James TN. The sinus node. *Am J Cardiol* 1977;40:965–986.

8. Warner MR, Levy MN. Sinus and atrioventricular nodal distribution of sympathetic fibers that contain neuropeptide Y. *Circ Res* 1990;67:713–721.

9. Kalman J, Lee R, Fisher W, et al. Radiofrequency catheter modification of sinus pacemaker function guided by intracardiac echocardiography. *Circulation* 1995;92:3070–3081.

10. Chu E, Kalman JM, Kwasman MA, et al. Intracardiac echocardiography during radiofrequency catheter ablation of cardiac arrhythmias in humans. *J Am Coll Cardiol* 1994;24(5):1351–1357.

11. Chu E, Fitzpatrick AP, Chin MC, et al. Radiofrequency catheter ablation guided by intracardiac echocardiography. *Circulation* 1994;89(3):1301–1305.

12. Olgin JE, Kalman JM, Fitzpatrick AP, et al. Role of right atrial endocardial structures as barriers to conduction during human type I atrial flutter: activation and entrainment mapping guided by intracardiac echocardiography. *Circulation* 1995;92(7):1839–1848.

13. Chorro FJ, Sanchis J, Lopez-Merino V, et al. Transcatheter ablation of the sinus node in dogs using high-frequency current. *Eur Heart J* 1990;11:82–89.

14. Hariman RJ, Hu DY, Beckman KJ, et al. Cryothermal mapping of the sinus node in dogs: a simple method of localising dominant and latent pacemakers. *Cardiovasc Res* 1989;23:231–238.

15. Littmann L, Svenson RH, Gallagher JJ, et al. Modification of sinus node function by epicardial laser irradiation in dogs. *Circulation* 1990;81:350–359.

16. Kalman J, Lee R, Fisher W, et al. Radiofrequency catheter modification of sinus node function guided by intracardiac echocardiography. *Circulation* 1995;92(9):3070–3081.

17. Shinbane J, Lesh M, Scheinman M, et al. Long term follow-up after radiofrequency sinus node modification for inappropriate sinus tachycardia. *J Am Coll Cardiol* 1977;29(2):199A.

Chapter 10

Ablation of Atrial Tachycardia within the Triangle of Koch

Ling-Ping Lai, MD, Jiunn-Lee Lin, MD,
Shoei K. Stephen Huang, M.D.

Atrial tachycardia is one of the possible mechanisms of supraventricular tachycardia.[1,2] It is less common than atrioventricular nodal reentrant tachycardia and atrioventricular reciprocating tachycardia. However, it is often refractory to pharmacological treatment and, therefore, ablative treatment is needed. A recent evolution in radiofrequency catheter ablation techniques has made it possible to cure atrial tachycardia with a high success rate.[3-8] Ablation of atrial tachycardia has been addressed in previous chapters. In this chapter, we focus upon ablation of atrial tachycardia within the triangle of Koch. Since there is atrial tissue within the triangle of Koch, it is possible that atrial tachycardia originates from this special location. This special subgroup of atrial tachycardia is worth noting because it raises 2 issues of concern. First, it may mimic atrioventricular nodal reentrant tachycardia (AVNRT) or atrioventricular reciprocating tachycardia (AVRT) incorporating a concealed right midseptal accessory pathway. Second, ablation of atrial tachycardia within the triangle of Koch may bear a potential risk of atrioventricular (AV) block. So far, there have been only 2 articles reporting on ablation of atrial tachycardia within the triangle of Koch. Lai et al[9] reported their experience in atrial tachycardia near the apex of Koch's triangle while Iesaka et al[10] reported atrial tachycardia from the AV nodal transitional area. Both articles report on atrial tachycardia within the triangle of Koch and their findings are very similar. Therefore, this tachycardia is a unique subgroup of atrial tachycardia and deserves description in a separate chapter.

From Huang SKS, Wilber DJ (eds.): *Radiofrequency Catheter Ablation of Cardiac Arrhythmias: Basic Concepts and Clinical Applications,* 2nd ed. Armonk, NY: Futura Publishing Company, Inc. ©2000.

Clinical Characteristics

The clinical characteristics of patients from both reports are listed in Table 1. The report by Iesaka et al included 11 patients (8 women and 3 men) with a mean age of 64.3±10.5 years (range 43 to 83). The other article, by Lai et al, included 6 patients (all women) with a mean age of 49.6±9.3 years (range 39 to 63). All patients were in the middle or older age group and there was a female predominance (14F:3M). The tachycardia cycle length was 363±51 milliseconds (range 270 to 440). Coexisting cardiac disease was present in more than half (13 of 17) of the patients. All the patients had paroxysms of supraventricular tachycardia. None of the patients had incessant tachycardia. The tachycardia could be terminated by verapamil 5 to 10 mg injection in all patients. Surface ECG analysis showed that the supraventricular tachycardia could have an RP interval greater than (long RP) or less than (short RP) the PR interval. The frontal plane P wave axis ranged from −90° to +30°; that is, the P wave could be either inverted or upright in the inferior leads (Figure 1).

Table 1

Clinical and electrocardiographic characteristics of 17 patients with atrial tachycardia within the triangle of Koch

Pt #	Age	Gender	TCL	Coexisting disease	Response to verapamil	Response to adenosine	P axis	Ref #
1	63	F	440	severe aortic regurgitation	NA	NA	−90	9
2	46	F	280	—	Termination	NA	+15	9
3	42	F	350	ventricular septal defect	Termination	NA	−90	9
4	39	F	420	—	NA	NA	+15	9
5	50	F	270	AV nodal reentrant tachycardia	NA	Termination	+30	9
6	58	F	330	coronary arteriovenous fistula	NA	NA	−45	9
7	70	F	330	hypertension	NA	Termination	NA	10
8	53	F	360	faciculoventricular bypass tract	NA	Termination	NA	10
9	60	F	320	hypertension	NA	Termination	NA	10
10	73	M	400	WPW syndrome	NA	Termination	NA	10
11	60	F	320	chronic renal failure	NA	Termination	NA	10
12	43	F	350	—	NA	Termination	NA	10
13	71	F	430	old inferior wall MI	NA	Termination	NA	10
14	57	F	420	—	NA	Termination	NA	10
15	67	M	390	WPW syndrome	NA	Termination	NA	10
16	70	F	400	hypertension	NA	Termination	NA	10
17	83	M	370	old inferior wall MI	NA	Termination	NA	10
	59±12	14F/3M	363±51					

F = female; M = male; MI = myocardial infarction; NA = not available; Pt = patient; Ref = reference; TCL = tachycardia cycle length in milliseconds.

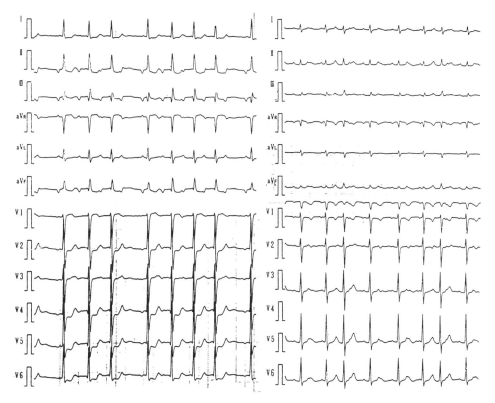

Figure 1. Surface ECGs from patient 1 (left) and patient 5 (right) (see Table 1) during tachycardia. The P wave was negative in II, III aVF in patient 1 but positive in patient 5. Weckebach type atrioventricular block (nodal block) was noted during the tachycardia in both patients.

Electrophysiological Characteristics

During the tachycardia, all patients had an atrial activation sequence different from that which occurred during sinus rhythm. The earliest atrial deflection was recorded near the AV junctional region. Dual AV nodal physiology was observed in 8 of the 17 patients. Tachycardia in all patients could be induced and terminated by an atrial premature beat. Isoproterenol was not required for the induction, and the tachycardia was initiated or terminated abruptly without gradual acceleration or deceleration of the rate in any patients. During the atrial extrastimulation study, induction of atrial tachycardia was associated with a longer extrastimulus-to-first-atrial-tachycardia-beat interval with progressive coupling prematurity in all patients. These findings suggest reentry as the mechanism although entrainment study was not performed in either study. The pathophysiology of this tachycardia remains unclear.

Atrial tachycardia within the triangle of Koch is sensitive to verapamil and adenosine. Verapamil and adenosine terminate the tachycardia either clinically or in the electrophysiological laboratory. These agents, when used in supraventricular tachycardia, can produce AV block.[11–13] Typical response of

AVRT and AVNRT to these agents is termination of the tachycardia because AV nodal conduction is part of the reentrant circuit. On the other hand, typical response of atrial tachycardia to these agents is the development of AV block while the tachycardia persists.[14] Adenosine sensitive atrial tachycardia has been reported and it has been proposed that these atrial tachycardias are due to trigger activity which is related to cAMP dependent calcium current.[15] However, both reports showed that atrial tachycardia within the triangle of Koch is likely due to reentry and this tachycardia could be terminated by adenosine. It is likely that other mechanisms may be operative. A possible explanation is that atrial tachycardia within the triangle of Koch may originate from transitional cells which are similar to AV nodal cells in their sensitivity to adenosine.

Diagnostic Problems with Atrial Tachycardia Within the Triangle of Koch

In general, atrial tachycardia can be diagnosed according to the following criteria:[16]

1. Atrial activation sequence different from that which occurs during sinus rhythm.
2. Changing PR interval and/or RP interval related to the tachycardia rate.
3. AV block may exist without affecting the tachycardia.

During an electrophysiological study, atrial tachycardia is suspected if the atrial activation sequence is different from that which occurs during ventricular pacing with ventriculoatrial conduction. However, atrial tachycardia with its focus near the triangle of Koch may mimic AVNRT or AVRT involving a septal accessory pathway because they all have the earliest atrial activation recorded near the AV junction. A reset study by delivering a ventricular premature beat during the His refractory period can help in differential diagnosis. AVRT incorporating a concealed right septal accessory pathway can usually be reset by right ventricular stimulation delivered during the His refractory period. Failure to reset the tachycardia by a ventricular premature beat makes the diagnosis of AVRT not likely. However, differentiation between AT and AVNRT is more difficult. The persistence of tachycardia independent of conduction block in the AV node may exclude AVNRT. However, this finding is not always observed and persistent 1:1 conduction during atrial tachycardia is very common. Adenosine and verapamil injection will not help in the differential diagnosis since both tachycardias may respond to either medication. However, the following findings favor the diagnosis of atrial tachycardia: the absence of dual AV nodal physiology; the presence of VA conduction block (either complete VA block or block at a relatively long ventricular pacing cycle length); the V-A-A-V sequence during initiation of tachycardia by ventricular pacing or ventricular extrastimulation. Diagnostic clues could also come from observing the VA conduction time during different episodes of the tachycardia. An AVNRT should have constant VA conduction time despite tachycardia rate variation. In contrast, the VA conduction time may change during AT rate variation since there is no ventriculoatrial conduction at all during the tachycardia. Pacing at the right atrium during sinus rhythm with a cycle length identical to that of the tachycardia will sometimes be useful. Man et al have reported that, in long RP supraventricular tachycardia, an AH interval during atrial pacing 40 milliseconds longer than that present during tachycardia favors the diagnosis of fast-slow AVNRT.[17] In contrast, atrial tachycardia has an AH interval during atrial pacing within 10 milliseconds from that present during tachycardia. However, the most important thing is the awareness and index of suspicion of this special subset of atrial tachycardia. Otherwise, these patients could be incorrectly treated as having AVNRT.

The incidence of atrial tachycardia within the Koch's triangle varies among different reports, ranging from 0 to 12% of the total number of patients with atrial tachycardia.[3–10] The discrepancy may be attributed to the difference in patient selection or study population. Because atrial tachycardia within the triangle of Koch may mimic AVNRT, a false attempt to treat AVNRT could have resulted in unintentional cure of the atrial tachycardia. This may account for another explanation for the discrepancy.

Catheter Ablation

Mapping and ablation of atrial tachycardia within the triangle of Koch is virtually the same as performed for atrial tachycardia in general. An endocardial activation map was used to find the earliest atrial activation site. The local electrogram at a successful ablation site is usually 30 to 60 milliseconds preceding the P wave on the surface ECG. However, a major concern about catheter ablation of atrial tachycardia within the triangle of Koch is the risk of AV block. Radiofrequency energy application near the His bundle or AV node has been reported to be associated with a high risk of AV block. Yeh et al reported a risk of up to 36% when ablating intermediate septal accessory pathways.[18] In a report by Iesaka et al, 2 patients developed transient AV block and one other patient developed permanent complete AV block during ablation of atrial tachycardia near the AV mode.[10] The atrial tachycardia was eliminated in 10 of the 11 patients (91%). In another smaller series by Lai et al, none of the 6 patients developed permanent complete AV block and one patient had transient AV block during ablation (Figure 2).[9] The success rate was 100% (6/6). In general, radiofrequency energy was applied during atrial tachycardia and the electrogram was continuously monitored. The power output was applied in a titrated manner,[19] beginning with 5 watts and increased by 5 watts for every 30 seconds of energy application until the tachycardia was eliminated or until the maximum of 40 watts was reached. If atrial tachycardia terminated at a given power level, the radiofrequency energy would be applied at that level for another 30 seconds. If the tachycardia did not terminate with 40 watts of output for 30 seconds, the catheter would be repositioned for further mapping. If an accelerated junctional rhythm occurred after atrial tachycardia termination, atrial overdrive pacing would be performed to monitor AV conduction.

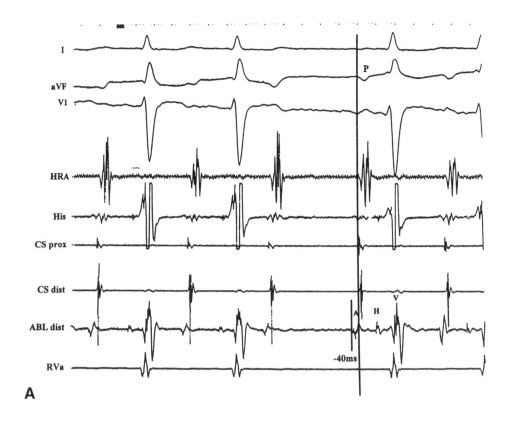

A

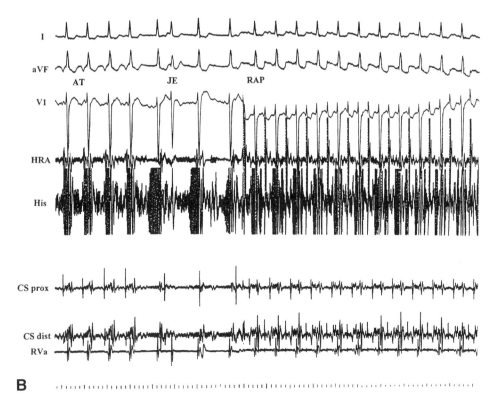

B

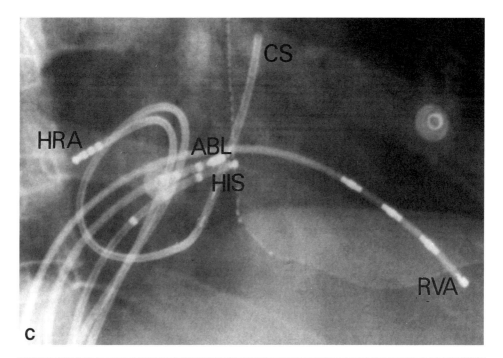

C

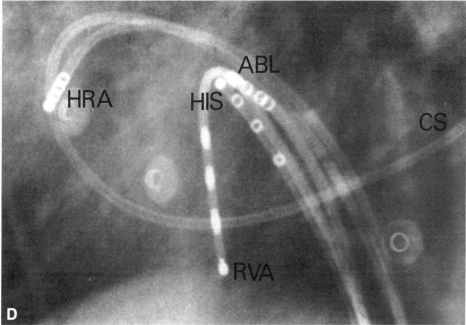

D

Figure 2. Local electrograms and fluoroscopic pictures during successful catheter ablation session in patient 1. (A) Local electrograms at the final successful ablation site (50 mm/sec). A discrete His bundle potential was recorded; the local atrial deflection was 40 milliseconds before P wave. (B) Local electrograms during energy application (12.5 mm/sec). The atrial tachycardia terminated and an accelerated junctional rhythm followed. Atrial overdrive pacing was initiated upon identification of the accelerated junctional rhythm for monitoring atrioventricular conduction. The radiofrequency interference in lead I, aVF and V1 has been erased for clarity. (C) RAO 30° and (D) LAO 60° fluoroscopic pictures of the successful catheter ablation site. A = atrial deflection; ABL = ablation catheter; AT = atrial tachycardia; CS = coronary sinus; dist = distal; H = His potential; HRA = high right atrium; JE = junctional ectopic rhythm; P = surface ECG P wave; prox = proximal; RAP = right atrial pacing; RVA = right ventricular apex; V = ventricular deflection.

2 important points must be reemphasized in order to avoid AV block: 1) use of a titrated radiofrequency energy output, and 2) use of overdrive atrial pacing to monitor AV conduction, should accelerated junctional rhythm occur.

One of the rationales for stressing a titrated output application is that the AV node or His bundle may be more deeply located relative to the atrial tachycardia focus, which may be more superficial.[20] A window zone of energy level should exist for a successful ablation of the atrial tachycardia focus without injury to the normal AV conduction system. By carefully titrating the energy output, one would be able to demonstrate the efficacy and safety of radiofrequency catheter ablation of atrial tachycardia within the Koch's triangle. Lai et al observed an occurrence of accelerated junctional rhythm in 67% of their patients.[9] Haissaguerre et al suggested immediate discontinuation of energy application upon identification of accelerated junctional rhythm during ablation of parahisian accessory pathways.[21] However, Lai et al found that radiofrequency energy could be safely continued during junctional rhythm as long as AV conduction could be monitored with overdrive atrial pacing. Transient AV block occurred in one patient without heralding accelerated junctional rhythm and the normal AV conduction was restored 12 seconds after cessation of the energy output. A report by Jentzer et al indicated that "prompt" discontinuation of energy output upon identification of heart block is usually associated with restoration of normal AV conduction.[22]

Conclusions

Atrial tachycardia within the triangle of Koch is a special subset of atrial tachycardia. This tachycardia should be differentiated from AVNRT or AVRT. Radiofrequency catheter ablation of atrial tachycardia within the Koch's triangle is feasible. However, the risk of AV block exists and careful monitoring of AV conduction during ablation is crucial for a safe ablative session.

References

1. Wu D, Amat-Y-Leon F, Denes P, et al. Demonstration of sustained sinus and atrial reentry as a mechanism of paroxysmal supraventricular tachycardia. *Circulation* 1975;51:234–243.
2. Scheinman MM, Basu D, Hollenberg M. Electrophysiological studies in patients with persistent atrial tachycardia. *Circulation* 1974;50:266–273.
3. Chen SA, Chiang CE, Yang CJ, et al. Radiofrequency catheter ablation of sustained intra-atrial reentrant tachycardia in adult patients: identification of electrophysiological characteristics and endocardial mapping techniques. *Circulation* 1993;88:578–587.
4. Kay GN, Chong F, Epstein AE, et al. Radiofrequency ablation for treatment of primary atrial tachycardias. *J Am Coll Cardiol* 1993;21:901–909.
5. Goldberger J, Kall J, Ehlert F, et al. Effectiveness of radiofrequency catheter ablation for treatment of atrial tachycardia. *Am J Cardiol* 1993;72:787–793.

6. Lesh MD, Van Hare GF, Epstein LM, et al. Radiofrequency catheter ablation of atrial arrhythmias results and mechanisms. *Circulation* 1994;89: 1074–1089.

7. Lau YR, Gillette PC, Wienecke MM, et al. Successful radiofrequency catheter ablation of an atrial ectopic tachycardia in an adolescent. *Am Heart J* 1992;123:1384–1386.

8. Walsh EP, Saul JP, Hulse JE, et al. Transcatheter ablation of ectopic atrial tachycardia in young patients using radiofrequency current. *Circulation* 1992;86:1138–1146.

9. Lai LP, Lin JL, Chen TF, et al. Clinical electrophysiological characteristics and radiofrequency catheter ablation of atrial tachycardia near the apex of Koch's triangle. *PACE* 1998;21:367–374.

10. Iesaka Y, Takahashi A, Goya M, et al. Adenosine-sensitive atrial reentrant tachycardia originating from the atrioventricular nodal transitional area. *J Cardiovasc Electrophysiol* 1997;8:854–864.

11. Belhassen B, Pelleg AA. Acute management of paroxysmal supraventricular tachycardia: verapamil, adenosine triphosphate or adenosine? *Am J Cardiol* 1984;54:225–227.

12. DiMacro JP, Sellers TD, Berne RM, et al. Adenosine: electrophysiological effects and therapeutic use for terminating paroxysmal supraventricular tachycardia. *Circulation* 1983;6:1254–1263.

13. Camm AJ, Garratt CJ. Adenosine and supraventricular tachycardia. *N Eng J Med* 1991;325:1621–1629.

14. DiMacro JP, Sellers TD, Lerman BB, et al. Diagnostic and therapeutic use of adenosine in patients with supraventricular tachyarrhythmias. *J Am Coll Cardiol* 1985;6:417–425.

15. Engelstein ED, Lippman N, Stein MK, et al. Mechanism-specific effects of adenosine on atrial tachycardia. *Circulation* 1994;89:2645–2654.

16. Josephson ME. Supraventricular tachycardia. In: Josephson ME, ed. *Clinical Cardiac Electrophysiology: Techniques and Interpretations,* 2nd ed. Philadelphia, PA: Lea & Febiger, 1992. pp 181–274.

17. Man KC, Niebauer M, Daoud E, et al. Comparison of atrial-His intervals during tachycardia and during atrial pacing in patients with long RP tachycardia. *J Cardiovasc Electrophysiol* 1995;6:700–710.

18. Yeh SJ, Wang CC, Wen MS, et al. Characteristics and radiofrequency ablation of intermediate septal accessory pathway. *Am J Cardiol* 1994;73: 50–56.

19. Langberg JJ, Harvey M, Calkins H, et al. Titration of power output during radiofrequency catheter ablation of atrioventricular nodal reentrant tachycardia. *PACE* 1993;16:465–470.

20. Dean JW, Ho SY, Rowland E, et al. Clinical anatomy of the atrioventricular junction. *J Am Coll Cardiol* 1994;24:1725–1731.

21. Haïssaguerre M, Marcus F, Poquet F, et al. Electrophysiological characteristics and catheter ablation of parahissian accessory pathways. *Circulation* 1994;90:1124–1128.

22. Jentzer JH, Goyal R, Williamson BD, et al. Analysis of junctional ectopy during radiofrequency ablation of the slow pathway in patients with atrioventricular nodal reentrant tachycardia. *Circulation* 1994;90:2820–2826.

Chapter 11

Reentrant Atrial Tachycardia Associated with Structural Heart Disease

George F. Van Hare, M.D.

Catheter ablation of atrial reentrant tachycardia may be the most attractive alternative for the treatment of the patient who has previously undergone surgery for congenital heart disease. With the exception of atrial flutter or fibrillation in the immediate postoperative period, such tachyarrhythmias are very unlikely to disappear spontaneously, and therefore, the need for antiarrhythmic therapy is likely to be lifelong. Because there is a high incidence of sinus node dysfunction in this patient population, the addition of antiarrhythmic agents may cause a patient with sinus node disease to experience new or more serious symptoms. These may include syncope, which may mandate implantation of a permanent pacemaker in order to continue antiarrhythmic therapy. Similarly, this patient population often has coexisting ventricular dysfunction. Many of the most effective agents for the control of tachyarrhythmias have the potential to worsen ventricular dysfunction, especially drugs, like the β-blockers, disopyramide, and sotolol. Even worse, the same patients are clearly at a much greater risk for the occurrence of proarrhythmia when treated with these agents, and in particular, flecainide, propafenone, and sotolol. Proarrhythmia may present as polymorphous ventricular tachycardia with syncope or sudden death. The prospect, therefore, of a curative procedure becomes very attractive, both for the purposes of patient acceptance and for patient safety. There are risks to any invasive procedure, however, and so the clinician needs to weigh these procedural risks, and weigh also the likelihood of success and of recurrence, against the difficulties of pharmacological management.

This chapter will discuss current techniques for mapping of atrial reentrant tachycardia in postoperative patients. The techniques for radiofrequency

From Huang SKS, Wilber DJ (eds.): *Radiofrequency Catheter Ablation of Cardiac Arrhythmias: Basic Concepts and Clinical Applications,* 2nd ed. Armonk, NY: Futura Publishing Company, Inc. ©2000.

catheter ablation, as well as post-ablation assessment, will be described. Lastly, the current results of these techniques will be reviewed.

Clinical Characteristics of Postoperative Atrial Flutter

In 1985, Garson et al[1] reported the findings of a multicenter study of 380 patients who had developed atrial flutter at ages between 12 months and 25 years. Among these 380 patients, seven diagnoses accounted for more than 75% of the patients. In order of frequency, they were D-transposition of the great arteries (20.5%); complex congenital heart disease (for example, single ventricle with or without pulmonary stenosis) (17.8%); atrial septal defect (12.1%); pulmonary stenosis (with or without ventricular septal defect), pulmonary atresia (with or without ventricular septal defect), and tetralogy of Fallot (7.9%); structurally normal (6.3%); dilated cardiomyopathy (5.8%); and complete atrioventricular canal defect (5.0%). Considering the relation to cardiac surgery, 60.4% of the patients had repaired congenital heart disease, 13.3% had congenital heart disease treated palliatively, and 7.6% had congenital heart disease not operated on. At least one cardiac operation had been performed in 75% of patients before the first episode of atrial flutter. The 5 most common repairs were the Mustard or Senning procedure (27.6%), the Blalock-Hanlon procedure for transposition (16.1%), surgical closure of an atrial septal defect (11.1%), repair of pulmonary atresia and/or tetralogy of Fallot (7.9%), and aorto-pulmonary shunt (6.6%).

Although currently the arterial switch procedure is performed for nearly all patients with D-transposition of the great arteries, a large number of previously repaired patients are followed who had the Senning or Mustard procedure ("atrial repair"). It has long been known that bradyarrhythmias are common following these procedures.[2,3] However, sudden deaths have been reported in patients with either type of repair.[4,5] To evaluate the mechanism of cardiac arrhythmias after the Mustard operation for transposition, Vetter et al performed invasive electrophysiological evaluations in 60 patients with transposition who had undergone a Mustard procedure.[6] Of these 60 patients, 55% had inducible atrial flutter, of whom roughly half had atrial flutter recognized clinically. Clearly, the substrate for atrial flutter seems inherent in the operation.

The actual incidence of serious arrhythmias in patients who have undergone the Senning or Mustard procedure may be higher than previously suspected. Bink-Boelkens et al[7] followed 50 patients who had had Mustard repair between 1969 and 1980. Roughly one quarter of the patients developed atrial flutter. There was a high late mortality: 8 of the 50 (16%) died suddenly, 2 of these despite having a functioning pacemaker. There was a notable relation between the type of arrhythmia and the occurrence of sudden death. For these 50 patients, the late mortality for those with sinus-node dysfunction was 19%, the junctional escape rhythm, 40%; and atrial flutter, 62%.

In a collaborative study of 372 patients after Mustard repair, Flinn et al[8] reported similar findings. Of 29 patients in whom the "dominant" arrhythmia was a supraventricular tachyarrhythmia, 64% had atrial flutter, and there was a significant association between the dominant arrhythmia and sudden death. Because of the increased risk of atrial flutter and poor outcome after the Mustard repair, Duster et al[9] has recommended that digoxin therapy be lifelong.

Patients who undergo anatomic correction (arterial switch) seem to be at a lower risk of atrial flutter.[10]

While atrial flutter is very common in patients who have undergone more complex forms of atrial surgery, there is an association between atrial septal defect repair and atrial flutter. Of the 380 patients with atrial flutter reported by Garson et al,[1] 47 (12.4%) had an atrial septal defect and 87% of these underwent repair. Bink-Boelkens et al[7] reported a series of 204 patients who underwent closure of a secundum atrial septal defect between 1967 and 1980. During the postoperative period, 18% of these patients developed atrial flutter and the only late (and sudden) death was of a patient with atrial flutter. The relatively high prevalence of adult patients who have undergone atrial septal defect repair as children in reported series of radiofrequency ablation[11] suggests that atrial flutter is more common in this group of patients than was previously recognized.

Patients who have congenital heart defects that are associated with an enlarged right atrium are thought to be more susceptible to the development of atrial flutter. Tricuspid atresia and Ebstein's abnormality of the tricuspid valve are 2 examples. In both conditions, an increased right atrial volume or pressure or both is thought to predispose to atrial flutter, requiring therapy.[12] Patients with tricuspid atresia who have undergone a Fontan procedure are at increased risk of atrial flutter both in the immediate postoperative period and over the long term.[13-17] According to Porter et al, approximately one quarter of these patients will develop a significant supraventricular tachyarrhythmia, predominantly atrial flutter, within 5 years after surgery.

Techniques for Mapping and Ablation of Intra-atrial Reentrant Tachycardia

The most common form of postoperative arrhythmia seen chronically is atrial flutter, also known in this patient population as intra-atrial reentrant tachycardia (IART). To understand the techniques used in mapping of large macro-reentrant circuits, several concepts must be reviewed: the concept of barriers to impulse propagation, and the concept of sites which are "in the circuit" versus sites that are "outside the circuit." These concepts were initially developed in the classic studies by Waldo et al[18] and were applied by various workers to the mapping and ablation of common atrial flutter in adults[18-25] as well as to ventricular tachycardia in patients with coronary artery disease[26–30] The techniques were subsequently extended for use in postoperative patients with atrial arrhythmias.[31–36] It is instructive, therefore, to briefly review what is now known about common ("Type 1") atrial flutter, and how this relates to the anatomic basis for reentry in the postoperative atrium.

Importance of Barriers to Intra-Atrial Conduction

Initial activation mapping studies of the typical form of atrial flutter in patients showed a counterclockwise reentrant activation in the right atrium when viewed from below,[37–39] with impulses spreading up the septum and down the right atrial freewall. From studies using the technique of concealed entrainment, as well as methods for the precise placement of ablative lesions, it is now well established that one critical element of the atrial flutter reentrant circuit is the isthmus between the IVC and the tricuspid valve annulus.[22] This area of tissue is protected by these 2 barriers to impulse propagation, which prevent the reentrant wave from circling back and catching the "tail of refractoriness," and thereby being extinguished. The situation is more complex, however, than simply a small isthmus of tissue between 2 small barriers. In fact, as shown by Olgin et al, and by Kalman et al, it is not the IVC per se but actually the crista terminalis, and its extension as the eustachian valve ridge, that act as the barrier to impulse propagation.[21,24] The crista terminalis is formed at the junction between the sinus venosus portion of the right atrium, which is smooth, and the "true" right atrium constituting the right atrial appendage and freewall, which is heavily trabeculated. The crista terminalis runs along the posterolateral aspect of the right atrium, coursing inferiorly. As it reaches the region of the IVC, it is extended by the eustachian valve ridge, which courses superiorly to the os of the coronary sinus to join with the valve of the coronary sinus to form the tendon of Todaro. In patients with common atrial flutter, it has been shown to act as a long line of intra-atrial block, and this block may either be anatomic and fixed, or may be functionally determined, in patients with clinical atrial flutter. The tricuspid annulus constitutes the "anterior barrier" in typical flutter and sites around the tricuspid annulus are activated sequentially and in a counterclockwise direction when viewed in the left anterior oblique projection. These 2 long barriers to impulse propagation form a funnel of conducting tissue in the right atrium, as described by Kalman et al.[24] This funnel forces atrial activation to the narrow isthmus between the tricuspid annulus and the IVC, where, because of the short distance, the reentrant circuit is most amenable to successful ablation.

It is interesting that in the otherwise normal human heart, despite the fact that there are numerous potential barriers to impulse propagation (IVC, SVC, coronary sinus os, tricuspid and mitral valve annuli, ostia of pulmonary veins, crista terminalis) most atrial reentrant arrhythmias are due to common counterclockwise or clockwise atrial flutter. This fact speaks to the importance of the crista terminalis and tricuspid annulus, and one would expect these structures to also be important in IART, which is seen following congenital heart disease surgery. The effect of extensive atrial surgery is complex, and may involve several elements that make IART more likely. First, the creation of a long atriotomy with subsequent suture closure may create a long line of block of impulse propagation, which is superimposed on the existing right atrial anatomy described above. Second, such an atriotomy may modify the typical flutter circuit by making it longer, thereby lengthening the tachycardia cycle length and slowing the atrial tachycardia rate. Third, the placement of an atriotomy near the crista terminalis, or the use of the crista terminalis for anchoring a suture line (as is done in the lateral Fontan modification) may cause the crista terminalis to begin to act as a line of conduction block.[40,41] Finally, extensive atrial surgery may cause slowing of conduction, making reentry more likely. At present, it is not known which of these possible mechanisms is most important. It is clear from clinical experience, however, that slow flutter involving the posterior flutter isthmus is very common in postoperative patients[32,33] but circuits which do not include the typical flutter zone, and so are due to reentry involving incisional suture lines, are also frequently seen.[35]

In preparation for mapping a patient with IART, it is important to carefully review the patient's cardiac anatomy, and in particular, the exact surgical approach that was used. This is facilitated by a review of the original operative report. The details of the exact placement of atriotomies, baffles, patches, and conduits will become important in the interpretation of the electrophysiological recordings and the results of mapping. If possible, the sites which are bounded by surgically-created and anatomic obstacles to impulse propagation should be identified, and several possible candidate sites for ablation should be determined prior to the study. For example, in patients who have undergone simple surgery, such as repair of an atrial septal defect, such sites might be a) the typical flutter isthmus, b) between an atriotomy and the tricuspid annulus, or c) between an atriotomy and the SVC. The cardiologist must combine an intimate knowledge of the patient's congenital defect with knowledge of the details of the surgical procedure to determine these sites.

Technical Points Regarding Access to the Heart

In performing the electrophysiological study, there are several technical issues to note. Patients who have had multiple prior procedures, or who have had long stays in the intensive care unit with indwelling lines, may have limited venous access, due to iliofemoral (or other venous) thrombosis. When bilateral, this problem may prevent a normal approach to the right atrium. Patients who have undergone the bidirectional Glenn procedure will have no direct access to the right atrium from the SVC, due to the direct connection of the SVC to the pulmonary artery. In both situations, one may consider approaching the right atrium from the other cava, for example from the SVC when there is bilateral iliofemoral thrombosis. Recent reports of the use of a trans-hepatic approach for diagnostic and interventional catheterization[42,43] suggest that this route might also be efficacious for catheter ablation. The left atrium or pulmonary venous atrium may be entered by a retrograde approach[44] (Figure 1) or after transseptal puncture, although the presence of atrial patch material or an intra-atrial baffle will make the later approach difficult or impossible. The existence of situs abnormalities can render a catheter ablation procedure potentially confusing, due to the nonstandard location of veins, arteries, and the heart itself, but these problems are not insurmountable if one possesses a knowledge of congenital cardiac pathology. Such abnormalities are unfortunately not limited to simple mirror-image arrangements. Standard fluoroscopy planes for normal anatomy may make little sense in the setting of situs abnormalities. When needed, transthoracic or transesophageal echocardiography may be used to confirm catheter tip locations.[45–47] Finally, patients with heterotaxy syndromes may have interruption of the IVC with azygous continuation. In such patients, a catheter passed from the femoral vein will traverse the azygous system to join the SVC and enter the atrium from above. In such pa-

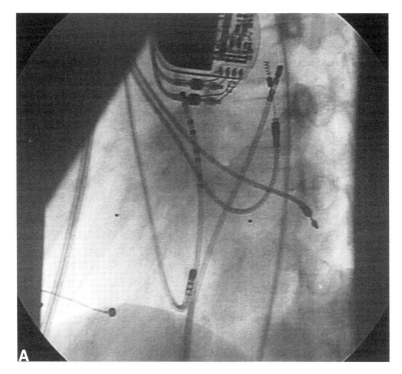

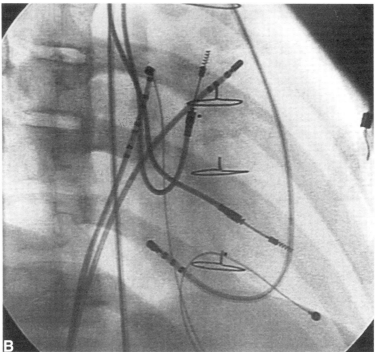

Figure 1. Fluoroscopy images of catheter positions in a patient with a Senning procedure for D-transposition, who also has a transvenous pacing system. The ablation catheter passes up the aorta, across the aortic valve, through the right ventricle, and through the tricuspid valve to sit on the "flutter isthmus" between the baffle and the tricuspid annulus. A: Left anterior oblique view. B: Right anterior oblique view. (From Van Hare GF. Catheter and surgical ablation. In: Gillette PC, Balaji S, Case CL, eds. *Cardiac Arrhythmias after Surgery for Congenital Heart Disease,* In press.)

tients, to facilitate catheter manipulation, one may instead choose to introduce an ablation catheter from the internal jugular or subclavian vein.

Methods for Mapping Macro-Reentrant Circuits

In general, methods for mapping clinical atrial arrhythmias have fallen into 3 broad categories: single site roving mapping, simultaneous multisite mapping, and "destructive" mapping. In practice, a typical procedure for ablation of atrial tachycardia incorporates elements of all 3. For single site mapping, a single steerable catheter is maneuvered throughout the atrium during tachycardia. Electrograms from various sites are recorded, and the map is constructed from these nonsimultaneous measurements. The advantage is that this technique uses few catheters and few amplifier channels, and does not require extensive computerization. The disadvantage is that it requires a great deal of time and fluoroscopy exposure. Most distressing, the tachycardia mechanism may change in the midst of a map, forcing the investigator to stop to reinduce the original rhythm. A new system has become available to make the process of constructing a nonsimultaneous multisite map faster.[48] This system utilizes an ultra-low magnetic field to determine the precise location of the mapping catheter tip in 3 dimensions and allows one to display both anatomic and electrical data together. This theoretically may allow for shorter fluoroscopy exposure times in the construction of the map, and certainly allows for more correct display of the electrical-anatomic relationships. It suffers from some of the same problems seen with other nonsimultaneous methods, namely the potential for sudden mid-map changes in tachycardia mechanism, and the inability to perturb the tachycardia by entrainment pacing and evaluate the results from one beat. The true utility of this system remains to be determined, but it is clearly the strongest in the mapping of focal automatic tachycardias, and may be helpful in the rapid detection of zones of slow conduction and in the assessment of lines of block following ablation.

Simultaneous multisite mapping involves various schemes for introducing large numbers of electrodes into or onto the heart. A standard four-wire electrophysiology study is a limited example of simultaneous multisite mapping. Research is ongoing at many centers with many systems. These include high electrode density catheters, basket catheters, and noncontact catheters, which record intracavitary potentials. For the latter method, sophisticated computer methods are used to reconstruct the endocardial activation pattern by solving the inverse problem.[49,50] The advantages include the potential to obtain a map on one beat of tachycardia, and to see the entire circuit. It is limited, however, by the basic inability to introduce electrodes in all parts of both atria in the catheterization laboratory. These systems also require many channels and are computer-intensive, requiring expensive equipment and large amounts of mass storage. Ultimately, even with many electrodes, resolution may not be adequate. Finally, areas which are "in the circuit" may not easily be identified and separated from those that are "out of the circuit" without the ability to perturb the system, for example by entrainment pacing.

To perform "destructive mapping" one places ablative lesions to achieve direct interruption of an area of conducting myocardium, with subsequent observation to determine whether the target rhythm has been eradicated. Intraoperatively, this can be done by "ice mapping," the creation of a nonpermanent injury with cryotherapy, or by direct surgical incision. In the catheterization laboratory, this may be done by the delivery of direct current or RF lesions (Figure 2). Ideally, such lesions are directed by the use of detailed maps to target these lesions. A successful RF lesion which eliminates a tachyarrhythmia is perhaps the best evidence that the site chosen for ablation was critical for maintenance of the arrhythmia. In 1914, Mines recognized the limitations of multisite mapping, saying in reference to atrial flutter that "the test for a circulating excitation is to cut through the ring at one point thereby terminating the flutter."[51] The advantage of this approach is that the lesion may very well be curative. The limitation, of course, is the potential for needless destruction of working myocardium which is not involved in the tachycardia, as well as the potential for lengthening the reentrant circuit, slowing the tachycardia, and making it more incessant. Finally, transient but not permanent block may be observed, and such an occurrence may be misleading, as it causes termination of the tachycardia but clearly is not sufficient for permanent cure.

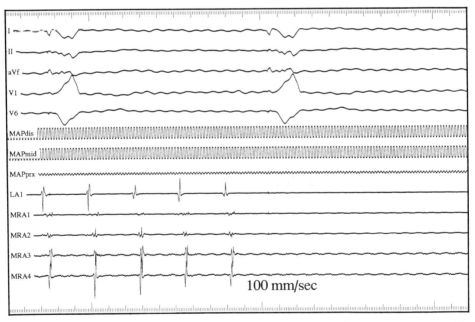

Figure 2. Intracardiac recordings during intra-atrial reentry tachycardia, in same patient as Figure 1, showing tachycardia termination coincident with delivery of radiofrequency energy. Abbreviations: LA = left atrium; MAP = mapping/ablation catheter; MRA = mid-right atrium; dis = distal electrode pair; Prx = proximal electrode pair. (From Van Hare GF. Catheter and surgical ablation. In: Gillette PC, Balaji S, Case CL, eds. *Cardiac Arrhythmias after Surgery for Congenital Heart Disease.* In press.)

Identification of Possible Lines of Conduction Block

During the electrophysiological study, the goal is to identify an isthmus of tissue which is bounded by 2 long barriers. For example, the tricuspid annulus often provides one important barrier in such patients. The identification and location of the tricuspid annulus is not challenging, as one has fluoroscopic landmarks as well as local atrial electrogram characteristics. Specifically, on the tricuspid annulus, one normally records both atrial and ventricular electrograms, and these are approximately equivalent in size when the catheter is resting on the annulus. Other sites of conduction block can be identified by the presence of double potentials, reflecting conduction up one side of the barrier and down the other side, with the bipolar electrogram recording both waves of atrial activation.[19,52] Such double potentials are easily recorded in patients with common atrial flutter along the crista terminalis and the eustachian valve ridge.[53] In patients who have undergone atrial surgery, the atriotomy may be identified along the anterior wall of the atrium, and may be followed along the atrial wall for some distance (Figure 3).[35] In patients after the Senning procedure for transposition, a long line of double potentials may be recorded along the edge of the baffle in the systemic venous atrium.[32]

It must be emphasized that the identification of a line of double potentials is not sufficient for the completion of the map, because such lines of double

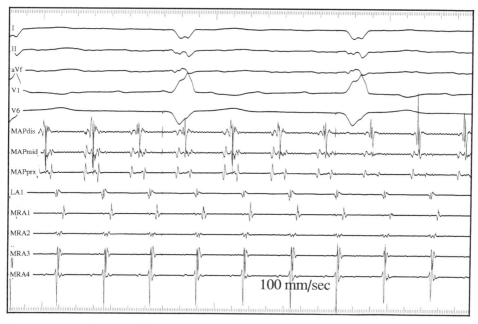

Figure 3. Intracardiac recordings during intra-atrial reentry tachycardia, in same patient as Figure 1, showing double potentials recorded from the anterior right atrial wall in the pulmonary venous atrium, most likely at the site of an atriotomy. Abbreviations: LA = left atrium; MAP = mapping/ablation catheter; MRA = mid-right atrium; dis = distal electrode pair; Prx = proximal electrode pair. (From Van Hare GF. Catheter and surgical ablation. In: Gillette PC, Balaji S, Case CL, eds. *Cardiac Arrhythmias after Surgery for Congenital Heart Disease.* In press.)

potentials are very common, and often are not associated in any way with the actual reentrant circuit. That is, both, one, or neither of the areas of atrial myocardium on either side of the line of block may be involved in the reentrant circuit. Areas that are uninvolved in the circuit are considered to be "bystander" areas. Confirmation that the line of block is critical for the tachycardia circuit must be obtained by entrainment pacing techniques.

The Use of Entrainment Principles in Mapping

Modern mapping techniques make use of the concept of transient entrainment, both for the documentation of the reentrant mechanism, as well as for identification of candidate sites for ablation. A full treatment of these concepts is beyond the scope of this chapter, and is covered more extensively elsewhere in this text.

The demonstration of transient entrainment has been used in the past for the determination that a given rhythm is reentrant, rather than automatic, in nature. As applied to atrial flutter by Waldo et al, one paces transiently in the atrium at a rate slightly faster than the atrial tachycardia rate and observes several features.[18] If one is pacing "upstream" from the critical protected zone of conduction, one observes acceleration to the paced tachycardia rate during pacing, constant fusion during any given pacing rate, progressive fusion at increasing pacing rates, and return to the tachycardia rate following termination of pacing. "Concealed entrainment" has been defined as the inability to demonstrate the usual characteristics of entrainment in an atrial rhythm that is known to be reentrant, despite demonstration of acceleration to the pacing rate and return to the tachycardia rate following pacing. One common cause for concealed entrainment is that one is pacing from within a protected zone of slow conduction. There is no fusion, because the retrograde wave of activation collides with the antegrade wave in the protected zone, and the atrial activation sequence changes little. There is latency between the pacing stimulus and the onset of the P wave due to conduction within this protected zone. Furthermore, the degree of latency from the stimulus to the P wave onset during entrainment pacing is similar to the latency, when not pacing, from the local electrogram at the pacing site to the onset of the P wave. Most importantly for the purposes of entrainment mapping, when one terminates pacing, the time necessary for return of the wave of activation to the pacing site, the post-pacing interval (PPI) is the same as the tachycardia cycle length (TCL). As pointed out by Stevenson with respect to ventricular tachycardia, the characteristic of PPI = TCL should be a reliable indication of whether a given site is within or outside of the reentry circuit.[29,54]

Unlike the situation of typical atrial flutter, in which the "protected slow zone" is restricted to the tricuspid-IVC isthmus, in patients with complex atrial surgery, there may be multiple areas of slow conduction and conduction block, which may or may not be part of the reentrant circuit. This situation is common in patients with the Senning or Mustard procedure for transposition, in whom a large section of lateral systemic venous atrium often acts as a bystander branch.[31,32] If one paces from a site in such a bystander area, it is clear that the PPI will be much longer than the TCL, as the return time to this site will equal the total of 1) conduction time into the circuit, 2) conduction time around the entire circuit, and 3) conduction time back to the pacing site in the side branch.

One may note in patients with complex atrial surgery that P waves are difficult to assess adequately, because they tend to have quite low voltage. Furthermore, they often lack sharp features, so that judging consistently the onset of the P wave in order to determine the latency, and assess for fusion, is difficult. This is particularly a problem with patients after the Senning or Mustard procedure, in which P waves are often nearly impossible to appreciate despite the presence of a sinus-like rhythm. For these reasons, one should rely more heavily on determination of the PPI and its comparison to TCL than on any measurement or assessment in which P wave morphology and timing are essential.

In practice, the standard ablation for intra-atrial reentrant tachycardia involves assessment of the circuit by all the methods described above. One starts with an understanding of the congenital cardiac anatomy and the superimposed surgical details in that particular patient. Reading the original operative report is invaluable in this respect. One then gets a rough idea, from roving and/or simultaneous multisite maps during tachycardia, of which areas are likely to be early in relation to the P wave and therefore may be candidate protected slow zones. Finally, using entrainment pacing, one tests each of these candidate sites and determines whether these sites are "in" or "out" of the circuit (Figures 4 and 5). This information is then related to the anatomic and sur-

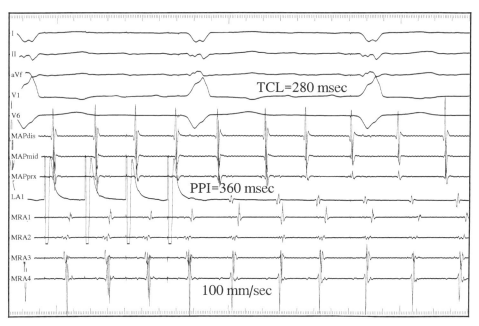

Figure 4. Intracardiac recordings during intra-atrial reentry tachycardia, in same patient as Figure 1, demonstrating entrainment pacing from the roof of the left atrium. Tachycardia cycle length (TCL) is 280 msec, the paced cycle length is 240 msecs, and the post-pacing interval (PPI) measured on the left atrial electrode pair is 360 msecs, indicating that this site is not in the circuit. Abbreviations: LA = left atrium; MAP = mapping/ablation catheter; MRA = mid-right atrium; dis = distal electrode pair; Prx = proximal electrode pair. (From Van Hare GF. Catheter and surgical ablation. In: Gillette PC, Balaji S, Case CL, eds. *Cardiac Arrhythmias after Surgery for Congenital Heart Disease.* In press.)

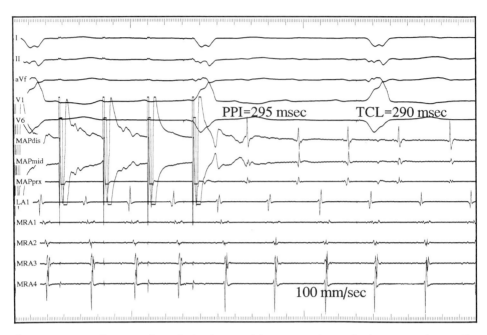

Figure 5. Intracardiac recordings during intra-atrial reentry tachycardia, in same patient as Figure 1, demonstrating entrainment pacing from the mapping catheter placed in the "flutter isthmus" after the catheter was introduced to the pulmonary venous atrium in a retrograde fashion. Note that PPI and TCL are nearly equivalent, indicating that this site is in the circuit. Abbreviations: LA = left atrium; MAP = mapping/ablation catheter; MRA = mid-right atrium; dis = distal electrode pair; Prx = proximal electrode pair. (From Van Hare GF. Catheter and surgical ablation. In: Gillette PC, Balaji S, Case CL, eds. *Cardiac Arrhythmias after Surgery for Congenital Heart Disease*. In press.)

gical details, and a plan is developed for attacking that particular substrate. This will involve placing a series of lesions in the atrial myocardium to sever the protected isthmus of atrial tissue in order to connect, by means of the radiofrequency lesions, 2 anatomic and/or surgical barriers.[11] For example, one might plan to place lesions which will "connect" the tricuspid annulus to an anterior atriotomy site. Currently, endocardial ablation of intra-atrial reentry and atrial flutter is best performed during tachycardia, until termination of tachycardia is observed. Retesting is carried out to test for inducibility, and additional lesions are placed as necessary.

Creation of a Transmural Lesion

Unfortunately, lesion formation using radiofrequency energy in patients who have postoperative arrhythmias is not as straightforward as in those whose hearts are otherwise normal. Patients who have atrial flutter in the setting of the modified Fontan procedure (atriopulmonary connection) often have an enlarged right atrium which interferes with energy delivery due to difficulty in achieving excellent catheter contact, as well as to the probable high convective heat loss associated with the large chamber volume. On the other hand, at times the target chosen for ablation turns out to be in an area of very low flow and as such, target temperature may be achieved at very low generator outputs, due to inadequate tip cooling, with consequent limited energy delivery. For macroreentrant rhythms, it is likely that larger lesions will be necessary to completely transect an isthmus of myocardium between 2 barriers, and this increases the difficulty of the procedure. Finally, it is apparent that some types of cardiac repair (such as atriopulmonary connection) are associated with significant myocardial hypertrophy and wall thickening, making the achievement of a transmural lesion difficult or impossible. Newer technology, which involves the use of catheter tip irrigation for cooling[55] will certainly influence the efficacy of these ablation procedures. The development of ablation catheters specifically designed to create long linear lesions will also doubtless contribute to improved efficacy.[56]

Assessment of Ablation Efficacy

Although it might seem to be a simple matter to determine whether or not a particular substrate for tachycardia has been successfully ablated, in practice the assessment of ablation efficacy is not at all straightforward in the postoperative patient. As will be seen, this problem stems from the large variability of macroreentrant circuits that may be seen in the electrophysiological laboratory.

In practice, there are 3 points of evidence that can be used to document a successful ablation. In order of increasing reliability, these are: 1) termination of tachycardia during radiofrequency energy application; 2) lack of tachycardia inducibility following ablation; and 3) documentation of block at a critical isthmus of conduction. These points are discussed below.

Tachycardia Termination During Application of Radiofrequency Energy

The sudden termination of an incessant tachycardia during application of radiofrequency energy is a dramatic event which strongly suggests that the lesion placed at the particular site has severed a critical isthmus of conducting tissue, or has destroyed an automatic focus (see Figure 2). In the latter case, in which an automatic focus tachycardia is mapped and ablated, it is likely that termination during RF application will be the only criteria that one may use to document success, as these tachycardias do not tend to be easily inducible, and they do not depend on conduction through a critical isthmus of tissue. In this circumstance, the focus is often responsive to medications such as isoproterenol or epinephrine, and administration of these medications after an appropriate, reasonable interval of 30–60 minutes constitutes the best that one can do to document success. In the former case, however, reliance upon RF termination as the sole criterion of a successful ablation is hazardous, for several reasons. First, such tachycardias may terminate spontaneously or in response to spontaneous premature atrial contractions, and termination may therefore be misleading. Second, RF application itself may be associated with induced premature atrial contractions, which may terminate the tachycardia without curing the substrate. Third, should termination occur during RF application, the sudden termination can be associated with catheter displacement from the critical site to another site, making it difficult to place additional lesions at the critical site. Finally, and most importantly, RF application may cause transient but not permanent block in the targeted isthmus of conducting tissue. Such block may last long enough to terminate the tachycardia by preventing conduction in a critical portion of the circuit, but may resolve after several seconds or minutes.

The observance of sudden termination may be very useful, however, in the course of a mapping procedure. Should the termination occur without premature beats which might be responsible for the termination, this finding provides evidence that the site is indeed critical to the maintenance of the tachycardia, and therefore should be targeted for additional lesions.

Lack of Inducibility of Intra-atrial Reentry

Intra-atrial reentry tachycardias are not always easily inducible at electrophysiological study, despite clearly being clinically symptomatic. Therefore, the inability to induce an arrhythmia after a possibly successful ablation is not as helpful as would be desirable, particularly if the initial induction of tachycardia was difficult or inconsistent. If one proposes to use the lack of inducibility as the primary criterion of success, it is important to spend a significant amount of time prior to the ablation documenting the best method of induction, demonstrating repeatedly that the tachycardia can be induced. Attempts at induction must include prolonged cycles of ramp pacing, consisting of atrial overdrive pacing at progressively shortening cycle lengths. In practice, one often observes patients in whom initial attempts at induction of atrial flutter by atrial burst pacing yield 2:1 capture at relatively long pacing cycle lengths, but in whom ramp pacing yields 1:1 capture at shorter cycle lengths and successful tachycardia induction. It may be that the act of ramp pacing shortens all atrial action potential durations and therefore shortens atrial refractory periods, allowing for sustained atrial reentry. Provided that such a complete and careful assessment of inducibility is performed prior to ablation, one considers the lack of inducibility following ablation, in the setting of easy inducibility prior to ablation, to be a better criterion of success than termination of tachycardia with RF ablation. Therefore, if one starts a procedure with the patient in the arrhythmia already, there is an advantage to terminating the arrhythmia by pacing, and then repeatedly reinducing the arrhythmia, prior to placing an RF ablation lesions.

Documentation of a Line of Block at a
Critical Isthmus of Conduction

In the treatment of common (Type 1) atrial flutter, with counterclockwise rotation around the tricuspid annulus, a major advance was made with the recognition that it was possible to assess the conduction patterns in the right atrium in the absence of atrial flutter, allowing assessment of the conduction through the critical isthmus between the tricuspid annulus and IVC.[57,58] This was a major advance, because it meant that one no longer needed to rely on the imperfect criteria mentioned above (termination during RF application, lack of inducibility) for documentation of success. Instead, one may now document bidirectional conduction in the isthmus before ablation, observe the development of isthmus block during RF application, and finally, demonstrate persisting bidirectional block following ablation. In this way, ablation of atrial flutter became technically similar to the ablation of, for example, an accessory pathway, in which signs of bidirectional accessory pathway block can be documented without relying on lack of tachycardia inducibility as the sole criterion of success. With the development of these techniques, reported long-term success rates for ablation of atrial flutter increased dramatically, due to the dramatically lower incidence of recurrence.[53,57,58]

Conduction in the atrial flutter isthmus may be documented in both directions. One may perform pacing from the mouth of the coronary sinus, ideally with a multipolar catheter advanced into the coronary sinus (CS) with pacing from the proximal pair of electrodes. Activation of the right atrium from this pacing site normally proceeds up the septum, as well as across the flutter isthmus to the low lateral right atrium. A 20-pole Halo catheter (Cordis-Webster, Baldwin Park, CA) positioned in the right atrium above the tricuspid annulus (Figure 6) records this pattern of activation with early activation of the low lateral right atrium and septum, and late activation at the site of collision of the 2 wave fronts (Figure 7). Following successful ablation, the septum activates normally, but the low lateral right atrium is activated much later, as the wave of activation must spread up the septum and down the lateral wall to reach the low lateral right atrium, rather than across the flutter isthmus (Figure 8).

Block in the opposite direction can be assessed by 3 methods. First, one may measure the conduction time with pacing from the low lateral right atrium to the CS os, and compare it to the conduction time from the low lateral right atrium to the atrial activation at the His bundle electrogram (HBE) site. Prior to ablation, conduction normally reaches the coronary sinus first, with the atrium at the HBE activating slightly later. Following successful ablation, the atrium at the HBE activates earlier than the CS os. Second, one may observe the morphology of the P wave with pacing from the low lateral right atrium. Prior to ablation, conduction proceeds rapidly via the flutter isthmus to activate the left atrium from below, giving rise to an inverted P wave in the inferior limb leads. Following successful ablation, the left atrium is only activated via Bachmann's bundle from above, giving rise to a different P wave morphology, with the terminal portion of the P wave being upright in the inferior leads.[59,60] Finally, one may observe the order of left atrial activation as recorded in the multipolar catheter placed in the coronary sinus during pacing of the low lateral right atrium. Prior to ablation, activation spreads from the proximal to the distal electrode pairs. Following ablation, activation can be observed to spread from the distal to the proximal pairs, again due to activation of the left atrium only via Bachmann's bundle from superior to inferior.

The use of these various maneuvers for assessing block in the flutter isth-

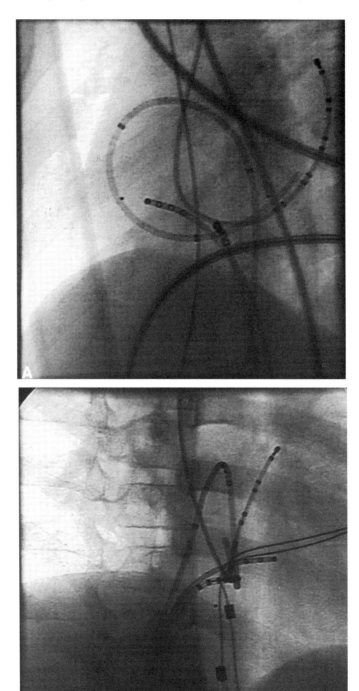

Figure 6. Fluoroscopy images of catheter positions in a patient with typical atrial flutter. Note that the coronary sinus is entered with a decapolar catheter, and a Halo catheter is deployed in the right atrium with the tip entering the coronary sinus. A: Left anterior oblique view. B: Right anterior oblique view. (From Van Hare GF. Catheter and surgical ablation. In: Gillette PC, Balaji S, Case CL, eds. *Cardiac Arrhythmias after Surgery for Congenital Heart Disease.* In press.)

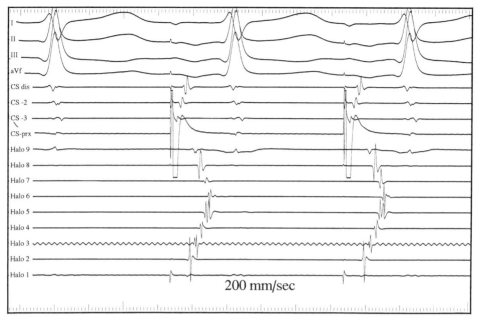

Figure 7. Intracardiac recordings during pacing of the proximal coronary sinus, in the same patient as in Figure 6, prior to radiofrequency ablation of atrial flutter. The tracing demonstrates early activation of the distal and the proximal Halo catheter electrode pairs, with later activation of the middle pairs, indicating intact conduction across the flutter isthmus.(From Van Hare GF. Catheter and surgical ablation. In: Gillette PC, Balaji S, Case CL, eds. *Cardiac Arrhythmias after Surgery for Congenital Heart Disease.* In press.)

mus makes the ablation procedure smoother, as one does not need to repeatedly induce atrial flutter after each lesion, and therefore avoids the risk of inducing atrial fibrillation inadvertently. One may continuously observe conduction via the isthmus during RF application, and can observe when block occurs in the isthmus, for example by pacing the low lateral right atrium and observing P wave morphology during RF application.

The adaptation of these techniques to the situation of the postoperative heart is challenging. As stated earlier, many patients with intra-atrial reentry essentially have the same circuit as patients with typical counterclockwise atrial flutter, proceeding either clockwise or counterclockwise.[32] Once the importance of the flutter isthmus is documented in such a patient, all of the above techniques can be used to assess conduction in the isthmus. This is straightforward in patients with atriopulmonary connections and those with simple defects such as atrial or ventricular septal defects, in which there is normal access to the right atrial structures. It is not as straightforward in patients in whom the morphologically right atrial structures are in the pulmonary venous atrium, such as patients who have undergone the Senning, Mustard, or lateral tunnel Fontan procedures. In such patients, it is unlikely that a multipolar catheter can be deployed in the pulmonary venous atrium. However, the morphology of paced P waves from the low lateral right atrium, as well as bidirectional conduction times through the isthmus, can certainly be assessed.

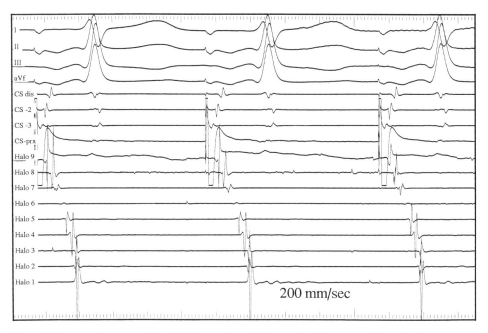

Figure 8. Intracardiac recordings during pacing of the proximal coronary sinus, in the same patient as in Figure 6, following radiofrequency ablation of atrial flutter. The tracings demonstrate early activation of only the proximal Halo catheter electrode pairs, with later activation of the distal pairs, indicating absent conduction across the flutter isthmus. (From Van Hare GF. Catheter and surgical ablation. In: Gillette PC, Balaji S, Case CL, eds. *Cardiac Arrhythmias after Surgery for Congenital Heart Disease.* In press.)

Results of Ablation Procedures in Patients Following Atrial Surgery

There are several reports of moderate-sized series of patients with intra-atrial reentry undergoing RF ablation procedures. In general, they have all shown moderately good acute success rates, with high recurrence rates, and long term success rates of no greater than 50%. Kalman et al reported the results of ablation procedures in 18 patients with 26 separate atrial tachycardias, all of whom were status post surgical repair of various forms of congenital heart disease.[35] Of these, 9 had had repair of a secundum atrial septal defect, and the rest were more complex. Initial success was achieved in 15 patients and 21 tachycardias. The highest success rates were in the patients with simple anatomy, for example atrial septal defects. At follow-up, only 9 of 18 were asymptomatic and off antiarrhythmic medications. With respect to the patients who had undergone repair of atrial septal defects, in all but one, the successful ablation site was related to an atriotomy. The atriotomy was "connected" via radiofrequency application to the tricuspid annulus in about half of tachycardias, to the IVC is about half, and rarely to the SVC.

Subsequently, Van Hare et al reported the experience of several centers with the ablation of intra-atrial reentry in 10 patients with either the Senning or the Mustard repair of transposition of the great vessels.[32] Initial success was reported in 10 of 13 tachycardias in 9 of 10 patients. In this series, it was interesting that the flutter circuit involved the flutter isthmus between the tricuspid annulus and the IVC in 8 of 13 tachycardias, and was located on the right atrial freewall in the remainder (Figure 9). Right atrial freewall circuits had to be approached by entering the right ventricle in a retrograde fashion and passing the catheter through the tricuspid valve and into the pulmonary venous atrium, where most of the original right atrial tissue is located in patients with this form of repair. Circuits that involved the flutter isthmus, in general, could be approached in an antegrade fashion via the IVC if the coronary sinus had been left to drain with the systemic venous atrium, but had to be approached in a retrograde fashion if the coronary sinus drained to the pulmonary venous atrium. Positioning of the catheter at the flutter isthmus, when introduced in a retrograde fashion, is straightforward in practice once the valve is crossed. However, maneuvering in the pulmonary venous atrium for mapping an ablation of right atrial freewall circuits is quite a bit more difficult.

Triedman et al reported findings in a group of 10 patients, most of whom had complex atrial anatomy and had undergone variations of the Fontan procedure.[33] At least one circuit was ablated in 8 of 10 patients, with recurrence documented at follow-up in 4 of 8. Subsequently, the same investigators re-

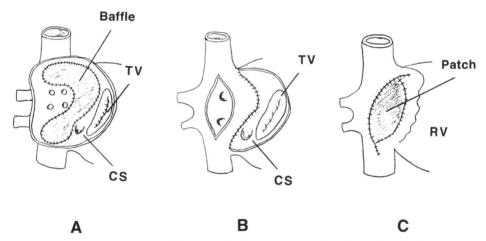

A   **B**   **C**

Figure 9. Most common surgically-created substrates for atrial tachycardia after the Senning and Mustard procedures. Panel A is a view of the Mustard procedure from pulmonary venous atrium, looking down on tricuspid valve annulus. Surgery involved resection of a large amount of atrium septum, leaving a rim of septum between the eventual baffle suture line and the coronary sinus os and tricuspid annulus. Panel B shows a view of the Senning procedure from the pulmonary venous atrium. The second suture line is shown where the right atrial wall is anastomosed to the ridge of atrial septum. Similar to the Mustard procedure, a rim of atrial septal tissue is left in the region of the mouth of the coronary sinus and tricuspid annulus. Panel C is a view of Senning procedure following final suture closure of pulmonary venous atrium, in which patch augmentation of the right atrium has been performed. This wide atrial incision leaves a rim of anterior right atrial wall bounded by the atriotomy on one side and the tricuspid annulus on the other side. (From Van Hare GF, Lesh MD, Ross BA, et al. Mapping and radiofrequency ablation of atrial tachyarrhythmias after the Senning or Mustard procedure for transposition of the great arteries. *Am J Cardiol* 1996;77:985–991.)

ported further experience with 55 procedures in 45 patients, with initial success of at least one circuit in 73%, and a 53% incidence of recurrence.[61] Often, clinical improvement was observed, based on a decreased incidence of tachycardia episodes, despite the recurrence of tachycardia. Sites of successful ablation were categorized by these investigators based on where sudden termination of tachycardia was observed during radiofrequency application, making the assumption that complete block at that site had been at least transiently achieved. While successful sites were reported throughout the atrium, these sites tended to cluster around the flutter zone, and along the lateral right atrial wall, both near the SVC junction and the IVC junction.

Finally, Baker et al reported their results in 14 patients with intra-atrial reentry following congenital heart disease surgery.[34] The patient group had primarily complex cardiac anatomy, with only 2 having had simple repair of an atrial septal defect. Of 31 tachycardias induced, 17 were targeted for ablation attempts, and successful ablation was achieved in 13 of 14 patients. In nearly all, the tachycardia was successfully ablated by placing lesions between the atriotomy and either the IVC or SVC. Recurrence was seen in 6 of 13 initially successful patients, all of whom underwent repeat ablation successfully.

Conclusion

In most cases of intra-atrial reentrant tachycardia in the setting of repaired congenital heart disease, definitive treatment should be preferable to long-term antiarrhythmic therapy, especially when one considers the numerous potential side effects of antiarrhythmic medication in this patient population. Unfortunately, to date the results of catheter ablation of atrial reentrant tachycardia are not as good as for ablation of more routine arrhythmias in the population of patients with otherwise normal hearts. While this may partly be due to a lack of understanding of the exact macroreentrant circuits that exist in each patient, and limitations in the ability to map with high resolution, it is more likely that the ability to make long linear and transmural lesions is suboptimal. Future progress in catheter and lesion formation technology, as well as further experience with surgical ablation, may allow more such patients to benefit from the advantages of definitive cure.

References

1. Garson AJ, Bink BM, Hesslein PS, et al. Atrial flutter in the young: a collaborative study of 380 cases. *J Am Coll Cardiol* 1985;6:871.
2. Champsaur GL, Sokol DM, Trusler GA, et al. Repair of transposition of the great arteries in 123 pediatric patients: Early and long-term results. *Circulation* 1973;47:1032.
3. Hagler DJ, Ritter DG, Mair DD, et al. Clinical, angiographic, and hemodynamic assessment of late results after Mustard operation. *Circulation* 1978;57:1214.

4. Gilljam T. Transposition of the great arteries in western Sweden 1964–83. Incidence, survival, complications and modes of death. *Acta Paediatr* 1996;85:825.

5. Gelatt M, Hamilton RM, McCrindle BW, et al. Arrhythmia and mortality after the Mustard procedure: a 30-year single-center experience. *J Am Coll Cardiol* 1997;29:194.

6. Vetter VL, Tanner CS, Horowitz LN. Inducible atrial flutter after the Mustard repair of complete transposition of the great arteries. *Am J Cardiol* 1988;61:428.

7. Bink-Boelkens MT, Velvis H, van der Heide JJ, et al. Dysrhythmias after atrial surgery in children. *Am Heart J* 1983;106:125.

8. Flinn CJ, Wolff GS, Dick MD, et al. Cardiac rhythm after the Mustard operation for complete transposition of the great arteries. *N Engl J Med* 1984;310:1635.

9. Duster MC, Bink-Boelkens MT, Wampler D, et al. Long-term follow-up of dysrhythmias following the Mustard procedure. *Am Heart J* 1985;109:1323.

10. Vetter VL, Tanner CS. Electrophysiological consequences of the arterial switch repair of d-transposition of the great arteries. *J Am Coll Cardiol* 1988;12:229.

11. Lesh MD, Van Hare GF, Epstein LM, et al. Radiofrequency catheter ablation of atrial arrhythmias: results and mechanisms. *Circulation* 1994;89:1074.

12. Alboliras ET, Porter CB, Danielson GK, et al. Results of the modified Fontan operation for congenital heart lesions in patients without preoperative sinus rhythm. *J Am Coll Cardiol* 1985;6:228.

13. Kurer CC, Tanner CS, Norwood WI, et al. Perioperative arrhythmias after Fontan repair. *Circulation* 1990;82:IV190.

14. Balaji S, Gewillig M, Bull C, et al. Arrhythmias after the Fontan procedure. Comparison of total cavopulmonary connection and atriopulmonary connection. *Circulation* 1991;84:III162.

15. Gewillig M, Wyse RK, de Leval MR, et al. Early and late arrhythmias after the Fontan operation: predisposing factors and clinical consequences [see comments]. *Br Heart J* 1992;67:72.

16. Porter CJ, Garson A. Incidence and management of dysrhythmias after Fontan procedure. *Herz* 1993;18:318.

17. Fishberger SB, Wernovsky G, Gentles TL, et al. Factors that influence the development of atrial flutter after the Fontan operation. *J Thorac Cardiovasc Surg* 1997;113:80.

18. Waldo AL, MacLean WA, Karp RB, et al. Entrainment and interruption of atrial flutter with atrial pacing: studies in man following open heart surgery. *Circulation* 1977;56:737.

19. Olshansky B, Okumura K, Henthorn RW, et al. Characterization of double potentials in human atrial flutter: studies during transient entrainment. *J Am Coll Cardiol* 1990;15:833.

20. Lesh MD, Van Hare GF, Fitzpatrick AP, et al. Curing reentrant atrial arrhythmias: targeting protected zones of slow conduction by catheter ablation. *J Electrocardiol* 1993;26:194.

21. Olgin JE, Kalman JM, Fitzpatrick AP, et al. Role of right atrial endocardial structures as barriers to conduction during human type I atrial flutter: ac-

tivation and entrainment mapping guided by intracardiac echocardiography. *Circulation* 1995;92:1839.

22. Feld GK. Catheter ablation for the treatment of atrial tachycardia. *Prog Cardiovasc Dis* 1995;37:205.

23. Poty H, Saoudi N, Nair M, et al. Radiofrequency catheter ablation of atrial flutter. Further insights into the various types of isthmus block: application to ablation during sinus rhythm. *Circulation* 1996;94:3204.

24. Kalman JM, Olgin JE, Saxon LA, et al. Activation and entrainment mapping defines the tricuspid annulus as the anterior barrier in typical atrial flutter [see comments]. *Circulation* 1996;94:398.

25. Olgin JE, Kalman JM, Saxon LA, et al. Mechanism of initiation of atrial flutter in humans: site of unidirectional block and direction of rotation. *J Am Coll Cardiol* 1997;29:376.

26. Waldo AL, Henthorn RW. Use of transient entrainment during ventricular tachycardia to localize a critical area in the reentry circuit for ablation. *PACE* 1989;12:231.

27. Fontaine G, Evans S, Frank R, et al. Ventricular tachycardia overdrive and entrainment with and without fusion: its relevance to the catheter ablation of ventricular tachycardia. *Clin Cardiol* 1990;13:797.

28. Morady F, Kadish A, Rosenheck S, et al. Concealed entrainment as a guide for catheter ablation of ventricular tachycardia in patients with prior myocardial infarction. *J Am Coll Cardiol* 1991;17:678.

29. Stevenson WG, Khan H, Sager P, et al. Identification of reentry circuit sites during catheter mapping and radiofrequency ablation of ventricular tachycardia late after myocardial infarction. *Circulation* 1993;88:1647.

30. Stevenson WG, Friedman PL, Sager PT, et al. Exploring postinfarction reentrant ventricular tachycardia with entrainment mapping. *J Am Coll Cardiol* 1997;29:1180.

31. Van Hare GF, Lesh MD, Stanger P. Radiofrequency catheter ablation of supraventricular arrhythmias in patients with congenital heart disease: results and technical considerations. *J Am Coll Cardiol* 1993;22:883.

32. Van Hare GF, Lesh MD, Ross BA, et al. Mapping and radiofrequency ablation of intraatrial reentrant tachycardia after the Senning or Mustard procedure for transposition of the great arteries. *Am J Cardiol* 1996;77:985.

33. Triedman JK, Saul JP, Weindling SN, et al. Radiofrequency ablation of intra-atrial reentrant tachycardia after surgical palliation of congenital heart disease. *Circulation* 1995;91:707.

34. Baker BM, Lindsay BD, Bromberg BI, et al. Catheter ablation of clinical intraatrial reentrant tachycardias resulting from previous atrial surgery: localizing and transecting the critical isthmus. *J Am Coll Cardiol* 1996;28:411.

35. Kalman JM, Van Hare GF, Olgin JE, et al. Ablation of "incisional" reentrant atrial tachycardia complicating surgery for congenital heart disease: use of entrainment to define a critical isthmus of conduction. *Circulation* 1996;93:502.

36. Triedman JK, Jenkins KJ, Colan SD, et al. Intra-atrial reentrant tachycardia after palliation of congenital heart disease: characterization of multiple macroreentrant circuits using fluoroscopically based three-dimensional endocardial mapping. *J Cardiovasc Electrophysiol* 1997;8:259.

37. Puech P. Le flutter et ses limites. *Arch Mal Coeur* 1970;61:116.
38. Cosio FC. Endocardial mapping of atrial flutter. In: Touboul P, Waldo AL, eds. *Atrial Arrhythmias.* St. Louis, MO: Mosby Year Book, 1990. pp 229.
39. Olshansky B, Okumura K, Hess PG, et al. Demonstration of an area of slow conduction in human atrial flutter. *J Am Coll Cardiol* 1990;16:1634.
40. Rodefeld MD, Bromberg BI, Schuessler RB, et al. Atrial flutter after lateral tunnel construction in the modified Fontan operation: a canine model. *J Thorac Cardiovasc Surg* 1996;111:514.
41. Gandhi SK, Bromberg BI, Rodefeld MD, et al. Lateral tunnel suture line variation reduces atrial flutter after the modified Fontan operation. *Ann Thorac Surg* 1996;61:1299.
42. Shim D, Lloyd TR, Cho KJ, et al. Transhepatic cardiac catheterization in children: evaluation of efficacy and safety. *Circulation* 1995;92:1526.
43. Sommer RJ, Golinko RJ, Mitty HA. Initial experience with percutaneous transhepatic cardiac catheterization in infants and children. *Am J Cardiol* 1995;75:1289.
44. Lesh MD, Van Hare GF, Scheinman MM, et al. Comparison of the retrograde and transseptal methods for ablation of left free wall accessory pathways. *J Am Coll Cardiol* 1993;22:542.
45. Lai WW, al-Khatib Y, Klitzner TS, et al. Biplanar transesophageal echocardiographic direction of radiofrequency catheter ablation in children and adolescents with the Wolff-Parkinson-White syndrome. *Am J Cardiol* 1993;71:872.
46. Drant SE, Klitzner TS, Shannon KM, et al. Guidance of radiofrequency catheter ablation by transesophageal echocardiography in children with palliated single ventricle. *Am J Cardiol* 1995;76:1311.
47. Tucker KJ, Curtis AB, Murphy J, et al. Transesophageal echocardiographic guidance of transseptal left heart catheterization during radiofrequency ablation of left-sided accessory pathways in humans. *PACE* 1996;19:272.
48. Shpun S, Gepstein L, Hayam G, et al. Guidance of radiofrequency endocardial ablation with real-time three-dimensional magnetic navigation system. *Circulation* 1997;96:2016.
49. Khoury DS, Taccardi B, Lux RL, et al. Reconstruction of endocardial potentials and activation sequences from intracavitary probe measurements. Localization of pacing sites and effects of myocardial structure. *Circulation* 1995;91:845.
50. Liu ZW, Jia P, Ershler PR, et al. Noncontact endocardial mapping: reconstruction of electrograms and isochrones from intracavitary probe potentials. *J Cardiovasc Electrophysiol* 1997;8:415.
51. Mines GR. On circulating excitation in heart muscles and their possible relations to tachycardia and fibrillation. *Trans R Soc Can* 1914;8 (ser III, sec IV):43.
52. Chinitz LA, Bernstein NE, O'Connor B, et al. Mapping reentry around atriotomy scars using double potentials. *PACE* 1996;19:1978.
53. Nakagawa H, Lazzara R, Khastgir T, et al. Role of the tricuspid annulus and the eustachian valve/ridge on atrial flutter: relevance to catheter ablation of the septal isthmus and a new technique for rapid identification of ablation success [see comments]. *Circulation* 1996;94:407.

54. Stevenson WG. Functional approach to site-by-site catheter mapping of ventricular reentry circuits in chronic infarctions. *J Electrocardiol* 1995;27 (suppl):130.

55. Nakagawa H, Yamanashi WS, Pitha JV, et al. Comparison of in vivo tissue temperature profile and lesion geometry for radiofrequency ablation with a saline-irrigated electrode versus temperature control in a canine thigh muscle preparation. *Circulation* 1995;91:2264.

56. Haïssaguerre M, Gencel L, Fischer B, et al. Successful catheter ablation of atrial fibrillation. *J Cardiovasc Electrophysiol* 1994;5:1045.

57. Poty H, Saoudi N, Abdel Aziz A, et al. Radiofrequency catheter ablation of type 1 atrial flutter. Prediction of late success by electrophysiological criteria. *Circulation* 1995;92:1389.

58. Cauchemez B, Haïssaguerre M, Fischer B, et al. Electrophysiological effects of catheter ablation of IVC-tricuspid annulus isthmus in common atrial flutter. *Circulation* 1996;93:284.

59. Mackall JA, Ozin B, Carlson MD, et al. A simple predictor of successful radiofrequency ablation of atrial flutter. *Circulation* 1996;94:I.

60. Hamdan MH, Kalman JM, Barron HV, et al. P wave morphology during right atrial pacing before and after atrial flutter ablation—a new marker for success. *Am J Cardiol* 1997;79:1417.

61. Triedman JK, Bergau DM, Saul JP, et al. Efficacy of radiofrequency ablation for control of intra-atrial reentrant tachycardia in patients with congenital heart disease. *J Am Coll Cardiol* 1997;30:1032.

Chapter 12

Radiofrequency Catheter Ablation for the Treatment of Type 1 Counterclockwise and Clockwise Atrial Flutter

Gregory K. Feld, M.D.,
Ulrika Birgersdotter-Green, M.D., and
Michael E. Mollerus, M.D.

Introduction

Atrial flutter is a relatively common arrhythmia which may cause significant symptoms, including palpitations, chest pain, shortness of breath, and even syncope. Potential serious complications associated with atrial flutter include embolic stroke, myocardial ischemia and infarction, and, rarely, a tachycardia-induced cardiomyopathy due to rapid atrioventricular (AV) conduction. Atrial flutter is relatively resistant to pharmacological suppression, and consequently alternative nonpharmacological treatments have been developed. Previously, antiarrhythmic surgery and AV node ablation with pacemaker implantation were performed, but more recently radiofrequency catheter ablation has been demonstrated to safely cure Type 1 atrial flutter, resulting in its rapid acceptance as first line therapy. Several techniques have been described for ablating atrial flutter, including first an electrophysiologically guided approach targeting the exits from an area of slow conduction in the low posterior right atrium, and subsequently anatomically guided approaches targeting the sub-eustachian (SE) isthmuses, including the tricuspid valve-inferior vena cava (TV-IVC) isthmus, or the tricuspid valve-coronary sinus (TV-CS) and coronary sinus-inferior vena cava (CS-IVC) isthmuses.[1-6] This chapter will review the

From Huang SKS, Wilber DJ (eds.): *Radiofrequency Catheter Ablation of Cardiac Arrhythmias: Basic Concepts and Clinical Applications,* 2nd ed. Armonk, NY: Futura Publishing Company, Inc. ©2000.

mechanism of human Type 1 atrial flutter, and techniques for its diagnosis, mapping, and ablation.

Mechanism of Atrial Flutter

The development of successful radiofrequency catheter ablation techniques for human Type 1 atrial flutter was dependent in part on the delineation of its electrophysiological mechanism. Through the use of advanced electrophysiological techniques, including intraoperative and transcatheter activation mapping,[1-9] Type 1 atrial flutter was determined to be due to a macro-reentrant circuit rotating in either a counterclockwise (common) or clockwise (uncommon) direction in the right atrium, with an area of relatively slow conduction velocity in the low posterior right atrium (Figure 1). This zone of slow conduction in the reentry circuit is located anatomically within the SE isthmus, through which conduction times may reach 80–100 milliseconds, or one-third to one-half the atrial flutter cycle length.[10] The SE isthmus is anatomically bounded by the inferior vena cava and eustachian ridge posteriorly and the tricuspid valve annulus anteriorly (see Figure 1), both of which form lines of conduction block or barriers creating a protected zone in the reentry circuit.[11] That the eustachian ridge forms a line of block[11-13] is suggested by the recording of double potentials along its length during atrial flutter (Figure 2A). Double potentials have also been recorded along the crista terminalis,[11-13] suggesting that it too forms a line of block separating the smooth septal right atrium from the trabeculated right atrial free wall (Figure 2B). Such lines of block (that is, either functional or anatomic) may be necessary to create an adequate path length for reentry to be sustained, even in the presence of an area of slow conduction.[14] The SE isthmus is anatomically contiguous with the interatrial septum near the coronary sinus ostium and with the low lateral right atrium near the inferior vena cava (see Figure 1), corresponding electrophysiologically to the exit and entrance to the zone of slow conduction, depending on whether the direction of reentry is counterclockwise or clockwise in the right atrium.[1] The path of the reentrant circuit outside the confines of the SE isthmus is controversial, but probably consists of a broad activation wavefront in the interatrial septum and right atrial free wall around the crista terminalis and around the tricuspid valve annulus (see Figure 1) in either a counterclockwise or clockwise direction depending on the direction of reentry through the SE isthmus.[11-12,15]

The slower conduction velocity in the SE isthmus, relative to the interatrial septum and right atrial free wall, may be caused by anisotropic fiber orientation.[10,14,16-17] This may also predispose to development of unidirectional block during rapid atrial pacing, and account for the observation that counterclockwise atrial flutter is more likely to be induced when pacing is performed from the coronary sinus ostium and conversely clockwise atrial flutter is more likely to be induced when pacing from the low lateral right atrium.[18] This is further supported by observations in animal studies which suggest that the direction of rotation of the reentrant wavefront during atrial flutter may be dependent on the direction of the paced wavefront producing unidirectional block at the time of its induction.[19] This area of slow conduction was presumed to be a critical zone

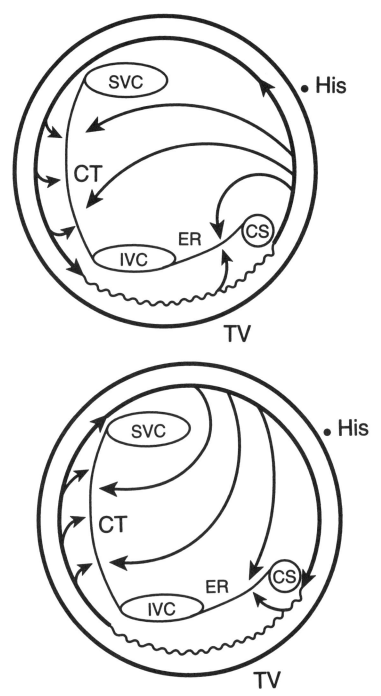

Figure 1. Schematic diagrams showing the activation patterns in common (panel A, top) and uncommon (panel B, bottom) forms of human Type 1 atrial flutter, as viewed from below the tricuspid valve annulus (TV) looking up into the right atrium. In the common form of Type 1 atrial flutter the reentrant wavefront rotates counterclockwise in the right atrium, whereas in the uncommon form reentry is clockwise. Note that the eustachian ridge (ER) and crista terminalis (CT) form lines of block, and that an area of slow conduction is present in the isthmus between the inferior vena cava and eustachian ridge and the tricuspid valve annulus. CS = coronary sinus ostium; His = His bundle; IVC and SVC = inferior and superior vena caval orifices; TV = tricuspid valve annulus.

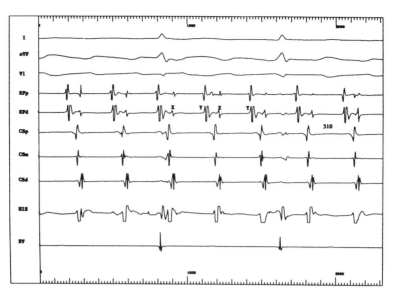

Figure 2A. Surface ECG leads I, aVF, and V$_1$, and endocardial electrograms in a patient with common Type 1 atrial flutter. An example of double potentials (XY) recorded along the eustachian ridge are shown (RFd). Note that the X and Y potentials straddle the onset of the initial down stroke of the F wave in lead aVF, indicating that the X potential is recorded immediately after the activation wavefront exits the SE isthmus and circulates around the coronary sinus above the eustachian ridge, while the Y potential is recorded after the activation wavefront rotates entirely around the atrium and is proceeding through the SE isthmus below the eustachian ridge. Double potentials may similarly be recorded along the crista terminalis.

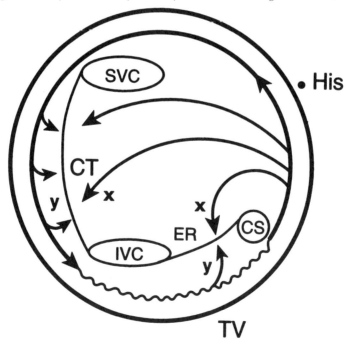

Figure 2B. A schematic diagram of the right atrium indicates where such double potentials (XY) may be recorded along the eustachian ridge and crista terminalis during common Type 1 atrial flutter. CSp,m,d = electrograms from the proximal, middle, and distal electrode pairs on a quadripolar catheter in the coronary sinus with the proximal pair at the ostium; His = electrogram from the His bundle catheter; RFp,d = electrograms from the proximal and distal electrode pairs of the mapping/ablation catheter with the distal pair positioned on the eustachian ridge.

in the reentry circuit, and was thus the target for ablation in the electrophysiologically guided approach first described for radiofrequency catheter ablation of atrial flutter.[1] It is now known that this area of slow conduction is located in the SE isthmus, which is the target for ablation in the currently preferred anatomically guided approach.[2-7]

Diagnosis and Mapping of Type 1 Atrial Flutter

The surface 12-lead ECG is helpful in establishing a diagnosis of Type 1 atrial flutter, at least the common form due to counterclockwise reentry in the right atrium. In common Type 1 atrial flutter an inverted F wave with a sawtooth pattern is observed in the inferior leads II, III, and aVF, with low amplitude biphasic F waves in leads I and aVL, an upright F wave in precordial lead V_1, with transition to an inverted F wave in lead V_6 (Figure 3A). In contrast, in the uncommon form of Type 1 atrial flutter the F wave pattern on the 12-lead ECG is less specific and variable (Figure 3B). However, since the common and uncommon forms of Type 1 atrial flutter use the same reentry circuit but in opposite directions, their rates are usually similar.

Despite the utility of the 12-lead ECG in making a presumptive diagnosis of Type 1 atrial flutter, an electrophysiological study with mapping and entrainment must be performed to confirm the underlying mechanism if radiofrequency catheter ablation is to be performed. For the electrophysiological study of atrial flutter, multi-electrode catheters are positioned in the right atrium, right ventricular apex, His bundle region, and coronary sinus using Seldinger percutaneous technique. In addition, to more precisely elucidate the endocardial activation sequence, a Halo 20-electrode mapping catheter (Cordis-Webster, Inc., Fremont, CA) or 2 steerable decapolar catheters are positioned around the tricuspid valve annulus or the interatrial septum and right atrial free wall, respectively (Figure 4).

In patients presenting in sustained atrial flutter, mapping may proceed immediately after positioning catheters in the heart. However, in patients presenting in sinus rhythm it is necessary to induce atrial flutter in order to confirm its mechanism. Induction of atrial flutter is accomplished by atrial programmed stimulation or burst pacing. Preferred pacing sites are the coronary sinus ostium and low lateral right atrium, since the type of atrial flutter induced may be dependent in part on the pacing site (counterclockwise or clockwise, respectively).

During electrophysiological study, a diagnosis of either the common or the uncommon form of Type 1 atrial flutter is suggested by observing a counterclockwise or clockwise activation pattern in the right atrium and around the tricuspid valve annulus, respectively. For example, as seen in Figure 5 in a patient with common Type 1 atrial flutter, the atrial electrogram recorded at the coronary sinus ostium is timed with the initial down stroke of the F wave in the inferior surface ECG leads, followed by caudal-to-cranial activation in the interatrial septum, and then cranial-to-caudal activation in the right atrial free wall, indicating that the underlying mechanism is a counterclockwise macro-reentry circuit with electrical activity encompassing the entire tachycardia cy-

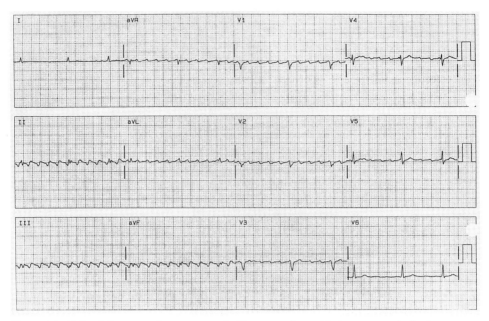

Figure 3A. 12-lead electrocardiogram recorded from a patient with the counterclockwise or common form of Type 1 atrial flutter. Note the typical saw-toothed pattern of inverted F waves in the inferior leads II, III, and aVF. Common Type 1 atrial flutter is also characterized by flat to biphasic F waves in I and aVL respectively, an upright F wave in V_1 and an inverted F wave in V_6.

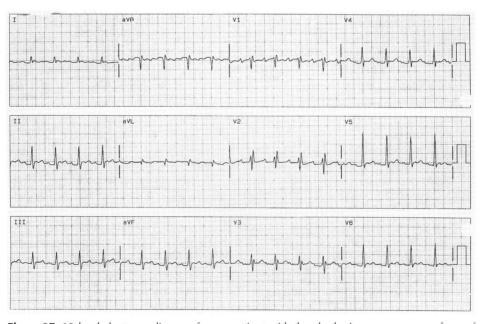

Figure 3B. 12-lead electrocardiogram from a patient with the clockwise or uncommon form of Type 1 atrial flutter. The F wave pattern in the uncommon form may occasionally manifest as the mirror image of the common form, but discrete F waves are often not seen and the pattern is variable from patient to patient. In this case the F waves are upright in the inferior leads II, III, aVF, biphasic in leads I, aVL and V_1, and upright in V_6.

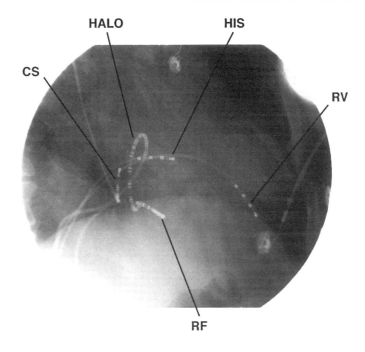

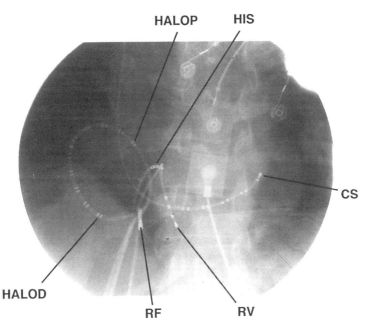

Figure 4. Right anterior oblique (panel A, top) and left anterior oblique (panel B, bottom) fluoroscopic projections showing the intracardiac positions of the right ventricular (RV), His bundle (HIS), coronary sinus (CS), Halo (HALO), and mapping/ablation catheter (RΓ). Note that the Halo catheter is positioned around the tricuspid valve annulus, with the proximal electrode pair (HALOP) at 1 o'clock and the distal electrode pair (HALOD) at 7 o'clock. The mapping/ablation catheter is positioned in the SE isthmus, midway between the interatrial septum and low lateral right atrium, with the distal ablation electrode near the tricuspid valve annulus.

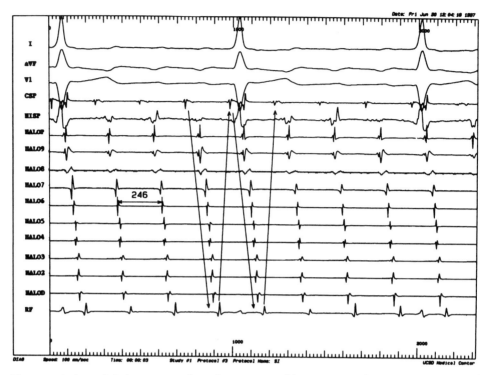

Figure 5. Endocardial electrograms from the mapping/ablation (RF), Halo, coronary sinus, and His bundle catheters, and surface ECG leads I, aVF, and V_1, demonstrating a counterclockwise rotation of activation in the right atrium in a patient with the common form of Type 1 atrial flutter. The atrial flutter cycle length was 246 milliseconds. Halo D-P = 10 bipolar electrograms recorded from the distal (low lateral right atrium) to proximal (high right atrium) poles of the 20 pole Halo catheter positioned around the tricuspid valve annulus with the proximal electrode pair at 1 o'clock and the distal electrode pair at 7 o'clock; CSP = electrograms recorded from the coronary sinus catheter proximal electrode pair positioned at the ostium; HISP = electrograms recorded from the proximal electrode pair of the His bundle catheter; RF = electrograms recorded from the mapping/ablation catheter positioned with the distal electrode pair in the SE isthmus.

cle length. Furthermore, confirmation that the reentry circuit uses the SE isthmus requires the demonstration of the classical criteria for entrainment, including concealed entrainment during pacing from the low posterior right atrium.[5] Criteria for demonstrating concealed entrainment of atrial flutter include tachycardia acceleration to the pacing cycle length without a change in the F wave pattern on surface ECG (Figure 6) or in the endocardial atrial activation pattern and electrogram morphology on intracardiac recordings, and the immediate resumption of the tachycardia at the original cycle length upon termination of pacing, including the first postpacing interval (Figure 7). When pacing entrainment is performed within the SE isthmus, the stimulus-to-F wave interval during pacing and the local electrogram-to-F wave interval during atrial flutter should be similar, when referenced to the initial down stroke of the inverted F wave in the inferior leads II, III and aVF on surface ECG (see Figure 7). Furthermore, during counterclockwise atrial flutter the stimulus-to-F wave and local electrogram-to-F wave intervals will be shorter when the pac-

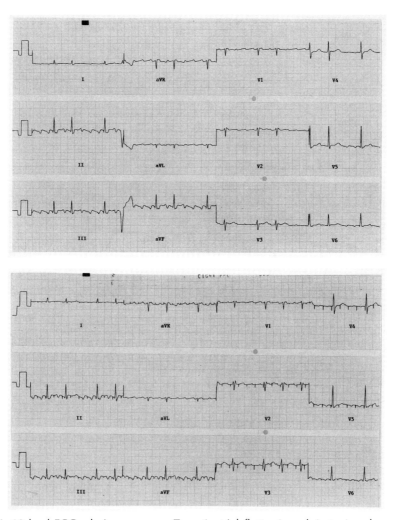

Figure 6. 12-lead ECGs during common Type 1 atrial flutter (panel A, top) and pacing entrainment (panel B, bottom) of common Type 1 atrial flutter. Note that the F wave morphology is unchanged during pacing compared to atrial flutter, indicating concealed entrainment. Furthermore, the stimulus-to-F wave interval is long, approximately 80 milliseconds, suggesting that the pacing site is relatively lateral in the SE isthmus resulting in a long conduction time through this area of slow conduction to the exit near the coronary sinus ostium.

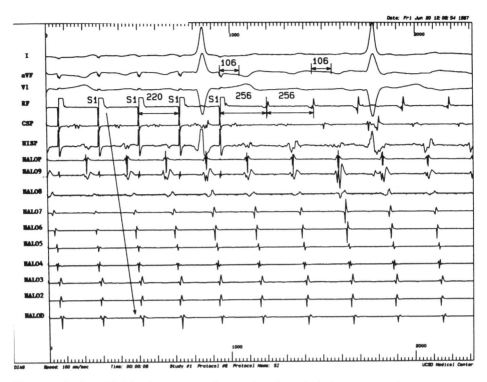

Figure 7. Surface ECG leads I, aVF, and V$_1$ and endocardial electrograms during pacing entrainment of common Type 1 atrial flutter via the mapping/ablation catheter (RF) positioned at the tricuspid valve-inferior vena cava (TV-IVC) isthmus. During pacing entrainment the tachycardia is accelerated to a cycle length of 220 milliseconds, but with termination of pacing there is immediate resumption of the tachycardia at a cycle length of 256 milliseconds on the first postpacing interval. Note that the F wave pattern on the surface ECG leads and the endocardial electrogram pattern are unchanged during pacing compared to those during atrial flutter, indicating concealed entrainment. During atrial flutter, local activation at the TV-IVC isthmus (RF) is approximately 106 milliseconds before the initial downstroke of the F wave in lead aVF. During pacing entrainment the stimulus-to-F wave interval is approximately 106 milliseconds as well. This suggests that the mapping/ablation catheter (RF) is located within the reentrant circuit. S1 = pacing stimulus artifact. All other abbreviations are the same as in previous figures.

ing site is medial near the exit from the SE isthmus (e.g. 30–50 milliseconds) and longer when the pacing site is lateral near the entrance to the SE isthmus (e.g. 80–100 milliseconds); during clockwise atrial flutter, the converse will be true. In contrast, pacing at sites outside the SE isthmus will result in overt entrainment of atrial flutter with variable degrees of constant fusion of the F wave pattern and endocardial atrial electrograms.

The uncommon form of Type 1 atrial flutter[6] is diagnosed electrophysiologically by demonstrating clockwise activation around the right atrium and tricuspid valve annulus, with cranial-to-caudal activation in the interatrial septum and caudal-to-cranial activation in the right atrial free wall, the opposite of that seen in the common form of Type 1 atrial flutter (Figure 8). In a manner similar to that described above for common Type 1 atrial flutter, entrainment may also be used in the uncommon form of Type 1 atrial flutter to confirm that the reentry circuit utilizes the SE isthmus, but in the opposite direction (Figure 9).

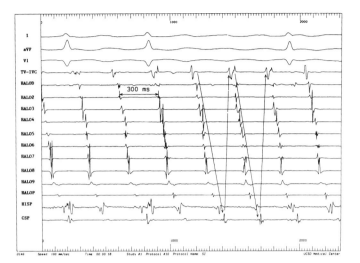

Figure 8. Surface ECG leads I, aVF, and V$_1$, and endocardial electrograms from the right atrial free wall, coronary sinus ostium, and His bundle region, demonstrating a clockwise rotation of activation in the right atrium in a patient with the uncommon form of Type 1 atrial flutter. The atrial flutter cycle length was 240 milliseconds. Halo D-P = bipolar electrograms from the distal to proximal electrode pairs on a 20-pole Halo catheter positioned along the right atrial free wall, with the distal pair positioned in the low lateral right atrium and the proximal pair in the high lateral right atrium. All other abbreviations are the same as in previous figures.

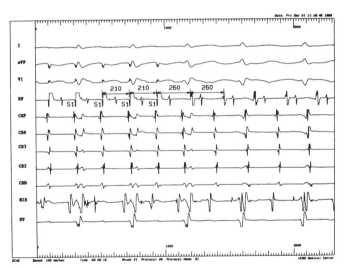

Figure 9. Surface ECG leads I, aVF, and V$_1$ and endocardial electrograms during pacing entrainment of uncommon Type 1 atrial flutter via the mapping/ablation catheter (RF) positioned at the lateral TV-IVC isthmus. During pacing entrainment the tachycardia is accelerated to a cycle length of 210 milliseconds, but with termination of pacing there is immediate resumption of the tachycardia at a cycle length of 260 milliseconds on the first postpacing interval. Note that the F wave pattern on the surface ECG leads and the endocardial electrogram pattern are unchanged during pacing compared to those during atrial flutter, indicating concealed entrainment. CSP,4,3,2,D = proximal to distal electrode pairs on a decapolar coronary sinus catheter, with the proximal electrode pair positioned at the ostium. All other abbreviations are the same as in previous figures.

Radiofrequency Catheter Ablation Techniques
for Cure of Atrial Flutter

Radiofrequency catheter ablation of Type 1 atrial flutter is performed with a steerable mapping/ablation catheter with a large distal ablation electrode 4–8 mm in length, positioned in the right atrium via a femoral vein.[1–6,20–23] The typical radiofrequency generator used by most laboratories is capable of automatically adjusting applied power (for instance, up to 50 watts) in order to achieve a tissue-electrode interface temperature that is programmed by the operator. Tissue temperature is monitored via a thermistor or thermocouple embedded in the distal ablation electrode. Automatic power control is important, since successful ablation requires a stable temperature of at least 50°C to 60°C, while temperatures in excess of 90°C may cause tissue vaporization and charring and formation of blood coagulum on the ablation electrode, resulting in a rise in impedance which limits energy delivery and lesion formation. A variety of mapping/ablation catheters and radiofrequency generators—e.g., EP Technologies, Inc. (Sunnyvale, CA) or Medtronic CardioRhythm, Inc. (Minneapolis, MN)—are currently available.

The currently preferred target for ablation is the TV-IVC isthmus, which can be localized using either a strictly anatomically guided approach or a combined electrophysiological and anatomically guided approach.[1–6,20-23] In an anatomically guided approach, a steerable mapping/ablation catheter is positioned using fluoroscopy alone (see Figure 4A and 4B) in the TV-IVC isthmus with the distal ablation electrode on or near the TV annulus in the right anterior oblique (RAO) view, midway between the interatrial septum and low right atrial free wall in the left anterior oblique view (LAO). In the combined electrophysiologically and anatomically guided approach, the ablation catheter is first positioned fluoroscopically in the midportion of the TV-IVC isthmus on or near the tricuspid valve annulus and its location is then confirmed electrophysiologically by demonstrating concealed entrainment, with a stimulus-to-F wave interval during pacing and local electrogram-to-F wave interval during atrial flutter of approximately 50–80 milliseconds, as described above. In addition, the ratio of atrial and ventricular electrogram amplitude may help localize the position of the ablation electrode in the TV-IVC isthmus, relative to the tricuspid valve annulus and inferior vena cava. For example, the AV ratio is typically 1:4 or less at the tricuspid valve annulus, 1: 2 to 1:1 within the TV-IVC isthmus, and 2:1 to 4:1 near the inferior vena cava.

With the anatomic or combined approach, after positioning the ablation catheter on or near the tricuspid valve annulus it is either gradually withdrawn toward the inferior vena cava during a continuous energy application, or in a stepwise manner with interrupted energy application.[2–6] Using a combined approach, electrogram recordings and pacing entrainment may be used in addition to fluoroscopy to ensure that the ablation electrode is in contact with viable tissue in the TV-IVC isthmus before each energy application.[1–6,20–23] Ablation of the entire TV-IVC isthmus (Figure 10) may require several sequential energy applications of 30–60 seconds during a stepwise catheter pullback, or a prolonged energy application of up to 120 seconds or more during a continuous catheter pullback. Alternatively, ablation of the TV-CS and CS-IVC isthmuses (see Figure 10)

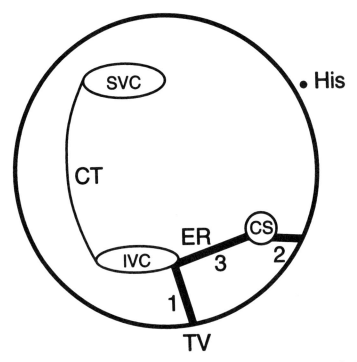

Figure 10. Schematic diagram of the right atrium showing the typical location for linear ablation of the TV-IVC isthmus (line 1), or the tricuspid valve-coronary sinus (line 2) and coronary sinus-inferior vena cava (line 3) isthmuses.

may be performed using an anatomic or combined approach in virtually an identical manner to that used to ablate the TV-IVC isthmus. However, for this approach to be successful it is probably necessary to ablate within the coronary sinus ostium as well.[1–6] It has also been recently reported that Type 1 atrial flutter may be cured by ablating between the tricuspid valve annulus and eustachian ridge, which is a narrower isthmus than the TV-IVC isthmus.[24]

In difficult cases in which the right atrium is enlarged, or the SE isthmus is very wide or deeply recessed, specially designed catheters with extra long curves, or specially designed long sheaths may be required to reach the target tissue or to stabilize the catheter position to ensure adequate tissue contact. A variety of custom catheter curves and guiding sheaths that may be used for this purpose are commercially available from most manufacturers of electrophysiology products.

Procedure Endpoints for Radiofrequency Catheter Ablation of Type 1 Atrial Flutter

Ablation may be performed during sustained atrial flutter or during sinus rhythm. If performed during atrial flutter the first endpoint is its terminates during energy application (Figure 11). If atrial flutter terminates during ablation, programmed stimulation and burst pacing should be performed im-

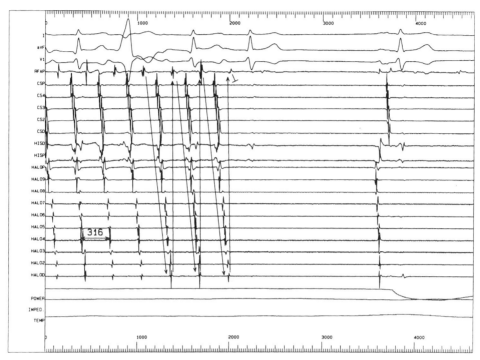

Figure 11. Termination of common Type 1 atrial flutter during radiofrequency energy application using an interrupted drag technique across the TV-IVC isthmus. Atrial flutter will usually terminate just as the distal ablation electrode on the mapping/ablation catheter (RF) approaches the inferior vena cava during a linear drag across the TV-IVC isthmus. Conduction fails at the SE isthmus as indicated by block developing between the low lateral right atrium (Halo D and RFAP) and coronary sinus (CSP) in the common form, and between the coronary sinus and the low lateral right atrium in the uncommon form (not shown). HRA = electrogram recording from a catheter positioned at the high right atrium; Imped. = impedance in ohms; Power = watts; RFAP = proximal electrode pair on radiofrequency ablation catheter; Temp = tissue temperature in degree centigrade. All other abbreviations are the same as in previous figures.

mediately and 30 minutes later to determine if either the common or uncommon form is still reinducible.[1-6] If atrial flutter is not terminated, or is reinducible after the first series of radiofrequency energy applications, ablation should be repeated. For an anatomic or combined approach, it may be necessary to rotate the ablation catheter away from the initial line of energy applications, either medially or laterally in the SE isthmus, in order to create new or additional lines of block.[2-6]

If atrial flutter is terminated and not reinducible after ablation, pace mapping should then be done to determine if there is bidirectional conduction block[20-22] in the SE isthmus (Figures 12–15). If ablation is done during sinus rhythm, pace mapping can be also done during energy application to monitor for the development of conduction block in the SE isthmus (Figure 16). The use of this recently described endpoint may be associated with a lower recurrence rate of atrial flutter during long-term follow-up.[20-22] Conduction in the

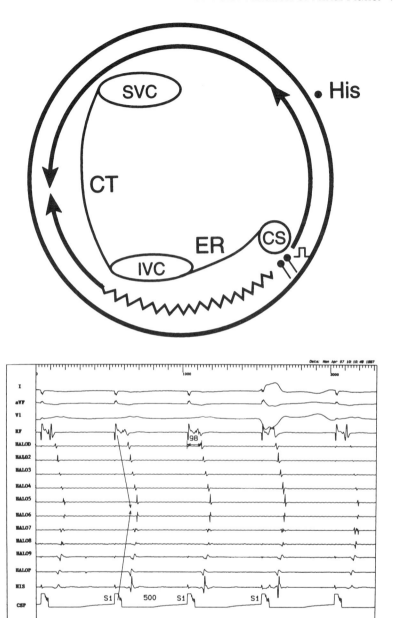

Figure 12. Panel A: A schematic diagram of the right atrium and, in panel B, surface ECG and right atrial endocardial electrograms during pacing in sinus rhythm from the coronary sinus ostium prior to ablation of the TV-IVC isthmus, in a patient with common Type 1 atrial flutter. Tracings include surface ECG leads I, aVF and V₁, and endocardial electrograms from the proximal coronary sinus (CSP), His bundle (HIS), tricuspid valve annulus at 1 o'clock (HaloP) to 7 o'clock (HaloD), and TV-IVC isthmus at 6 o'clock (RF). Note that the activation pattern during coronary sinus pacing is caudal to cranial in the interatrial septum and low right atrium, with collision of the septal and right atrial wavefronts in the mid-lateral right atrium. Activation time from the coronary sinus ostium to the low lateral right atrium through the SE isthmus is 98 milliseconds in this patient.

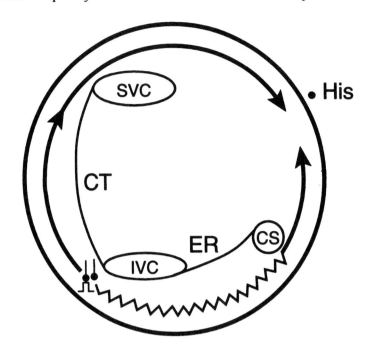

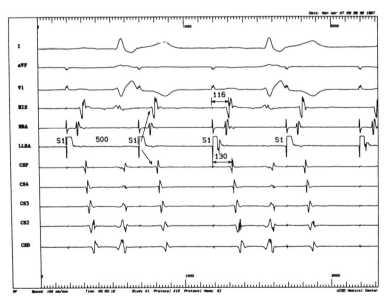

Figure 13. Panel A: A schematic diagram of the right atrium and, in panel B, surface ECG and right atrial endocardial electrograms during pacing in sinus rhythm from the low lateral right, prior to ablation of the TV-IVC isthmus atrium (same patient as in Figure 13). Tracing includes surface ECG leads I, aVF, and V$_1$ and endocardial electrograms from the low lateral right atrium (LLRA), high right atrium (HRA), proximal coronary sinus (CSP), and His bundle catheter (HIS). Note that the activation pattern during low right atrial pacing is caudal to cranial in the lateral right atrium, and interatrial septum, with collision of wavefronts in the mid septum. Consequently, activation times from the low lateral right atrium to the coronary sinus ostium (130 milliseconds) and His bundle (116 milliseconds) are similar.

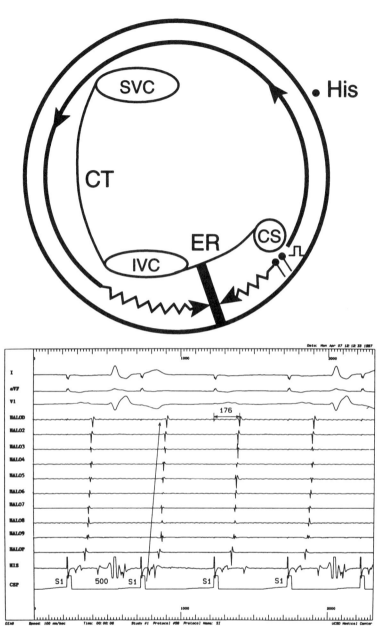

Figure 14. Panel A: A schematic diagram of the right atrium and, in panel B, surface ECG and right atrial endocardial activation patterns during pacing in sinus rhythm from the coronary sinus ostium, following linear ablation of the TV-IVC isthmus about halfway between 5 and 6 o'clock (same patient as in Figure 13). Tracing includes surface ECG leads I, aVF and V_1, and endocardial electrograms from the proximal coronary sinus (CSP), His bundle (HIS), tricuspid valve annulus at 1 o'clock (HaloP) to 7 o'clock (HaloD). Note that the activation pattern during coronary sinus pacing is still caudal to cranial in the interatrial septum, but the lateral right atrium is now activated in a strictly cranial to caudal pattern (i.e. counterclockwise), indicating complete clockwise conduction block in the SE isthmus. Consequently, the activation time from the coronary sinus ostium to the low lateral right atrium through the SE isthmus is increased from 98 to 176 milliseconds.

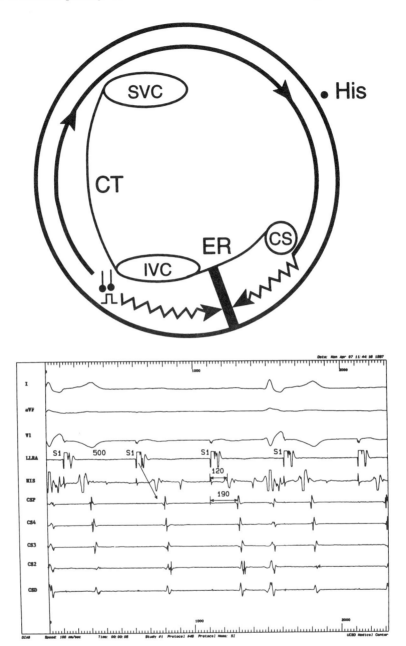

Figure 15. Panel A: A schematic diagram of the right atrium and, in panel B, surface ECG and right atrial endocardial electrograms during pacing in sinus rhythm from the low lateral right atrium, following linear ablation of the TV-IVC isthmus about halfway between 5 and 6 o'clock (same patient as in Figure 13). Tracing includes surface ECG leads I, aVF and V₁ and endocardial electrograms from the low lateral right atrium (LLRA), high right atrium (HRA), proximal coronary sinus (CSP), and His bundle catheter (HIS). Note that the activation pattern during low right atrial pacing is still caudal to cranial in the lateral right atrium, but the interatrial septum is now activated in a strictly cranial to caudal pattern (i.e. clockwise), indicating complete counterclockwise conduction block in the SE isthmus. Consequently, the activation time from the low lateral right atrium to the coronary sinus ostium is increased from 130 to 190 milliseconds, whereas the activation time to the His bundle is essentially unchanged at 120 milliseconds.

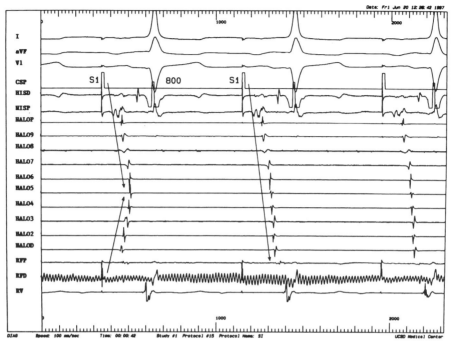

Figure 16. Surface ECG leads I, aVF and V$_1$, and endocardial electrograms from the coronary sinus, His bundle, Halo, mapping/ablation (RF), and right ventricular catheters during radiofrequency catheter ablation of the TV-IVC isthmus, while pacing from the coronary sinus ostium. Note the change in activation of the right atrium on the Halo catheter from a bidirectional to a unidirectional pattern after the first beat, indicating the development of clockwise block in the SE isthmus. This was associated with simultaneous development of counterclockwise block (i.e. bidirectional block), which was subsequently demonstrated during low right atrial pacing (not shown). HISd = electrogram from the distal electrode pair of the His bundle catheter. All other abbreviations are the same as in previous figures.

SE isthmus is evaluated by comparing activation patterns in the right atrial free wall and interatrial septum or around the tricuspid valve annulus, while pacing during sinus rhythm at slow rates (i.e., cycle lengths ≥600 milliseconds) from the low lateral right atrium and coronary sinus ostium, before and after ablation. Bidirectional conduction block in the SE isthmus is confirmed by demonstrating a change from a bidirectional wavefront with collision in the right atrial free wall or interatrial septum prior to ablation (see Figure 12 and Figure 13), to a strictly cranial to caudal activation sequence following ablation (see Figure 14 and Figure 15), during pacing from the coronary sinus ostium or low lateral right atrium, respectively. Bidirectional conduction block is further supported by prolongation of activation time from the low lateral right atrium to the coronary sinus ostium or from the coronary sinus ostium to the low lateral right atrium, during pacing from the contralateral site, respectively (see Figures 12–15). In addition, the recording of double potentials at the site of linear ablation in the SE isthmus during pacing from the low lateral right atrium or coronary sinus ostium indicates the presence of conduction block (Figure 17).

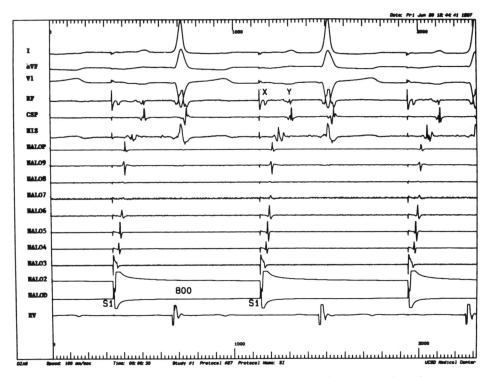

Figure 17. Surface ECG leads I, aVF and V$_1$, and endocardial electrograms from the coronary sinus, His bundle, Halo, mapping/ablation (RF), and right ventricular catheters during pacing from the distal electrode pair on the Halo catheter in the low lateral right atrium, following linear ablation of the TV-IVC isthmus. Note the double potentials (XY) recorded on the distal electrode pair of the mapping/ablation catheter (RF) positioned in the TV-IVC isthmus, indicating the presence of a line of block at the ablation site. In addition, there is strictly caudal-cranial activation of the right atrial free wall and cranial-caudal activation of the interatrial septum (i.e. clockwise). All abbreviations are the same as in previous figures.

Outcomes and Follow-up

Radiofrequency catheter ablation of atrial flutter is relatively safe, but serious complications can rarely occur, including heart block, cardiac tamponade, and stroke. Although conversion of atrial flutter to sinus rhythm is less likely (compared to atrial fibrillation) to cause thromboembolic complications such as stroke, anticoagulation prior to ablation must be considered in patients with chronic atrial flutter, particularly those with depressed left ventricular function, mitral valve disease, and left atrial enlargement with left atrial thrombus or spontaneous contrast (i.e., smoke) on echocardiography.[25]

Early reports[1–6] of radiofrequency catheter ablation of atrial flutter revealed high initial success rates, but with recurrence rates of 20–45% (Table 1). However, as experience with radiofrequency catheter ablation of atrial flutter has increased, more recent reports[20–23] suggest that recurrence rates may be reduced to 10% or less (see Table 1). Contributing to these improved results has been the introduction of bidirectional conduction block in the TV-IVC isthmus as an endpoint for successful radiofrequency catheter ablation of atrial flutter.[20–22] For ex-

Table 1
Success Rates for Radiofrequency Catheter Ablation of Atrial Flutter

Author	# Pts	% Acute Success	F/U in Mos	% Recurrence
Feld et al, 1992[1]	16	100	4 ± 2	17
Cosio et al, 1993[2]	9	100	$2 - 18$	44
Kirkorian et al, 1994[3]	22	86	8 ± 13	16
Fischer et al, 1995[4]	80	73	20 ± 8	19
Poty et al, 1995[20]	12	100	9 ± 3	8
Schwartzman et al, 1996[21]	35	100	$1 - 21$	8
Chauchemez et al, 1996[22]	20	100	8 ± 2	20
Chen et al, 1996[23]	65	93	20 ± 11	8

Pts = number of patients studied; % Acute Success = termination of atrial flutter during ablation or demonstration of isthmus block following ablation; F/U in Mos = duration of follow-up in months; % Recurrence = % of patients in whom Type 1 atrial flutter recurred during follow-up.

ample, in our laboratory we compared the efficacy of radiofrequency catheter ablation in 52 consecutive patients with Type 1 atrial flutter (common and uncommon forms) using either an electrophysiologically guided approach targeting the exits from the area of slow conduction in 25 patients (group 1), or a combined anatomically and electrophysiologically guided approach targeting the TV-IVC isthmus in 27 patients (group 2). Both acute success in terminating and preventing reinduction of atrial flutter (that is, 100% in group 2 versus 84% in group 1) and long-term success in preventing recurrence of atrial flutter (93% in group 2 versus 64% in group 1 at more than 24 months mean follow-up) were significantly better using a combined anatomically and electrophysiologically guided approach compared to an electrophysiologically guided approach alone.

Summary

Radiofrequency catheter ablation has rapidly become a first line treatment for Type 1 atrial flutter. The most effective approach, and that preferred by most laboratories, is an anatomically guided or a combined anatomically and electrophysiologically guided ablation of the SE isthmus, with procedure endpoints of arrhythmia noninducibility and bidirectional isthmus conduction block. Future advances for radiofrequency catheter ablation of Type 1 atrial flutter may include the use of superlong (8–10 mm) ablation electrodes, high output generators (up to 100 watts), and alternate energy sources (e.g., microwave) to reduce procedure time and the number of energy applications required for cure.[26]

References

1. Feld GK, Fleck RP, Chen PS, et al. Radiofrequency catheter ablation for the treatment of human Type 1 atrial flutter: identification of a critical zone in the reentrant circuit by endocardial mapping techniques. Circulation 1992;86:1233–1240.

2. Cosio FG, Lopez-Gil M, Goicolea A, et al. Radiofrequency ablation of the inferior vena cava-tricuspid valve isthmus in common atrial flutter. *Am J Cardiol* 1993;71:705–709.

3. Kirkorian G, Moncada E, Chevalier P, et al. Radiofrequency ablation of atrial flutter: efficacy of an anatomically guided approach. *Circulation* 1994;90:2804–2814.

4. Fischer B, Haïssaguerre M, Garrigues S, et al. Radiofrequency catheter ablation of atrial flutter in 80 patients. *J Am Coll Cardiol* 1995;25:1365–1372.

5. Calkins H, Leon AR, Deam G, et al. Catheter ablation of atrial flutter using radiofrequency energy. *Am J Cardiol* 1994;73:353–356.

6. Lesh MD, Van Hare GF, Epstein LM, et al. Radiofrequency catheter ablation of atrial arrhythmias: results and mechanisms. *Circulation* 1994;89:1074–1089.

7. Klein GJ, Guiradon GM, Sharma AD, et al. Demonstration of macroreentry and feasibility of operative therapy in the common type of atrial flutter. *Am J Cardiol* 1986;57:587–591.

8. Olshansky B, Okumura K, Gess PG, et al. Demonstration of an area of slow conduction in human atrial flutter. *J Am Coll Cardiol* 1990;16:1639–1648.

9. Cosio FG, Goicolea A, Lopez-Gil M, et al. Atrial endocardial mapping in the rare form of atrial flutter. *Am J Cardiol* 1990;66:715–720.

10. Feld GK, Birgersdotter-Green U, Fujimura O, et al. Conduction velocity in the right atrium and IVC-TVC isthmus is slower in patients with atrial flutter compared to those without atrial flutter. *J Am Coll Cardiol* 1997;29:358A.

11. Olgin JE, Kalman JM, Fizpatrick AP, et al. Role of right atrial endocardial structures as barriers to conduction during human Type 1 atrial flutter: activation and entrainment mapping guided by intracardiac echocardiography. *Circulation* 1995;92:1839–1848.

12. Olgin JE, Kalman JM, Lesh MD. Conduction barriers in human atrial flutter: correlation of electrophysiology and anatomy. *J Cardiovasc Electrophysiol* 1996;7:1112–1126.

13. Feld GK, Shahandeh-Rad F. Mechanism of double potentials recorded during sustained atrial flutter in the canine right atrial crush-injury model. *Circulation* 1992;86:628–641.

14. Cha YM, Wales A, Wolf P, et al. Electrophysiologic effects of the new class III antiarrhythmic drug dofetilide compared to the class Ia antiarrhythmic drug quinidine in experimental canine atrial flutter: role of dispersion of refractoriness in antiarrhythmic efficacy. *J Cardiovasc Electrophysiol* 1996;7:809–827.

15. Kalman, JM, Olgin JE, Saxon LA, et al. Activation and entrainment mapping defines the tricuspid annulus as the anterior barrier in typical atrial flutter. *Circulation* 1996;94:398–406.

16. Spach MS, Miller WT III, Dolber PC, et al. The functional role of structural complexities in the propagation of depolarization in the atrium of the dog: cardiac conduction disturbances due to discontinuities of effective axial resistivity. *Circ Res* 1982;50:175–191.

17. Spach MS, Dolber PS, Heidlage JF. Influence of the passive anisotropic properties on directional differences in propagation following modification

of sodium conductance in human atrial muscle: A model of reentry based on anisotropic discontinuous propagation. *Circ Res* 1988;62:811–832.

18. Olgin JE, Kalman JM, Saxon LA, et al. Mechanisms of initiation of atrial flutter in humans: site of unidirectional block and direction of rotation. *J Am Coll Cardiol* 1997;29:376–384.

19. Feld GK, Shahandeh-Rad F. Activation patterns in experimental canine atrial flutter produced by right atrial crush injury. *J Am Coll Cardiol* 1992;20:441–451.

20. Poty H, Saoudi N, Aziz AA, et al. Radiofrequency catheter ablation of type 1 atrial flutter. Prediction of late success by electrophysiologic criteria. *Circulation* 1995;92:1389–1392.

21. Schwartzman D, Callans D, Gottlieb CD, et al. Conduction block in the inferior caval-tricuspid valve isthmus: association with outcome of radiofrequency ablation of type 1 atrial flutter. *J Am Coll Cardiol* 1996;28:1519–1531.

22. Cuachemez B, Haïssaguerre M, Fischer B, et al. Electrophysiologic effects of catheter ablation of the inferior vena cava-tricuspid annulus isthmus in common atrial flutter. *Circulation* 1996;93:284–294.

23. Chen SA, Chiang CE, Wu TJ, et al. Radiofrequency catheter ablation of common atrial flutter: comparison of electrophysiologically guided focal ablation technique and linear ablation technique. *J Am Coll Cardiol* 1996;27:860–868.

24. Nakagawa H, Imai S, Schleinkofer M, et al. Linear ablation from tricuspid annulus to eustachian valve and ridge is adequate for patients with atrial flutter: extending ablation line to the inferior vena cava is not necessary. *J Am Coll Cardiol* 1997;29:199A.

25. Prater S, Wades M, Reynerston S, et al. Incidence of atrial thrombus in patients with type 1 atrial flutter undergoing catheter ablation. *Circulation* 1996;94:I-728.

26. Feld GK, Fujimura O, Green R, et al. Radiofrequency catheter ablation of human type 1 atrial flutter: comparison of results with 8 mm versus 4 mm tip ablation catheter. *J Am Coll Cardiol* 1995;169A.

Chapter 13

Ablation of Atypical Atrial Flutter

John G. Kall, M.D., David J. Wilber, M.D.

Recent developments in interventional electrophysiology have led to the recognition of multiple mechanisms of reentrant atrial tachycardia in humans. The electrophysiological characteristics and ablation of typical (Type 1, common) atrial flutter, the prototypical macro-reentrant atrial tachycardia, have been well described.[1–25] In addition, many macro-reentrant atrial tachycardias observed after reparative surgery for congenital heart disease ("incisional" or "postatriotomy" reentrant atrial tachycardias) may be mapped using conventional electrophysiological techniques and effectively treated with radiofrequency catheter ablation.[24,26] While mapping data obtained from experimental models of atrial flutter indicate that macroreentry may originate in sites remote from the tricuspid valve annulus-eustachian ridge isthmus (traditionally referred to as the tricuspid valve annulus-inferior vena cava isthmus or sub-eustachian isthmus)[27–44] only limited data has been reported characterizing these tachycardias in humans. This chapter will discuss some relevant clinical aspects of atypical forms of atrial flutter, review our preliminary experience with mapping and ablation of atypical atrial flutter originating in the right atrial free wall (RAFW), and preview future directions of investigation.

Classification and Nomenclature

The principal difficulties with the traditional classification and nomenclature of atrial tachycardias and flutter have been summarized recently by Lesh et al.[45] In this chapter, we use the term macro-reentrant atrial tachycardia interchangeably with atrial flutter, mainly because of the historical significance and the popular use of atrial flutter as a descriptive term. For the purposes of

From Huang SKS, Wilber DJ (eds.): *Radiofrequency Catheter Ablation of Cardiac Arrhythmias: Basic Concepts and Clinical Applications,* 2nd ed. Armonk, NY: Futura Publishing Company, Inc. ©2000.

this discussion, atypical atrial flutter will be considered any macro-reentrant atrial tachycardia which 1) does not utilize the tricuspid annulus-eustachian ridge (TA-ER) isthmus as a critical component of a tachycardia circuit (i.e., not counterclockwise or clockwise typical atrial flutter), and 2) is not associated with reentry around a surgical scar. These latter tachycardias are discussed elsewhere in this volume.

Macro-reentrant atrial tachycardias may be described in terms of the type of reentrant circuit (single-loop or double-loop), the location of the reentrant circuit, the relation of the circuit to anatomic, surgical, and/or functional barriers to conduction, and the direction of activation within the reentrant circuit. Where possible, a more complete characterization of these parameters will facilitate communication and comparisons between individual investigators and clinicians.

Experimental Data

Both single-loop and double-loop macro-reentrant circuits not incorporating the TA-ER isthmus as a critical component have been described in atrial incisional (intercaval and right atrial crush injury, atrial surgery/congenital heart disease surgery), right atrial enlargement (tricuspid insufficiency/pulmonary stenosis), left atrial enlargement (subclavian arterial/pulmonary venous shunt), and sterile pericarditis models.[27-44] In some cases these macro-reentrant tachycardias represent transitional rhythms between atrial flutter and fibrillation, particularly in models in which atrial fibrillation is the predominant rhythm. Autonomic tone may also be important in this regard.[47] While data from experimental models of atrial flutter suggest that atypical atrial flutter represents a heterogenous group of arrhythmias, isolated atypical atrial flutter circuits are identified occasionally in individual experimental preparations. Thus, it is not surprising that single atypical atrial flutter circuits can and do account for clinical tachycardia in some patients.

Several observations relevant to the mapping of macro-reentrant atrial tachycardias in humans were first described in animal models. Experimental data indicate that functional conduction block plays a critical role in the genesis of many of these tachycardias.[32,33,36,37,41-44] In several models, the RAFW has been demonstrated to be a frequent site for the development of both functional central lines of conduction block and atrial flutter.[32-34,36,38,41-43] Double potentials are recorded from the center of the atrial flutter reentrant circuit, irrespective of whether the circuit utilizes a fixed (as with the right atrial crush model of atrial flutter)[39,40] or an entirely functional central line of conduction block (as observed in the sterile pericarditis and atrial enlargement models)[34,35,43] In addition, studies in some experimental models of atrial flutter indicate that the production of conduction block across a critical isthmus within the tachycardia circuit results in the termination and/or elimination of tachycardia.[27,44] However, as demonstrated in a surgical model simulating reparative surgery for congenital heart disease, ablative procedures intended to eliminate one tachycardia may also result in the development of additional tachycardias.[46]

Incidence of Atypical Atrial Flutter

The incidence of atypical atrial flutter in an otherwise unselected patient population is unknown. The surface electrocardiographic findings of atrial flutter are often not specific to a tachycardia mechanism, making analysis of atrial flutter based solely on 12-lead electrocardiograms problematic.[17] Reports of programmed electrical stimulation performed systematically in large numbers of patients predisposed to atrial flutter are limited. The clinical significance of atypical atrial flutter induced in the electrophysiology laboratory in patients presenting with other arrhythmias (including typical atrial flutter) is uncertain, and correlation to specific myocardial pathology has not been characterized.

We performed atrial programmed stimulation prospectively in 160 patients referred for ablation of typical atrial flutter. All patients had symptomatic atrial flutter and presented with electrocardiograms suggesting the presence of counterclockwise and/or clockwise typical atrial flutter. Incremental burst pacing was performed for at least 10 beats at cycle lengths at an initial cycle length of ~300 milliseconds. Pacing cycle length was then decremented by 10 milliseconds per burst until induction of atrial flutter (or atrial fibrillation) or 2:1 atrial capture. The induction protocol was performed from the coronary sinus (CS) os (medial TA-ER isthmus) and the lateral right atrium adjacent to the TA (lateral isthmus) in all patients. Stimulation at these sites permits the selective induction of counterclockwise (with pacing from the medial TA-ER isthmus) and clockwise (with pacing from the lateral isthmus) atrial flutter for further evaluation and comparison with the clinical tachycardias, and allows for the baseline assessment conduction across the TA-ER isthmus.[14] Burst pacing from the high lateral right atrium was completed in an additional 45 patients. Tachycardias were arbitrarily considered to be sustained if atrial flutter was stable and persistent for more than 60 seconds following induction.

In this group of 160 patients, atrial burst pacing resulted in the induction of a sustained atypical atrial flutter in 36 patients (23%). The putative location of each tachycardia was determined by analysis of atrial activation sequence and response to pacing including determination of the post-pacing interval (PPI) and the ability to entrain the tachycardia from multiple atrial sites.[9,10,48–50] The atypical atrial flutters were mapped to the left atrium in 22 of 36 patients (61%) and to the anterior RAFW in 6 patients. Localization was indeterminate in the remaining 8 patients due either to insufficient mapping data (6 patients) or the presence of multiple tachycardias or atrial fibrillation (2 patients).

The patients with atrial flutter localized to the RAFW underwent further detailed mapping and ablation. Characterization of the tachycardias in these 6 patients is presented to illustrate approaches to the evaluation and ablation of atypical atrial flutter.

Atypical Atrial Flutter Originating in the Right Atrial Free Wall

Patient Characteristics

Five patients were male, age 67 to 74 years, with structural heart disease. One additional patient was a 49-year-old female with no evidence of structural heart disease or pulmonary or systemic hypertension. Three patients had coronary artery disease including right coronary artery involvement and inferior infarction. Coronary artery disease was present in 3 patients; one had idiopathic dilated cardiomyopathy and one had mitral valvular disease. In 5 patients, there was no prior history of cardiac surgery or pericarditis. One patient had undergone mitral valve replacement for mitral incompetency 11 years prior to development of atrial flutter. Review of operative records (and subsequent direct pathological examination) indicated no RAFW atriotomy (see the section headed Anatomic Correlation, below).

Electrophysiological Assessment

The electrophysiological testing protocol used in our laboratory for patients with typical atrial flutter has been previously described.[51] Briefly, a decapolar catheter (2-mm intra-electrode and 5-mm interelectrode pair spacing) was positioned in the coronary sinus such that the proximal electrode pairs bracketed the CS os. An octapolar (1.5 mm interelectrode spacing) 6F electrode catheter (Biosense Webster, Inc., Baldwin Park, CA) was inserted into a femoral vein and positioned to record from the low septal right atrial and His bundle regions. A deflectable quadripolar catheter (2-5-2-mm interelectrode spacing) was used to record and pace at selected right atrial sites. These catheters are used in our standard protocol for electrophysiological assessment prior to typical atrial flutter ablation. Additionally, in the first 3 patients, one or 2 custom (Biosense Webster) deflectable 18-electrode 7F catheters (1.5-mm intra-electrode and 10-mm interelectrode pair spacing) were used to survey regional right atrial activation. Catheter positions were assessed with biplane fluoroscopy. Intracardiac electrograms and simultaneous 12-lead electrocardiograms were acquired continuously with data stored on optical disk (CardioLab, Prucka Engineering, Inc., Houston, TX).

In the last 3 patients, activation sequence was determined from high-density maps (100–400 right atrial recording sites) obtained using a magnetic electroanatomic mapping system (Carto, Biosense Webster, Inc., Tirat HaCarmel, Israel and Marlton, NJ, USA). The operation and accuracy of this nonfluoroscopic catheter navigation and mapping system have been described previously.[51] Mapping was performed using catheters with 2-5-2-mm interelectrode spacing and 4-mm distal electrodes. Distances and conduction velocities within the reentrant circuit (as well as right atrial volumes) were determined from high-density electroanatomic maps.[12] Ablation sites may be "tagged" to permit visualization of the ablation line on the electroanatomic map. This system also permits delineation of local anatomy which may be of importance when planning an ablation approach. Direct visualization of the reentrant circuit is particularly helpful when isoelectric flutter waves or difficulty obtaining atrial capture from multiple sites during entrainment mapping complicate conventional mapping techniques.

For each spontaneous or induced sustained atypical atrial flutter, flutter cycle length (FCL), standard 12-lead ECG, atrial activation pattern, and response to pacing at multiple right atrial sites were examined. During atypical atrial flutter in the first 3 patients, one or 2 18-electrode mapping catheters were positioned systematically at multiple right atrial locations to survey for double or fractionated potentials indicating the possible presence of conduction delay or block. In all 6 patients, entrainment pace mapping was used to identify sites within the atypical atrial flutter circuit.[9–11,49] During entrainment mapping, bipolar pacing (2-mm interelectrode spacing) was performed at current threshold for at least 10 beats at cycle lengths 10 to 30 milliseconds less than the FCL. Any change in atrial activation during entrainment compared to baseline tachycardia as determined by analysis of all available surface and intracardiac electrocardiographic recordings was considered to represent manifest fusion. Concealed entrainment was considered to be present if pacing resulted in entrainment with no change in atrial endocardial activation or surface F wave morphology.

Induction and Electrocardiographic Characteristics of Atypical Atrial Flutter

In each patient, sustained atypical atrial flutter could be induced reliably with burst pacing at cycle lengths of 200 to 240 milliseconds from the CS os at baseline. In each case, atrial fibrillation was not observed as an intermediate rhythm and additional sustained atypical atrial flutters were not induced. Most episodes of spontaneous and/or induced tachycardia persisted from several minutes to hours and required overdrive pacing for termination. Spontaneous transitions between atypical and typical atrial flutter were observed in 2 patients.

There was no statistical difference in the FCL of typical versus atypical atrial flutter. The FCL of atypical atrial flutter in the study patients ranged from 215 to 330 milliseconds. In the 5 patients in which TA-ER isthmus ablation was performed prior to atypical atrial flutter ablation, ablation across the TA-ER isthmus did not affect the inducibility, cycle length, or, interestingly, F wave morphology of atypical atrial flutter. The presence of a "negative F wave" RAFW flutter after confirmation of persistent bidirectional TA-ER isthmus block (as demonstrated in 4 patients) suggests that the activation wavefront engages the crista terminalis at the level of the RAFW. Histoanatomic studies of the inferior right atrium in human autopsy specimens suggest division of the inferior crista into anterior and posterior eustachian ridge components.[54] Activation of the left atrium via a posterior eustachian ridge connection may explain the persistence of a "negative F wave" RAFW flutter despite bidirectional TA-ER isthmus block (versus transition to a "positive F wave" flutter coincident with TA-ER isthmus block).

In all patients, a predominantly negative F wave was displayed in the inferior surface ECG leads. In 3 cases, the F wave morphology was virtually identical to that of counterclockwise typical atrial flutter induced in the same patient. These findings indicate that the electrocardiographic pattern of counterclockwise typical atrial flutter is not specific for typical atrial flutter. Similar observations have been reported previously by Kalman et al.[17] These observations concur with the experimental findings of Waldo and Okumura et al indicating that the polarity of the F wave alone cannot be used to localize or to predict the location of or direction of rotation within an intra-atrial reentrant circuit.[31,35] Representative electrocardiograms are presented in Figure 1. In 2 patients, spontaneous transitions in F wave polarity between negative and positive (or isoelectric) in the inferior leads during otherwise stable atypical atrial flutter were observed.

Activation and Entrainment Mapping

Analysis of the activation sequence revealed right to left (proximal to distal CS) atrial activation during atypical atrial flutter. Detailed mapping of the midlateral RAFW identified a discrete vertical line of widely split double potentials at the center of the reentrant circuit (Figure 2). Counterclockwise (described in an epicardial view of the right atrium) and clockwise rotation around the central line of double potentials was observed in 3 patients each.

Electroanatomic mapping of the right atrium during atypical atrial flutter provided definitive demonstration of the reentrant circuit and its relation to right

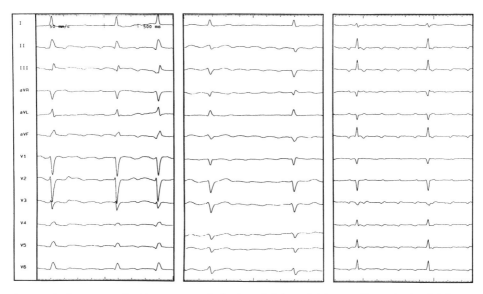

Figure 1A. Representative F wave morphologies of right atrial free wall atypical atrial flutter. An atypical atrial flutter with negative F wave polarity in the inferior leads was observed in each patient (counterclockwise rotation was demonstrated in the right atrial free wall in the first 2 panels on the left and clockwise rotation in the far right panel).[72]

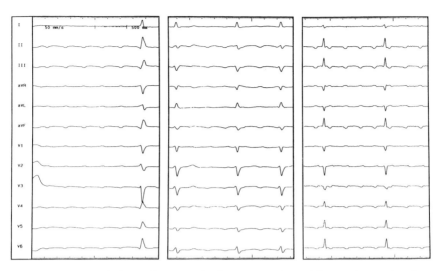

Figure 1B. F wave morphology of counterclockwise typical atrial flutter observed in the same patients whose data appears in Figure 1A. Note the similarity of the F wave morphology of counterclockwise typical atrial flutter with that of negative F wave RAFW atypical atrial flutter in each patient.[72]

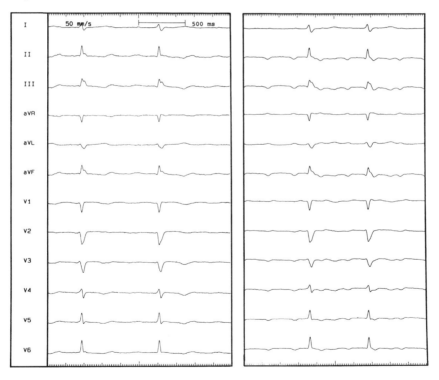

Figure 1C. Additional representative (in the inferior surface ECG leads) positive F wave morphology of right atrial free wall atypical atrial flutter (left panel). Spontaneous transition in F wave polarity between negative (as seen in the panel at the right) and positive in the inferior leads was observed. Transitions in F wave polarity were not rate-dependent. A shift in early activation from the inferior (displaying negative F wave polarity in the inferior leads) to the superior (with positive F wave polarity) interatrial septum during stable right atrial free wall activation coincided with the change in polarity. This phenomenon is reminiscent of similar behavior observed in the canine sterile pericarditis model of atrial flutter.[31,35]

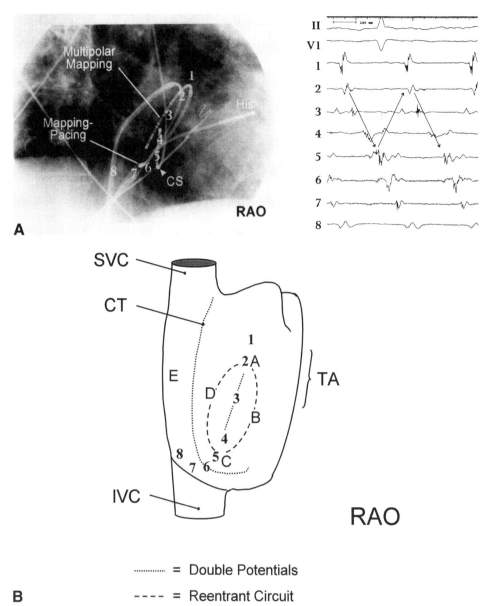

= Double Potentials

= Reentrant Circuit

Figure 2. Activation mapping of the right atrial free wall during atypical atrial flutter. A: The 30° right anterior oblique (RAO) fluoroscopic view demonstrates the position of a multipolar mapping catheter relative to a CS catheter and octapolar catheter in the His bundle position. A deflectable catheter for mapping and pacing is positioned at the lateral aspect of the inferior vena cava-right atrial junction. The numerical designations signify lateral right atrial recording sites with the corresponding electrograms displayed in the composite activation map. Analysis of entrainment mapping data indicated at sites 2–5 were within the reentrant circuit. Note the double potentials recorded from sites 3 and 4 and fractionated electrograms from site 5. Counterclockwise rotation (described in the right lateral epicardial view) around the central line of double potentials (discrete from the crista terminalis) was observed. B: Schematic of the right atrium (right anterior oblique view) illustrates the relative location of the recording sites within the reentrant circuit. Entrainment with short postpacing intervals was demonstrated at sites A, B, C, and D, but not E. An additional line of double potentials was recorded from along the expected anatomic course of the crista terminalis. Radiofrequency energy application to sites 4–7 resulted in termination and inability to reinduce the tachycardia.[72]

atrial anatomy. A representative activation map is presented in Figure 3. The presence of a central discrete vertical line of double potentials in the midlateral right atrium (small olive circular tags in Figure 3) was confirmed. This discrete line of double potentials was clearly separate from an additional line of double potentials identified along the expected anatomic course of the crista terminalis from the superior right atrium to the eustachian ridge. The discrete central line of double potentials was located from 1.0 to 1.5 cm anterior to the crista terminalis. The approximate length of the these central lines of conduction block ranged from 2 to 2.5 cm. The proximity of the central line of double potentials to the crista terminalis emphasizes the need for precise mapping, particularly when conventional mapping techniques are utilized. In the present cases, electroanatomic mapping facilitated the identification of relatively short central lines of double potentials which were located very close to the crista terminalis by readily providing high-density activation maps. Rotation within the RAFW was counterclockwise (Figure 4). In 2 additional patients undergoing electroanatomic mapping,

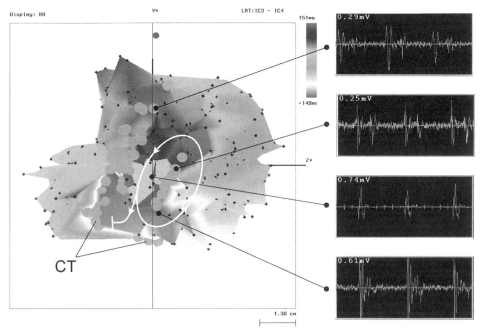

Figure 3. A representative electroanatomic right atrial activation map during atypical atrial flutter (410 recording sites; right lateral view). This patient had a history of inferior infarction (right coronary artery occlusion) and no prior cardiothoracic surgery. Activation sequence is color-coded with red indicating relatively early activation and purple indicating late activation (gray indicates a software solution for adjacent sites demonstrating very early and very late activation times, respectively. A line of double potentials (olive pips) was demonstrated along the expected anatomic course of the crista terminalis. An additional discrete line (approximately 1.5 cm in length) of double potentials was identified just anterosuperior to the crista terminalis. Activation was noted to occur in counterclockwise fashion around the discrete line of double potentials. Note block from the reentrant circuit to the inferior interatrial septum at the crista terminalis. The atrium located septal to the crista terminalis is activated passively (see text, Activation and Entrainment Mapping). Electrograms recorded from specific lateral right atrial sites are shown in the panels at the far right (electrogram amplitude in the upper left corner of each panel). See color plate.

clockwise activation was demonstrated in a similar reentrant circuit in the mid-anterior RAFW adjacent to the crista terminalis. Atrial volumes determined from the electroanatomic maps confirmed echocardiographic estimates of right atrial volume in all 3 patients (133 cc and 170 cc in the 2 patients with echocardiographic right atrial enlargement and 53 cc in the remaining patient with normal right atrial size; normal right atrial volume is approximately 40–80 cc). In each patient, analysis of the isochronal maps (a representative isochronal map is presented in Figure 5) indicated multiple (in this case 3) discrete areas of slow conduction (con-

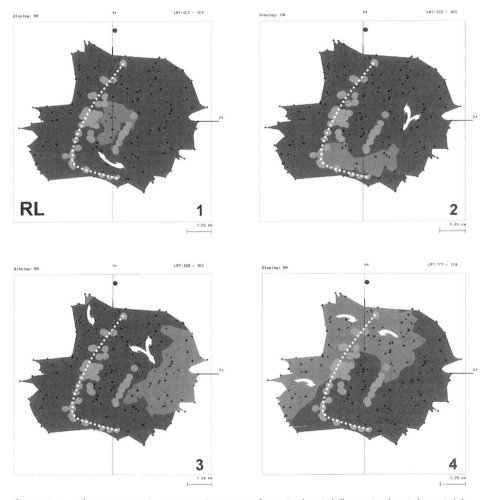

Figure 4. An electroanatomic propagation map of atypical atrial flutter in the right atrial free wall (right lateral view). The same tachycardia is depicted in Figure 3. Locations of double potentials are represented by olive pips. The activation wavefront (red) is observed to rotate (arrows) within a midlateral right atrial reentrant circuit in counterlockwise fashion around a discrete central line of double potentials located approximately 2 cm anterior to the crista terminalis (broken white line). Note late (passive) activation of portions of the right atrium (including the interatrial septum) posterior and septal to the crista terminalis. Clockwise rotation around a central line of double potentials in the midlateral free wall was demonstrated with electroanatomic mapping in 2 additional patients. See color plate.

duction velocity <0.5 meters per second) within the reentrant circuit. While these findings may not necessarily be extrapolated to atypical atrial flutter arising in other locations, they should be considered when interpreting activation and entrainment maps of atypical atrial flutter.

Spontaneous transitions in F wave polarity from negative (F wave morphology indistinguishable from that of counterclockwise typical atrial flutter) to positive (or isoelectric) in the inferior ECG leads were observed in 2 patients. Reversal in F wave polarity from negative to positive was associated with a change in early activation from the inferior posteroseptum (CS os) to the superior right atrium, and with a reversal in the inferior posteroseptal electrogram polarity. Based on experimental data reported previously, these observations suggested that the interatrial septum and left atrium were passively activated during atypical atrial flutter.[31,35] Transitions in F wave polarity were not rate dependent.

Pacing at sites immediately anterior or inferior to the line of double potentials resulted in concealed entrainment with PPI-FCL intervals of <30 milliseconds. The presence of concealed entrainment is best explained by the location of the pacing site relative to barriers to conduction including the central line of conduction block, the inferior crista terminalis or lateral margin of the IVC os inferiorly, and the anterolateral TA anteriorly. Pacing at other relatively "unprotected" sites adjacent to the line of double potentials (sites superior to the central line of conduction block within the trabeculated portion of the right atrium) resulted in PPI-FCL intervals of <30 milliseconds with manifest fusion (as indicated by changes in local activation despite no discernible change in surface F wave morphology). Pacing from the inter-atrial septum or from sites within the TA-ER isthmus resulted in manifest fusion with PPI-FCL intervals of >30 milliseconds indicating that these sites were outside of the flutter circuit.

Catheter Ablation of RAFW Flutter

Ablation of RAFW flutter was performed at the time of primary electrophysiology study in all 6 patients and after typical atrial flutter ablation (with confirmation of bidirectional TA-ER isthmus conduction block) in 5 patients. We hypothesized that interruption of conduction across a critical isthmus between an anatomic barrier (the IVC os) and a central barrier (a line of block in the midlateral right atrium) would result in termination and prevent induction of tachycardia. Of several potential ablation lines, a line between the lateral margin of the IVC os and the central line of double potentials was selected because of technical considerations (available guiding sheaths were particularly suited for catheter positioning in the inferolateral right atrium) and lesions avoided the phrenic nerve and major components of the conduction system. It should be noted that currently available guiding sheaths are not optimally designed for positioning catheters along the inferolateral or inferoposterior right atrium, and frequently deflect anteriorly and toward the septum as the catheter is advanced. In the first 3 patients, we used modified Daig SR3 and SR4 guiding sheaths (Daig Corporation, Minnetonka, MN, USA) to optimize ablation electrode positioning and contact. Radiofrequency energy (Radionics, Inc., RFG-3D, Burlington, MA, or Medtronic CardioRhythm, Inc., Sunnyvale, CA, lesion generators) was applied using an 8-mm tip electrode of a 7F quadripolar mapping and ablation catheter (EP Technologies, Inc., Sunnyvale, CA, or Medtronic CardioRhythm) and 2 posterior chest cutaneous patch electrodes (~420 cm² total area). Power was regulated to produce an ablation electrode temperature of 50°C to 60°C in 2 patients.

Radiofrequency energy was applied during sustained atypical atrial flutter. Discrete radiofrequency energy applications (10–40 watts, 45–60 seconds per application) delivered sequentially to produce a linear lesion from the lateral margin of the IVC os superiorly toward the midlateral right atrial double potentials resulted in the termination and subsequent inability to reinduce atrial flutter. Fluoroscopic views of the ablation line are presented in Figure 6.

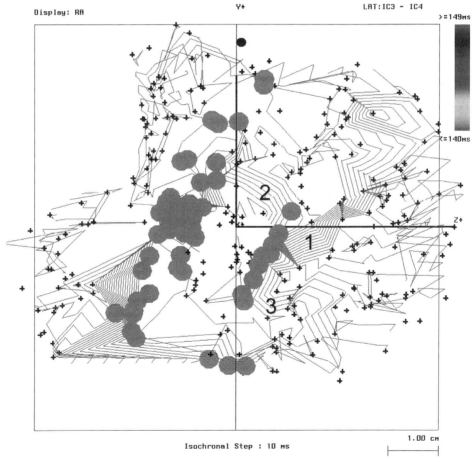

Figure 5. An electroanatomic isochronal map of atypical atrial flutter in the right atrial free wall (right lateral view; same patient as in Figure 3). Note crowding of the 10 ms isochrones at several sites (sites 1, 2, and 3) indicating multiple discrete areas of slow conduction (conduction velocities of <0.5 meters per second) within the reentrant circuit. The possible presence of multiple areas of slow conduction within a reentrant circuit should be considered when interpreting activation and entrainment mapping data obtained using conventional mapping techniques. See color plate.[72]

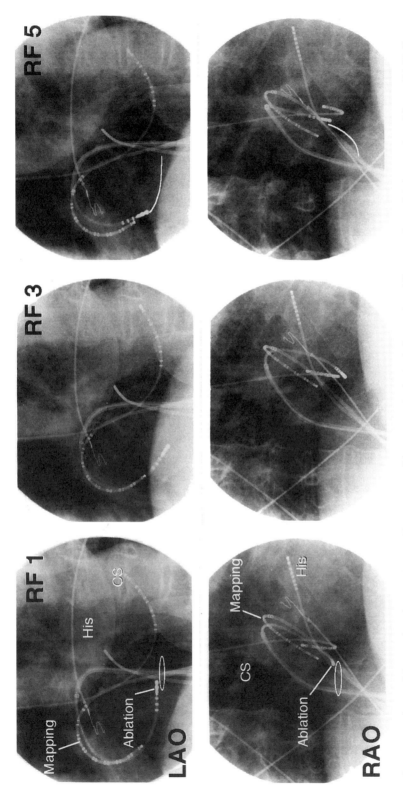

Figure 6. Catheter ablation (first three patients). The upper and lower panels depict left anterior oblique (LAO) and right anterior oblique (RAO) fluoroscopic views, respectively. Radiofrequency (RF) energy was applied sequentially from the IVC os (RF 1) superiorly towards the central line of double potentials (the solid white lines in the final panels indicate the ablation line). Atrial flutter terminated during RF #5. Ablation was guided using electroanatomical maps to generate similar ablation lines in the final three patients. Analysis of right atrial activation at the time of termination was consistent with block at the ablation site.

In the final 3 patients, ablation was guided using the electroanatomic mapping and navigation system. Ablation was performed using Biosense Webster mapping/ablation catheters with a 4-mm tip electrode. Guiding sheaths were not used. Radiofrequency energy was also applied during sustained tachycardia. Interestingly, in these 3 cases, radiofrequency energy applications near the central line of double potentials resulted in immediate termination of tachycardia in each of the 3 patients. However, tachycardia remained inducible in each case. Using the electroanatomic map, subsequent radiofrequency energy applications were delivered sequentially toward the IVC os (or, as delineated by the electroanatomic map, the inferolateral portion of the crista terminalis). In each case, no tachycardia was inducible following completion of the planned ablation line. In 5 patients, termination of atrial flutter during energy application occurred without a change in FCL. Progressive cycle length prolongation without oscillation was observed during final radiofrequency energy applications prior to flutter termination in only one patient. The mean number of radiofrequency energy applications was 8 using the 8-mm tip electrode and 13 using the 4-mm tip electrode with electroanatomic map guidance. Analysis of right atrial activation during termination of flutter demonstrated block at the site of radiofrequency energy application in the inferolateral right atrium. Following ablation, burst pacing protocols from at least 2 right atrial sites including the CS os and the lateral right atrium failed repeatedly to induce any sustained atrial flutter in each patient. There were no complications.

All patients were initially followed off antiarrhythmic drugs. One patient developed atrial fibrillation at one month follow-up and was treated with amiodarone (with a subsequent follow-up of 3 months without recurrent atrial flutter or fibrillation). The one patient in whom TA-ER isthmus ablation was not performed at the time of atypical atrial flutter ablation developed typical atrial flutter 8 months later and underwent ablation directed at the TA-ER isthmus. At that time of the second procedure, RAFW flutter remained noninducible. This patient has subsequently remained free of any atrial flutter recurrence. Since lesions contiguous with anatomic barriers may generate or extend a line of conduction block, thus potentially creating the substrate for other tachycardias and/or facilitating their occurrence, it is possible the RAFW ablation line could have facilitated the occurrence of typical atrial flutter. This possibility should be considered when planning ablation in patients presenting with only atypical atrial flutter. In the remaining 5 patients, there has been no recurrence of any atrial flutter for a mean of 18±17 months (range 3–40 months).

The consistent response to catheter ablation observed in these patients confirms that the inferolateral right atrium is a critical component of the RAFW reentrant circuit. It should be stressed that termination of atrial flutter during radiofrequency energy application and subsequent non-inducibility may not always be a sufficient ablation protocol end point.[13] However, in each of these patients, RAFW flutter was reproducibly initiated by atrial pacing prior to ablation. In addition, all have remained free of spontaneous RAFW flutter during follow-up. It is possible that a different anatomic approach (possibly targeting the narrow isthmus between the central line of double potentials and the crista terminalis) may have been equally effective.

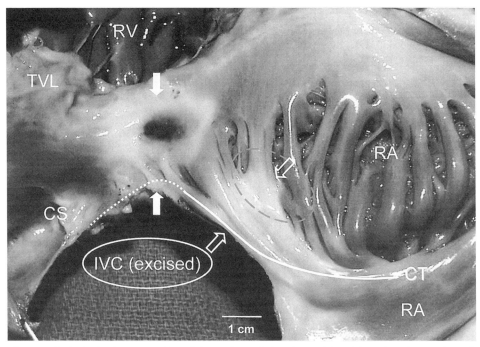

Figure 7. Pathological examination of the endocardial surface of the right atrium in a patient after radiofrequency ablation of both typical and right atrial free wall atypical atrial flutter. The heart was obtained following cardiac transplantation. The solid white line indicates the location of the crista terminalis and the adjoining white broken line indicates the eustachian ridge. Note the presence of a typical atrial flutter ablation lesion between the tricuspid valve annulus and the eustachian ridge (solid arrows). An additional lesion (open arrows) is present in the inferior aspect of the right atrial free wall and originates at the the inferior vena cava-right atrial junction, crosses the inferior crista terminalis, and extends into the pectinate musculature. Application of radiofrequency energy was guided using the Biosense electroanatomic mapping and catheter navigation system. Microscopic examination indicated only moderate atrial myocyte hypertrophy and mild interstitial fibrosis. No distinct scar was identified in the right atrium. The putative location of the reentrant circuit based upon analysis of the electroanatomic map superimposed on the right atrial anatomy is indicated by the red broken line. CS = coronary sinus; IVC = inferior vena cava; RA = right atrium; TVL = tricuspid valve leaflet. See color plate.

Anatomic Correlation

The presence of coronary artery disease with right coronary artery involvement in 3 of the 6 patients studied is of some interest. It is reasonable to speculate that right atrial infarction following proximal right coronary occlusion contributed to the generation of an arrhythmic substrate. Direct pathological evidence is lacking at this time and no comparable experimental models have been reported.

One patient underwent cardiac transplantation 7.5 months after catheter ablation of atypical atrial flutter arising in the RAFW. This patient had undergone mitral valve replacement for mitral incompetency eleven years prior to the development of atrial flutter. Review of operative records indicated no atriotomy in the RAFW. Gross examination of the heart disclosed a mitral valve prosthesis with left atriotomy in the atrial appendage, severe left and moderate right ventricular enlargement, and mild biatrial enlargement. The lateral right atrium was free of gross scarring. Histological examination of the lateral right atrium disclosed moderate myocyte hypertrophy with mild, diffuse interstitial fibrosis.

Examination of the right atrial endocardial surface disclosed 2 prior (chronic) ablation lesions, one across the TA-ER isthmus and a second originating at the lateral aspect of the IVC-right atrial junction, and extending across the inferolateral aspect of the crista terminalis and about 1.5 cm into the pectinate musculature of the inferolateral RAFW (see Figure 7). The anatomic location of the RAFW ablation lesion correlated with the location as indicated on the electroanatomic map. The putative location of the reentrant circuit based upon analysis of the electroanatomic map is depicted in Figure 8. The discrete areas of slow conduction identified on an isochronal map (see Figure 5) appear to correlate with conduction across prominent pectinate muscle bundles. These pathologic findings provide further evidence that the reentrant circuit incorporates pectinate musculature adjacent to the inferolateral crista terminalis. However, histopathological examination failed to establish definitively the anatomic substrate for the central line of conduction block. Further pathoanatomic correlation is required to definitively characterize the anatomic basis for macroreentry in the RAFW.

Clinical Implications

Within this select group of patients with typical atrial flutter, macroreentry within the RAFW was identified (either as a spontaneous rhythm or induced during electrophysiological evaluation) in a small number of patients (about 4%). These tachycardias may be characterized using conventional activation and entrainment mapping techniques. However, precise mapping is required to distinguish the relatively small central lines of double potentials (lines of conduction block constituting central obstacles), which are located in close proximity to the crista terminalis, from the crista terminalis itself. Areas of slow conduction (typically multiple and discrete) within the circuit appear to correlate with conduction across pectinate musculature within the RAFW. Similar tachycardias have also been described recently by Bogun et al.[55] It is likely that other regions of the right atrium are capable of supporting macroreentry in susceptible patients.

Although controlled data are not available, it should be noted that ablation in the pectinate musculature may be potentially complicated. Pericardial effusion may develop following energy delivery to extremely thin areas of myocardium between pectinate muscle bundles. Also, high energy outputs and/or "unconventional" ablation catheters (such as 8 mm tip and irrigated-tip catheters) may be required to effect successful ablation when areas with particularly thick pectinate muscle bundles are encountered. Since at least some of these tachycardias appear to utilize the pectinate portions of the atrium, these factors should be considered when contemplating ablation in these areas. The risk of systemic thromboembolism inherent to left atrial procedures, particularly linear ablation within the left atrium, remains a substantial and persistent clinical problem. The use of ablation electrode temperature monitoring and "temperature-controlled" radiofrequency energy delivery appears to reduce the incidence of adverse impedance rises, particularly during energy application in low flow areas and in atria subject to low flow states. Further investigation is required to define the role of cooled-tip or irrigated-tip ablation catheters in left atrial ablation procedures.[56]

Other Forms of Atypical Atrial Flutter

Little additional data is currently available that describes the clinical and electrophysiological characteristics of atrial flutters arising in other areas of the right atrium.[17,57–59] Only preliminary data on atrial flutters arising in the left atrium has been reported.[17,60–63] Jais et al recently characterized left atrial flutter in 13 patients.[62] Structural heart disease (predominantly left heart disease) was present in 11 of 13 patients (mitral valvular disease in 8 patients, and aortic valvular disease, hypertrophic cardiomyopathy, and ischemic cardiomyopathy in one patient each). Spontaneous atrial fibrillation, as well as additional morphologies of atypical atrial flutter, was observed in several of the patients studied. Interestingly, in 10 of 13 patients, an electrically silent area was identified in the left atrium by conventional and/or electroanatomic mapping techniques. Electrically silent areas were identified in the posterior left atrium in 6 patients, in the anterior left atrium in one patient, and in multiple areas in the left atrium in 3 patients. These electrically silent areas were also present during sinus rhythm. A variety of electrocardiographic (flutter wave) morphologies were observed. Analysis of electroanatomic maps of the left atrium obtained during left atrial flutter disclosed anatomic or functional lines of conduction block of varying lengths, in some cases in conjunction with an electrically silent area. A variety of reentrant circuits utilizing the electrically silent areas alone or in combination with additional anatomic (pulmonary veins and mitral valve annulus) or functional lines of conduction block were identified. Radiofrequency catheter ablation directed at a critical isthmus between an electrically silent area and an anatomic barrier (most commonly the mitral valve annulus) was successful in 10 of 13 patients. Those patients undergoing successful ablation remained in sinus rhythm (in the absence of antiarrhythmic drugs in 7 patients) over a follow-up period of 10 ± 4 months. Similar findings in patients with left atrial flutter have been reported recently by Natale et al.[63]

An electroanatomic map of a spontaneous left atrial flutter occurring in a 76-year-old man with no demonstrable structural heart disease (aside from echocardiographic evidence of moderate biatrial enlargement) is presented in Figure 7. Pacing from perimitral valve annular sites resulted in PPIs identical to the FCL. A broad electrically silent area (highlighted by the broken line in Figure 7) in the posterior left atrium was demonstrated during atrial flutter and during sinus rhythm. Conduction velocities within the reentrant circuit (and mitral annular dimensions) were determined from the electroanatomic map prior to radiofrequency energy application. A region of slow conduction (conduction velocity ≤ 0.5 meters per second) was located along the inferolat-

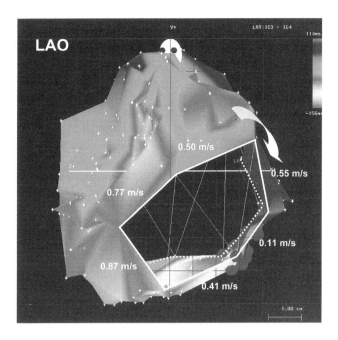

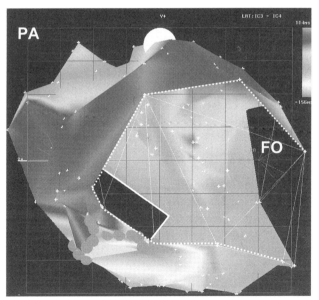

Figure 8. Electroanatomic activation maps of left atrial flutter. 7A: Left anterior oblique (LAO) projection. 7B: Posterior-anterior (PA) projection. The results of entrainment mapping indicated that perimitral annular sites were within the reentrant circuit. The electroanatomic map demonstrates clockwise activation around the mitral annulus (visualized best in the LAO view). An extensive electrically silent area was demonstrated in the posterior left atrium (outlined by a broken white line in each view). The electrically silent area was also present during sinus rhythm. Conduction velocities along the mitral annulus are presented in the LAO view. A region of slow conduction (conduction velocity <0.5 meters per second) was identified along the inferolateral aspect of the mitral annulus. Radiofrequency energy application from the electrically silent area to the inferolateral mitral valve annulus resulted in the termination and subsequent inability to reinduce this tachycardia. The ablation line (brown pips) along the inferolateral left atrium was documented using the Biosense mapping system. MVA = mitral valve annulus; FO = fossa ovalis; LAO = left anterior oblique view; PA = posteroanterior view; L LAT = left lateral view. See color plate.

eral and lateral mitral annulus. Circuit length (along the mitral annulus) was determined to be approximately 14.5 cm. Radiofrequency energy applied from the inferolateral mitral annulus to the posterior left atrial electrically silent area near the left lower pulmonary vein ostium (individual ablation sites were tagged producing the ablation line indicated by the brown area in Figure 7) resulted in termination and prevented the reinduction of this tachycardia. Left atrial volume as determined from the electroanatomic map was approximately 136 cc. Note the clear three-dimensional graphical depiction of the ablation line on the electroanatomic map shown in Figure 7.

A unique mechanism of atypical atrial flutter occurring in a 47-year-old patient without structural heart disease has recently been described by Olgin et al.[64] A macro-reentrant circuit incorporating a critical isthmus in the proximal coronary sinus was mapped using conventional activation and entrainment mapping techniques. The activation wavefront was mapped exiting the coronary sinus in the lateral left atrium and returning to the CS os via the left atrium and interatrial septum. Circumferential radiofrequency ablation within the proximal coronary sinus (approximately 1–2 cm distal to the coronary sinus os) resulted in termination and prevented reinitiation of the tachycardia. Bidirectional block at the ablation target site was confirmed with multipolar recordings. These findings, as well as additional anatomic studies and endocardial mapping data in both canines and in humans, indicate electrical isolation or poor coupling of the posterior mitral annulus/proximal coronary sinus complex from the left atrium in at least some patients.[65–68]

Conclusions

Due to the complexity of mapping required to completely characterize many atypical atrial flutters, and the frequency of multiple tachycardias and atrial fibrillation, systems capable of rapidly acquiring and multiplexing data may be required to facilitate the mapping of these tachycardias. The Biosense electroanatomic mapping system provides important anatomic information as well as providing precise localization of the ablation catheter and three-dimensional graphical presentation of the ablation line. Additional investigational mapping systems including multielectrode basket catheters and non-contact multielectrode mapping arrays are currently under development. Preliminary investigations that use these systems in the right atrium are promising.[69–71] Endocardial voltage mapping may also provide additional useful information by facilitating the localization of high voltage structures such as prominent pectinate musculature, or low-voltage structures such as infarcted or scarred myocardium.

Most clinical, electrophysiological, and pathoanatomic aspects of atypical atrial flutter remain incompletely characterized. The presence of multiple reentrant circuits and/or atrial fibrillation remains a substantial clinical problem and may hinder the ability to define the relevant reentrant circuits in some, if not many, patients at this time. However, isolated, stable atypical atrial flutter does account for clinical arrhythmias in some patients. While conventional mapping and ablation systems may be successfully used in selected cases, advanced multisite mapping systems facilitate characterization of these tachycardias. Currently available electroanatomic mapping systems may be used to map and guide the ablation of stable tachycardias. However, mapping systems that are capable of rapidly acquiring and multiplexing data simultaneously from a large number of sites are likely to grow in importance as multiple and/or unstable tachycardias are targeted for ablation. Anatomic approaches and ablation catheter/guiding sheath systems require further development to optimize and standardize treatment of these tachycardias. Finally, further clinical experience is required to define subsets of patients who are most likely to benefit from ablation of atypical atrial flutter.

References

1. Puech P, LaTour H, Grolleau R. Le flutter et ses limites. *Arch Mal Coeur* 1970;63:116–144.
2. Disertori M, Inama G, Vergara G, et al. Evidence of a reentry circuit in the common type of atrial flutter in man. *Circulation* 1983;67:434–440.
3. Klein SJ, Guiradon GM, Sharma AD, et al. Demonstration of macro-reentry and feasibility of operative therapy in the common type of atrial flutter. *Am J Cardiol* 1986;57:587–591.
4. Cosio FG, Giocolea A, Lopez-Gil M. Fragmented electrograms and continuous electrical activity in atrial flutter. *Am J Cardiol* 1986;57:1309–1314.
5. Cosio FG, Arribas F, Barbero JM. Validation of double spike electrograms as markers of conduction delay or block in atrial flutter. *Am J Cardiol* 1988;61:775–780.
6. Olshansky B, Okumura K, Henthorn RW, et al. Characterization of double potentials in human atrial flutter: studies during transient entrainment. *J Am Coll Cardiol* 1990;15:833–841.
7. Cosio FG, Lopez-Gil M, Arribas F, et al. Mechanisms of entrainment of human common flutter studied with multiple endocardial recordings. *Circulation* 1994;89:2117–2125.
8. Waldo AL. Transient entrainment of atrial flutter. In: Waldo AL, Touboul P, eds. *Atrial Flutter*. Armonk, NY: Futura Publishing Co.,1996:241–258.
9. Kalman JM, Olgin JE, Saxon LA, et al. Activation and entrainment mapping defines the tricuspid annulus as the anterior barrier in typical atrial flutter. *Circulation* 1996;94:398–406.
10. Olgin JE, Kalman JM, Fitzpatrick AP, et al. Role of right atrial endocardial structures as barriers to conduction during human Type 1 atrial flutter: activation and entrainment mapping guided by intracardiac echocardiography. *Circulation* 1995;92:1839–1848.
11. Nakagawa H, Lazzara R, Khastgir T, et al. Role of the tricuspid annulus and the eustachian valve/ridge on atrial flutter: relevance to catheter ablation of the septal isthmus and a new technique for rapid identification of ablation success. *Circulation* 1996;94:407–424.
12. Wilber DJ, Rubenstein D, Burke MC, et al. Global activation patterns during high-density electro-anatomical mapping of atrial flutter [abstract]. *J Am Coll Cardiol* 1997;29:331A.

13. Olgin JE, Kalman JM, Saxon LA, et al. Mechanism of initiation of atrial flutter in humans: site of unidirectional block and direction of rotation. *J Am Coll Cardiol* 1997;29:376–384.

14. Kinder C, Kall J, Kopp D, et al. Conduction properties of the inferior vena cava-tricuspid annular isthmus in patients with typical atrial flutter. *J Cardiovasc Electrophysiol* 1997;8:727–737.

15. Cosio FG, Lopez-Gil M, Goicolea A, et al. Atrial endocardial mapping in the rare form of atrial flutter. *Am J Cardiol* 1990;66:715–720.

16. Saoudi N, Nair M, Abdelazziz A, et al. Electrocardiographic patterns and results of radiofrequency catheter ablation of clockwise Type I atrial flutter. *J Cardiovasc Electrophysiol* 1996;7:931–942.

17. Kalman JM, Olgin JE, Saxon LA, et al. Electrocardiographic and electrophysiologic characterization of atypical atrial flutter in man. *J Cardiovasc Electrophysiol* 1997;8:121–144.

18. Chauvin M, Brechenmacher C. A clinical study of the application of endocardial fulguration in the treatment of recurrent atrial flutter. *PACE* 1989;12:219–224.

19. Saoudi N, Atallah G, Kirkorian G, et al. Catheter ablation of the atrial myocardium in human type 1 atrial flutter. *Circulation* 1990;81:762–771.

20. Feld GK, Fleck RP, Chen PS, et al. Radiofrequency catheter ablation for the treatment of human type 1 atrial flutter. *Circulation* 1992;86:1233–1240.

21. Cosio F, Lopez-Gil M, Goicolea A, et al. Radiofrequency ablation of the inferior vena cava-tricuspid valve isthmus in common atrial flutter. *Am J Cardiol* 1993;71:705–709.

22. Calkins H, Leon AR, Deam AG, et al. Catheter ablation of atrial flutter using radiofrequency energy. *Am J Cardiol* 1994;73:353–356.

23. Kirkorian G, Moncada E, Chevalier P, et al. Radiofrequency ablation of atrial flutter: efficacy of an anatomically guided approach. *Circulation* 1994;90:2804–2814.

24. Lesh MD, Van Hare GF, Epstein LM, et al. Radiofrequency catheter ablation of atrial arrhythmias: results and mechanisms. *Circulation* 1994;89:1074–1089.

25. Poty H, Saoudi N, Aziz AA, et al. Radiofrequency catheter ablation of Type 1 atrial flutter: prediction of late success by electrophysiologic criteria. *Circulation* 1995;92:1389–1392.

26. Kalman JM, Van Hare GF, Olgin JE, et al. Ablation of "incisional" reentrant atrial tachycardia complicating surgery for congenital heart disease: use of entrainment to define a critical isthmus of conduction. *Circulation* 1996;93:502–512.

27. Frame LH, Page RL, Hoffman BF. Atrial reentry around an anatomic barrier with a partially refractory excitable gap: a canine model of atrial flutter. *Circ Res* 1986;58:495–511.

28. Frame LH, Page PL, Boyden PA, et al. Circus movement in the canine atrium around the tricuspid ring during experimental atrial flutter and during reentry in vitro. *Circulation* 1987;76:1155–1175.

29. Rosenblueth A, Garcia Ramos J. Studies of artifical obstacles on experimental auricular flutter. *Am Heart J* 1947;33:677–684.

30. Boineau JP, Schuessler RB, Mooney CR, et al. Natural and evoked atrial flutter due to circus movement in dogs. *Am J Cardiol* 1980;45:1167–1181.

31. Waldo AL, Hoffman BF, James TN. The relationship of atrial activation to P wave polarity and morphology. In: Little RC, ed. *Physiology of Atrial Pacemakers and Conductive Tissue.* Mt. Kisco, NY: Futura Publishing Co., 1980. pp 261–289.

32. Page PL, Plumb VJ, Okumura K, et al. A new animal model of atrial flutter. *J Am Coll Cardiol* 1986;8:872–879.

33. Boyden PA. Activation sequence during atrial flutter in dogs with surgically induced right atrial enlargement. I: Observations during sustained rhythms. *Circ Res* 1988;62:596–608.

34. Schoels W, Gough WB, Restivo M, et al. Circus movement atrial flutter in the sterile pericarditis model: activation patterns during initiation, termination and sustained reentry in vivo. *Circ Res* 1990;67:35–50.

35. Okumura K, Plumb VJ, Page PL, et al. Atrial activation sequence during atrial flutter in the canine sterile pericarditis model and its effects on the polarity of the flutter wave in the electrocardiogram. *J Am Coll Cardiol* 1991;17:509–518.

36. Shimizu A, Nozaki A, Rudy Y, et al. Onset of induced atrial flutter in the canine pericarditis model. *J Am Coll Cardiol* 1991;17:1223–1234.

37. Shimizu A, Nozaki A, Rudy Y, et al. Multiplexing studies of effects of rapid atrial pacing on the area of slow conduction during atrial flutter in canine sterile pericarditis model. *Circulation* 1991;83:983–994.

38. Schoels W, Restivoe M, Caref EB, et al. Circus movement atrial flutter in a canine sterile pericarditis model: activation patterns during entrainment and termination of single-loop reentry in vivo. *Circulation* 1991;83:1716–1730.

39. Feld GK, Shahandeh-Rad F. Activation patterns in experimental canine atrial flutter produced by right atrial crush injury. *J Am Coll Cardiol* 1992;20:441–451.

40. Feld GK, Shahandeh-Rad F. Mechanism of double potentials recorded during sustained atrial flutter in the canine right atrial crush injury model. *Circulation* 1992;86:628–641.

41. Waldo AL. The canine sterile pericarditis model of atrial flutter. In: Waldo AL, Touboul P, eds. *Atrial Flutter.* Armonk, NY: Futura Publishing Co., 1996. pp 173–192.

42. Schoels W, Kuebler W, Yang H, et al. A unified functional-anatomic substrate for circus movement atrial flutter: activation and refractory patterns in the canine right atrial enlargement model. *J Am Coll Cardiol* 1993;21:73–84.

43. Shimuzu A, Nozaki A, Rudy Y, et al. Characterization of double potentials in a functionally determined reentrant circuit: multiplexing studies during interruption of atrial flutter in the canine sterile pericarditis model. *J Am Coll Cardiol* 1993;22:2022–2032.

44. Isber N, Restivo M, Gough WB, Yang H, El-Sherif N. Circus movement atrial flutter in the canine sterile pericarditis model: cryothermal termination from the epicardial site of the slow zone of the reentrant circuit. *Circulation.* 1993;87:1649–1660.

45. Lesh MD, Kalman JM. To fumble or tackle "tach"?: toward updated classifiers for atrial tachyarrhythmias. *J Cardiovasc Electrophysiol* 1996;7:460–466.
46. Yamauchi S, Schuessler RB, Kawamoto T, et al. Use of intraoperative mapping to optimize surgical ablation of atrial flutter. *Ann Thorac Surg* 1993;56:337–342.
47. Haj-Darwish YM, Baerman JM, Kall JG, et al. Atrial fibrillation induced by vagal stimulation of atrial flutter: insights from an animal model [abstract]. *J Am Coll Cardiol* 1993;21:184A.
48. Arenal A, Almendral J, San Roman D, et al. Frequency and implications of resetting and entrainment with right atrial stimulation in atrial flutter. *Am J Cardiol* 1992;70:1292–1298.
49. Stevenson WG, Khan H, Sager P, et al. Identification of reentry circuit sites during catheter mapping and radiofrequency ablation of ventricular tachycardia late after myocardial infarction. *Circulation* 1993;88:1647–1670.
50. Della Bella P, Marenzi G, Tondo C, et al. Usefulness of the excitable gap and pattern of resetting in atrial flutter for determining reentry circuit location. *Am J Cardiol* 1991;68:492–497.
51. Paydak H, Kall JG, Burke MC, et al. Atrial fibrillation after radiofrequency ablation of Type 1 atrial flutter: time to onset, determinants, and clinical course. *Circulation* 1998;98:315–322.
52. Gepstein L, Hayam G, Ben-Haim SA. A novel method for nonfluoroscopic catheter-based electroanatomical mapping of the heart: in vitro and in vivo accuracy results. *Circulation* 1997;95:1611–1622.
53. Uno K, Kumagai K, Khrestian C, et al. New insights regarding the atrial flutter reentrant circuit in the canine sterile pericarditis model [abstract]. *J Am Coll Cardiol* 1997;29:254A.
54. Wang Z, Jorge A, Jo W, et al. Anatomic variability of the human eustachian ridge [abstract]. *PACE* 1996;19:724.
55. Bogun F, Bender B, Li Y-G, et al. Concealed entrainment in radiofrequency catheter ablation of atypical atrial flutter in patients without prior cardiac surgery [abstract]. *J Am Coll Cardiol* 1996;33:116 A.
56. Jais P, Haïssaguerre M, Shah DC, et al. Successful irrigated-tip catheter ablation of atrial flutter resistant to conventional radiofrequency ablation. *Circulation* 1998;98:835–838.
57. Gomes JA, Santoni-Rugiu F, Mehta D, et al. Uncommon atrial flutter: characteristics, mechanisms, and results of ablative therapy. *PACE* 1998;21:2029–2042.
58. Cheng J, Cabeen WR, Scheinman MM. Mechanisms and anatomic substrates of atypical atrial flutter in the right atrium [abstract]. *PACE* 1998;21:795.
59. Cheng J, Scheinman MM. Acceleration of typical atrial flutter due to double-wave reentry induced by programmed electrical stimulation. *Circulation* 1998;97:1589–1596.
60. Nunez A, Arribas F, Lopez Gil M, et al. A study of the mechanism of atrial flutter and atrial tachycardia in adults by mapping and pacing [abstract]. *PACE* 1995;18:803.
61. Cosio FG, Arribas F, Lopez Gil M, et al. Atrial flutter mapping and ablation

I. Studying atrial flutter mechanisms by mapping and entrainment. *PACE* 1996;19:841–853.

62. Jais P, Haïssaguerre M, Shah D, et al. A new electrophysiological substrate for spontaneous left atrial flutters [abstract]. *Circulation* 1998;98:I-19.

63. Natale A, Richey M, Tomassoni GF, et al. Clinical characteristics and ablation of left side atrial flutter [abstract]. *J Am Coll Cardiol* 1999;33:116 A.

64. Olgin JE, Jayachandran V, Engelstein E, et al. Atrial macroreentry involving the myocardium of the coronary sinus: a unique mechanism for atypical flutter. *J Cardiovasc Electrophysiol* 1998;9:1094–1099.

65. Antz M, Otomo K, Arruda M, et al. Does the coronary sinus form an electrical connection between the left atrium and the right atrium? [abstract] *PACE* 1997;20:1200.

66. Arruda M, Widman L, Antz M, et al. Myocardial continuity between the right atrium and left atrium via the coronary sinus [abstract]. *J Am Coll Cardiol* 1997;29:358A-359A.

67. Cheng J, Ursell PC, Dorostkar PC, et al. Electrophysiologic and anatomic correlates of protected conduction in the posterior mitral annular vestibule [abstract]. *PACE* 1998;21:795.

68. Chauvin M, Marcellin L, Douchet M-P, et al. Muscular connections between right and left atria in the coronary sinus region in humans: anatomo-pathologic observations [abstract]. *PACE* 1998;21:816.

69. Goyal R, Zivin A, Souza J, et al. Endocardial mapping of typical atrial flutter using a non-contact mapping system [abstract]. *Circulation* 1998;98:I-73.

70. Zrenner B, Panescu D, Karch M, et al. Initial experience with a novel multielectrode simultaneous-mapping and ablation navigation system in right atrial tachyarrhythmias [abstract]. *Circulation* 1998;98:I-282.

71. Kadish A, Hauck J, Pederson B, et al. Accuracy of geometric localization using non-contact multielectrode array in the right atrium [abstract]. *J Am Coll Cardiol* 1999;33:122A.

72. Kall JG, Rubenstein DS, Kopp DE, et al. Atypical atrial flutter originating in the right atrial free wall. *Circulation* 2000;101:270–279.

Chapter 14

Anatomic Structures and Barriers in the Ablation of Atrial Tachycardia and Flutter: The Role of Intracardiac Echocardiography

Jeffrey E. Olgin, M.D. and Michael D. Lesh, M.D.

The invasive electrophysiology era has led to a better understanding of the substrate, mechanism, and types of atrial flutter. Detailed mapping and novel imaging techniques have yielded a better understanding of the anatomy of the atria and have allowed the correlation of this anatomy to electrophysiological properties. This has in turn led to an appreciation of the anatomic substrate of many atrial arrhythmias. This review will focus on these anatomic correlates as related to atrial flutter.

Atrial Endocardial Anatomy

The right atrial endocardial surface is comprised of many orifices and embryonic remnants, accounting for an irregular, complex surface. This complex endocardial anatomy provides several potential areas around which reentry could occur if these anatomic structures translated to electrophysiological barriers. Orifices of the 2 vena cavae lie in the superior and inferior aspects of the right atrium, respectively. The tricuspid annulus lies anteriorly to the body of the right atrium. The right atrial endocardium is architecturally divided into the anterior trabeculated right atrium, derived from the true embryonic right atrium, and the posterior smooth-walled right atrium, derived from the em-

From Huang SKS, Wilber DJ (eds.): *Radiofrequency Catheter Ablation of Cardiac Arrhythmias: Basic Concepts and Clinical Applications,* 2nd ed. Armonk, NY: Futura Publishing Company, Inc. ©2000.

bryonic sinus venosus.[1] These distinct anatomic regions of the right atrium are separated by the crista terminalis on the lateral wall and the eustachian ridge in the inferior aspect. The crista terminalis extends from the high septum, anterior to the orifice of the superior vena cava superiorly, and courses caudally along the posterolateral wall. In its inferior extent, it courses anteriorly to the orifice of the inferior vena cava. The eustachian ridge is the remnant of the embryonic sinus venosus valve and extends from the orifice of the inferior vena cava to the coronary sinus (CS) os along the floor of the right atrium. The inferior portion of the tricuspid annulus lies a short distance anterior (approximately 1–4 centimeters) to the eustachian ridge, though its course varies among individuals. In some patients it may bifurcate and may terminate anterior or posterior to the CS os. The CS os lies medial to the orifice of the inferior vena cava, as the floor of the right atrium becomes the septum. On the lower third of the interatrial septum lies the fossa ovalis.

Definitions

Prior to the current era of catheter ablation, the nomenclature used to define the term "atrial flutter" was somewhat confusing. However, since the only therapy at that time was drugs, the distinction between the various types of atrial flutter mattered less. In the catheter ablation era, on the other hand, this distinction is critical to the operator attempting specific curative ablation. Thus, "atrial flutter" is a term that has been used both specifically and nonspecifically to describe a variety of different atrial tachycardias. What is sometimes referred to as atrial flutter occurring after reparative surgery for congenital heart disease (Mustard, Senning, or Fontan operations, atrial septal defect repair, etc.) is a different tachycardia than the "typical," "classic," "common," "usual," "Type 1," "Type A," or "orthodromic" atrial flutter involving counterclockwise reentry (in the frontal plane) through an isthmus in the low right atrium. Such "typical atrial flutter" is seen in patients with or without heart disease, but does not require prior surgical incisions in the atrium. Though typical atrial flutter has been defined by electrocardiographers as a regular atrial tachycardia with an atrial rate between 250 and 350 beats per minute and a sawtooth pattern on ECG, flutter can be considerably slower in some patients, particularly those on antiarrhythmic drugs or with abnormal atria.

Even more confusing, perhaps, is the division of "atrial flutter" into subtypes based variously on rate; surface ECG morphology; ability to terminate with overdrive pacing from the high right atrium; and/or endocardial activation sequence. Thus, we have "atypical," "uncommon," "rare," "antedromic," "clockwise," "Type 2," "Type B," "unusual," "fast," "slow," "left atrial," and "reverse" "atrial flutter." Lesh and Kalman have suggested an updated nomenclature which is adopted here in Table 1.[2] Figure 1 demonstrates the characteristic 12-lead ECG of counterclockwise and clockwise typical atrial flutter. Figure 2 demonstrates the activation sequence around the tricuspid annulus in clockwise and counterclockwise flutter.

Table 1
Classification of atrial flutter.

TYPE	ECG	CHARACTERISTICS	CIRCUIT	MAPPING TECHNIQUES	ABLATION SITE
Typical Atrial Flutter					
Counterclockwise	Negative Fl waves II, III, aVF; Predominantly negative V$_6$	Macroreentrant in right atrium with regular rate (usually 250–350 bpm)	Around tricuspid annulus anterior to CT and ER	Anatomic, activation and entrainment to confirm critical isthmus	TA to IVC (ER)
Clockwise	Positive/notched Fl waves in II, III, aVF; Predominantly positive in V$_6$	Rate, regularity and circuit same as counterclockwise but opposite rotation around TA	Around tricuspid annulus anterior to CT and ER	Anatomic, activation and entrainment to confirm critical isthmus	TA or IVC (ER)
Atypical Flutter	Variable	Rate usually faster than typical, often more irregular	Unknown (pulmonary veins, portion of CT, functional barriers)	Activation sequence inconsistent with typical flutter; often difficult to entrain	???
Incisional Reentry (atrial tachycardia in repaired congenital heart disease)	Variable	After surgical repair of congenital heart disease. Rates variable depending on barriers, atrial disease and length of circuit	Repair of congenital defects. Circuit often involves surgical scars or prosthetic material. May also involve subeustachian isthmus.	Identify lines of block with split potentials; activation mapping to identify early sites; entrainment mapping to identify critical isthmus	Variable, but must sever an isthmus from one barrier (surgical or anatomic) to another.

CT = crista terminalis; ER = eustachian ridge; TA = tricuspid annulus; IVC = inferior vena cava

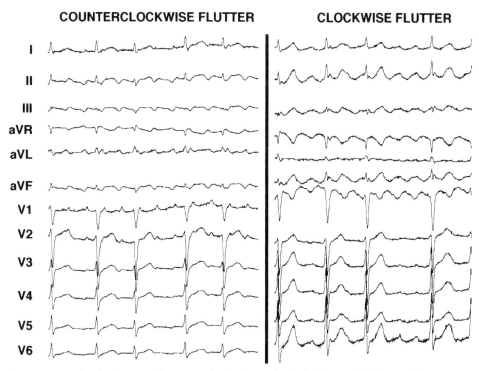

Figure 1. Twelve-lead ECG of counterclockwise and clockwise typical flutter. For counterclockwise flutter, the characteristic negative flutter waves in leads II, III, aVF and V¹ are seen. In clockwise flutter, the upright and notched flutter waves in II, III and aVF are seen as well as the positive flutter wave in V⁶.

The common feature of these tachycardias is that they involve a macroreentrant circuit somewhere in the atria and generally (though not always) involve structural barriers which define the reentrant path. What varies is the specific nature and location of those barriers. In addition, given a potential reentrant circuit, actual reentrant excitation can revolve in 1 of 2 possible directions.

Typical Atrial Flutter

Typical atrial flutter has a characteristic pattern on 12-lead ECG, with superiorly directed flutter waves and rates in a range of 200–300 beats per minute (Figure 1). The uniformity of these characteristics among patients in whom cardiac pathology varies suggests a common substrate for the arrhythmia. It is now well established that atrial flutter is a reentrant arrhythmia confined to the right atrium.[3–5] The unique endocardial anatomy of the right atrium, with its many orifices and distinct structures around which reentry can occur, likely explains the consistency of atrial flutter from patient to patient.

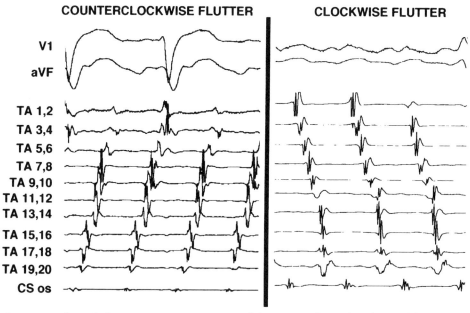

Figure 2. Endocardial activation sequence around the tricuspid annulus obtained from a halo catheter during counterclockwise and clockwise atrial flutter. Halo poles TA 1, 2 are positioned in the low lateral right atrium and poles TA 19, 20 are position on the septum near the His position. In counterclockwise flutter, the activation is seen to procede from the CS os up the septum to TA 19, 20 in a counterclockwise fashion to TA 1, 2. For clockwise flutter, the activation sequence is the opposite, with activation from the CS os proceding first to TA 1, 2 on the low lateral right atrium then in a clockwise fashion toward the TA 19, 20. Notice that in both cases the tricuspid annulus is activated in a sequential manner.

Animal Models of Atrial Flutter

Much of our current understanding of the role of barriers in atrial flutter has come from animal models. Rosenblueth and Garcia-Ramos developed a canine model of atrial flutter by creating a crush lesion between the orifices of the venae cavae.[6] This lesion produced an atrial tachycardia which was identical to atrial flutter in both rate and morphology.[6] When this lesion was extended laterally, the cycle length of the tachycardia lengthened.[6] When the lesion was extended to the tricuspid annulus, the tachycardia terminated.[6] Although these data suggest that the tachycardia was due to reentry set up by these artificial obstacles, the study was limited by its method of sequential mapping and did not define the entire circuit. This model is the basis for most of the subsequent reliable animal models of atrial flutter and unequivocally demonstrated the necessity of barriers to maintain atrial flutter.

Frame et al used a model of atrial flutter similar to that of Rosenblueth and Garcia-Ramos with a Y-shaped lesion in the right atrium, between the venae cavae, and a connecting lesion extending toward the right atrial appendage.[7,8] Mapping revealed that reentry occurred around the tricuspid annulus and not around the lesion itself.[7,8] The Y-shaped lesion served as a barrier to conduction, protecting the tissue between the lesion and the tricuspid annulus from excitation from an inferiorly spreading wavefront, thus remaining excitable when the reentrant wavefront arrived. These studies have demonstrated the importance of not 1, but 2 barriers between which reentry can occur, with a second barrier to "protect" the circuit from excitation by wavefronts other than the reentrant wavefront (that is, short circuiting).

In a dog with spontaneous atrial reentry, Boineau et al found hypoplasia of the crista terminalis and atrophic pectinate muscle.[9] From this observation he and others used ligation of the crista terminalis as a model of atrial flutter in dogs.[9–11] In this model, atrial reentry around the crista terminalis occurs with characteristics similar to human atrial flutter.[10,11] From these experiments, it was suggested that the crista terminalis might play a role as an obstacle in human atrial flutter.[11]

Feld et al utilized a single crush lesion in the right atrial free wall to produce atrial reentry in dogs.[12,13] Activation mapping suggested that reentry occurred around the crush lesion; however, the role of other barriers (such as the tricuspid annulus and crista terminalis) was not studied.[12,13]

Other animal models not involving artificial obstacles include sterile pericarditis[14–16] and right atrial enlargement secondary to tricuspid avulsion.[17,18] Both functional and anatomic obstacles have been found in these models of atrial flutter.[14,17,18] Debate continues as to what role, if any, is played by functional barriers in human typical atrial flutter.

Mapping of Human Atrial Flutter

Activation Mapping

Multi-electrode endocardial activation maps have been performed in human flutter and have provided valuable information about the general location of the reentrant circuit. Indeed, independent of mapping technique, there has been remarkable similarity among the mapping studies of human atrial flutter, from that of Lewis in 1921 using vectorcardiography[19] to more recent studies utilizing multisite endocardial and epicardial mapping[3,4,20–23]—a counterclockwise rotation in the frontal plane of the right atrium.

Using multisite endocardial mapping in patients with atrial flutter, Puech et al found that the septal wall of the right atrium is activated inferior-to-superior while the anterolateral (free) wall of the right atrium is activated superior to inferior.[21] Klein et al studied 2 patients with atrial flutter using epicardial mapping and found that the coronary sinus ostium was the earliest site of activation in relation to the flutter wave.[4] Activation in the right atrium spreads superiorly from the CS os, up to the septum and down the lateral right atrial wall.[4] A critical area of conduction was identified between the CS os, the tricuspid valve ring, and the inferior vena cava.[4] Endocardial mapping with multisite, multipolar recording by Olshansky et al, Cosio et al, and

Feld et al have confirmed this counterclockwise rotation of typical flutter (Figure 1).[3,20,23] Although a critical area of conduction was identified between the tricuspid annulus, the CS os, and the inferior vena cava in these studies, the basis for the disparate activation patterns of the septum and free wall were not addressed.

Double Potentials

During activation mapping of atrial flutter, double, or "split" potentials, defined as discrete electrograms separated by an isoelectric phase, have been frequently recorded during atrial flutter.[3,20–26] While controversy exists as to whether isolated double potentials may indicate disparate endocardial and epicardial activation or merely slowed conduction, in many cases they undoubtedly indicate activation on either side of a line of block.[12,24,25,27] The anatomic basis and precise location of lines of block represented by these split potentials recorded during atrial flutter were not identified in early studies. Moreover, these lines of block may occur at sites which are not within the primary reentrant circuit, and thus are not necessary for reentry. This was not addressed in these early studies.

Entrainment Mapping

Entrainment has also been used to interrogate the atrial flutter circuit. Waldo et al first described transient entrainment to demonstrate that atrial flutter was indeed a reentrant arrhythmia.[28] Subsequently, Okumura et al described concealed entrainment, which was defined as paced acceleration of a tachycardia (for which manifest entrainment can be shown during pacing from a different site) without demonstration of surface fusion.[29] Concealed entrainment has been demonstrated in the low right atrium and at the CS os during atrial flutter.[13,22,23,30,31]

It has also been observed that the postpacing interval, defined as the interval from the last entrained beat to the first spontaneous beat measured at the pacing site, is useful to evaluate components of a reentrant circuit.[10,23,32] Comparing the postpacing interval at the pacing site to the spontaneous tachycardia cycle length indicates whether a site is inside or outside of the reentrant circuit.[32–34]

Barriers in Typical Atrial Flutter

From activation and entrainment mapping obtained in recent studies whose specific aims were to identify barriers, and from extensive previous investigation, a more complete understanding of the human atrial flutter circuit can now be constructed. Figure 3 shows the typical atrial flutter circuit. As predicted by the results obtained in studies of animal models of flutter, there are 2 barriers, generally anteriorly and posteriorly located.

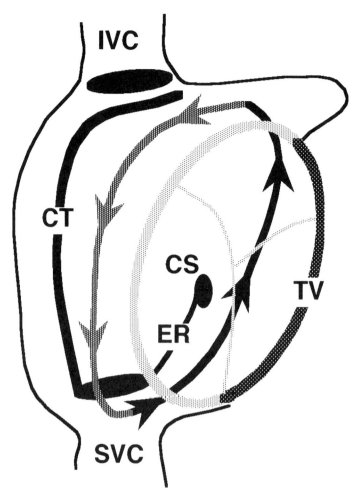

Figure 3. Diagram of the barriers in the reentrant circuit of typical flutter. The broad wavefront rotates around the tricuspid annulus, between it (as the anterior barrier) and the crista terminalis/eustachian ridge as the posterior barrier. The narrow isthmus is between the tricuspid annulus and the eustachian ridge, which lies just anterior to the inferior vena cava. IVC = inferior vena cava; SVC = superior vena cava; CT = crista terminalis; ER = eustachian ridge; CS = coronary sinus; TV = tricuspid valve.

Anterior Barrier (Tricuspid Annulus)

Cosio et al have previously demonstrated sequential activation around the tricuspid annulus during typical atrial flutter.[3] Using activation and entrainment mapping from the closely spaced sites around the tricuspid annulus during human typical atrial flutter, Kalman et al have confirmed that the flutter wave proceeds in a counterclockwise fashion around the tricuspid annulus (Figures 4 and 5).[35] Activation around the entire tricuspid annulus accounts for 100% of the flutter cycle length.[35] Using entrainment mapping, all sites around the circumference of the tricuspid annulus were determined to be a part of the

A

B

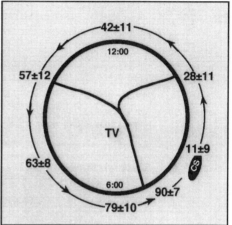

Figure 4. Panel A: Activation times at sites on either side of the crista terminalis and eustachian ridge.[22] Panel B: Activation times at sites around the tricuspid annulus.[35] Values are expressed as mean ± standard deviation activation times from the CS os electrogram as a percent of the flutter cycle length. In panel A, sites at which activation times are shown on either side of the crista terminalis and eustachian ridge were determined with intracardiac echo.[22] Sites posterior to the crista terminalis and eustachian ridge are activated significantly earlier than sites anterior to these structures. Statistical comparisons were made to sites just opposite the crista terminalis or eustachian ridge.[22] In panel B, activation times around the tricuspid annulus demonstrate that 100% of the flutter cycle length is accounted for and proceeds in a counterclockwise fashion, sequentially around the annulus.[35] (Modified from *Circulation* with permission from American Heart Association. Pathology specimen courtesy of R. H. Anderson and A. E. Becker.) *$P < 0.02$ SVC = superior vena cava; IVC = inferior vena cava; CT = crista terminalis; FO = fossa ovalis; CS = coronary sinus; TV = tricuspid valve.

flutter reentrant circuit, since the postpacing interval was equal to the flutter cycle length.[35] These findings were confirmed by Nakagawa et al in a similar study in 30 patients using both activation and entrainment mapping.[26] Thus the tricuspid annulus is the anterior barrier in atrial flutter, and is, of course, fixed.

Posterior Barriers (Crista Terminalis and Eustachian Ridge)

Since the atrial endocardial structures are not seen on fluoroscopy, intracardiac echocardiography has been used to directly visualize and map specific anatomic structures during atrial flutter.[22] Using multisite mapping in relation to the crista terminalis and eustachian ridge, Olgin et al determined that the trabeculated right atrium—anterior to the crista terminalis and eustachian ridge—was activated superior-to-inferior (Figure 4). The smooth-walled right atrium (septum)—posterior to the crista terminalis and eustachian ridge—was activated inferior-to-superior (Figure 4).[22]

In addition, using intracardiac echocardiograpy to place a multipolar

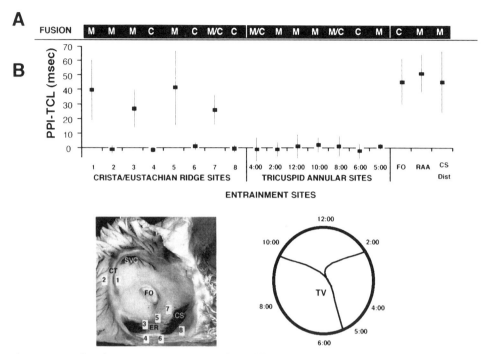

Figure 5. Results of entrainment mapping of atrial flutter from sites in the right atrium on either side of the crista terminalis and eustachian ridge, under ICE guidance[22] and around the tricuspid annulus.[35] The anatomic location of the sites are shown in the diagrams at the bottom of the figure. The sites on either side of the CT/ER are labeled 1–8. The sites around the tricuspid annulus are labeled as clock face. Values are mean ± standard deviation. **A)** The presence of surface fusion is shown as either manifest (M) or concealed (C). Concealed fusion was observed only at sites between the eustachian ridge and tricuspid annulus, indicating that this is a protected isthmus.[22,35] **B)** The postpacing interval minus the flutter cycle length for each site is shown. Sites where the postpacing interval is equal to the flutter cycle length are within the reentrant circuit.[22] These sites included all sites anterior to the crista terminalis and eustachian ridge.[22] Sites posterior to these structures are not within the circuit.[22] All sites along the tricuspid annulus demonstrated a postpacing interval equal to the flutter cycle length and are thus within the reentrant circuit.[35] The fossa ovalis, tip of the right atrial appendage, and distal coronary sinus were not within the reentrant circuit.[22,35] (Modified from *Circulation* with permission from American Heart Association. Pathology specimen courtesy of R. H. Anderson and A. E. Becker.) M = manifest; C = concealed; PPI = postpacing interval; FCL = flutter cycle length; Stim Time = stimulus time; Act Time = activation time; SVC = superior vena cava; IVC = inferior vena cava; CT = crista terminalis; FO = fossa ovalis; ER = eustachian ridge; CS = coronary sinus; TA = tricuspid annulus; RAA = right atrial appendage.

catheter along the length of the crista terminalis and eustachian ridge, split potentials can be recorded along these structures with disparate activation sequences of each component (Figure 6).[22] Nakagawa also demonstrated split potentials along the length of a multipolar catheter placed along the eustachian ridge (Figure 7).[26] The recording of split potentials with opposite activation sequences along the entire length of the crista terminalis and its extension as the eustachian ridge is strong evidence of these structures forming a line of block.

CLOCKWISE　　　　　**COUNTERCLOCKWISE**

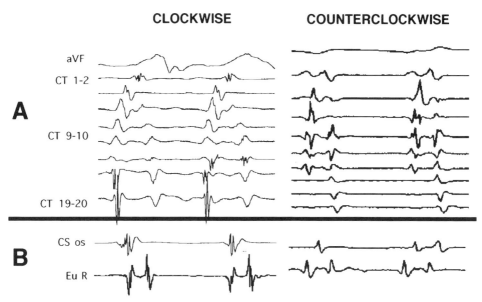

Figure 6. Split potentials recorded along the crista terminalis (**A**) and eustachian ridge (**B**) in counterclockwise and clockwise (typical) flutter. These structures were mapped under intracardiac echo guidance to ensure catheter location. Each component of the split potentials along the crista is activated in opposite sequence.

Moreover, entrainment can be used to demonstrate that one component of the split potential is within the reentrant circuit while the other is not.[26] If the split components were merely due to slowed conduction across a region, the individual components would not be differently entrained.[25,27]

Similarly, using ICE-guided entrainment, it was demonstrated that entrainment at any site along the radius from the tricuspid annulus anteriorly to the crista terminalis or eustachian ridge posteriorly yields a postpacing interval equal to the flutter cycle length, indicating that the entire trabeculated right atrium is within the reentrant circuit of flutter (Figure 5).[22,26] Entrainment from sites just posterior to these structures yields a postpacing interval significantly greater than the flutter cycle length, indicating that areas of the smooth right atrium are not within the flutter reentrant circuit.[22]

Although the crista terminalis and eustachian ridge are a part of the posterior barriers, there appears to be an anatomic "gap" in what must be the continuation of this posterior barrier from the CS os to the superior-medial aspect of the crista terminalis. The interatrial septum has been shown by activation mapping and entrainment not to be within the reentrant circuit, except for the septum immediately adjacent to the annulus.[22] Therefore, there must be an additional barrier from the end of the eustachian ridge at the CS os to the medial aspect of the crista terminalis. It is possible that this portion of the posterior barrier is completed as a functional, alternate pathway barrier described by Boyden.[36] Thus, the most "direct" pathway for the flutter circuit to take from the CS os is along the tricuspid annulus, superiorly towards the medial aspect of the crista terminalis. Activation away from the annulus on the septum,

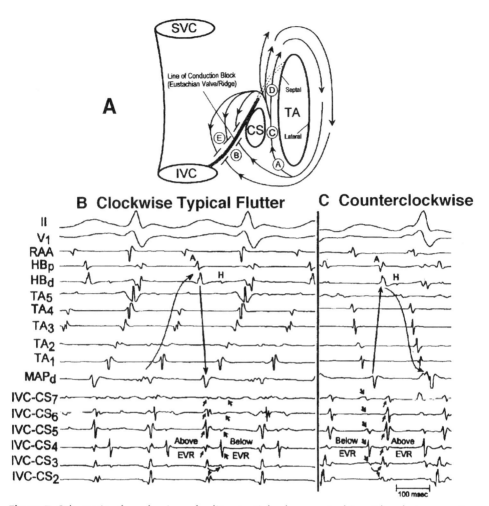

Figure 7. Schematic of mechanism of split potentials along eustachian ridge during counterclockwise flutter (A) and demonstration of split potentials along the eustachian ridge during clockwise atrial flutter (B) and during counterclockwise flutter (C).[26] [Modified from *Circulation* with permission from the American Heart Association.] RAA = right atrial appendage; HB = His bundle; TA = tricuspid annulus; IVC-CS = catheter along eustachian ridge.

because it is a longer path (either physically or due to slow conduction), would not arrive at the medial crista terminalis in time to "short circuit" the reentrant wave. In fact, if there was a continuous fixed barrier between the CS os and the medial crista terminalis, the septum would be activated very late, after the left atrium. Activation mapping has shown that indeed the septum is activated just after the CS os, suggesting that the alternate pathway explanation is likely. There have been reports of associations between atrioventricular nodal reentry tachycardia and atrial flutter. it is intriguing to postulate that the flutter circuit continues from the CS os through preferential pathways (that is, slow and fast pathways of atrioventricular nodal reentry tachycardia) to the medial crista terminalis. Another possibility is that the tendon of Todaro, which is the fibrous extension of the eustachian ridge, is an anatomic barrier. The structure, however, lies below the atrial endocardium and does not grossly or microscopically interrupt the atrial muscle fibers, at least in normal hearts. Its structure, specifically in patients with atrial flutter, has not been explored.

It is also not known how the reentrant wavefront proceeds in the superiomedial aspect of the right atrium. Several studies have demonstrated that the upper turn around point of the flutter circuit is near the superior vena cava, between the crista terminalis (which lies just anterior to the superior vena cava) and the tricuspid annulus.[22,35,37] The tip of the right atrial appendage has been demonstrated not to be a part of the circuit.[35] However, the course of the wavefront at the base of the right atrial appendage is not known. Most likely the wavefront proceeds through 1 side of the base, with the other side as a longer alternate pathway. This, however, has yet to be demonstrated.

Whether the crista terminalis is a fixed or functional barrier is not known with certainty, but strong evidence suggests that it is fixed in the majority of patients with typical flutter. Saffitz et al have shown that the crista terminalis preferentially conducts longitudinally wit poor transverse conduction.[38] The basis for this was a disparate distribution of gap junctions with fewer gap junctions in the transverse (side to side) orientation.[38] In patients with atrial flutter, split potentials have been recorded along the crista terminalis both during atrial flutter and during slow pacing in sinus rhythm (Figure 8). Using intracardiac echo to ensure placement of a 20-pole catheter along the length of the crista terminalis, split po-

PACING FROM INTRA-ATRIAL SEPTUM DURING SINUS RHYTHM

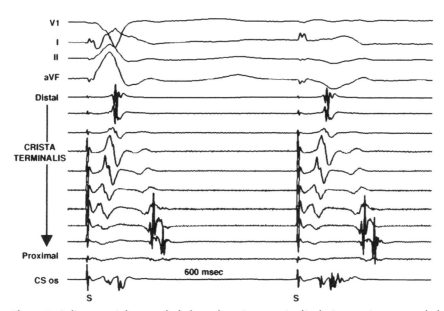

Figure 8. Split potentials recorded along the crista terminalis during pacing at a cycle length of 600 milliseconds from the mid-right atrial septum during sinus rhythm in a patient referred for ablation of atrial flutter. As in atrial flutter, disparate activation of each component of the split potentials during pacing suggests that the crista terminalis is a fixed barrier to conduction. Split potentials were not seen during sinus rhythm, since the crista terminalis is the location of the sinus mechanism, with activation spread on either side of the crista in a high-to-low sequence.

tentials with disparate activation sequences have been recorded during pacing at slow rates from the low right atrial septum.[39] Nakagawa et al demonstrated split potentials along the eustachian ridge during pacing at slow rates.[26] While this is not proof of a fixed line of block, it is suggestive. Another piece of evidence that the crista terminalis and eustachian ridge are fixed lines of block is provided by the technique of demonstrating successful radiofrequency ablation by pacing on either side of the radiofrequency lesion between the inferior vena cava and tricuspid annulus (Figure 9).[26,40–42] With the technique, after ablation, a bidirectional line of block is demonstrated at the ablation site by pacing just lateral to and then just medial to the lesion during sinus rhythm (Figures 10 and 11). Pacing laterally to the lesion yields an altered activation sequence in the atrium, compared to preablation which proceeded from the low lateral right atrium, up the lateral wall, down the septum and to the CS os (Figure 11). If the crista terminalis and eustachian ridge were not fixed lines of block, the septum and lateral wall would be activated in unison rather than in sequence, even if a lesion were placed in the low right atrium. Whether these lines of block are fixed in all people is currently unknown. It is intriguing to speculate that the fixed nature of these lines of block may be the requisite anatomic substrate for flutter, which is at least 1 factor separating those patients who have flutter from those who do not. A trigger, often atrial fibrillation, is also required. Not all patients with the

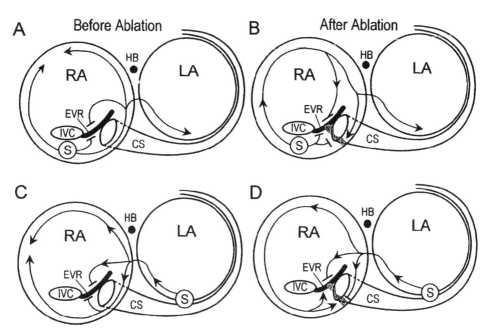

Figure 9. Schematic illustrating technique of confirming bidirectional conduction block in the isthmus following ablation.[26] **A)** Pacing from the low lateral right atrium prior to ablation results in activation around the tricuspid annulus in both clockwise and counterclockwise directions. **B)** Following ablation, pacing from the low lateral right atrium results in activation only in the clockwise direction. **C)** Pacing from the coronary sinus prior to ablation results in activation around the tricuspid annulus in both clockwise and counterclockwise directions. **D)** Following ablation, CS pacing results in only counterclockwise activation. [Modified from *Circulation* with permission from the American Heart Association.]

PACING FROM THE CS OS DURING RADIOFREQUENCY ABLATION

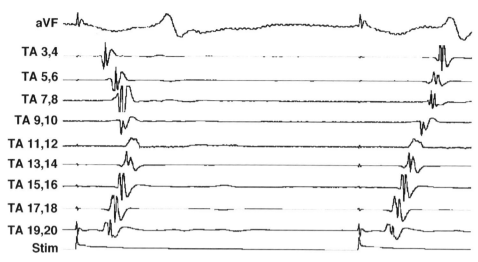

Figure 10. Demonstration of isthmus block during radiofrequency ablation of a patient with atrial flutter. After flutter was terminated, pacing from the CS os was performed during radiofrequency ablation. Two paced beats are shown during radiofrequency energy application. On the beat on the left, activation of the halo catheter procedes in both the clockwise and counterclockwise direction with fusion of the wavefronts near TA 11, 12. On the next beat, conduction block in the isthmus had been completed as evidenced by activation of the halo catheter in a counterclockwise direction only.

PACING FROM THE LOW LATERAL RIGHT ATRIUM

A   **B**

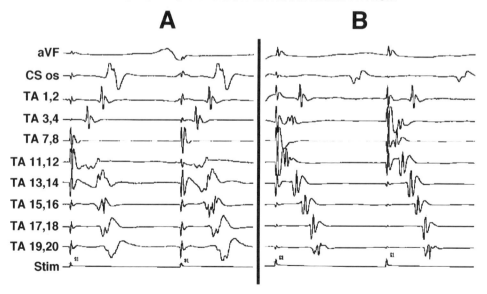

Figure 11. Demonstration of bidirectional block in the patient shown in Figure 5. Pacing from the low lateral right atrium in the region of TA 5, 6 prior to ablation **(A)** demonstrates activation of the CS os through the flutter isthmus (TA 1, 2, which is activated before CS os). **B)** Following ablation, pacing from the low lateral right atrium demonstrates that the CS os is activated after TA 19, 20, confirming block in the flutter isthmus.

anatomic substrate necessarily have clinical atrial flutter if the conditions for initiation, including a proper trigger, are not met.

Critical Isthmus

Many investigators have identified an isthmus of conduction in the low right atrium.[20,23,31,43] Concealed entrainment has been demonstrated in the area between the tricuspid annulus and the inferior vena cava.[20,31] Feld et al has further demonstrated concealed entrainment near the inferior vena cava (between it and the tricuspid annulus) producing a long activation time from stimulus to flutter wave (>40 milliseconds), and near the CS os (between it and the tricuspid annulus) producing a short activation time from stimulus to flutter wave (<40 milliseconds), suggesting that the inferior vena cava is near the entrance and that the CS os is the exit of an isthmus.[20] Using intracardiac echo to guide entrainment mapping, we have determined that this isthmus in the low lateral right atrium is bordered by the tricuspid annulus and the eustachian ridge.[22] This was confirmed by the study by Nakagawa et al.[26]

Other Forms of Atrial Flutter

Clockwise Flutter

It has recently been recognized that 1 form of what had been termed "atypical atrial flutter" is simply clockwise rotation in the frontal plane of the flutter wave that uses the same barriers as counterclockwise typical flutter (Figures 1 and 2).[44–46] Split potentials can be recorded along the crista terminalis and eustachian ridge during clockwise flutter (Figure 6).[26,44] In addition, clockwise activation can be demonstrated around the tricuspid annulus. Entrainment techniques, similar to those described above, have been used to demonstrate that this form of flutter uses the same isthmus in the low right atrium bordered by the tricuspid annulus and eustachian ridge.[26,44] For this reason, this form of flutter is ablated in the same way as typical (counterclockwise) atrial flutter.[26,44,46]

Atypical Flutter

Other forms of atypical atrial flutter do not appear to use the same circuit as typical atrial flutter. The rates and endocardial activation are inconsistent with either clockwise or counterclockwise flutter. Although the barriers are unknown for this type of atypical flutter, there is preliminary data to suggest that at least some of these arrhythmias are due to reentry around a portion of the crista terminalis.[44] Other forms of atypical flutter may be due to macroreentry in the left atrium, where the role of anatomic barriers such as the pulmonary veins or mitral annulus has yet to be completely explored.

Incisional Reentry

Incisional atrial reentry, which occurs following surgical repair of congenital heart disease, is similar to atrial flutter except that at least 1 of the barriers are surgically placed—either a surgical scar or prosthetic material (such as an atrial septal defect patch). These forms of atrial reentry have been modeled in dogs and extensively mapped in a patient to demonstrate that, indeed, surgical scars serve as barriers.[47–49] This form of atrial reentry may be more akin to some of the animal models of atrial flutter since an artificial object, surgically placed, is responsible for the reentry, either as the central barrier or as a second barrier. Because the barriers are variable among patients and isthmuses can be wide at points, both entrainment mapping and recording of split potentials are useful to define barriers in individual patients.[50,51] Using these mapping techniques, incisional reentry is readily cured with catheter ablation by severing a critical isthmus between barriers.[50,51] In addition, extending these suture lines to barriers such as the inferior vena cava and tricuspid annulus at the time of surgery will prevent many of these incisional reentrant arrhythmias.

Clinical Implications

Induction of Flutter

Oftentimes, patients who are referred for atrial flutter ablation present to the laboratory in sinus rhythm. Although ablation can be performed in sinus rhythm (see below), it is often useful to confirm the diagnosis of typical atrial flutter and perform endocardial mapping to guide ablation. Because the circuit for both counterclockwise and clockwise flutter are the same, the site from which flutter is induced with programmed stimulation determines in which direction the flutter rotates.[52] Pacing from the smooth right atrium posterior to the crista terminalis and eustachian ridge induces counterclockwise flutter while pacing from the trabeculated right atrium anterior to these structures produces clockwise flutter.[52] This site dependence exists because the initiating unidirectional block occurs in the sub-eustachian isthmus.[52]

Ablation

Atrial flutter is now readily cured with catheter ablation.[20,41–43,53–58] This is performed by creating a lesion from the tricuspid annulus to the eustachian ridge (which is the anterior aspect of the inferior vena cava), severing the narrow isthmus.[43,56] With the identification of the barriers in the flutter circuit, many have taken a purely "anatomic" approach to ablating flutter with equal success rates to that of an electrophysiological mapping approach.[55] This region is used because it is the narrowest region between the known barriers of the reentrant circuit. However, it would be possible in theory to cure atrial flutter using any lesion that bridged the 2 barriers—the anterolateral tricuspid annulus to the lateral crista terminalis, for example, if a lesion could be made of that length.

There was in the early experience a fairly high recurrence rate after atrial flutter ablation (20–30%).[20,41–43,53–58] Most recurrences likely represented a failure in end point testing of the ablation. An apparent acute success may result from an inability to reinduce atrial flutter after attempted lesion placement.[52] It is clear from the knowledge of barriers in atrial flutter that 2 barriers must be bridged by the ablation lesion for long-term success. Local edema and transient changes in conduction properties in the area of ablation may terminate atrial flutter and make it difficult to reinduce immediately after energy delivery. This may occur without having permanently severed the isthmus between the eustachian ridge and tricuspid annulus.

Poty et al first described a technique to confirm that ablation in the isthmus creates a line of block in the sub-eustachian isthmus with pacing techniques.[41] By pacing from the CS os and then from the low lateral right atrium, they demonstrated that the activation sequence through the isthmus and around the tricuspid annulus is changed after successful ablation.[41] This demonstration of conduction block predicted long-term success better than lack of reinducibility of flutter.[41] Several other studies have confirmed this finding and have demonstrated that rate-independent, bidirectional block is a good predictor of long-term success (Figures 9, 10, 11).[26,40–42]

Conclusions

The importance of anatomically-based conduction barriers in atrial flutter has been borne out in human flutter, as was first suggested by early studies and animal models. Not only has the identification of these anatomic barriers led to a better understanding of the substrate for atrial flutter, it has also led to improved techniques for ablation of typical flutter and enabled assessment of a proper end point. Continued efforts to correlate electrophysiology with anatomy may lead to a better understanding of atypical flutter and atrial fibrillation.

References

1. Anderson R, Becker A. The development of the heart. In: Anderson R, Becker A, eds. *Cardiac Anatomy*. London: Gower Medical Publishing, 1980. pp 10–17.
2. Lesh M, Kalman J. To fumble flutter or tackle tach? Toward updated classifiers for atrial tachyarrhythmias. *J Cardiovasc Electrophysiol* 1996;7: 460–466.
3. Cosio FG, Lopez GM, Goicolea A, et al. Electrophysiologic studies in atrial flutter. *Clin Cardiol* 1992;15:667–673.

4. Klein G, Giraudon G, Sharma A, et al. Demonstration of macroreentry and feasibility of operative therapy in the common type of atrial flutter. *Am J Cardiol* 1986;57:587–591.

5. Olshansky B, Wilber DJ, Hariman RJ. Atrial flutter—update on the mechanism and treatment. *PACE* 1992;15:2308–2335.

6. Rosenblueth A, Garcia-Ramos J. The influence of artificial obstacles on experimental auricular flutter. *Am Heart J* 1947;33:677–684.

7. Frame L, Page R, Hoffman B. Atrial reentry around an anatomic barrier with a partially refractory excitable gap: a canine model of atrial flutter. *Circ Res* 1986;58:495–511.

8. Frame LH, Page RL, Boyden PA, et al. Circus movement in the canine atrium around the tricuspid ring during experimental atrial flutter and during reentry in vitro. *Circulation* 1987;76:1155–1175.

9. Boineau JP, Schuessler RB, Mooney CR, et al. Natural and evoked atrial flutter due to circus movement in dogs: role of abnormal atrial pathways, slow conduction, nonuniform refractory period distribution and premature beats. *Am J Cardiol* 1980;45:1167–1181.

10. Inoue H, Toda I, Saihara S, et al. Further observations on entrainment of atrial flutter in the dog. *Am Heart J* 1989;118:467–474.

11. Yamashita T, Inoue H, Nozaki A. et al. Role of anatomic architecture in sustained atrial reentry and double potentials. *Am Heart J* 1992;124:938–946.

12. Feld GK, Shahandeh RF. Mechanism of double potentials recorded during sustained atrial flutter in the canine right atrial crush-injury model. *Circulation* 1992;86:628–641.

13. Feld GK, Shahandeh RF. Activation patterns in experimental canine atrial flutter produced by right atrial crush injury. *J Am Coll Cardiol* 1992;20:441–451.

14. Schoels W, Gough WB, Restivo M. et al. Circus movement atrial flutter in the canine sterile pericarditis model: activation patterns during initiation, termination, and sustained reentry in vivo. *Circ Res* 1990;67:35–50.

15. Shimizu A, Nozaki A, Rudy Y, et al. Onset of induced atrial flutter in the canine pericarditis model [see comments]. *J Am Coll Cardiol* 1991;17:1223–1234.

16. Okumura K, Plumb VJ, Page PL, et al. Atrial activation sequence during atrial flutter in the canine pericarditis model and its effects on the polarity of the flutter wave in the electrocardiogram. *J Am Coll Cardiol* 1991;17:509–518.

17. Boyden PA, Frame LH, Hoffman BF. Activation mapping of reentry around an anatomic barrier in the canine atrium: observations during entrainment and termination. *Circulation* 1989;79:406–416.

18. Schoels W, Kuebler W, Yang H, et al. A unified functional/anatomic substrate for circus movement atrial flutter: activation and refractory patterns in the canine right atrial enlargement model. *J Am Coll Cardiol* 1993;21:73–84.

19. Lewis T. Observations upon flutter and fibrillation as it occurs in patients. *Heart* 1921;8:193.

20. Feld GK, Fleck RP, Chen PS, et al. Radiofrequency catheter ablation for the treatment of human type 1 atrial flutter: identification of a critical zone in

the reentrant circuit by endocardial mapping techniques. *Circulation* 1992;86:1233–1240.

21. Puech P, Latour H, Grolleau R. Le flutter et ses limites. *Arch Mal Coeur* 1970;63:116–144.
22. Olgin J, Kalman J, Fitzpatrick A, et al. The role of right atrial endocardial structures as barriers to conduction during human type I atrial flutter: activation and entrainment mapping guided by intracardiac echocardiography. *Circulation* 1995;92:1893–1848.
23. Olshansky B, Okumura K, Hess PG, et al. Demonstration of an area of slow conduction in human atrial flutter. *J Am Coll Cardiol* 1990;16:1639–1648.
24. Cosio F, Arribas F, Barbero J, et al. Validation of double spike electrograms as markers of conduction delay or block in atrial flutter. *Am J Cardiol* 1988;61:775–780.
25. Olshansky B, Okumura K, Henthorn RW, et al. Characterization of double potentials in human atrial flutter: studies during transient entrainment. *J Am Coll Cardiol* 1990;15:833–841.
26. Nakagawa H, Lazzara R, Khastgir T, et al. Role of the tricuspid annulus and the eustachian valve/ridge on atrial flutter: relevance to catheter ablation of the septal isthmus and a new technique for rapid identification of ablation success. *Circulation* 996;94:407–424.
27. Olshansky B, Moreira D, Waldo AL. Characterization of double potentials during ventricular tachycardia: studies during transient entrainment. *Circulation* 1993;87:373–381.
28. Waldo AL, McLean WAH, Karp RB, et al. Entrainment and interruption of atrial flutter with atrial pacing: studies in man following open heart surgery. *Circulation* 1977;56:737–745.
29. Okumura K, Henthorn RW, Epstein AE, et al. Further observations on transient entrainment: importance of pacing site and properties of the components of the reentry circuit. *Circulation* 1985;72:1293–1307.
30. Fujimoto T, Inoue T, Fukuzaki H. Characterization of slow conduction in the common type of atrial flutter—using transient entrainment. *Jpn Circ J* 1990;54:21–31.
31. Cosio FG, Lopez GM, Arribas F, et al. Mechanisms of entrainment of human common flutter studied with multiple endocardial recordings. *Circulation* 1994;89:2117–2125.
32. Stevenson W, Khan H, Sager P, et al. Identification of reentry circuit sites during catheter mapping and radiofrequency ablation of ventricular tachycardia late after myocardial infarction. *Circulation* 1993;88:1647–1670.
33. Stevenson W, Sager P, Friedman P. Entrainment techniques for mapping atrial and ventricular tachycardias. *J Cardiovasc Electrophysiol* 1995;6:201–216.
34. Waldo A, Carlson M, Biblo L, et al. The role of transient entrainment in atrial flutter. In: Waldo A, ed. *Atrial Arrhythmias,* 1993, pp 210–228.
35. Kalman J, Olgin J, Saxon L, et al. Activation and entrainment mapping defines the tricuspid annulus as the anterior barrier in typical atrial flutter. *Circulation* 1996;94:398–406.
36. Boyden PA. Models of atrial reentry. *J Cardiac Electrophysiol* 1995;6:313–324.

37. Arribas F, Lopex-Gil M, Nunez A, et al. The upper link of the common atrial flutter circuit [abstract]. *Circulation* 1994;90:I–376.
38. Saffitz J, Kanter L, Green K, et al. Tissue-specific determinants of anisotropic conduction velocity in canine atrial and ventricular myocardium. *Circ Res* 1994;74:1065–1070.
39. Kalman J, Olgin J, Saxon L, et al. Electrophysiology of the crista terminalis in normal human atria. *PACE* 1996;19:578.
40. Cauchemez B, Haïssaguerre M, Fischer B, et al. Electrophysiological effects of catheter ablation of inferior vena cava-tricuspid annulus isthmus in common atrial flutter. *Circulation* 1996;93:284–294.
41. Poty H, Saoudi N, Abdel Aziz A, et al. Radiofrequency catheter ablation of type 1 atrial flutter: prediction of late success by electrophysiological criteria. *Circulation* 1995;92:1389–1392.
42. Poty H, Saoudi N, Nair M, et al. Radiofrequency catheter ablation of atrial flutter—further insights into the various types of isthmus block: application to ablation during sinus rhythm. *Circulation* 1996;94:3204–3213.
43. Cosio FG, Lopez GM, Goicolea A, et al. Radiofrequency ablation of the inferior vena cava-tricuspid valve isthmus in common atrial flutter. *Am J Cardiol* 1993;71:705–709.
44. Kalman J, Olgin J, Saxon L, et al. Electrocardiographic and electrophysiologic characterization of atypical atrial flutter in man: use of activation and entrainment mapping and implications for catheter ablation. *J Cardiovasc Electrophysiol* 1997;8:121–144.
45. Kall J, Glascock D, Kopp D, et al. Characterization and catheter ablation of the antidromic form of typical atrial flutter [abstract]. *Circulation* 1995;92:I–84.
46. Tai C, Chen S, Chiang C, et al. Electrophysiologic characteristics and radiofrequency catheter ablation in patients in clockwise atrial flutter. *J Cardiovasc Electrophysiol* 1997;8:24–34.
47. Canavan TE, Schuessler RB, Cain ME, et al. Computerized global electrophysiological mapping of the atrium in a patient with multiple supraventricular tachyarrhythmias. *Ann Thorac Surg* 1988;46:232–235.
48. Cronin CS, Nitta T, Mitsuno M, et al. Characterization and surgical ablation of acute atrial flutter following the Mustard procedure: a canine model. *Circulation* 1993;88:II461–471.
49. Rodefeld M, Bromberg B, Schuessler R, et al. Atrial flutter after lateral tunnel construction in the modified fontan operation: a canine model. *J Thorac Cardiovasc Surg* 996; 111:514–526.
50. Kalman JM, Van Hare GF, Olgin JE, et al. Ablation of "incisional" reentrant atrial tachycardia complicating surgery for congenital heart disease: use of entrainment to define a critical isthmus of conduction. *Circulation* 1996; 93:502–512.
51. Lesh MD, Van Hare GF, Fitzpatrick AP, et al. Curing reentrant atrial arrhythmias: targeting protected zones of slow conduction by catheter ablation. *J Electrocardiol* 1993:194–203.
52. Olgin J, Kalman J, Saxon L. et al. Induction of atrial flutter in man: site dependence and site of unidirectional block. *J Am Coll Cardiol* 1997;29: 376–384.

53. Saoudi N, Derumeaux G, Cribier A, et al. The role of catheter ablation techniques in the treatment of classic (type 1) atrial flutter. *PACE* 1991; 14(11):2002–2027.

54. Calkins H, Leon AR, Deam AG, et al. Catheter ablation of atrial flutter using radiofrequency energy. *Am J Cardiol* 1994;73:353–356.

55. Kirkorian G, Moncada E, Chevalier P, et al. Radiofrequency ablation of atrial flutter: efficacy of an anatomically guided approach. *Circulation* 1994;90:2804–2814.

56. Fischer B, Haïssaguerre M, Garrigues S, et al. Radiofrequency catheter ablation of common atrial flutter in 80 patients. *J Am Coll Cardiol* 1995; 25:1365–1372.

57. Steinberg JS, Prasher S, Zelenkofske S, et al. Radiofrequency catheter ablation of atrial flutter: procedural success and long-term outcome. *Am Heart J* 1995;130:85–92.

58. Saxon LA, Kalman JM, Olgin JE, et al. Results of radiofrequency catheter ablation for atrial flutter. *Am J Cardiol* 1996;77:1014–1016.

Part III

Radiofrequency Catheter Ablation for Control of Atrial Fibrillation

Chapter 15

Complete Atrioventricular Junction Ablation for Control of Symptomatic Drug-Resistant Atrial Fibrillation

Shoei K. Stephen Huang, M.D., Ling-Ping Lai, M.D., Jiunn-Lee Lin, M.D.

Introduction

Atrial fibrillation is by far the most common tachyarrhythmia in humans. Although the primary goal of treatment is to keep the patient in sinus rhythm, restoration of sinus rhythm and prevention of atrial fibrillation recurrence are sometimes difficult, even with vigorous antiarrhythmic drug therapy. The secondary goal is to maintain a good control of ventricular rate during atrial fibrillation. The traditional way of achieving ventricular rate control is the use of atrioventricular (AV) nodal blocking agents including β-blockers, calcium channel blockers, and digitalis. With the advent of modern catheter ablation technique, AV junction ablation has evolved as an important and effective means to achieve ventricular rate control in patients with atrial fibrillation. In this chapter, we describe the techniques, benefits, and shortcomings, together with clinical follow-up data with regard to AV junction ablation for ventricular rate control in symptomatic, drug-resistant atrial fibrillation.

Techniques of Complete AV Junction Ablation

Early works on AV junction ablation were achieved by direct current (DC) shock.[1,2] Nowadays, radiofrequency energy has almost completely replaced DC shock as the energy source for catheter ablation of the AV junction.[3–11]

From Huang SKS, Wilber DJ (eds.): *Radiofrequency Catheter Ablation of Cardiac Arrhythmias: Basic Concepts and Clinical Applications,* 2nd ed. Armonk, NY: Futura Publishing Company, Inc. ©2000.

Typically, a right side approach is used. The procedure can be performed using an electrogram-guided approach or an anatomically guided approach. For His bundle ablation, an electrogram-guided approach can be used. The ablation catheter is positioned at the AV junction where a His bundle potential can be clearly recorded. For AV nodal ablation, an anatomically guided approach can be used. The ablation catheter is placed at a midseptal position where the His bundle potential is barely visible and the atrial to ventricular electrogram amplitude ratio is ≥ 1.0. A backup pacing catheter is positioned at the right ventricular apex before the application of radiofrequency energy. During the energy application, right ventricular pacing is used after complete AV block is achieved (Figure 1). A permanent pacemaker is then implanted during the same session. A left side approach can be used as an alternative if the right heart approach is undesirable or unsuccessful.[12,13]

The overall success rate for AV junction ablation is approaching 100% in recent reports. In rare circumstances in which standard right heart and left heart approaches are both unsuccessful, energy delivery to the region of the noncoronary aortic cusp where the His bundle potential is recorded may lead to complete AV block (Figure 2).[14]

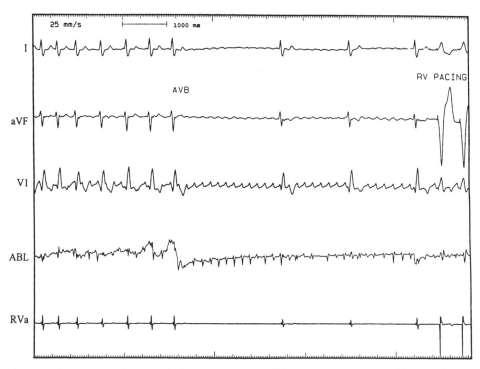

Figure 1. Electrograms during radiofrequency energy delivery for AV junction ablation. The patient had atrial fibrillation throughout the procedure. The ventricular rate was about 150/min initially. After a gradual decrease of ventricular rate, complete AV block with junctional escape beats developed. Pacing from a backup right ventricular electrode catheter was performed thereafter. ABL = ablation catheter; Rva = right ventricular apex.

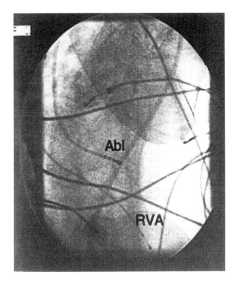 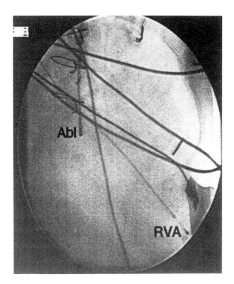

LAO 30°   RAO 30°

Figure 2A. Right anterior oblique (RAO 30°) and left anterior oblique (LAO 30°) fluoroscopic frames showing the location of the ablation catheter (ABL) in the supravalvular region of the non-coronary cusp of the aortic valve and a temporary pacing catheter in the right ventricular apex.

Benefits

Complete ablation of the AV junction plus pacemaker therapy is effective for ventricular rate control.[3,4] This approach is devoid of the adverse effects of AV nodal blocking drugs. Brignole et al has performed a multicenter, randomized study in 43 patients to compare AV junction versus pharmacological treatment in patients with symptomatic atrial fibrillation.[5] The report showed that AV junction ablation with pacemaker implantation was superior in controlling symptoms related to palpitations, dyspnea, and exercise tolerance in a 6-month follow-up period. The improvement of quality of life was also greater in the ablation group. Similar results have been shown in another noncontrolled but larger series of 107 patients.[6] In the latter series, not only did the quality of life improve, the number of doctor visits, hospital admissions, and episodes of heart failure were all significantly decreased. Thus, the medical costs were substantially reduced. With regular R-R intervals, the cardiac output and overall cardiac performance as well as exercise capacity can be improved.[7,8] A reduction of left ventricular dimension and increase of contractility have also been shown 6 months after the ablation.[9]

Shortcomings

There are several shortcomings in the ablation/pacemaker approach. First, the procedure is invasive with inherent complications, although the procedure-

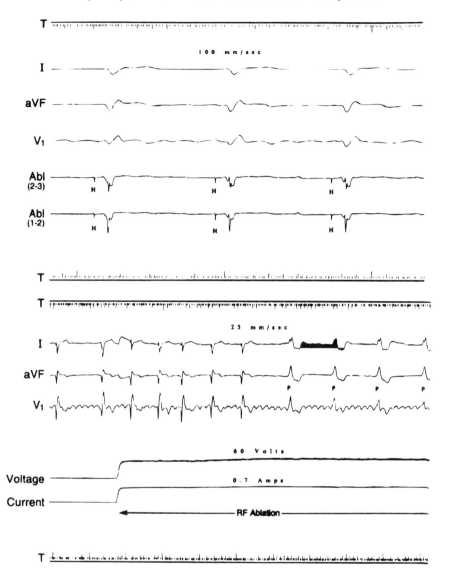

Figure 2B. Simultaneous recordings of surface ECG lead I, aVF and V_1; and electrograms recorded at the ablation site (upper panel). His bundle potential was clearly visible at the Abl (1–2) and Abl (2–3) with an HV interval of 60 milliseconds. During radiofrequency energy application, complete AV block developed (lower panel).

related complications are reportedly low. Second, the implantation of a permanent pacemaker is associated with a possible risk, although minimal, of pacemaker and/or lead malfunction. The need for battery replacement in the future should also be considered in patients with a long life expectancy. Third, it has been reported that sudden death due to ventricular tachycardia/fibrillation might occur after AV junction ablation (Figure 3). This is a major concern and will be discussed separately in the next section.

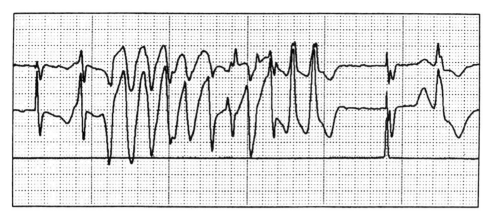

Figure 3. A representative rhythm strip obtained from a follow-up ambulatory ECG recording after AV junction ablation. The rhythm shows atrial fibrillation with a run of polymorphic ventricular tachycardia.

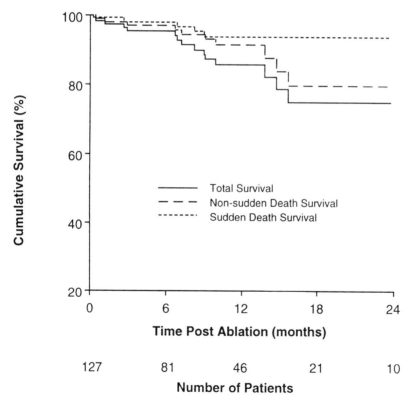

Figure 4. Kaplan-Meier survival curves showing the cumulative percentage of survival (vertical axis) over time after AV junction ablation (horizontal axis) in the group of patients with total death, sudden and non-sudden death.

Sudden cardiac death after AV junction ablation

Early studies described sudden death in patients undergoing AV junction ablation with the use of DC shock.[1,2] Although a definite correlation between the procedure and the sudden death is not clear, sudden death is still a concern. A prospective, multicenter study was conducted in the United States in this respect.[10] This study included 127 patients in 13 centers. There were 63 men and 64 women. Their mean age was 63±11 years (±standard deviation; range 12–90). Figure 4 shows the Kaplan-Meier survival curves in the group of patients with total death, sudden and non-sudden death. There were 5 patients with sudden cardiac death in a cohort of 127 patients with a mean follow-up period of 10.2 months. Table 1 shows the clinical characteristics of the 5 patients with sudden cardiac death. The 5 patients were all male and 4 of them had organic heart disease. The sudden death occurred from 7–272 days after the ablation. Severe left ventricular dysfunction was found in 3 (ejection fraction 10–21%). All 5 patients had persistent atrial fibrillation with frequent ventricular ectopies before and after the ablation. In the study, a comparison of the clinical characteristics between the sudden death group (n = 5) and non-sudden death group (n = 11) was made. Table 2 shows that there was a trend toward a lower ejection fraction (27±22% versus 49±19%, $P<0.13$) and a higher number of radiofrequency applications (16±11 versus 5±5, $P<0.094$) in the sudden death group.

Table 1
Clinical characteristics of 5 patients with sudden death

Characteristics	Patient number				
	1	2	3	4	5*
Age (years)	74	69	48	69	69
Gender	male	male	male	male	male
Cardiac diagnosis	CAD HCVD	CAD HCVD	DCM	none (COPD)	DCM
CHF (NYHA class)	II	II	IV	no	III
LVEF (%)	17	21	10	60	unknown
Presenting arrhythmia	AFib	AFib	AFib	AFib	AFib
Ablation approach	right	right	right & left	right	right
RF applications	3	18	30	20	9
Pacemaker type	VVI	VVIR	VVI	VVIR	unknown
Pacemaker lowest rate	70/min	90/min	70/min	90/min	unknown
Specific antiarrhythmics after ablation	none (digoxin)	none (digoxin)	none (digoxin)	none (β-blocker)	none
Time to death postablation	7 days	272 days	209 days	81 days	250 days
Ventricular arrhythmias preablation	PVC, nsVT	PVC, nsVT	PVC, nsVT	PVC	unknown
postablation	PVC, nsVT	PVC, nsVT	PVC, nsVT	PVC	PVC, nsVT syncope

*Patient 5 was an unwitnessed sudden death. Afib = atrial fibrillation; CAD = coronary artery disease; CHF = congestive heart failure; COPD = chronic obstructive pulmonary disease; DCM = dilated cardiomyopathy; HCVD = hypertensive cardiovascular disease; LVEF = left ventricular ejection fraction; NYHA = New York Heart Association; nsVT = nonsustained ventricular tachycardia; PVC = premature

Table 2
Comparison of clinical characteristics between patients with sudden and non-sudden death

	Gender	Age	LVEF (%)	RF Applications
Sudden death (n = 5)	5M	66±10 (range 48–74)	27±22 (range 10–60)	16±11 (range 3–30)
Non-sudden death (n = 11)	6M, 5F	61±12 (range 41–78)	49±19 (range 15–65)	5±5 (range 1–15)
P value	0.22	0.48	0.13	0.094

F = female; LVEF = left ventricular ejection fraction; M = male

In Europe, another large scale multicenter study was conducted in which the incidence of sudden cardiac death was 5% (11 out of 220 patients).[11] The etiology of sudden death in the 11 patients was acute myocardial infarction in 5. In the remaining 6 patients, extensive coronary artery disease was found in 1, severe heart failure in 1, cardiac hypertrophy in 1, and no identifiable etiology of sudden death in 3. From these 2 multicenter studies, a definite causal relationship between AV junction ablation and sudden cardiac death does not appear to exist.

Conclusions

Complete AV junction ablation plus pacemaker implantation for ventricular rate control in refractory atrial fibrillation is an effective and relatively safe procedure. Its potential benefits have made it an alternate therapeutic choice to drug therapy. Nevertheless, it is an invasive undertaking and should be considered after overall risk and benefit evaluation.

References

1. Evans T, Scheinman M, Zipes D, et al. The percutaneous cardiac mapping and ablation registry: final summary of results. *PACE* 1988;11:1621–1626.
2. Evans T, Scheinman M, Bardy G, et al. Predictors of in-hospital mortality after direct current catheter ablation of atrioventricular junction: results of a prospective, international, multicenter study. *Circulation* 1991;84:1924–1937.
3. Brignole M, Menozzi C. Control of rapid heart rate in patients with atrial fibrillation: drugs or ablation? *PACE* 1996;19:348–356.
4. Jensen SM, Bergfeldt L, Rosenqvist M. Long-term follow-up of patients treated by radiofrequency ablation of the atrioventricular junction. *PACE* 1995;18:1609–1614.
5. Brignole M, Gianfranchi L, Menozzi C, et al. Assessment of atrioventricular junction ablation and DDDR mode-switching pacemaker versus pharmacological treatment in patients with severely symptomatic paroxysmal atrial fibrillation a randomized controlled study. *Circulation* 1997;96:2617–2624.
6. Fitzpatrick AP, Kourouyan HD, Siu A, et al. Quality of life and outcomes

after radiofrequency His-bundle catheter ablation and permanent pacemaker implantation: impact of treatment in paroxysmal and established atrial fibrillation. *Am Heart J* 1996;131:499–507.

7. Natale A, Zimerman L, Tomassoni G, et al. Impact on ventricular function and quality of life of transcatheter ablation of the atrioventricular junction in chronic atrial fibrillation with a normal ventricular response. *Am J Cardiol* 1996;78:1431–1433.

8. Buys EM, Hemel NM, Kelder JC, et al. Exercise capacity after His bundle ablation and rate response ventricular pacing for drug refractory chronic atrial fibrillation. *Heart* 1997;77:238–241.

9. Geelen P, Goethals M, Bruyne BD et al. A prospective hemodynamic evaluation of patients with chronic atrial fibrillation undergoing radiofrequency catheter ablation of the atrioventricular junction. *Am J Cardiol* 1997;80:1606–1609.

10. Huang SKS, Wagshal AB, Mittleman RS, et al. Sudden cardiac death after complete radiofrequency catheter ablation of the atrioventricular junction: a multicenter prospective study [abstract]. *Circulation* 1994;90:I–335.

11. Darpo B, Walfridsson H, Aunes M, et al. Incidence of sudden death after radiofrequency ablation of the atrioventricular junction for atrial fibrillation. *Am J Cardiol* 1997;80:1174–1177.

12. Sousa J, El-Atassi R, Rosenheck S, et al. Radiofrequency catheter ablation of the atrioventricular junction from the left ventricle. *Circulation* 1991;84:567–571.

13. Sousa O, Gursoy S, Simonis F, et al. Right-sided versus left-sided radiofrequency ablation of the His bundle. *PACE* 1992;15:1454–1459.

14. Cuello C, Huang SKS, Wagshal AB, et al. Radiofrequency catheter ablation of the atrioventricular junction by a supravalvular non-coronary aortic cusp approach. *PACE* 1994;17:1182–1185.

Chapter 16

Modification of Atrioventricular Conduction for Control of Symptomatic Drug Resistant Atrial Fibrillation

Shih-Ann Chen, M.D., Shih-Huang Lee, M.D., Mau-Song Chang, M.D.

Introduction

Although class I and class III antiarrhythmic drugs might be effective in preventing and suppressing atrial fibrillation, and AV node-blocking drugs might be effective in decreasing the ventricular response rate, they also may produce side effects and proarrhythmias.[1,2] Furthermore, pharmacological control of rapid ventricular response to paroxysmal atrial fibrillation may be difficult in some patients with normal or enhanced atrioventricular (AV) node conduction. Alternative treatments include surgical Maze procedure or linear catheter ablation of atrial wall to eliminate atrial fibrillation circuits, and catheter ablation or modification of AV junction to prevent rapid ventricular response during atrial fibrillation. However, the risk and morbidity in surgical procedure, long fluoroscopic time, high complication rate with low success rate in catheter linear ablation, the development of lifetime pacemaker dependency, loss of physiologic AV activation sequence, and risk of sudden death after complete AV junction ablation have been the major limitations of these procedures.[3–9]

From Huang SKS, Wilber DJ (eds.): *Radiofrequency Catheter Ablation of Cardiac Arrhythmias: Basic Concepts and Clinical Applications,* 2nd ed. Armonk, NY: Futura Publishing Company, Inc. ©2000.

Techniques Used for Modification of AV Junction

The conventional target sites for complete ablation or modification of the AV junction were located anteriorly and superiorly on the tricuspid annulus. [6–9] Huang et al performed radiofrequency modification of AV junction in a canine model by an anterior approach and Duckeck et al used the same method in human study.[9,14] Although the purpose of these 2 studies was to decrease ventricular rate during atrial pacing or atrial fibrillation, the results were disappointing because of a high incidence of AV block (immediate or late) and low clinical efficiency with high incidence of delayed recurrence during the follow-up studies.

Recently, several reports demonstrated that application of radiofrequency energy to the right posteroseptal and/or midseptal area could decrease the ventricular rate during atrial fibrillation. The benefit of this approach is lower risk of complete AV block. Most of the patients had preservation of AV node conduction.[10–13] The right atrial septum adjacent to the septal leaflet of the tricuspid valve and extending from the ostium of the coronary sinus to the recording site at the His bundle was divided into posterior, medial and anterior regions, then each of these 3 regions was further divided into 3, 2, and 2 subsections, respectively.[13] They were: posterior-1 (P1), posterior-2 (P2), posterior-3 (P3) (around the coronary sinus ostium), medial-1 (M1), medial-2 (M2), anterior-1 (A1) and anterior-2 (A2) (Figure 1). Recording of slow pathway potential (high-low or low-high frequency potential) during clinical electrophysiological study and detailed endocardial mapping of the AV junction using multiple electrodes during cardiac surgery demonstrated that the fast pathway was located anterior and the slow pathway was located posterior to the compact AV node, respectively.[15–20] Thus the P level and lower part of M level might be the posterior input area, whereas the upper part of M level might be the compact node area. In this laboratory, among the 36 patients who had no dual pathway physiology but had successful modification, radiofrequency energy was delivered to 1 site (16 patients, 44%), multiple close sites within 1 subsection level (8 patients, 23%) or multiple close sites on more than 1 subsection level (12 patients, 33%). Of the 8 patients with transient AV block, the ablation sites with transient AV block were 1 in P2 and 7 in M2 levels. Of the 2 patients with immediate complete AV block, the ablation sites were M2 levels. Among the 10 patients with dual pathway physiology, the sites with successful elimination of slow pathway were 3 in P1, 5 in P2 and 2 in M1 areas. The 4 patients who still had rapid ventricular rate after successful elimination of slow pathway received the second modification session, and the effective ablation sites were in the higher subsection levels (Figure 2). Feld et al and Williamson et al also reported that some patients had successful modification after delivering radiofrequency energy to the M level.[10,11]

Possible Mechanisms in Successful Modification of AV Node Conduction

The determinants of ventricular rate during atrial fibrillation were controversial. In vitro studies showed that asynchronous conduction, concealed

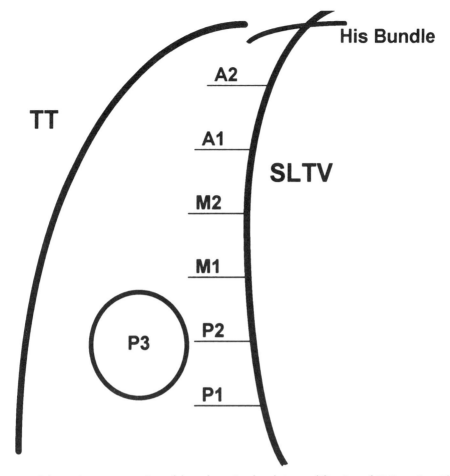

Figure 1. Schematic representation of the subsection levels in modification of AV junction. The right atrial septum adjacent to the septal leaflet of the tricuspid valve and extending from the ostium of the coronary sinus to the recording site at the His bundle was divided into posterior, medial and anterior regions, then each of these 3 regions was divided again into 3, 2, and 2 subsections, respectively. They were: posterior-1 (P1), posterior-2 (P2), posterior-3 (P3) (around the coronary sinus ostium), medial-1 (M1), medial-2 (M2), anterior-1 (A1), and anterior-2 (A2). The ostium of coronary sinus was defined by coronary sinus venography. T = tendon of Todaro; SLTV = septal leaflet of tricuspid valve. (Reproduced from Chen et al, Electrophysiological mechanisms in successful radiofrequency catheter modification of atrioventricular junction for patients with medically refractory paroxysmal atrial fibrillation. *Circulation* 1996;93:1690)

conduction, summation, cancellation of wave fronts, rate and irregularities of atrial impulses, local reentry, pacemaker activity of the nodal cells, electronic modulation, and the electrophysiological parameters of AV node function may all contribute.[21–30] Human studies showed that the mean ventricular rate during atrial fibrillation correlated significantly with AV node conduction properties.[3,31–34] Thus far, no model has incorporated all these different elements to account for the ventricular response rate in atrial fibrillation.

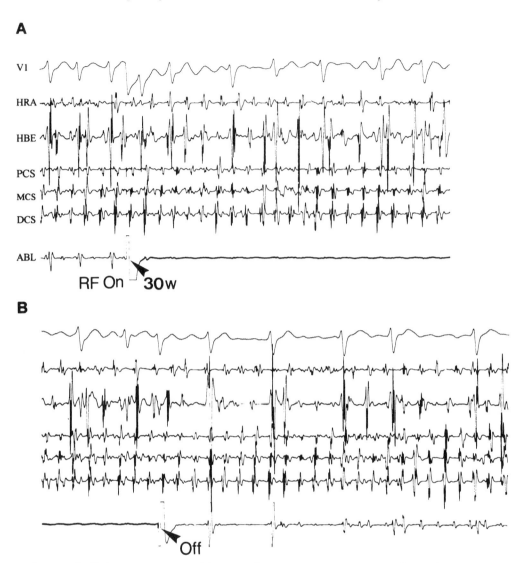

Figure 2. Radiofrequency (RF) modification of AV junction in a patient with rapid ventricular rate during atrial fibrillation. After delivery of RF energy, the ventricular rate decelerated. (Reproduced from Chen et al, Electrophysiological mechanisms in successful radiofrequency catheter modification of atrioventricular junction for patients with medically refractory paroxysmal atrial fibrillation. *Circulation 1996;93:1690*)

Possible Elimination of Posterior Input

During atrial pacing from a single site, the impulses penetrate the AV node from the same direction, through either the anterior or posterior AV nodal input. During atrial fibrillation, both inputs may be used randomly.[24] In the isolated AV junctional preparation of the rabbit heart, Janse compared the functional properties of both inputs and found that AV conduction through the anterior input was blocked at lower atrial pacing rates than when the posterior input was used.[24] Mazgalev et al obtained similar results during premature atrial stimulation.[26] They also demonstrated that during atrial fibrillation, AV conduction could be modulated by "summation" or "inhibition" of atrial impulses entering the AV junction from different inputs. In contrast to the experiments of Janse and Mazgalev et al Chorro et al did not find significant differences in ventricular response rate during incremental atrial pacing from either site.[28] A possible explanation for this difference might be that in isolated superfused AV junctional preparations, when subjected to high pacing rates the interstitial fluid in the center of the AV node is not adequately refreshed. A change in electrolyte composition in the extracellular space might affect the conduction properties of the AV node during high atrial rates.[28]

Previous studies demonstrated that radiofrequency modification of the right posteroseptal or midseptal area in patients with AV node reentrant tachycardia could eliminate the slow pathway with cure of this tachycardia.[18–20] Furthermore, the follow-up electrophysiological study after eliminating slow pathway conduction showed that the fast pathway with its long Wenckebach block cycle length and effective refractory period was preserved.[18–20,35,36] Thus, the ventricular rate would be controlled by the ablation of some or all of these posterior atrionodal inputs if conduction was poorer through the anterior atrionodal inputs than through the posterior inputs.[10–12,31] However, if the properties of the anterior and posterior atrionodal inputs were similar, the decrease in ventricular rate would be smaller after ablation of the posterior input. This laboratory showed that the patients with dual pathway physiology had marked decrease of ventricular rate than occurred in patients with larger changes of the effective refractory period and Wenckebach block cycle length (larger difference between the electrophysiological properties of fast and slow pathways.[13] Blanck et al and Markowitz et al also demonstrated that the mechanism of decrease in ventricular response to pacing-induced atrial fibrillation after ablation of the slow pathway in patients with AV node reentrant tachycardia could be mostly explained by elimination of posterior input.[31,33] However, Strickberger et al showed that the mechanism of decrease in ventricular response rate could not be explained exclusively by elimination of posterior input: they found that decrease of ventricular response was present only during total autonomic blockade, and it was absent during isoproterenol infusion.[32]

In the patients without dual AV node physiology, the possible presence of posterior input could not be excluded. Because some patients might have better conduction properties of anterior input than posterior input (shorter refractory period of anterior input, without AH jump), the AH interval, AV node effective refractory period, and Wenckebach block cycle length would not change after elimination of posterior input.[35,36] Decrease of ventricular rate after modification might result from destruction of the summation effects from both the posterior and anterior inputs.[23] Furthermore, some patients might have a little overlapping of conduction properties between the anterior and posterior inputs (shorter refractory period of posterior input, without AH jump), and the AV node effective refractory period and Wenckebach block cycle length would increase after elimination of posterior input (without change of AH interval).[35,36] These mechanisms are possible in patients without dual pathway physiology. This lab-

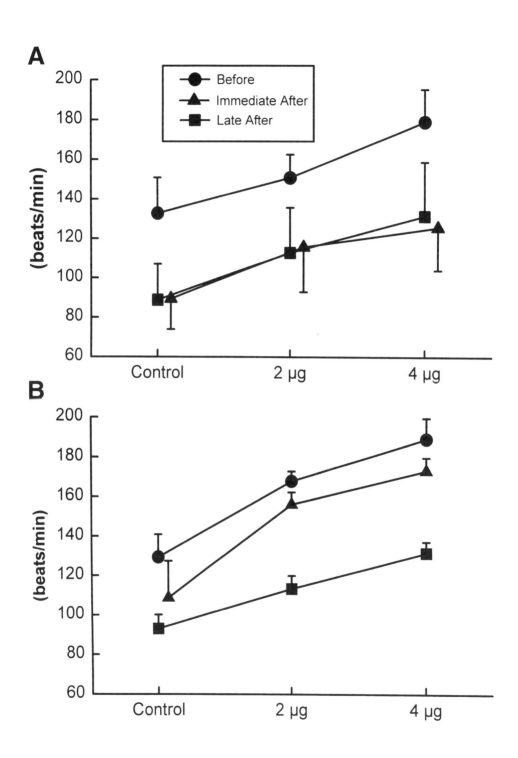

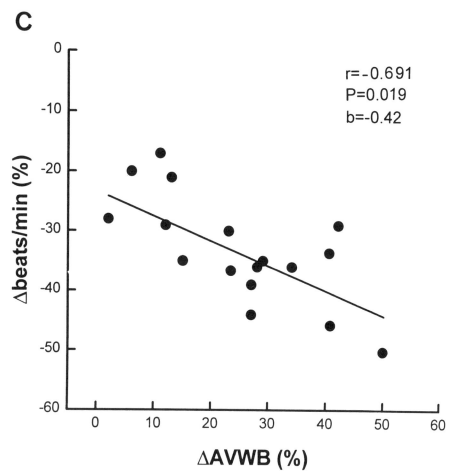

Figure 3. Modification of AV junction in patients without dual pathway physiology. Panel A: Average ventricular rate during atrial fibrillation before, immediately after, and late after radiofrequency modification of AV junction in patients with successful outcome. C = baseline ventricular rate; 2 μg, 4μg = ventricular rate during different doses of intravenous administration of isoproterenol (2 μg/min, 4 μg/min). Panel B: Serial change of ventricular rate in three patients who had unsuccessful results (partial effects) immediately after modification but they had delayed successful outcome. Panel C: Correlation between percentage changes (Δ%) of ventricular rate (beats/min) and AV Wenckebach block cycle length (AVWB) after successful modification; b = quantitative slope. (Reproduced from Chen et al, Electrophysiological mechanisms in successful radiofrequency catheter modification of atrioventricular junction for patients with medically refractory paroxysmal atrial fibrillation. *Circulation* 1996;93,1690).

oratory also demonstrated that the change in ventricular rate had a closer relationship to change in AV Wenckebach block cycle length than to change in AV node effective refractory period and the relationship between change in AV Wenchebach block cycle length and AV node effective refractory period is not 1:1. Thus, these findings may support an argument for additional effects of radiofrequency ablation of slow pathway or AV nodal input, such as reduction of summation rather than simple prolongation of overall AV nodal effective refractory period, as a mechanism for ventricular rate control (Figures 3 and 4).

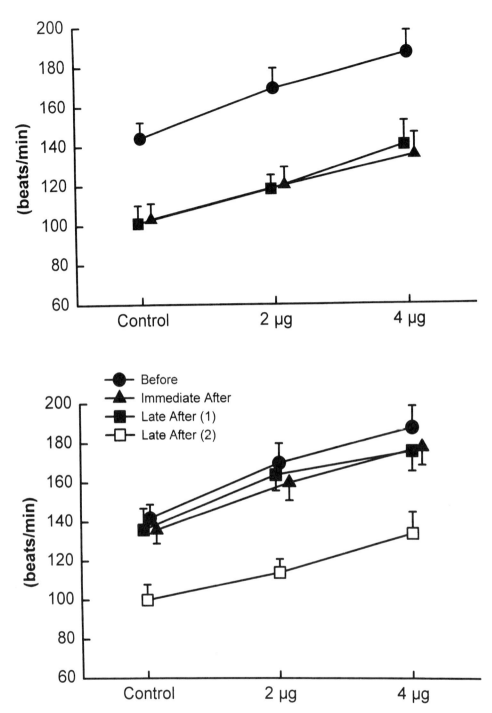

Figure 4. Modification of AF junction in patients with dual pathway physiology. Panel A: Average ventricular rate during atrial fibrillation before, immediately after, and late after elimination of slow AV node pathway in 6 patients with significant decrease of ventricular rate. Panel B: Serial change of ventricular rate in 4 patients without significant decrease of ventricular rate after elimination of slow AV node pathway. Further modification of AV junction decreased the ventricular rate significantly. (1) = first modification session; (2) = second modification session with modification sites in the higher subsection levels. (Reproduced from Chen et al, Electrophysiological mechanisms in successful radiofrequency catheter modification of atrioventricular junction for patients with medically refractory paroxysmal atrial fibrillation. *Circulation* 1996;93:1690)

Possible Injury to the Compact Node

Several investigators have demonstrated that successful ablation of the slow AV node pathway with a posterior approach might be accompanied with inadvertent ablation of the fast AV node pathway. Jackman et al reported injury to the fast pathway in one patient after delivering radiofrequency energy at the coronary sinus ostium.[18] Langberg et al reported that 14% of patients had unintended injury of the fast pathway during slow pathway ablation with a posterior approach.[37] Williamson et al reported that transient or permanent third-degree AV block occurred in 6 of the 19 patients who received radiofrequency modification of AV junction, and suggested that target sites near the orifice of the coronary sinus may be close enough to the compact node to injure that structure.[11] This laboratory also showed that sites with successful outcome were in the same locations as sites with transient AV block.[13] Strickberger et al also showed that partial injury to the compact node was possible in successful modification of AV junction to decrease ventricular response rate.[33] It may be that the rate was controlled, at least in some patients, by partial injury to the compact node.

In the patients with dual pathway physiology who had greater difference of conduction properties between the fast and slow pathways, simple elimination of slow pathway could significantly decrease ventricular rate. However, in the patients with similar conduction properties between the fast and slow pathways, significant decrease of ventricular rate was achieved after further modification of AV junction in the multiple sites of higher subsection levels. Therefore, pathological lesions in these might include injury to the compact node in addition to the slow pathway (Figure 5).[10,11,13,33]

Other Possible Mechanisms

Change of electronic modulation or concealment within the AV junction due to radiofrequency energy, possible anatomic differences of AV node, or different sensitivity of AV node to thermal effects of radiofrequency energy must be considered. Injury to the His bundle is an unlikely explanation for control of the ventricular rate, because His bundle depolarization was not visible in the target-site electrograms and the location of transient or permanent AV block was always away from the His bundle.

Consideration of AV Block in Modification Procedures

Despite the absence of a His bundle depolarization in the electrograms at the target sites and the posterior position of the target sites relative to the AV node, the delivery of radiofrequency energy resulted at times in transient or permanent AV block.[10,11,13] In an attempt to avoid AV block, radiofrequency energy was used as a step-up method, discontinuing application of the energy whenever there was a sudden slowing in the ventricular rate or appearance of accelerating junctional tachyarrhythmia.[10,11,13] Williamson et al reported that about two-

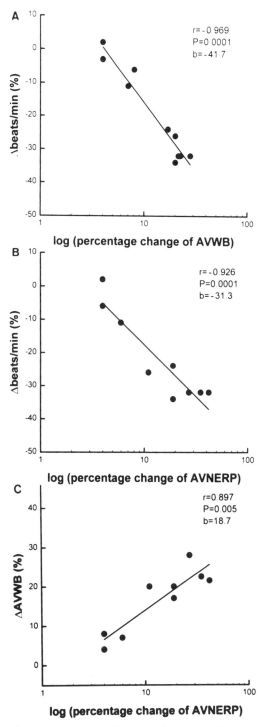

Figure 5. Correlation between changes of ventricular rate and AV Wenckebach block cycle length (AVWB) (Panel A), correlation between changes of ventricular rate and AV node effective refractory period (AVNERP) (Panel B), and correlation between changes of AVWB and AVNERP (Panel C) after successful modification in patients who had dual pathway physiology. (Reproduced from Chen et al, Electrophysiological mechanisms in successful radiofrequency catheter modification of atrioventricular junction for patients with medically refractory paroxysmal atrial fibrillation. *Circulation* 1996;93;1690)

thirds of the patients with transient AV block had delayed onset of persistent AV block about 36 to 72 hours after the procedure.[11] This laboratory showed that 5 of the 8 patients with transient AV block had delayed occurrence of AV block within 16 hours after the procedure, and 4 patients had recovery of AV conduction.[13] It is possible that transient thermal injury to the AV conduction system results in an inflammatory reaction that is responsible for the delayed occurrence of AV block. Although this laboratory showed that the 4 patients had recovery of AV conduction, long-term follow-up is necessary. Furthermore, most of the ablation sites with transient or persistent AV block were in the M2 level, so care should be taken when radiofrequency energy is delivered in a higher level.[11,13] If transient AV block occurs during an attempt to modify AV conduction, continuous electrocardiographic monitoring on an inpatient basis is appropriate for a period of 3–4 days to watch for a delayed recurrence of AV block.

Accidental AV block with lifetime pacemaker dependency and loss of physiological AV activation sequence during sinus rhythm were the major limitation for the modification or complete ablation of AV junction.[6–9] Considering the transient and delayed AV block, and the possibility of late sudden death in patients receiving the modification procedure, more efforts would be necessary to decrease the radiofrequency pulse number and pathological area to decrease the possibility of late complication. In addition, this procedure should be reserved for patients with atrial fibrillation who are symptomatic enough to justify ablation of the AV junction and implantation of a permanent pacemaker.

Late Outcome

In this laboratory, although the average ventricular rates during atrial fibrillation decreased significantly immediate after the modification procedure, the ventricular rate obtained from baseline condition and isoproterenol infusion increased slightly during late follow-up study.[13] The ventricular rate increased during the late follow-up study; compared with the immediate result, this may reflect partial recovery of AV conduction from the immediate effects of radiofrequency energy. Nevertheless, the average ventricular rate during high dose isoproterenol in the late follow-up study was still approximately 25% lower than at baseline level, a degree of attenuation adequate for the persistent resolution of symptoms. This change was similar to the other reports about modification of AV junction for patients with chronic atrial fibrillation.[11] Furthermore, the late follow-up ventricular rate did not differ significantly from the data immediately after modification procedure. Thus, these results demonstrated that immediate success could predict the late effects in most of the patients. Morady et al also showed that about 70% of patients had improvement of symptoms after AV junction modification procedure in the long term follow-up study.[38]

Compared with AV junction modification, AV junction ablation with permanent pacing had the advantages of better control of rapid ventricular rate and regularization of heart rhythm; however, it had the disadvantages of asynergic ventricular contraction and the loss of AV synchrony during sinus rhythm in patients with paroxysmal atrial fibrillation. Several recent studies have emphasized that right ventricular apical pacing might make LV function worse in patients with baseline depressed LV function.[38,39] Some studies have demonstrated that irregularity of the ventricular rhythm, independent of the ventricular rate, might also contribute to impairment of cardiac function during atrial fibrillation.[40,41] In this laboratory, 60 patients with medically refractory atrial fibrillation were randomly assigned to receive complete AV junction ablation with permanent pacing or AV junction modification. We found that after complete AV junction ablation or modification, the patients had a significantly greater improvement in the general quality of life, frequency of significant symptoms and symptoms during attacks, left ventricular systolic function, and activity capacity. Furthermore, all the improvements after ablation or modification procedure were maintained over the 6 months follow-up. However, a larger-population study would be necessary to compare the morbidity, mortality, and long-term effects in complete ablation or modification of AV junction for a longer follow-up period.

Conclusion

It may be appropriate to attempt first to modify AV conduction in patients with medication-refractory paroxysmal atrial fibrillation and rapid ventricular rates who are appropriate candidates for ablation of the AV junction. The mechanisms of successful modification might be elimination of posterior input and/or partial injury of compact node. Furthermore, simple elimination of slow pathway might be inadequate for control of ventricular rate in patients with smaller difference of conduction properties between fast and slow pathways.

References

1. Flaker GC, Blackshear JL, McBride R, et al. Antiarrhythmic drug therapy and cardiac mortality in atrial fibrillation. *J Am Coll Cardiol* 1992;20: 527–532.
2. Falk RH. Proarrhythmia in patients treated for atrial fibrillation or flutter. *Ann Intern Med* 1992;117:141–150.
3. Cox JL, Boineau JP, Scheussler RB, et al. Operations for atrial fibrillation. *Clin Cardiol* 1991;14:827–834.
4. Swartz JF, Pellersels G, Silvers J, et al. A catheter-based curative approach to atrial fibrillation in humans. *Circulation* 1994;90(Part 2):I–335.
5. Haïssaguerre M, Jaïs P, Shan DC, et al. Right and left atrial radiofrequency catheter therapy of paroxysmal atrial fibrillation. *J Cardiovasc Electrophysiol* 1996;7:1132–1144.
6. Langberg JJ, Chin MC, Rosenqvist M, et al. Catheter ablation of the atrioventricular junction with radiofrequency energy. *Circulation* 1989;80: 1527–1535.
7. Jackman WM, Wang X, Friday KJ, et al. Catheter ablation of atrioventricular junction using radiofrequency current in 17 patients: comparison of standard and large-tip catheter electrodes. *Circulation* 1991;83: 1562–1576.
8. Olgin JE, Scheinman MM. Comparison of high energy current and ra-

diofrequency catheter ablation of the atrioventricular junction. *J Am Coll Cardiol* 1993;21:557–564.

9. Duckeck W, Engelstein ED, Kuck KH, Radiofrequency current therapy in atrial tachyarrhythmias: modulation versus ablation of atrioventricular nodal conduction. *PACE* 1993;16:629–636.

10. Feld GK, Fleck RP, Fujimura O, et al. Control of rapid ventricular response by radiofrequency catheter modification of the AV node in patients with medically refractory atrial fibrillation. *Circulation* 1994;90:2299–2307.

11. Williamson BD, Strickberger SA, Hummel JD, et al. Radiofrequency catheter modification of atrioventricular conduction to control the ventricular rate during atrial fibrillation. *N Engl J Med* 1994;331:910–917.

12. Della Bella P, Carbucicchio C, Tondo C, et al. Modulation of atrioventricular conduction by ablation of the slow atrioventricular node pathway in patients with drug-refractory atrial fibrillation or flutter. *J Am Coll Cardiol* 1995;25:39–46.

13. Chen SA, Lee SH, Chiang CE, et al. Electrophysiological mechanisms in successful radiofrequency catheter modification of atrioventricular junction for patients with medically refractory paroxysmal atrial fibrillation. *Circulation* 1996;93:1690–1701.

14. Huang SK, Bharati S, Graham AR, et al. Closed chest catheter desiccation of the atrioventricular junction using radiofrequency energy; a new method of catheter ablation. *J Am Coll Cardiol* 1987;9:349–58.

15. Sung RJ, Waxman HL, Saksena S, et al. Sequence of retrograde atrial activation in patients with dual atrioventricular nodal pathways. *Circulation* 1983;54:1059–1067.

16. Ross DL, Johnson DC, Denniss AR, et al. Curative surgery for atrioventricular junctional ("AV nodal") reentrant tachycardia. *J Am Coll Cardiol* 1985;6:1383–1392.

17. Keim S, Werner P, Jazayeri M, et al. Localization of the fast and slow pathways in atrioventricular nodal reentrant tachycardia by intraoperative ice mapping. *Circulation* 1992;86:919–925.

18. Jackman WM, Beckman KJ, McCleland JH, et al. Treatment of supraventricular tachycardia due to atrioventricular nodal reentry by radiofrequency catheter ablation of slow-pathway conduction. *N Engl J Med* 1992;327:313–318.

19. Haïssaguerre M, Gaita F, Fischer B, et al. Elimination of atrioventricular nodal reentrant tachycardia using discrete slow potentials to guide application of radiofrequency. *Circulation* 1992;85:2162–2175.

20. Jazayeri MR, Sra JS, Deshpande SS, et al. Electrophysiologic spectrum of atrioventricular nodal behavior in patients with atrioventricular nodal reentrant tachycardia undergoing selective fast or slow pathway ablation. *J Cardiovasc Electrophysiol* 1993;4:99–111.

21. Moe GK, Abildskov JA. Observations on the ventricular dysrhythmia associated with atrial fibrillation in the dog heart. *Cir Res* 1964;14:447–460.

22. Langendorf R, Pick A, Katz LN. Ventricular response in atrial fibrillation: role of concealed conduction in the AV node. *Circulation* 1965;32:69–75.

23. Zipes DP, Mendez C, Moe GK. Evidence for summation and voltage dependency in rabbit atrioventricular nodal fibers. *Circ Res* 1973;32:170–177.

24. Janse MJ. Influence of the direction of the atrial wave front on AV nodal transmission in isolated hearts of rabbit. *Circ Res* 1969;25:439–449.

25. Billette J, Nadeau RA, Roberge F. Relation between the minimum RR interval during atrial fibrillation and the functional refractory period of the AV junction. *Cardiovasc Res* 1974;8:347–351.

26. Mazgalev T, Dreifus LS, Bianchi J, et al. Atrioventricular nodal conduction during atrial fibrillation in rabbit heart. *Am J Physiol* 1982;243: H754–H760.

27. Wittkampf FHM, De Jongste MJL, Meijler FL. Competitive anterograde and retrograde atrioventricular junctional activation in atrial fibrillation. *J Cardiovasc Electrophysiol* 1990;1:448–456.

28. Chorro FJ, Kirchhof CJHJ, Brugada J, et al. Ventricular response during irregular atrial pacing and atrial fibrillation. *Am J Physiol* 1990;259: H1015–21.

29. Lesh MD, Gibb WJ, Epstein L. Electronic interaction between dual AV nodal pathways: evidence from RF ablation and a computer model [abstract]. *Circulation* 1992;86(suppl1):I–30.

30. Toivonen , Kadish A, Kou W, et al. Determinants of the ventricular rate during atrial fibrillation. *J Am Coll Cardiol* 1990;16:1194–1200.

31. Blanck Z, Dhala A, Sra J, et al. Characterization of AV nodal behavior and ventricular response during atrial fibrillation before and after a selective slow-pathway ablation. *Circulation* 1995;91:1086–1094.

32. Strickberger SA, Weiss R, Daoud EG, et al. Ventricular rate during atrial fibrillation before and after slow-pathway ablation: effects of autonomic blockade and β-adrenergic stimulation. *Circulation* 1996;94:1023–1026.

33. Markowitz SM, Stein KM, Lerman BB. Mechanism of ventricular rate control after radiofrequency modification of atrioventricular conduction in patients with atrial fibrillation. *Circulation* 1996;94:2856–2864

34. Kreiner G, Heinz G, Siostrzonek P, et al. Effect of slow pathway ablation on ventricular rate during atrial fibrillation: dependence on electrophysiological properties of the fast pathway. *Circulation* 1996;93:277–283.

35. Jazayeri MR, Sra JS, Deshpande SS, et al. Electrophysiologic spectrum of atrioventricular nodal behavior in patients with atrioventricular nodal reentrant tachycardia undergoing selective fast or slow pathway ablation. *J Cardiovasc Electrophysiol* 1993;4:99–111.

36. Tai CT, Chen SA, Chiang CE, et al. Complex electrophysiological characteristics in atrioventricular nodal reentrant tachycardia with continuous atrioventricular node function curves. *Circulation* 1997;95:2541–2547.

37. Langberg JJ, Leon A, Borganelli M. A randomized prospective comparison of anterior and posterior approaches to radiofrequency catheter ablation of atrioventricular nodal reentry tachycardia. *Circulation* 1993;87:1551–1556.

38. Morady F, Hasse C, Strickberger SA, et al. Long-term follow-up after radiofrequency modification of the atrioventricular node in patients with atrial fibrillation. *J Am Coll Cardiol* 1997;27:113–121.

39. Rosenqvist M, Isaaz K. Botvinick E, et al. Relative importance of activation sequence compared to AV synchrony in left ventricular function. *Am J Cardiol* 1991;67:148–156.

40. Betocchi S, Piscione F, Villari B, et al. Effects of induced asynchrony on left

ventricular diastolic function in patients with coronary artery disease. *J Am Coll Cardiol* 1993;21:1124–1131.

41. Chorro FJ, Kirchhof HJ, Brugada J, et al. Ventricular response during irregular atrial pacing and atrial fibrillation. *Am J Physiol* 1990;28:H1015–H1021.

42. Daoud EG, Weiss R, Bahu M, et al. Effect of an irregular ventricular rhythm on cardiac output. *Am J Cardiol* 1996:78:1433–1436.

Chapter 17

Catheter Ablation of Paroxysmal Atrial Fibrillation: Results in 234 Patients

Michel Haïssaguerre, M.D., Pierre Jaïs, M.D., Dipen C. Shah, M.D., Thomas Lavergne, M.D., Mélèze Hocini, M.D., Atsushi Takahashi, M.D., Serge S. Barold, M.D., Jacques Clémenty, M.D.

Introduction

Atrial fibrillation (AF) is the most common sustained cardiac rhythm disturbance. Its prevalence increases rapidly with age to 5.9% over the age of 65[1–3] and is associated with manifestations ranging from palpitations to cardiac failure. The most dreaded complication is stroke, with 30% of cases over the age of 65[2] due to AF. Catheter techniques for ventricular rate control (atrioventricular junction ablation, atrioventricular nodal modification)[4–7] have been shown to be effective, but the persistence of AF and the frequent requirement for a permanent pacemaker are significant disadvantages. Curative therapies are currently being developed both by surgeons[8–13] and cardiologists based on studies demonstrating the simultaneous existence of several reentrant wavelets in a critical mass of atrial tissue being necessary for perpetuating AF[14–59] and the role of triggering foci for the initiation of AF.[60–69] This review will focus on the results of catheter ablation of paroxysmal AF using radiofrequency (RF) energy, based on an experience of 234 patients.

From Huang SKS, Wilber DJ (eds.): *Radiofrequency Catheter Ablation of Cardiac Arrhythmias: Basic Concepts and Clinical Applications,* 2nd ed. Armonk, NY: Futura Publishing Company, Inc. ©2000.

The Atrial Fibrillatory Substrate: Spatial Disparities in Fibrillatory Activity

Atrial fibrillation is considered to be maintained by shifting leading circle and random reentry as initially hypothesized by Moe[14] and confirmed later by Allessie.[15] Their experimental data suggest that wavelets occurring during AF are homogeneously distributed in the atria.

Jaïs et al have reported the spatial and temporal distribution of complex electrical activity during human AF, defined as continuous electrical activity or electrograms with FF intervals less than 100 milliseconds.[31] The duration of complex activity was assessed for 60 seconds (expressed as a percentage of time) using a 14-pole catheter sequentially positioned in different regions. Twenty-five males and 2 females (mean age 49±11 years) suffering from paroxysmal AF were studied. Except for amiodarone, all antiarrhythmic drugs were discontinued for 5 half-lives before the mapping study. The results illustrated in Figure 1 indicate that trabeculated regions (lateral: 22±23% and anterior: 21±26%) in the right atrium had less frequently complex electrograms than the nontrabeculated regions extending to the crista terminalis region (septum: 74±32% and intercaval: 63±33%). Holm et al also found an organization of atrial activity, sometimes centrifugal, during surgical mapping of chronic AF.[32] In contrast, electrograms recorded from the majority of the left atrium (LA) were complex for 87±11% of time except near the appendage (18±14%), again a trabeculated region. The band of atrial tissue bordering the anatomic boundary of the mitral annulus (and the coronary sinus) was sometimes organized in

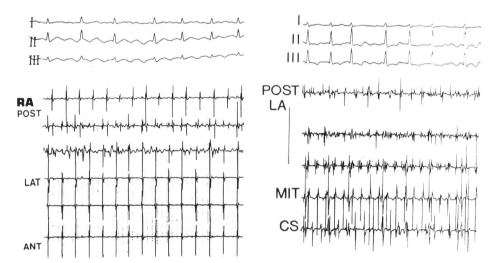

Figure 1. Left panel: Electrical activity recorded from a multipolar catheter placed horizontally across the anterior (ANT), lateral (LAT) and posterior regions of the right atrium (RA POST). The posterior RA exhibits complex activity whereas the trabeculated lateral and anterior segments are organized. Right panel: The vast majority of the LA also exhibits complex electrical activity with short FF intervals and intermittent continuous electrical activity, except the paramitral band (MIT) and adjoining coronary sinus (CS). RA = right atrium; LA = left atrium. Paper speed: 25 mm/sec.

contrast with the remainder of the LA probably because the annulus allowed penetration of wavelets only from one direction. Whereas the proximal (septal) coronary sinus was usually fibrillating, its posterior and lateral distal parts could be organized in spite of fibrillating activity in the neighboring endocardial region showing that regular coronary sinus activity is not a reliable indicator of left atrial activity.

Li et al also demonstrated spatial disparities in disorganized electrical activity with the smooth intercaval region exhibiting more complex electrograms than the trabeculated right atrium. The posterior wall exhibited Type III AF that reorganized anteriorly toward a Type I AF. Somewhat paradoxically, the shortest FF intervals were associated in fact with the longest refractory periods.[33] Other authors confirmed these data in chronic AF and showed that activation in the trabeculated right atrium may follow a consistent pattern.[34,35]

It is likely that the regions exhibiting the temporally maximal complex electrical activity are preferentially arrhythmogenic and/or associated with the most pathologically affected tissues.[36] Because the interindividual differences in fibrillatory activity are minor (septum and LA dominantly fibrillating), they do not required prior mapping and can be anatomically targeted for ablation. Individualized mapping to guide ablation may be useful for unusual cases where an ectopic focus or a single stable reentrant circuit are the determinant of AF.

Ablation of Atrial Fibrillation in Experimental Models

Different animal models of AF have been recently developed, including creation of tricuspid or mitral regurgitation, sterile pericarditis, or chronic rapid atrial pacing mainly in the canine heart.[33,36-44] One significant limitation of animal models is the small size and thickness of the atria, particularly in dogs. This renders induction of fibrillation more difficult and, more importantly, makes termination easier (i.e., with smaller lesions)—and therefore hampers extrapolation to the clinical context. Also, there is no currently available in vivo model with a reproducible and spontaneous initiation of AF to allow study of triggering events except one described in a preliminary paper by Fenelon et al.[45]

In various dog models of AF, linear transmural atrial lesions produced mainly by endocardial RF current application have been shown to reduce the inducibility and duration of AF (Table 1). The majority of these have been in the right atrium and have been based upon the anatomic approach. Thus, with few exceptions, none of these studies have used mapping data obtained during AF to guide placement of atrial lesions. The results of right atrial ablation in these models have been quite good with success rates varying from 57% to 100%.[33,38–42] High success rates with relatively localized and directed ablation in the right atrium have also been reported. Tondo et al described the efficiency of a single midseptal line in normal dogs.[43] In the sterile pericarditis model, Nakagawa et al and Uno et al performed successful ablation in the region of Bachman's bundle after mapping data from Waldo's group suggested that about half of reentrant wavelets traversed this area.[41,46,47] The consequences for interatrial conduction and LA hemodynamics were however not evaluated. Li et al[33] used 2 different canine models of AF and showed that linear right atrial ab-

Table 1
Summary of experimental results using energy applications to prevent
induction of sustained AF.

Study	Model of AF	Target site(s)	Success
Avitall et al[35]	Sterile pericarditis	RA: SVC to IVC SVC to tricuspid valve	6/6 (100%)
Elvan et al[36]	Vagal stimulation	RA + LA + coronary sinus	23/23 (100%)*
Li et al[32]	Sterile pericarditis	RA: SVC to IVC	4/7 (57%)
	Chronic rapid pacing	RA: SVC to IVC	1/6 (17%)
Tondo et al[37]	Normal dogs	Right atrial septum	8/9 (89%)
Nakagawa et al[38]	Sterile pericarditis	Bachman's bundle	8/9 (89%)
Uno et al[42]	Sterile pericarditis	Bachman's bundle	8/9 (89%)
Morillo et al[34]	Chronic rapid pacing	Left atrial posterior wall	9/11 (82%)
Haines et al[39]	Mitral regurgitation	RA	0/7 (0%)
		LA	4/7 (57%)

Definition of noninducibility and success varies in the different studies.
*At low-level vagal stimulation.
AF = atrial fibrillation; IVC = inferior vena cava; LA = left atrium; RA = right atrium; SVC = superior vena cava.

lation in the posterior intercaval right atrium (which was shown to have mainly disorganized electrograms but the longest ERP) abolished or greatly attenuated the duration of induced AF.

Right atrial ablation rendered AF noninducible in 4 of 7 dogs (57%) with sterile pericarditis versus 1 of 6 dogs (17%) of the rapid pacing model. Also, Morillo et al terminated AF in the rapid pacing model by cryosurgical applications confined to the left posterior atrium[37] where the shortest AF cycle length was recorded. In the mitral regurgitation model in sheep, Haines et al[40] observed that successful ablation was only achieved by left atrial lines. Right atrial lines increased the right but not left atrial cycle length. In contrast, left atrial lines increased both left and right atrial cycle lengths until termination of the arrhythmia. Elvan et al and Kalman et al eliminated sustained AF in half of dogs by right atrial ablation whereas both atria needed to be targeted in the other half.[48,49] Thus experimental results seem to depend also upon the specific animal model. Some of the previous studies support the concept of targeting discrete anatomic structures—Bachman's bundle, septum—in contrast to the surgical strategy employed for the Maze procedure. Others indicate the possible role of the AF model and animal species in determining the efficacy of ablation. Ablation in the right atrium seems sufficient in either normal dogs or those with sterile pericarditis while ablation in the LA seems to be required in about half of cases in the rapid pacing and mitral regurgitation models.

The mechanism by which atrial lines alter AF was studied by Sih et al.[50] They reported that refractoriness, conduction velocity, and the number, size, and complexity of wavelets did not change, whereas AF cycle length increased with the number of linear lesions. The same group reported that the intercellular gap junction protein connexin 43 was absent in ablated areas but also reduced in the nearby areas 1 to 2 cm away.[49]

Lastly, one feature that has been relatively consistently described is the "proarrhythmic" effect of certain locations and kinds of lesions resulting in the induction of "new" atrial flutters. Avitall et al found that discontinuous lesions were as frequently associated with this phenomenon as full linear lesions;[44] also, linear intercaval lesions have been found to stabilize and prolong macroreentrant right atrial flutters.[33] The clinical experience in the right as well as the LA also demonstrates the proarrhythmic effects of incomplete lines[21,51] sometimes linked to a single small residual gap.[52]

Linear Ablation Targeting Atrial Substrate in Humans

Paroxysms of AFs have been shown to be frequently preceded by atrial ectopics—natural triggers—and the duration of these episodes is thought to correlate with the extent of atrial pathology or electrical remodelling.

After 2 case reports in 1994 demonstrating the feasibility of catheter linear ablation of AF in humans, different lesions restricted to the right atrium or mimicking a catheter biatrial Maze procedure were investigated.

Linear Right Atrial Ablation

The efficacy of linear ablation limited to the right atrium was reported in 45 patients with daily paroxysmal AF (mean duration = 379 minutes per day) using a 14-pole catheter. Three groups of 15 patients each underwent increasingly complex lesion patterns in the right atrium. Ablation led to stable sinus rhythm during the procedure in 18 patients (40%) but noninducibility of AF using burst pacing was achieved in only 5 patients (11%). The lesions produced linear conduction block in only 4 out of a total of 90 lines (5%). Final success rates with all 3 types of lesion patterns were similar: 6 patients (13%) without drug, increasing to 15 (33%) in combination with antiarrhythmic drug therapy. Further deterioration was observed during long-term assessment (Figure 2). Previously undocumented typical atrial flutter was observed in the initial patients after linear ablation in the right atrium requiring subsequent ablation targeting the cavotricuspid isthmus[24] and this line was later performed systematically. The factors predictive of clinical success using right atrial lines were the successful ablation of an arrhythmogenic focus or extension of lines to the LA (in 10 patients); both are unrelated to linear right atrial ablation.

Gaïta et al reported another series of catheter ablation in the right atrium with concordant limited results that also worsened after a longer follow-up. Disorganized atrial activity in the right atrial free wall was associated with unsuccessful acute outcome.[54] The Carto system (Biosense Webster, Inc., Tirat HaCarmel, Israel and Marlton, NJ, USA) has been proposed to reproducibly make several ablation passages on the same line and achieve complete linear block. Right atrial linear lesions were created by Kuck et al with a dragging technique and produced complete conduction block to the extent of producing intraatrial dissociation. However, most patients, including all 4 with right atrial isolation, continued to have episodes of ectopics and fibrillation pointing

Success rate after right atrial linear ablation

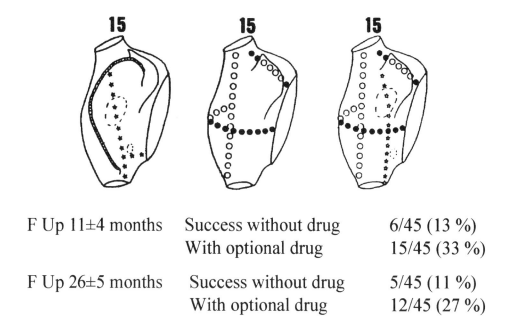

F Up 11±4 months	Success without drug	6/45 (13 %)
	With optional drug	15/45 (33 %)
F Up 26±5 months	Success without drug	5/45 (11 %)
	With optional drug	12/45 (27 %)

Success rate after septal + left atrial ablation

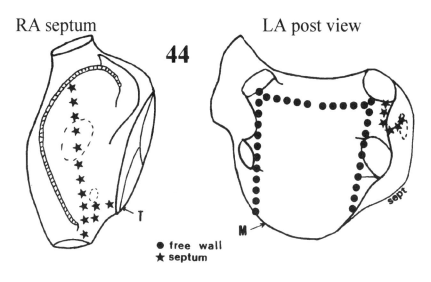

| F Up 11±5 months | Success without drug | 25/44 (57 %) |
| | With optional drug | 37/44 (84 %) |

Figure 2. Schema of ablation lines performed in 2 successive series of 45 and 40 patients.

to the initiating and driving role of the LA.[55] Intracardiac ultrasound imaging has also been studied in animals in order to improve the quality of linear lesions and avoid proarrhythmic discontinuities.[56] Although these right atrial procedures were relatively safe (main risks being the effect on cardiac conduction and phrenic nerve), the subset of patients who could benefit on a long-term basis from a right atrial approach only, with or without additional drug therapy, is limited and cannot presently be clearly defined prospectively.

A substantial proportion of patients referred for ablation of common atrial flutter also have episodes of AF. Several studies reported a decrease in the incidence of AF after successful ablation of the cavotricuspid isthmus indicating that AF resulted from flutter. In patients followed after isthmus ablation, 8% to 15% of patients without previous AF had "new"AF whereas 38% to 86% with previously documented AF had recurrence of AF. The presence of structural heart disease, frequent AF episodes or the presence of P on T ectopy were predictive of AF recurrence.[62,65,66] When flutter results from the conversion of AF by class I or III antiarrhythmic drugs, isthmus ablation followed by drug therapy maintains sinus rhythm in 73% of patients.

Linear Left Atrial Ablation

The combination of a right septal (as well as isthmus) and 3 left atrial lines performed through transeptal access were assessed in a total series of 44 patients—38 men, 6 women, 54 ± 8 years; the initial 9 patients underwent an additional left septal line.[59] The lines in the LA attempted to create a rectangle with the mitral annulus as its base on the posterior wall with a gap left in one segment to avoid isolation of the posterior LA. Anatomic structural blocks (the pulmonary veins [PV], mitral annulus) were connected together to minimize the lines and avoid peri-incisional reentry. The procedures were performed under full heparinization (partial thromboplastin time 60 to 90 seconds) and after transoesophageal echocardiography confirmed the absence of preexisting thrombi. A drag technique with a thermocouple-equipped catheter and a maximal target temperature of 54°C to 57°C (to eliminate clot formation) was used to perform the lines and repeated in an attempt to produce linear conduction block. If this was unsuccessful, an irrigated-tip ablation catheter was used with a protocol[53] proven to be safe in animals (that of target temperature = 50°C, power limit = 45–50 watts, static ablation duration = 40 seconds).

Stable sinus rhythm was obtained in 37 patients whereas AF or left atrial flutters persisted in 7 at the end of the session. Inducibility was tested using high rate biatrial pacing and one impressive finding was that sustained AF (more than 3 minutes) was rendered noninducible in 70% of patients. However, left atrial flutters appeared secondarily in 31 patients, despite their noninducibility in most cases at the end of the session indicating "remodeling" of linear lesions leaving gaps. These secondary left atrial flutters represented a major problem because they needed extensive 3-dimensional mapping to reconstruct the circuit, had multiple morphologies and required repeated sessions to be eliminated (Figure 3). For lines connected to the mitral annulus, the

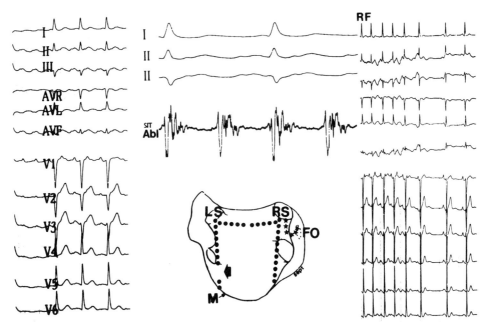

Figure 3. Left panel: Twelve-lead surface ECG of atypical left flutter (A) occurring after biatrial linear RF ablation for atrial fibrillation. Middle panel: This flutter was found to propagate through a gap (arrow) in the left superior PV (LS) to mitral (M) line. The ablation site (SIT Abl) exhibits fractionated and long-duration electrograms straddling the interval of double potentials recorded above and below the gap. Right panel: RF ablation delivered at this site interrupted the flutter. RS = right superior PV; FO = fossa ovalis.

coronary sinus provided an ideal and convenient site to easily assess the presence and width of double potentials and thus differentiate complete from incomplete linear block. This is illustrated in Figure 4. Gaps were encountered at any point of the 4 left atrial lines but most frequently at the bottom of the right superior PV-mitral line; although, obviously, 2 gaps were obligatory in the rectangular schema to allow macroreentry around anatomic obstacles. Extremely discrete gaps were sufficient to maintain left atrial flutters and could be interrupted within a few seconds by a single punctiform pulse; while prolonged and multiple RF pulses were necessary in the thickest parts of the LA along the mitral annulus from both the endocardium and epicardium via the coronary sinus. Therefore multiple ablation sessions (for flutter or arrhythmogenic foci) were required in 37 patients and the 120 procedures were complicated by the following side effects: pericardial effusion in 5 (3 requiring drainage), pulmonary embolism, inferior myocardial infarction, a reversible neurological deficit, and left PV thrombosis in one patient each. A complete line of block could be created in only 18 patients; in 16, an irrigated-tip catheter was required (see Figure 2). The procedures were prolonged, lasting 280±101 minutes with 78±37 minutes of fluoroscopy time and a total RF delivery duration of 85±49 minutes.

During a follow-up of 24±5 months (after the last session), ablation was successful in 37 patients. Twenty-five were cured without drug (57%) and 12

Assessment of left atrial lines from the coronary sinus electrograms

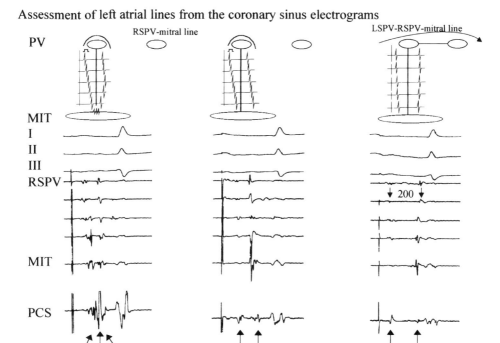

Figure 4. Progressive achievement of complete linear block in the LA. Left panel: A decapolar catheter placed all along the line from the RSPV to the mitral annulus records double potentials all along its length during right atrial pacing. However, the second potential is not sufficiently delayed and the double potential configuration converging downward is not compatible with a linear block. A gap at the bottom of the line is confirmed by the recording of a continuous fractionated electrogram occupying the isoelectric interval of adjacent double potentials from within the coronary sinus (indicated by 3 closely spaced arrows). After ablation at the gap, wide double potentials are recorded along the right superior PV-mitral annulus line (middle panel) and the double potential interval increased after creation of a second (right panel) complete line of block between both superior PVs. The delays in activation times are 100 or 160 milliseconds respectively, both endocardially and epicardially from within the coronary sinus (PCS)

with a previously ineffective drug (see Figure 2). In most unsuccessfully treated patients, the recurrent arrhythmias were left atrial flutters. Three variables were predictive of success: achievement of at least one complete line of block (18 of 37 versus 0 of 7), successful ablation of an arrhythmogenic focus (20 of 37 versus 0 of 7) and smaller longitudinal left atrial diameter (53 ± 7 millimeters versus 60 ± 6 millimeters). Fourteen of the 18 patients with at least one complete line of block had no inducible arrhythmias, no documentation of AF on Holter recordings, and total elimination of symptoms without drug ($P < 0.05$). When one of these patients underwent coronary bypass surgery 11 months after ablation, examination of the endocardial aspect of the LA showed that the area of the line of block between the right superior PV and the mitral annulus was visually indistinguishable from other areas and covered by normal appearing endothelium. On palpation, however, there was induration along the line.

In a series of 34 patients with chronic AF, Swartz et al achieved a success rate of 80% with a progressively modified biatrial (predominantly left atrial) ablation schema with most patients being free of drug therapy. Packer et al performed a similar procedure including 5 linear lesions in the LA. Acute conversion in sinus rhythm was obtained in 15 of 18 patients and maintained in 4 and 10 with and without an antiarrhythmic drug. Maloney et al achieved long-term success without drug in 9 out of 15 patients.[58] Kuck et al and Pappone et al performed a circular line encircling the PV using the Carto system. Half the patients were improved, usually with a drug; the absence of complete linear block was obvious based on persistent 1:1 activation of the posterior LA.[55,57] Nademanee et al reported a 55% success rate in 32 patients including those with additional drug therapy. All the procedures of linear ablation in the LA were prolonged, lasting 12 hours, sometimes under general anesthesia. Despite strict anticoagulation and temperature-controlled ablation, embolic events have occurred, notably when conventional (nonirrigated) catheters are used. Furthermore RF applications have been delivered inside the PVs without limiting the delivered RF power and probably as a result, PV stenosis has been reported.[59,63]

The predictive value of linear block as well as the high incidence of left atrial flutters caused by recovery/remodeling of ablated tissue indicates that new catheter technologies are needed to optimize lesion characteristics at the index procedure, prevent the need for further ablation sessions, and thus improve efficiency of linear ablation.

Ablation of Triggers Initiating AF in Humans

Arrhythmogenic foci are critical for patients with paroxysmal AF. Either they represent the sole abnormality in a small subset of patients in whom the focus discharges for long periods (focal AF) or, more commonly, foci trigger episodes of AF that subsequently continue independently of the initiating event (focally initiated AF).[19,61,64]

Mapping of Triggering Foci

These foci have a characteristically predominant anatomic location in the PVs, and unusual properties including long conduction time to the LA, unpredictable firing, and frequent occurrence of focal discharges confined within the vein. In Holter recordings, either multiple daily bouts of varying duration may be recorded or only isolated ectopics at other times, or only AF without any isolated ectopics because discharges from the focus occur only in rapid and/or prolonged trains, every train inducing AF. The first ectopic P wave, whether isolated or initiating AF, is superimposed on the T wave of the previous QRS complex producing a P on T pattern recognizable at first sight.

The same focus produces different types of atrial arrhythmias. Single discharges manifest as isolated extrasystoles, repetitive discharges with long cycle lengths as an automatic rhythm; shorter cycles result in organized monomorphic tachycardia or a pattern of focal flutter (Figure 5) whereas at short cycle

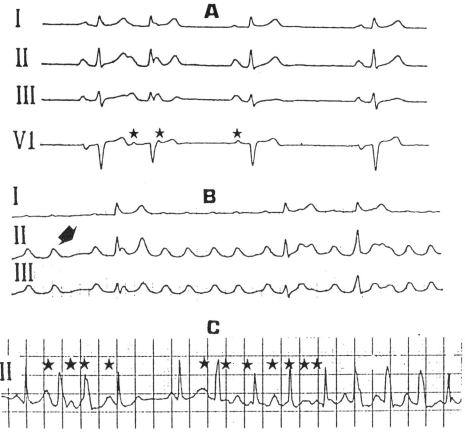

Figure 5. Surface ECG recordings of various manifestations of atrial focus. Panel A: Isolated extrasystoles (stars) with contours similar to the atrial tachycardia in panel B. Note the irregular cycle length from one beat to the other (arrow). Panel C: Recording of incessant salvos from the same focal source separated by a single intervening sinus beat.

lengths an ECG pattern (a rapid and irregular tachycardia without discrete P waves of AF) is produced (focal AF). Sudden variations (up to 350 milliseconds beat to beat) in the focus discharge rate were also responsible for the irregular cycle lengths (see Figure 5). True intracardiac AF was initiated when the focus abruptly discharged a very rapid train with a cycle length of 182 ± 57 milliseconds (330 beats per minute) leading to chaotic atrial activity. The source of isolated extrasystoles was also the same, and initiation was therefore the result of sudden transformation of benign isolated extrasystoles into a malignant train of rapid discharges acting as a natural fibrillator. Initiation of common atrial flutter, its degeneration into AF and its interruption were also the result of PV discharges.

In our center, a total of 135 patients have been investigated, including 33 with structural heart disease; none have undergone left atrial ablation. In patients with frequent ectopics and nonsustained AF, a single catheter was introduced in the LA for vein by vein mapping. In patients with few ectopics and/or sustained AF, 2 roving ablation catheters with different radius curves

(Biosense Webster yellow and blue) were used simultaneously. Of triggering foci, 96% originated from the PVs for a total of 265 arrhythmogenic PV: 32 % and 68% of patients has single or multiple PV respectively. In the PVs, specific activity was marked by spikes (the PV potentials = PVP) reflecting atrial muscular bundles extending 2 (inferior PVs) to 4 cm (superior PVs) from the LA into the PVs. The PVP was identified during sinus rhythm in right PV but may require left atrial or coronary sinus pacing in left PV to be highlighted at the end of the multicomponent atrial activity (Figure 6). The atrial electrogram-PVP sequence inverted during extrasystoles (or repetitive focal tachycardia) in the source vein of ectopy whereas in other veins, the same activation sequence as in sinus rhythm indicated passive (bystander) activation (Figure 7). This potential could be tracked from its source inside the veins to its atrial exit. The source of ectopy marked by the earliest PVP was very discrete in contrast to the ostial exit where a synchronous PVP could be recorded in wide sectors. A lower amplitude far-field PVP (< 0.1 mV) could also be recorded from contiguous branches or the corresponding PV trunk or a neighboring PV trunk. A local high frequency PVP could be recorded simultaneously in other parts of the same vein, but with a later timing, indicating progression towards the ostium and its left atrial exit. Considerably later conduction could also be recorded in different parts of the same vein so that recording late activity in one sector of the PV

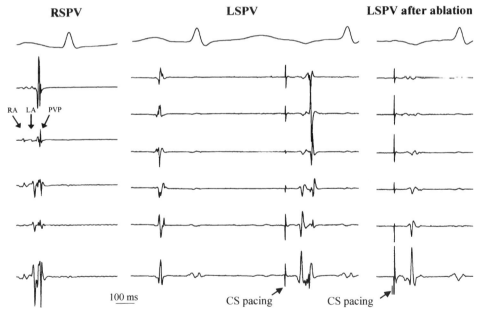

Figure 6. Multipolar cirfumferential recordings from the PV. In the right panel, local PV potentials (PVP) are usually obvious during sinus rhythm in the right superior pulmonary vein (RSPV) at the terminal part of multicomponent bipolar electrograms. The first 2 "far-field" deflections are the right atrial (RA) and left atrial (LA) potentials respectively. The bipolar tracings on the middle panel show 2 beats into the LSPV, a sinus beat followed by another during pacing from the distal coronary sinus. Though the electrograms during sinus rhythm do not show evident local PV potentials, characteristic sharp potentials distinct from the initial far-field potential are recorded during pacing. The electrograms after ablation in the same recording sites in the left panel show abolition of PVP and unchanged LA potentials.

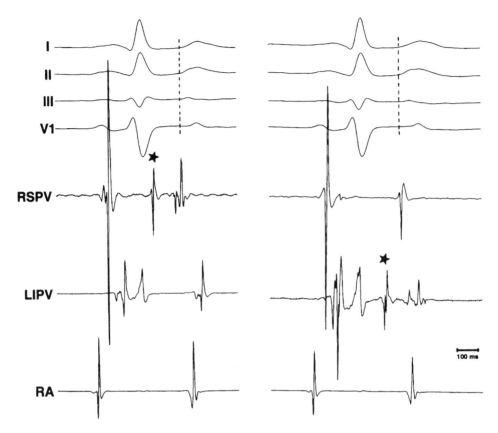

Figure 7. Documentation of 2 different arrhythmogenic PV in the same patient. In the right panel, a sharp deflection (\\) in the RSPV is followed by the atrial electrogram, which is coincident with the surface P wave onset (broken line). The activation sequence is unchanged in the LIPV. The second panel shows an ectopy originating from the LIPV.

during ectopy did not exclude an origin in another part of the same vein. Importantly, plurifocal sources could be found in the same PV often corresponding to different tributaries. The same source could also produce ectopy with different activation patterns in the complex muscle architecture clearly indicating multiple potential sources or "pathways." These phenomena could be clearly demonstrated by multielectrode catheters stably positioned within the PV (Figure 8). The conduction time to the LA was long, up to 160 milliseconds, and exhibited decremental conduction with increasing prematurity. Ectopics closely coupled to the previous sinus beat were not conducted to the LA (i.e., were confined within the vein) and this was documented in 42% to 70% of arrhythmogenic PVs often as a "concealed venous bigeminal rhythm." Such PV discharges resulted in ectopic PVP usually synchronous with the local ventricular electrogram which could be distinguished by its intermittent occurrence or disappearance with atrial pacing. A slightly longer coupling interval (5 to 10 milliseconds) and/or isoproterenol infusion was sufficient to allow conduction to the LA so that even isolated concealed discharges were enough to identify an arrhythmogenic PV.

Different AF initiation patterns from the same PV (LIPV)

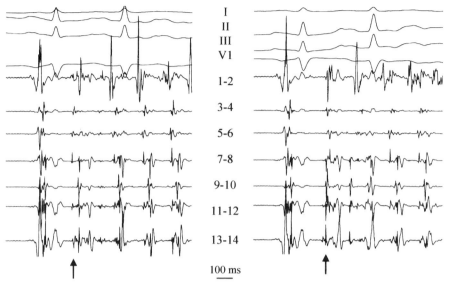

Figure 8. Multielectrode recordings of 2 different initiation patterns of AF from the same vein (LIPV). A multipolar catheter recording circumferentially inside the LIPV shows multicomponent electrograms with terminal spikes representing local PV muscle activation. Identical electrograms during sinus rhythm in both panels indicate the stability of recording sites. The initial activation within the PV (arrows) shows 2 different patterns inducing AF.

Limitations in Effective Mapping of PV Foci

1. The spontaneous occurrence of ectopy was unpredictable, and provocative maneuvers are often necessary in eliciting ectopy. Isoproterenol infusion produced ectopy in half the patients (during or after infusion), notably in those having arrhythmias during or just after effort. In other patients, volume infusion, vagal maneuvers (deep breathing, Valsalva, ATP injection), and/or atrial pacing could reproducibly elicit ectopy occurring just after the postpacing pause. Rapid pacing was significantly more provocative than slow rate pacing, and the combination of pacing and isoproterenol was the most sensitive method.

2. Ectopy could induce AF lasting for minutes or hours, forcing prolonged waiting periods for its spontaneous interruption, for which external or internal electrical cardioversions (sometimes multiple) were required. The use of a low energy cardioversion catheter allowed repetitive shocks to be delivered without general anesthesia during the procedure, particularly in patients in whom every PV focus discharge initiated AF.

3. Mechanically produced beats ("vulnerability") were often observed in the arrhythmogenic and nonarrhythmogenic PV, confusing mapping data and requiring comparison of their ECG morphology, coupling interval, and intra-atrial sequence with those of spontaneous ectopy.

4. Spontaneous or provoked ectopy obtained and ablated in one ablation session did not exclude the possibility of other foci appearing later from another part of the targeted PV or different PV which will require further ablation.

These limitations may be overcome by prior identification of ectopic P wave morphologies from surface ECG techniques, recognition of arrhythmogenic PV from electrogram characteristics, and more efficient multielectrode mapping catheters. Ultimately an anatomically guided approach to ablation of PV may be appropriate.

RF Ablation of PV Foci

RF ablation could be performed at the site of earliest spike activity (source) or along its intravenous course or at its ostial exit into the LA. The substrate at the ostium was wider than distally but ablation had a lower risk of inducing significant stenosis. Obviously, the procedural end point of acute arrhythmia suppression was only evident in the situation of frequent ectopy. In patients with rare ectopy, a systematic elimination of PVP in the PVs was performed by sequential RF applications at the ostium targeting the PVP during sinus rhythm or left atrial pacing. It has the considerable advantage of avoiding further mapping and risk-inducing AF, besides providing a direct assessment of the local PV substrate. A few seconds of RF energy application were sufficient at some sites to eliminate both ostial and downstream PV muscle activity (Figures 9 and 10) whereas repeated and prolonged RF application was required in others. Abolition of all PVP was confirmed by inability to capture the LA by pacing from the

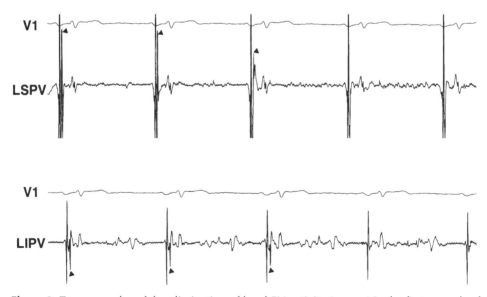

Figure 9. Two examples of the elimination of local PV activity (arrows) in the first seconds of RF delivery.

RF eliminates PV potentials

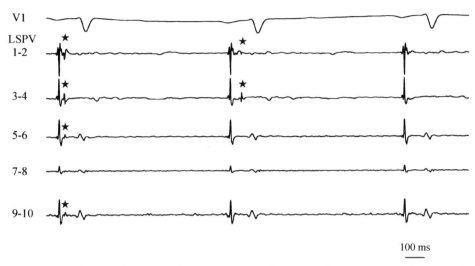

Figure 10. Final RF application at the LSPV ostium eliminates all PV activity as shown in the circumferential bipolar recordings within the vein.

PV. Successful ablation of the foci producing elimination of AF paroxysms (and eventually atrial flutter) was strongly associated with disappearance of all local PV potentials in sinus rhythm (see Figures 6, 9 and 10). Persistent discrete PVP was sufficient to initiate AF. The success rate—that is, the elimination of AF—was 90% when all PVP were abolished, whereas persistence or recovery of the PVP was associated with a 55% risk of arrhythmia recurrence.

PV stenosis, defined as a diameter reduction $\geq$ 50%, was observed in 6 cases (2.5 %) but only 2 patients had symptoms. PV stenosis occurred acutely (immediately at the end of ablation) and few changes were observed later. No patient had pulmonary hypertension. The left inferior PV, a distal ablation site (close to PV branching) and the use of RF power reaching 45–50 watts were predictive factors. Without limitation of RF power,[69] some authors reported up to 42% of PV stenosis indicated by a significant PV flow acceleration. In our experience, with a limitation of RF power below 30 watts, no PV stenosis occurred at the ostia although a longer-term follow-up is probably necessary. This power was associated with low "achieved" temperature in the PV (42°C) owing to the local high cooling blood flow mimicking an irrigated-tip catheter.

With a follow-up of 8±4 months (including repeated Holter recordings), ablation of the initiating triggers alone produces complete elimination of AF with a success rate depending on the number of arrhythmogenic PV: 92% success in patients with a single arrhythmogenic PV, 73% with 2 PV, and 44% when more PV were involved. PV angiograms were performed in 72 patients 3 to 20 months after ablation and have not revealed new PV stenosis. Anticoagulants were interrupted in all successfully treated patients.

Ablation targeted to arrhythmogenic pulmonary veins is therefore a curative technique for paroxysmal AF. The main caveat to mapping guided PV ablation is the unpredictable occurrence of ectopics and their inconsistent inducibility. Complete elimination of PVP is the most effective end point, applicable even when ectopics are rare or absent, but this is difficult to achieve in multiple PV.

Indications

In view of the difficulties in linear lesion making and multiple PV ablation, we offer this procedure to multidrug-resistant, symptomatic patients with paroxysmal AF as an alternative to AV junctional ablation. A history of thromboembolic phenomena or tachycardia-mediated heart failure, as a testimonial of AF morbidity, strengthens the indication for the procedure. Patients with infrequent episodes should not be presently considered for linear ablation since incomplete lines may organize atrial activity and render arrhythmia more frequent or more prolonged. On the other hand, proarrhythmia phenomena have not yet been encountered with PV ablation alone.

It is anticipated that continued technological developments will optimize and facilitate these complex techniques. Ultimately it may become a widespread procedure provided that further studies demonstrate a favorable risk/benefit ratio; notably, maintained improvement of symptoms, better survival, and decreased risk of embolic events compared to alternative treatments.

Acknowledgment

The authors would like to acknowledge their appreciation of the secretarial assistance of Joëlle Bassibey.

References

1. Feinberg WM, Blackshear JL, Laupacis A, et al. Prevalence, age distribution, and gender of patients with atrial fibrillation: analysis and implications. *Arch Intern Med* 1995;155:469–473.
2. Wolf PA, Abbott RD, Kannel WB. Atrial fibrillation, a major contributor to stroke in the elderly: the Framingham Study. *Arch Intern Med* 1987;147: 1561–1564.
3. Lévy S, Breithardt G, Campbell RWF, et al. Atrial fibrillation: current knowledge and recommendations for management. *Eur Heart J* 1998;19: 1294–1320.
4. Scheinman MM, Morady F, Hess DS, et al. Catheter-induced ablation of atrioventricular junction to control refractory supraventricular arrhythmias. *JAMA* 1982;248:855–861.
5. Langberg JJ, Chin M, Schamp DJ, et al. Ablation of the atrioventricular junction with radiofrequency current energy using a new electrode catheter. *Am J Cardiol* 1991;67:142–147.
6. Huang SK, Bharati S, Graham AR, et al. Closed chest catheter dessication

of the atrioventricular junction using radiofrequency energy: a new method of catheter ablation. *J Am Coll Cardiol* 1987;9:349–358.

7. Williamson BD, Man KC, Daoud E, et al. Radiofrequency catheter modification of atrioventricular conduction to control the ventricular rate during atrial fibrillation. *N Engl J Med* 1994;331:910–917.

8. Williams JM, Ungerleider RM, Lofland GK, et al. Left atrial isolation: a new technique for the treatment of supraventricular arrhythmias. *J Thorac Cardiovasc Surg* 1980;80:373–380.

9. Cox JL, Canavan TE, Schuessler RB, et al. The surgical treatment of atrial fibrillation II: intraoperative electrophysiologic mapping and description of the electrophysiologic basis of atrial flutter and fibrillation. *J Thorac Cardiovasc Surg* 1991;101:406–426.

10. Cox JL, Boineau JP, Schuessler RB, et al. Five-year experience with the Maze procedure for atrial fibrillation. *Ann Thorac Surg* 1993;56:814–824.

11. Defauw JJ, Guiraudon GM, Van Hemel NM, et al. Surgical therapy of paroxysmal atrial fibrillation with the corridor operation. *Ann Thorac Surg* 1992;53:564–571.

12. Shyu KG, Cheng JJ, Chen JJ, et al. Recovery of atrial function after atrial compartment operation for chronic atrial fibrillation in mitral valve disease. *J Am Coll Cardiol* 1994;24:392–398.

13. Kosakai Y, Kawaguchi AT, Isobe F, et al. Modified Maze procedure for patients with atrial fibrillation undergoing simultaneous open heart surgery. *Circulation* 1995;92(suppl 9):II359–364.

14. Moe GK, Rheinboldt WC, Abildskov JA. A computer model of atrial fibrillation. *Am Heart J* 1964;200–220.

15. Allessie MA, Lammers WJEP, Bonke FIM, et al. Experimental evaluation of Moe's multiple wavelet hypothesis of atrial fibrillation. In Zipes DP, Jalife J, eds. *Cardiac Electrophysiology and Arrhythmias.* Orlando, FL: Grune & Stratton, 1985. pp 265–276.

16. Cox JL, Canavan TE, Scheussler RB, et al. The surgical treatment of atrial fibrillation II: intraoperative mapping and description of the electrophysiologic basis of atrial flutter and atrial fibrillation. *J Thorac Cardiovasc Surg* 1991;101:402–426.

17. Konings KTS, Kirchhof CJHJ, Smeets JRLM, et al. High density mapping of electrically induced atrial fibrillation in humans. *Circulation* 1994;89:1665–1680.

18. Misier ARR, Opthof T, Van Hemel NM, et al. Increased dispersion of refractoriness in patients with idiopathic paroxysmal atrial fibrillation. *J Am Coll Cardiol* 1992;19:1531–1535.

19. Haïssaguerre M, Gencel L, Fischer B, et al. Successful catheter ablation of atrial fibrillation. *J Cardiovasc Electrophysiol* 1994;5:1045–1052.

20. Swartz JF, Pellersels G, Silvers J, et al. A catheter-based curative approach to atrial fibrillation in humans. *Circulation* 1994;90 (4) part 2:I-335.

21. Haïssaguerre M, Jaïs P, Shah DC, et al. Right and left atrial radiofrequency catheter therapy of paroxysmal atrial fibrillation. *J Cardiovasc Electrophysiol* 1996;12:1132–1144.

22. Ching Man K, Daoud E, Knight B, et al. Right atrial-radiofrequency catheter ablation of paroxysmal atrial fibrillation. *J Am Coll Cardiol* 1996;188A.

23. Natale A, Tomassoni G, Kearney MM, et al. Catheter ablation approach on the right side only for paroxysmal atrial fibrillation therapy. *Circulation* 1996;92:I-266.

24. Cosio FG, Lopez-Gil M, Goicolea A, et al. Radiofrequency ablation of the inferior vena cava-tricuspid valve isthmus in common atrial flutter. *Am J Cardiol* 1993;71:705–709.

25. Lesh MD, Van Hare GF, Epstein LM, et al. Radiofrequency catheter ablation of atrial arrhythmias: results and mechanisms. *Circulation* 1994;89: 1074–1089.

26. Scheinman MM, Olgin J. Catheter ablation of cardiac arrhythmias of atrial origin. In: Zipes DP, ed. *Catheter Ablation of Arrhythmias*. Armonk, NY: Futura Publishing Co., 1994. pp 129–149.

27. Fischer B, Haïssaguerre M, Garrigues S, et al. Radiofrequency catheter ablation of common atrial flutter in 80 patients. *J Am Coll Cardiol* 1995;25: 1365–1372.

28. Shoda M, Kajimoto K, Matsuda N, et al. A novel mechanism of human atrial fibrillation: single macro-reentry with intra-atrial conduction block. *PACE* 1997;20 (part II):1065.

29. Wang J, Liu L, Feng J, et al. Regional and functional factors determining induction and maintenance of atrial fibrillation in dogs. *Am J Physiol* 1996;271:148–158.

30. Gaïta F, Riccardi R, Lamberti F, et al. Right atrium radiofrequency catheter ablation in idiopathic vagal atrial fibrillation. *Eur Heart J* 1996;17:301.

31. Jaïs P, Haïssaguerre M, Shah DC, et al. Regional disparities of endocardial atrial activation in paroxysmal atrial fibrillation. *PACE* 1996;19(part II): 1998–2003.

32. Holm M, Johansson R, Brandt J, et al. Epicardial right atrial free wall mapping in chronic atrial fibrillation. Documentation of repetitive activation with a focal spread, a hitherto unrecognized phenomenon in man. *Eur Heart J* 1997;18:290–310.

33. Li H, Hare J, Mughal K, et al. Distribution of atrial electrogram types during atrial fibrillation: effect of rapid atrial pacing and intercaval junction ablation. J Am Coll Cardiol 1996;27:1713–1721.

34. Steiner PR, Kalman JN, Karch MR, et al. Regional anatomic differences in atrial fibrillation organization in the canine right atrium [abstract]. *Circulation* 1996;94(8):352.

35. Gepstein L, Hayam G, Shpun S, et al. 3D spatial dispersion of cycle length histograms during atrial fibrillation in the chronic goat model. *Circulation* 1997;96:236.

36. Avitall B, Hartz R, Bharati S, et al. The correlation of local histology with fractionated local electrical activity during atrial fibrillation in patients undergoing the Maze procedure and mitral valve replacement [abstract]. *PACE* 1996;19(part II):725.

37. Morillo CA, Klein GJ, Jones DL, et al. Chronic rapid atrial pacing: structural, functional and electrophysiologic characteristics of a new model of sustained atrial fibrillation. *Circulation* 1995;91:1588–1595.

38. Avitall B, Helms RW, Chiang W, et al. Nonlinear atrial radiofrequency lesions are arrhythmogenic: a study of skipped lesions in the normal atria. *Circulation* 1995;92:I-265.

39. Elvan A, Pride HP, Eble JN, et al. Radiofrequency catheter ablation of the atria reduces inducibility and duration of atrial fibrillation in dogs. *Circulation* 1995;91:2235–2244.

40. Haines DE, McRury IA. Primary atrial fibrillation ablation (PAFA) in a chronic atrial fibrillation model. *Circulation* 1995;92:I-265.

41. Nakagawa H, Kumagai K, Imai S, et al. Catheter ablation of Bachmann's bundle from the right atrium eliminates atrial fibrillation in a canine sterile pericarditis model. *PACE* 1996;19:581.

42. Olgin J, Kalman JM, Maguire M, et al. Electrophysiologic effects of long linear atrial lesions placed under intracardiac echo guidance. *Circulation* 1997;96:2715–2721.

43. Tondo C, Scherlag BJ, Otomo K, et al. Critical atrial site for ablation of pacing-induced atrial fibrillation in the normal dog heart. *J Cardiovasc Electrophysiol* 1997;8:1255–1265.

44. Avitall B, Helms RW, Chiang W, et al. Nonlinear atrial radiofrequency lesions are arrhythmogenic: a study of skipped lesions in the normal atria. *Circulation* 1995;92:I-265.

45. Fenelon G, Shepard RK, Turner A, et al. Evidence of a focal origin as the mechanism of atrial tachycardia in dogs with ventricular pacing-induced congestive heart failure. *PACE* 1997;20 (part II):1095.

46. Uno K, Kumagai K, Krestian CM, et al. New radiofrequency ablative cure of atrial flutter [abstract]. *PACE* 1997;20(part II):1234.

47. Kumagai K, Krestian C, Waldo AL. Simultaneous multisite mapping studies during induced atrial fibrillation in the sterile pericarditis model. Insights into the mechanism of its maintenance. *Circulation* 1997;95:511–521.

48. Kalman J, Olgin J, Karch M, et al. Are linear lesions needed in both atria to prevent atrial fibrillation in a canine model? *Circulation* 1996;94:I-555.

49. Elvan A, Huang W, Pressler M, et al. Radiofrequency catheter ablation of the atria eliminates pacing-induced sustained atrial fibrillation and reduces connexin 43 in dogs. *Circulation* 1997;96:1675–1685.

50. Sih HJ, Berbari EJ, Zipes DP. Epicardial maps of atrial fibrillation after linear ablation lesions. *J Cardiovasc Electrophysiol* 1997;8:1046–1054.

51. Jaïs P, Haïssaguerre M, Shah DC, et al. Catheter therapy of multiple left atrial flutters following atrial fibrillation ablation. *PACE* 1997;20(part II):1181.

52. Shah DC, Jaïs P, Haïssaguerre M, et al. Simplified electrophysiologically directed catheter ablation of recurrent common atrial flutter. *Circulation* 1997;96:2505–2508.

53. Lavergne T, Jaïs P, Haïssaguerre M, et al. Evaluation of a single passage RF ablation line in animal atria using an irrigated tip catheter. *Circulation* 1997;96:259.

54. Gaïta F, Riccardi R, Lamberti F, et al. Right atrium radiofrequency catheter ablation in idiopathic vagal atrial fibrillation. *Circulation* 1998;97:2136–2145.

55. Kuck KH, Ernst S, Khanedani A, et al. Clinical follow-up after primary catheter-based ablation of atrial fibrillation using the CARTO system [abstract]. *PACE* 1998;21(part II):868.

56. Packer DL, Johnson SB, Pederson B, et al. The utility of non-contact map-

ping in identifying and rectifying discontinuity: mediated atrial proarrhythmia accompanying linear lesion creation. *PACE* 1998;21(part II):867.

57. Pappone C, Lamberti F, Rillo M, et al. Catheter ablation of atrial fibrillation using a nonfluoroscopic system [abstract]. *J Am Coll Cardiol* 1998; 31:202A.

58. Maloney JD, Milner L, Barold SS, et al. Two-staged biatrial linear and focal ablation to restore sinus rhythm in patients with refractory chronic atrial fibrillation: procedure experience and follow-up beyond one year. *PACE* 1998;21(part II):2527–2532.

59. Jaïs P, Shah DC, Haïssaguerre M, et al. Septal and left atrial linear ablation for atrial fibrillation: efficacy and safety. *Am J Cardiol* (in press).

60. Haïssaguerre M, Marcus FI, Fischer B, et al. Radiofrequency catheter ablation in unusual mechanisms of atrial fibrillation: report of three cases. *J Cardiovasc Electrophysiol* 1994;5:743–751.

61. Jaïs P, Haïssaguerre M, Shah DC, et al. A focal source of atrial fibrillation treated by discrete radiofrequency ablation. *Circulation* 1997;95:572–576.

62. Haïssaguerre M, Jaïs P, Shah DC, et al. Predominant origin of atrial panarrhythmic triggers in the pulmonary veins: a distinct electrophysiologic entity. *PACE* 1997;20(part II):1065.

63. Robbins IM, Colvin EV, Doyle TP, et al. Pulmonary vein stenosis after catheter ablation of atrial fibrillation. *Circulation* 1998;98:1769–1775.

64. Haïssaguerre M, Jaïs P, Shah DC, et al. Spontaneous initiation of atrial fibrillation by ectopic beats originating in the pulmonary veins. *N Engl J Med* 1998;339:659–666.

65. Paydak H, Kall JG, Burke MC, et al. Atrial fibrillation after radiofrequency ablation of type I atrial flutter: time to onset, determinant and clinical course. *Circulation* 1998;98:315–322.

66. Nabar A, Rodriguez ML, Timermans C, et al. Effect of right atrial isthmus ablation in the occurrence of atrial fibrillation: observations in 4 patient groups having type 2 atrial flutter with or without associated atrial fibrillation. *Circulation* 1999;99:1441–1445.

67. Lau CP, Tse HF, Ayers GM. Defibrillation-guided radiofrequency ablation of atrial fibrillation secondary to an atrial focus. *J Am Coll Cardiol* 1999;33:1217–1226.

68. Hwang C, Karagueuzian HS, Chen PS. Idiopathic paroxysmal atrial fibrillation induced by a focal discharge mechanism in the left superior pulmonary vein: possible roles of the ligament of Marshall. *J Cardiovasc Electrophysiol* 1999;10:636–648.

69. Tsai CF, Chen SA, Tai CT, et al. Bezold-Jarisch-like reflex during radiofrequency ablation of the pulmonary vein tissues in patients with paroxysmal focal atrial fibrillation. *J Cardiovasc Electrophysiol* 1999;10:27–35.

Chapter 18

Experimental Studies of Catheter-Based Linear Lesions for Ablation of Atrial Fibrillation

Boaz Avitall, M.D., Ph.D., F.A.C.C.,
Ray W. Helms, B.S.E., Gopal N. Gupta, B.S.

Introduction

Prevalence

Chronic atrial fibrillation (AF) is the most common arrhythmia in humans and can be found in 0.3–0.4 % of the adult population.[1] The prevalence of this rhythm disorder increases with age from 2–4% in people over the age of 60[2] to 11.6 % in those over the age of 75.[3] AF is also very common in patients with overt congestive failure, where its prevalence is as high as 40%.[4,5] Many medical complications are associated with AF including loss of the "atrial kick" and impaired autonomic control over the heart rate during exercise and rest. The most catastrophic complication associated with AF is embolic stroke, which may be incapacitating or fatal. In fact, AF has been identified in over 50% of all instances of systemic thromboembolism from the heart.[6]

Pharmacological Intervention

Current pharmacological treatment of AF in many patients is not adequate[7]. In some cases chronic antiarrhythmic therapy can be complicated by proarrhythmia, which may lead to syncope or sudden death. Treatment of AF

From Huang SKS, Wilber DJ (eds.): *Radiofrequency Catheter Ablation of Cardiac Arrhythmias: Basic Concepts and Clinical Applications,* 2nd ed. Armonk, NY: Futura Publishing Company, Inc. ©2000.

with Class Ia and Class III antiarryhthmic drugs can prolong the QT interval and cause unstable polymorphic ventricular tachycardia, while therapy with Class Ic drugs has been documented to cause a threefold increase in mortality in post-myocardial infarction patients.[8] Both Class Ia and Ic drugs have been associated with the inception or exacerbation of congestive heart failure. Long-term evaluation of treatment with Class III drugs has shown that at 3 years only 53% of patients are able to maintain sinus rhythm.[9]

Surgical Intervention

In the absence of safe and effective antiarrhythmic drug therapy for the maintenance of sinus rhythm, several invasive approaches have been developed. The procedures currently used require extensive open-heart surgery, are technically demanding, and involve considerable intra- and perioperative morbidity. The long-term results of surgical procedures have been encouraging, with a low risk of severe complications in selected patients.[10,11] Currently, the Maze operation is considered the most effective treatment of AF with the highest long-term success rate, over 90% in selected series.[12] This operation grew out of intraoperative mapping of AF that demonstrated multiple reentrant circuits rather than truly disorganized electrical activity. The procedure involves the placement of multiple linear incisions in a very specific pattern to modify conduction without completely electrically isolating atrial tissues. All the incisions are sutured closed, thus creating a maze-like pattern. This procedure divides atrial tissues into separate territories that are smaller than the critical area needed to sustain AF. The atria appear to function well, with sinoatrial (SA) and atrioventricular (AV) nodal function preserved in most instances and a low risk for embolization after the postoperative course.[10] Unfortunately, many physicians are reluctant to use this approach for the correction of AF alone because of the inherent expense and morbidity that thoracic surgery entails.[13] In addition, many patients are not candidates for this approach due to the presence of contraindications to extensive surgery.

Catheter Ablation

It would be extremely attractive to reproduce the Maze procedure results with a minimally invasive technique capable of electrophysiologically dividing atrial tissue into separate, functional territories. In recent years we have witnessed the expanding use of transcatheter ablation to replace surgical therapy for arrhythmias. Transcatheter application of radiofrequency (RF) power to cardiac tissue destroys the tissue's electrical properties and causes conduction decoupling, as demonstrated by the ablation of accessory pathways. A percutaneous transvascular catheter approach to ablate AF by separating atrial tissue with linear RF lesions, if effective even in a select patient population, would be a significant achievement in the treatment of this highly prevalent disorder.

Based on the work of Cox et al,[10,12] the ablation of AF is likely to require lesions that are linear, contiguous, and transmural, similar to those created via the surgical Maze procedure. The lesions must terminate in a manner that prevents the formation of atrial flutter. The currently accepted catheter and RF technology is unlikely to allow the design flexibility capable of creating lesions similar to the surgical Maze without inflating production costs, compounding complexity, and compromising safety. In pursuing such an ablation system, we further assume that not every patient with AF requires a full set of Maze lesions. In addition, a successful AF ablation system may not totally eliminate the arrhythmia but may provide an increase in susceptibility to drugs, a decrease in the length of time and incidence of paroxysmal AF, or conversion of sustained AF to paroxysmal AF. Since there is much to be learned about the mechanism of AF, a simple, safe technology that provides the operator with mapping and ablation capability should be used initially. Such a technology will maximize the information input and increase our understanding of this arrhythmia.

Assumptions and Goals for Catheter-based Ablation of AF

Technique

The primary guiding forces for developing and evaluating catheter technology must be safety, and to a lesser extent efficacy. The most devastating nonfatal complication of an ablation procedure is the development of thromboembolic stroke, which may totally disable a patient who was functional before the intervention. A stroke may result from excessive catheter dragging, which could dislodge an existing fibrin clot, or from overheating tissues and blood causing the formation of char that is loosely adherent to the ablating electrode and/or the endocardium. Once the catheter is moved, this material may be dislodged and could cause a stroke, a myocardial infarct, or a peripheral infarct. Another cause for a stroke may be air emboli introduced via guiding sheaths during catheter and sheath exchanges or via the infusion of fluids.

There are many other complications that must be avoided, including:

· Perforation leading to tamponade
· Injury to the AV valves, ventricular tissues, or coronary arteries
· Sinus node injury/dysfunction
· AV node and/or His ablation requiring the insertion of a permanent pacemaker
· Excessive radiation exposure to both the patient and operator
· Development of a new rhythm disturbance, such as incessant atrial flutter, which may be more difficult to treat than the AF for which the patient initially received the intervention

To justify exposing the patient to this procedure, the recovery of atrial mechanical function after the procedure is imperative. Theoretically, AF can be terminated by ablating the majority of the atrial tissue. Though rate control may be achieved, no mechanical benefit will be provided to the patient. Without the restoration of atrial mechanical function, the risk of thromboembolic stroke will remain high and may require continuous anticoagulation. If this is the outcome of a catheter-based AF intervention, AV node modification or ablation of the AV node or His followed by permanent pacemaker insertion and continued anticoagulation may be more appropriate in highly symptomatic patients in whom pharmacological therapy has failed. These techniques offer minimal acute risk and are often rewarding.[14]

Thus, the goal of catheter-based ablation of AF should be safe minimal tissue destruction allowing for the restoration of sinus rhythm under autonomic nervous system control with recovery of atrial mechanical transport to prevent thromboembolic complications and provide hemodynamic benefits.

Technology

Recently several investigations have reported that chronic AF can be ablated via transcatheter lesion generation in humans.[15–17] Based on the success rate achieved by Cox et al,[12] the current assumption is that a modified Maze-type procedure is required to ablate AF successfully. When subjecting a patient to an extensive surgical procedure, the goal is to achieve a very high rate of cure since a repeat procedure is unlikely. This is especially true for those patients in whom AF is the only indication for surgery. An extensive surgical procedure that requires thoracotomy may not allow for repeat surgery if the AF recurs. Thus, an extensive complete Maze procedure is required in every surgical patient to ensure the desired outcome. However, with transcutaneous catheter-based lesion generation, minimally invasive follow-up procedures are feasible.

Cox's studies concluded that completely linear, continuous, and transmural lesions are needed to terminate and prevent the re-initiation of AF (atrial fibrillation) and/or atrial flutter. However, the recent experience by Haïssaguerre et al[15,16] and Swartz and associates[17] suggests that such conditions may not be absolutely necessary, since it is unlikely that the catheter drag technique is capable of creating perfectly linear, contiguous lesions in all cases. Perhaps the most important conclusion that can be drawn from these studies is that, despite the technological limitations and the uncertainty of the character of the lesions, the investigators were able to successfully terminate AF.

The most important factor involved in the creation of an effective linear lesion with RF power is the contact between the ablating electrode(s) and the tissue. Based on this primary principle, a safe and effective catheter-based system to ablate AF must meet various design goals including:

- Ability of the catheter to adapt to the curvature of the atrium to establish and maintain good continuous contact with the atrial tissues while delivering energy or recording electrical activity.
- Ability to deliver RF energy to create transmural, continuous linear lesions with *minimal excessive tissue destruction*
- Minimization of the need for catheter manipulation, so as to reduce throm-

boembolic risk and radiation exposure
- Ease in placement of the catheter in specific anatomic orientations, with effective control over the degree and direction of deflection
- ˙RF power titration using closed-loop temperature control and local electrical activity monitoring to define effective lesion formation and prevent overheating and char formation
- Ability to retrieve discrete localized recordings from multiple electrodes to assess electrophysiological changes during energy application
- Simplicity of construction and operation to ensure safety

Having multiple ablation electrodes on a single shaft can minimize catheter manipulation and may reduce both thromboembolic risk and radiation exposure. A catheter should have a tip that is soft enough to avoid perforations and structural injuries. It should not become hooked on atrial tissues or valvular structures. Finally, during the current era of cost consciousness, with severe limits being placed on medical expenditures, the design of an ablation system must be simple to construct, and the overall cost of the procedure must be minimized.

Experimental AF Models

The inducibility of AF, via burst pacing or programmed electrical stimulation, is commonly used to gauge the effectiveness of pharmacological or ablative interventions. Induced AF is commonly categorized by its duration and is referred to as "sustained" or "nonsustained." Unfortunately, there is no standard for this classification. The word "sustained" has been used to describe AF runs of 30 or 45 seconds;[18,19] one,[20] 3,[21] 5,[22] 10,[23] or 30[24,25] minutes; and 24 hours[26] by different investigators.

A variety of experimental techniques have been used to create acute AF in animals including burst pacing, sterile pericarditis, vagal stimulation, and drugs such as acetylcholine and methacholine. Each of these can increase the inducibility of AF, while a combination of techniques can further increase the likelihood of long runs of sustained AF.

There are 2 methods commonly used to create chronic AF in animal models. The mitral regurgitation model was developed to investigate surgical interventions for AF.[27] Chronic rapid atrial pacing is currently the primary model used to test RF AF ablation technologies. Mitral regurgitation and chronic rapid atrial pacing have also been used concurrently to create chronic AF.[28]

Acute Models of AF

Sterile Pericarditis

The sterile pericarditis model was developed to simulate the AF that commonly occurs after cardiac surgery. This technique involves opening the chest to expose the pericardium, applying sterile talcum powder to the epicardial surface, suturing the chest closed, and allowing the animal to recover for at least 24 hours. After 24 hours, the inducibility of atrial arrhythmias, including AF (atrial fibrillation) and atrial flutter, via burst pacing is significantly increased.

In a study of sterile pericarditis in 12 dogs performed by Ortiz and associates,[29] sustained AF (>5 minutes) was inducible in 12 of 12 dogs on days 1 and 2, but only 9 of 12 on day 3. On day 4, only brief episodes of AF were inducible in 3 dogs and sustained AF in 3 more. The episodes of AF lasted longer on days 1 and 2 (36±4 minutes) than on day 3 (18±4 minutes). Mapping studies on the fourth day found 1–4 activation wavefronts in the right atrium (RA) and 1–3 in the left atrium (LA). Unstable reentrant circuits were found only in the RA free wall, and no ectopic foci were identified.

Kumagai and colleagues[22] used epicardial plaques and intracardiac catheters to record atrial activity in the sterile pericarditis model. Their mapping studies led to the conclusion that, in the sterile pericarditis model, unstable reentrant circuits generate multiple wavefronts that are continuously re-forming reentrant circuits of shorter cycle length, therefore maintaining AF. During sustained AF, they recorded an average of 6.4 total wavefronts in the atria (3.8 in the RA and 2.6 in the LA). Multiple (up to 4 per 100 ms window) unstable reentrant circuits of relatively short cycle length were present, but no fixed reentrant circuits were identified. In addition, they concluded that wavefronts from the atrial septum play an important role in reactivating tissue and reforming unstable reentrant circuits. At least one reentrant circuit was always present during AF, and it circulated for several rotations.

Vagal Stimulation

Rapid stimulation of the isolated vagal trunks increases the variability in atrial refractoriness in different regions of the atria,[30] which increases the inducibility of AF.[31] In a multisite mapping study of both atria, Wang and associates[32] concluded that vagally induced AF consists of several coexistent "apparent" reentry circuits of relatively small diameter.

Drugs

Methacholine and acetylcholine have been used to create experimental models of acute AF. They both increase cholinergic drive causing a shortening of the refractory period. This leads to a shortening of the wavelength of conduction by as much as 30–40% [33] and, therefore, increases susceptibility to AF.

Chronic Models of AF

Sterile pericarditis, vagal stimulation, and drug infusion are acute models that use normal hearts, in which the morphological changes associated with human AF are absent. Therefore, investigators have developed chronic models of AF that more closely resemble the presentation of chronic AF in humans.

Mitral Regurgitation

Cox and associates developed the mitral regurgitation (MR) model of chronic AF to simulate the AF seen in humans with mitral valve disorders.[27] To create the model, they threaded a special tool into the heart to cut the chordae tendonae of the mitral valve, therefore elevating the LA pressure to 10–12 mm Hg from a baseline level of 2–4 mm Hg. The resultant mitral regurgitation and increased LA pressure cause the left atrium to dilate over time and increase the inducibility of AF. In a study of 25 dogs, Cox and colleagues[27] found that after a minimum of 3 months' recovery, 3 of 25 dogs had spontaneous AF and 19 of 25 had inducible AF and/or atrial flutter. Epicardial mapping studies were performed on 15 of 19 dogs with AF and/or atrial flutter, and sustained AF was inducible via programmed electrical stimulation in 5 of the 15 dogs. Mapping studies of both atria led them to conclude that reentry is the principal mechanism of AF and that AF could be caused either by a single reentrant circuit or by multiple reentrant circuits. Increasing complexity and duration of AF were associated with increasing atrial enlargement. Animals with sustained AF had

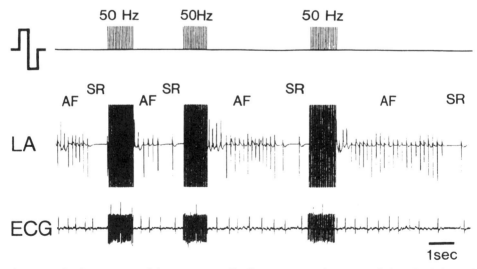

Figure 1. The functioning of the automatic fibrillation pacemaker. A single bipolar left atrial electrogram was sensed continuously for the occurrence of an isoelectrical segment of longer than 300 ms. As soon as a long isoelectrical segment was detected (sinus rhythm), the pacemaker automatically delivered a 1-second burst of stimuli (interval 20 ms, 4 × threshold) and AF was promptly reinduced. In this example the fibrillation pacemaker had just been turned on and only short episodes of self-terminating AF were produced. LA = left atrial bipolar electrogram; ECG = precordial surface ECG; AF = atrial fibrillation; SR = sinus rhythm. (From Wijffels, et al. Atrial fibrillation begets atrial fibrillation: a study in awake chronically instrumented goats. *Circulation* 1995; 92(7):1954–1968.)

a grossly enlarged LA, while those with nonsustained AF had a more modest atrial enlargement.

Chronic Burst Pacing

In a study of chronically instrumented goats, Wijffels and colleagues[26] used a pacing system to maintain chronic AF in 11 goats via short burst pacing. A computer was used to monitor electrical activity recorded from surgically implanted electrodes. After recording any conversion to sinus rhythm, a 1-second burst was applied to convert the heart back to AF (Figure 1). The system kept track of the duration of AF between sinus conversions. The duration of AF between sinus conversions increased over time (Figure 2). Initially, the hearts converted within a few seconds, but the AF episodes lasted about 20 seconds after 24 hours. After 7.1 ± 4.8 days, 10 of 11 goats were in sustained AF, lasting more than 24 hours. After 2 weeks, the electrograms had a lower amplitude and a higher degree of fragmentation with fewer steep deflections (Figure 3). The authors concluded that artificial maintenance of AF leads to a marked shortening of atrial effective refractory period (Figures 4 and 5); a reversion of physiological rate adaptation; and an increase in the rate, inducibility, and stability of AF. In 5 dogs, the burst pacing system was

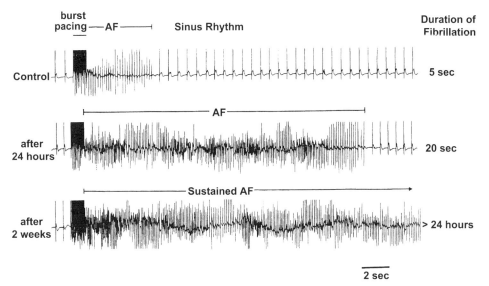

Figure 2. Prolongation of the duration of episodes of electrically induced AF after maintaining AF for 24 hours and 2 weeks, respectively. The 3 tracings show a single atrial electrogram recorded from the same goat during induction of AF by a 1-second burst (50 Hz, 4 × threshold). In the upper tracing the goat has been in sinus rhythm continuously and AF self-terminated within 5 seconds. The second tracing was recorded after the goat had been connected to the fibrillation pacemaker for 24 hours showing a clear prolongation of the duration of AF to 20 seconds. The third tracing was recorded after 2 weeks of electrically maintained AF. After induction of AF, this episode became sustained and did not terminate. AF = atrial fibrillation. (From Wijffels, et al. Atrial fibrillation begets atrial fibrillation: a study in awake chronically instrumented goats. *Circulation* 1995; 92(7):1954–1968.)

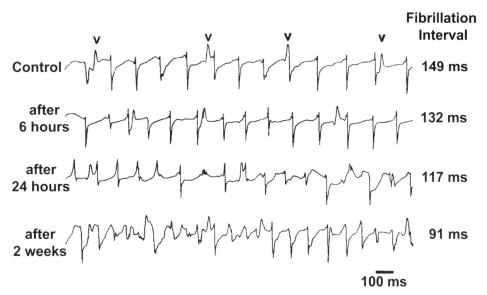

Figure 3. Unipolar atrial electrograms recorded from the left atrial appendage during different stages of AF. At the right-hand side of the tracings, the corresponding median fibrillation intervals, as measured from these short samples of AF, are plotted. As can be seen from the electrograms and the calculated median fibrillation intervals, the atrial rate clearly increased during the initial phase of AF. Also, the morphology of the atrial electrograms changed in the course of AF. Whereas during recent onset fibrillation the electrograms mostly showed single deflections of high amplitude separated by an isoelectric segment (upper tracing), after 2 weeks of AF the electrograms were of lower amplitude and showed a higher degree of fragmentation (lower tracing). V = ventricular complex. (From Wijffels, et al. Atrial fibrillation begets atrial fibrillation: a study in awake chronically instrumented goats. *Circulation* 1995; 92(7):1954–1968.)

turned off after developing sustained AF during 2–4 weeks of AF maintenance. After 24 hours of sinus rhythm, only short episodes of AF could be induced via burst pacing, lasting 6±4 seconds. After 1 week of sinus rhythm, the atrial effective refractory period and the inducibility of AF returned to baseline levels. These results suggest that sustained rapid atrial rates alter atrial electrophysiological function and decrease the ability to maintain an organized rhythm. Ausma and associates described the structural changes to atrial myocardium in this same model. After maintaining chronic AF in 13 goats for 9–31 weeks, atrial myocytes were observed to be depleted of contractile material and showed accumulation of glycogen (Figure 6). Though the myocytes were enlarged, myolysis was present at the perinuclear area and often extended toward the plasma membrane. Longitudinal sections (Figure 7) revealed altered profiles of sarcoplasmic reticulum and abnormally shaped mitochondria.

Single Lead Rapid Atrial Pacing

Rapidly pacing the RA over an extended period can increase the inducibility of AF and cause a decrease in atrial effective refractory period. In

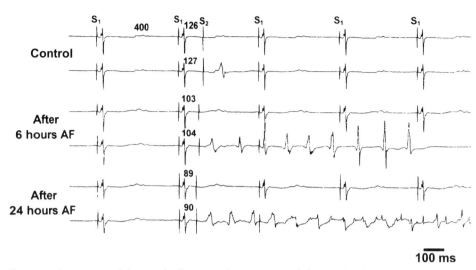

Figure 4. Shortening of the atrial effective refractory period during the first 24 hours of electrically maintained AF. The atrial effective refractory period (AERP) was determined by an interpolated stimulus during pacing at a fixed interval of 400 ms. While during control (upper 2 tracings) a premature stimulus given after 126 ms still fell in the refractory period, a stimulus with a coupling interval of 127 ms evoked a premature atrial response. After 6 hours of AF (middle tracings) the AERP already had decreased to 104 ms. After 24 hours of AF (lower tracings) the AERP had become as short as 90 ms. While during control no arrhythmias were induced by a single premature stimulus, after 6 and 24 hours of AF short runs of AF were induced. S_1 = basic stimulus; S_2 = extra stimulus. (From Wijffels, et al. Atrial fibrillation begets atrial fibrillation: a study in awake chronically instrumented goats. *Circulation* 1995; 92(7):1954–1968.)

some cases, AF is chronically present when the rapid pacing is terminated. In a patient with atrial tachycardia and rapid ventricular response resistant to pharmacological therapy, Moriera and colleagues[33] used rapid pacing to cause sustained AF. A pacemaker paced the patient's right atrium at 375 beats per minute for 11 months, after which stable AF remained for 72 months until the patient's death. Morillo and associates[34] paced the right atrial appendage (RAA) at 400 beats per minute for 6 weeks in 22 dogs. Immediately after the cessation of pacing, 18% (4/22) of the dogs were spontaneously in AF. Sustained AF (> 15 minutes) was inducible in 82% (18/22) of the dogs via extrastimulus and burst-pacing techniques. The remaining 4 dogs (9%) had only nonsustained AF induced. The RA effective refractory period, measured at cycle lengths of 400 and 300 milliseconds, was significantly shortened after pacing from 150±8 to 127±10 milliseconds and from 147±11 to 123±12 milliseconds, respectively. The AF cycle length was measured at the 10 sites shown in Figure 8. The graph in Figure 9 shows that the AF cycle length was increased at sites with a higher mean effective refractory period. The decrease in refractory period was highly predictive of AF inducibility (90%). Electron microscopic observation (Figure 10) revealed changes in atrial architecture including fiber disarray and early hypertrophy, which may con-

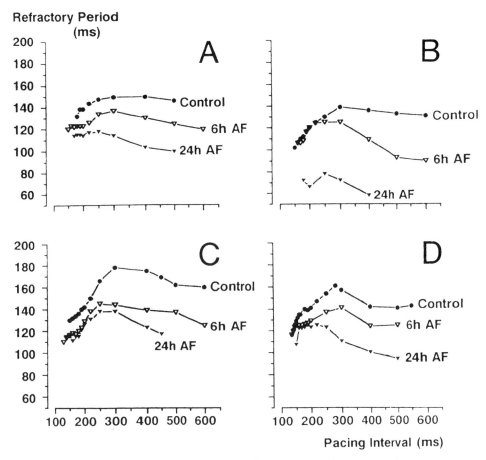

Figure 5. Refractory period versus pacing interval (3 time periods, 4 goats). These are 4 examples of changes in atrial refractoriness in the course of the first 24 hours of fibrillation. In all goats, the refractory period shortened markedly at all pacing intervals. In general the amount of shortening was higher at slow heart rates. As a result, the normal physiological rate adaptation of the refractory period was either reversed (panels A and B) or attenuated (panel D). AF = atrial fibrillation. (From Wijffels, et al. Atrial fibrillation begets atrial fibrillation: a study in awake chronically instrumented goats. *Circulation* 1995; 92(7):1954–1968.)

tribute to the maintenance of AF. Two-dimensional echocardiographic evaluation of atrial areas showed that a 40% increase in atrial area was strongly correlated with the ability to induce sustained AF. Studies by Goette[35] and Elvan[36] and their colleagues documented significant decreases in atrial effective refractory period after rapid pacing for 7 hours and 2–6 weeks, respectively (Figure 11 and Figure 12). Both experiments noted a reversal toward baseline effective refractory period values after conversion to sinus rhythm. Figure 13 from Elvan's study shows that with rapid atrial pacing, the duration of AF increased over time. The relationship between the duration of AF and the effective refractory period is shown in Figure 14. Longer runs of AF

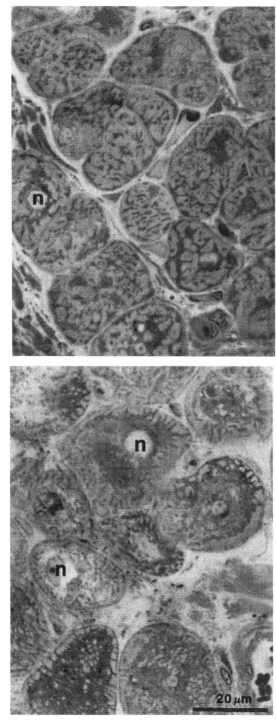

Figure 6. Light microscopy of sections 2 μm thick from goat atrial myocardium. Panel 1a: Atrial myocardium sections from goat in sinus rhythm with normally structured cardiomyocytes. PAS staining is almost absent in these cardiomyocytes. Sarcomeres stained with toluidine blue are present throughout cytoplasm of cardiomyocytes. Panel 1b: Section from goat in chronic AF showing severe myolysis. Central part of myocytes is free of sarcomeres and contains abundant glycogen (PAS-positive staining). Magnification × 500. n = nucleus. (From Ausma J, et al. Structural changes of atrial myocardium due to sustained AF in the goat. *Circulation* 1997;96(9):3157–3163.)

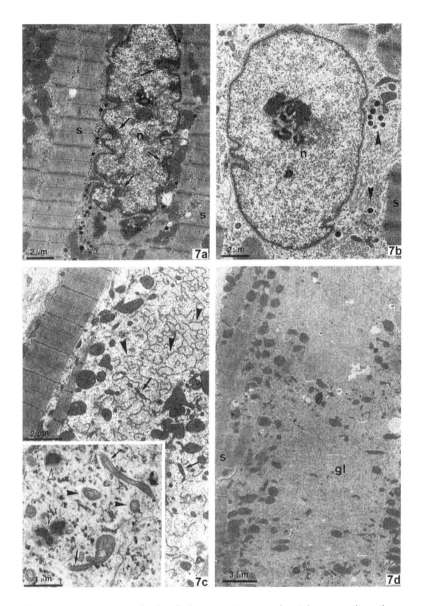

Figure 7. Electron microscopy of subcellular organization of atrial myocardium from goats in sinus rhythm (panel 3a) and after prolonged AF (panels 3b through 3d). Panel 3a: Detail of normal atrial cardiomyocyte from control animal showing regularly structured sarcomeres (s) surrounding nucleus (n) in which heterochromatin (arrows) is clustered near nuclear membrane. Magnification × 3125. Panel 3b: Detail of nuclear area from chronically fibrillating myocardium showing dispersion of heterochromatin throughout nucleus. In vicinity of nucleus, sarcomeres are dissolved and glycogen is present. Some remnants of sarcomeres can still be seen. Atrial granules (arrowheads) are found in vicinity of nucleus. Magnification × 3125.
Panel 3c: Longitudinal section of part of atrial cardiomyocyte from chronically fibrillating atrial myocardium showing altered profiles of sarcoplasmic reticulum membranes (arrowheads) and abnormally shaped mitochondria (arrows). Magnification × 4160. Inset shows slender elongated mitochondria with longitudinally oriented cristae (arrows), which appear as small, doughnut-shaped structures on cross section (arrowheads). Clumps of Z-band material (open arrowheads) represent remnants of sarcomeres. Magnification × 8050. Panel 3d: Severely affected myolytic atrial cardiomyocyte from chronically fibrillating atrial myocardium with huge amounts of glycogen (gl) present in myolytic area. Only a rim of sarcomeres is still present at border of cell. Magnification × 2425. (From Ausma J, et al. Structural changes of atrial myocardium due to sustained atrial fibrillation in the goat. *Circulation* 1997;96(9):3157–3163.)

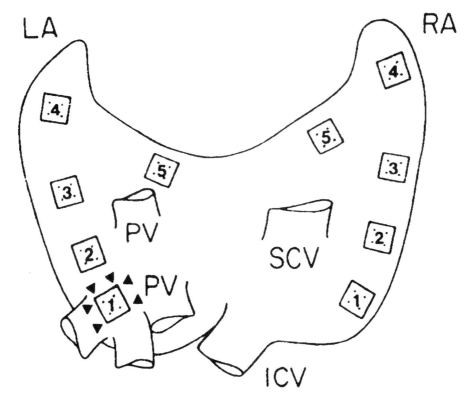

Figure 8. Location of atrial epicardial electrodes and cryoablation target. This posterior view depicts the location and distribution of the atrial epicardial electrodes. Four quadripolar plaque electrodes (diameter, 1.5 mm; interelectrode distance, 10 mm) were sutured to the right atrial (RA) and left atrial (LA) walls from the posterior wall toward the atrial appendages (electrodes 1 through 4). Two quadripolar plaque electrodes were also sutured to the right and left Bachman bundles. Cryoablation was directed to the area with the shortest AF cycle length, which was consistently localized to the left inferoposterior atrium (arrowheads). ICV = inferior caval vein, PV = pulmonary veins, and SCV = superior caval vein. (From Morillo CA, et al. Chronic rapid atrial pacing. *Circulation* 1995;91(5):1588–1595.)

were induced when the effective refractory period was reduced. Elvan and associates also noted an increase in corrected sinus node recovery time and P wave duration, suggesting that chronic rapid atrial pacing may adversely affect sinus node function.

Avitall and associates[37] collected tissues from specific anatomic areas in patients with mitral valve disease who were undergoing the Maze procedure. Similar specimens were obtained from dogs that had developed chronic AF due to rapid atrial pacing. Similar histopathologic observations included the presence of fat infiltration and fibroelastosis. The changes were most prominent in the LA appendages and near the pulmonary veins, suggesting that these areas might be critical targets in attempting to ablate AF.

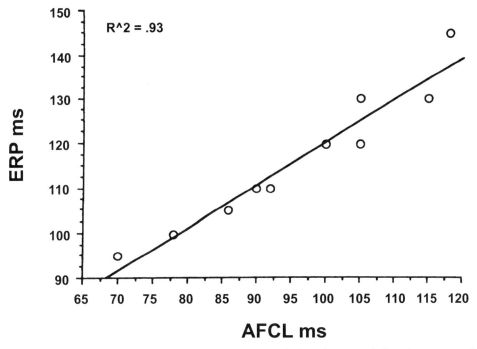

Figure 9. Atrial effective refractory period versus AF cycle length. AF cycle length (AFCL) and atrial effective refractory period (ERP) were determined by the extrastimulus technique at a basic cycle length of 400 ms at 10 epicardial sites in eight dogs with sustained AF. A high correlation coefficient (R^2 =0.93) was achieved between AFCL and ERP. (From Morillo CA, et al. Chronic rapid atrial pacing. *Circulation* 1995;91(5):1588–1595.)

Single Lead Rapid Atrial Pacing with Mitral Regurgitation

Haines and colleagues[28] used a combination of rapid atrial pacing and mitral regurgitation in an attempt to create AF in 13 dogs. A wire-hook catheter was inserted retrogradely into the LV and used to cut chordae tendonae until the mean wedge pressure increased 4–6 mm Hg. Single lead rapid atrial pacing (SLRAP) was then employed for more than 8 weeks. Five of the 13 dogs died during this period due to tamponade (n=3), severe MR (n=1), and pacing lead dislodgment (n=2). Sustained AF was induced in 75% (6/8) of the remaining dogs. A repeat hook-wire catheter procedure yielded sustained AF after 8 additional weeks of pacing in one of the 2 dogs in which the initial procedure failed.

Dual Lead Rapid Atrial Pacing

Kotov and colleagues[38] developed a rapid pacing model of AF that uses dual-site RA pacing to increase the yield of spontaneous AF. In 22 mongrel dogs

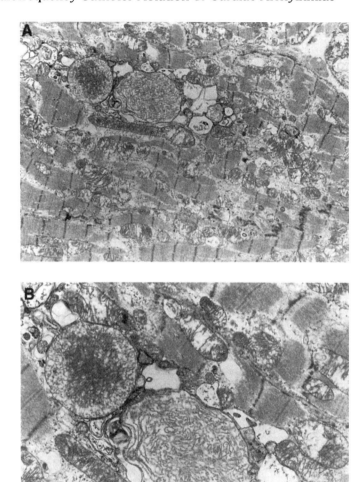

Figure 10. Electron microscopy of right atrial tissue from dog after 6 weeks of rapid atrial pacing. Panel A: Low-power electron microscopy (× 900) of right atrial tissue showing enlarged and disarrayed fibers and giant mitochondria. Moderate dilation of the rough endoplasmic reticulum is also shown. Panel B: High-power electron microscopy (× 2100) of the same sample, showing giant mitochondria with disintegrated crystae and an anarchic pattern. These findings are consistent with hypertrophy and perturbation of metabolic activity. (From Morillo CA, et al. Chronic rapid atrial pacing. *Circulation* 1995;91(5):1588–1595.)

(27–32 kg), pacemakers (SX-2FAST, Pacesetter, Los Angeles, CA) were implanted. In 5 dogs a single lead was fixed in the RAA, and in 17 dogs 2 leads were placed, one in the RAA and another in the low RA. In both groups, the RAA was paced at 400 beats per minute. In the second group, an extra stimulus was delivered to the low RA after every fourth stimulus of the RAA. Surface and endocardial electrograms were examined weekly while pacing and with the pacemaker off. Echocardiographic assessment of cardiac chamber size and

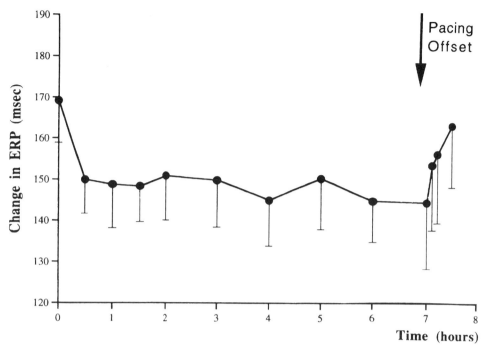

Figure 11. Change in effective refractory period versus time. The effects of continuous rapid atrial pacing on atrial effective refractory period (ERP) in 5 dogs receiving 7 hours of continuous rapid atrial pacing who were pretreated with atropine and propanolol. The pattern of electrical remodeling appears to be bimodal, with an initial rapid drop followed by a more gradual decline during hours 1 through 7. The ERP recovered quickly after cessation of pacing, with a return to within 97% of baseline after 30 minutes. (From Goette A, et al. Electrical remodeling in atrial fibrillation. *Circulation* 1996;94(11):2968–2974.)

function was performed before and after completion of the pacing protocol. Atrial tissues were then obtained for histological evaluation.

Only 2 of the 5 single-site pacing dogs (40%) developed AF after pacing for 151 ± 124 days. All 17 of the dual-site pacing dogs (100%) developed spontaneous AF within 41 ± 19 days ($P<0.05$ versus single-site pacing). In 11 of these dogs, pacing was continued for 58 ± 21 days after the onset of AF. The pacemaker was then turned off for 76 ± 40 days during which the AF persisted. Echocardiography showed that the development of AF correlated with severe atrial enlargement and ventricular dysfunction. RA size increased from 20 ± 2 to 27 ± 5 mm, LA size increased from 32 ± 3 to 43 ± 9 mm, and LVEF decreased from $50\pm10\%$ to $24\pm7\%$. Development of AF was associated with severe dilatation of both atria and with atrial tissue changes such as fat infiltration, fibrosis, fibroelastosis, and myocardial disarray. Dual-site pacing causes severe atrial myopathy more rapidly and with a higher yield of spontaneous sustained AF than single-site pacing.

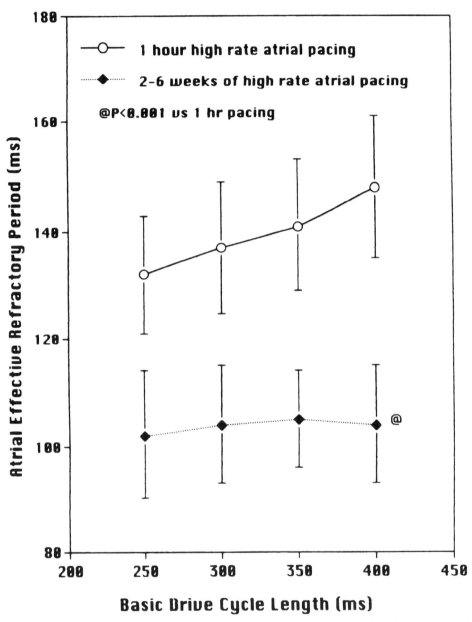

Figure 12. Atrial effective refractory period versus basic drive cycle length. After 2 to 6 weeks of rapid atrial pacing, atrial ERP was markedly shortened and became independent of basic drive cycle length duration. (From Elvan, et al. Pacing-induced chronic atrial fibrillation impairs sinus node function in dogs. *Circulation* 1996;94(11):2953–2960.)

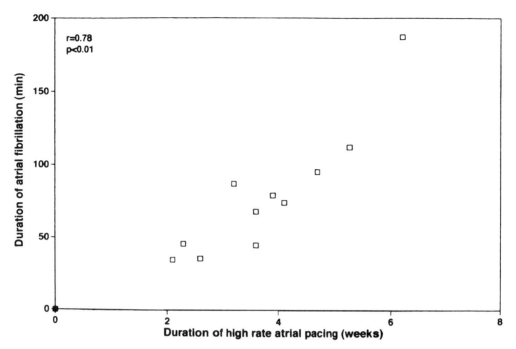

Figure 13. Duration of AF versus duration of rapid atrial pacing. Solid square denotes duration of AF in all dogs after 1 hour of rapid atrial pacing. Open squares denote duration of AF for each animal obtained at second EPS after 2 to 6 weeks of AF. The duration of AF increased with the duration of rapid atrial pacing. (From Elvan, et al. Pacing-induced chronic atrial fibrillation impairs sinus node function in dogs. *Circulation* 1996;94(11):2953–2960.)

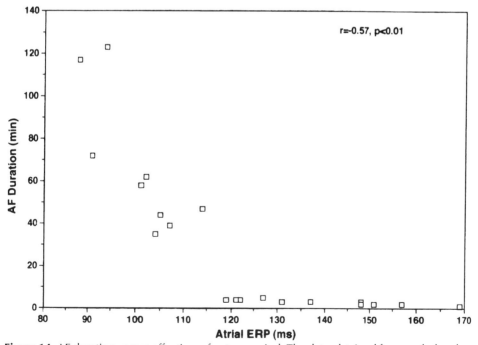

Figure 14. AF duration versus effective refractory period. The data obtained from each dog during 2 electrophysiological studies shows that atrial ERP shortening (ERP <120 ms) was associated with significantly longer episodes of AF. (From Elvan, et al. Pacing-induced chronic atrial fibrillation impairs sinus node function in dogs. *Circulation* 1996;94(11):2953–2960.)

Experimental Ablation of AF in Animals

Acute models often require less intervention than chronic models to reverse proarrhythmic effects.

Burst Pacing

A single lesion at the intra-atrial septum can eliminate burst pacing induced AF in normal hearts. Tondo and associates[18] used burst pacing (cycle length = 100 milliseconds) in the high RA to induce episodes of sustained AF (> 30 seconds) in 11 dogs. After creation of a single lesion across the midatrial septum, AF was no longer inducible in 10/11 dogs. In the remaining dog, the duration of induced AF was significantly reduced, from 54 seconds to 8 seconds.

Sterile Pericarditis

Right atrial lesions alone can ablate AF in the sterile pericarditis model. In 2 studies, Avitall and colleagues[39,40] were able to ablate sustained AF in the sterile pericarditis model by creating long linear radiofrequency lesions. Epicardial linear lesions were created in the RA and LA and converted sustained AF to sustained atrial flutter in 4 of 6 dogs.[40] After creating LA lesions from the pulmonary veins to the mitral valve, sustained AF was still inducible. Subsequent generation of RA lesions produced conversions from AF. In a second study,[39] a catheter with 20 4-mm electrodes was used to create endocardial lesions in only the RA. These RA lesions were made in locations similar to those used in the epicardial study: from the SVC along the posterolateral RA to the IVC and then from the SVC along the anterior RA to the IVC. Prior to creating the lesions, sustained AF (> 3 minutes) was inducible in 6 of 7 dogs. Following ablation, AF could not be induced in any of the dogs during 10 attempts of burst pacing. Thus, ablation of the RA is critical in attempting to ablate AF in the sterile pericarditis model.

Several investigations have concluded that AF in the sterile pericarditis model can be ablated by creating single lesions in the anterior RA septum at Bachmann's bundle. Kumagai and colleagues[22] successfully ablated sustained AF in the sterile pericarditis model via Bachmann's bundle ablation in 3 dogs. Nakagawa and associates[25] used a catheter with a 5 mm irrigated tip to ablate Bachmann's bundle in 9 closed-chest dog studies. Before ablation, sustained AF (57±50 minutes) was inducible in all 9 dogs. After ablation, only AF of less than 10 seconds in duration could be induced in 8 of 9 dogs. After 11 lesions in the remaining dog, AF lasting 10 minutes was still inducible.

Vagal Stimulation

Chiou and colleagues[41] evaluated AF inducibility during vagal stimulation before and after they used a 4 mm electrode to create epicardial lesions in the

RA and LA. In doing so, they were able to describe the anatomy of the vagal innervation of the atria. According to their study, most efferent vagal fibers to the atria travel through a fat pad between the medial SVC and aortic root (SVC-Ao fat pad). They then project to both atria via a fat pad at the IVC-LA junction (IVC-LA) or a right pulmonary vein-atrial junction (RPV) fat pad. A few fibers bypass the SVC-Ao pad and extend directly through the IVC-LA and RPV fat pads. Figure 15 shows the anatomic locations of these 3 fat pads. After vagal denervation of the RA or both atria via ablation of these fat pads (Figure 16), sustained AF (> 30 minutes) was no longer inducible in 42 dogs.

Avitall and associates[21] created 2 linear lesions in the RA to ablate AF induced during stimulation of the right and left vagal trunks. Before any lesions were created, the threshold voltage of vagal stimulation needed to induce spontaneous AF was measured for the right and left vagal trunks (right = 6±3 volts, left = 5±2 volts). The voltages were set at 75% threshold and AF lasting 28±17 seconds could be induced via single decremental premature atrial beats. No significant change in AF inducibility was noted after creating a lesion from the SVC to the IVC. After generating a second lesion from the SVC to the tricuspid ring (TR), AF lasting only 4±2 seconds could be induced with higher voltage vagal stimulation (over 10 volts).

In attempting to ablate AF induced during vagal stimulation, Elvan and colleagues[24] created epicardial lesions in 5 locations: around the RAA, around the left atrial appendage (LAA), from the SVC to the IVC laterally, from the SVC medially to the RAA, and in the coronary sinus (Figure 17). In 5 dogs, sustained AF (> 30 minutes) was inducible via burst pacing or multiple premature atrial stimuli at baseline with low-level vagal stimulation (right = 2 volts, 8 Hz; left = 3 volts, 8 Hz). After creating the 5 lesions, the duration of induced AF decreased to 5.6±4.1 minutes during high-level vagal stimulation (right = 5 volts, 20 Hz; left = 8 volts, 20 Hz) and burst pacing. The shortening of effective refractory period induced via high or low level vagal stimulation was significantly diminished after ablation as shown in panels A and B of Figure 18.

Avitall and associates[42] developed a thoracoscopic epicardial technique to ablate AF induced during vagal stimulation. Thoracoscopic ports were placed in the fourth and fifth left intercostal spaces, the pericardium was opened along the phrenic nerve, and a radiofrequency probe was placed on the epicardial. Four lesions were created: encircling the RAA, encircling the LAA, from the SVC to the IVC laterally, and from the SVC across the medial RAA to the tricuspid ring. At baseline, sustained AF (> 3 minutes) was recorded in each of the 4 dogs. After generation of the 4 lesions, sustained AF was no longer inducible.

Drugs

The direct application of topical acetylcholine and the infusion of methacholine have been used to evaluate the efficacy of linear lesions in reducing AF inducibility. Seifert and colleagues[19] used a topical 4% acetylcholine solution applied for 1–3 minutes to evaluate AF inducibility via burst pacing before and

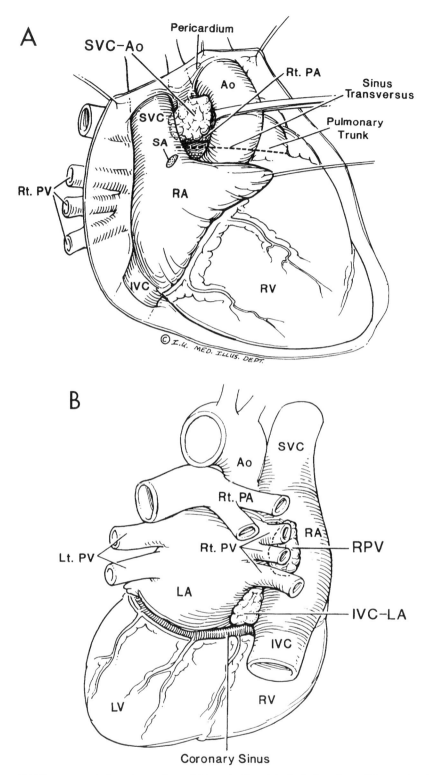

Figure 15. The anatomic locations of vagal fat pads. Panel A: Anterior view of the canine heart showing the SVC-Ao fat pad located between the medial SVC and aortic root superior to the right pulmonary artery. This fat pad did not include the fat tissue surrounding the aortic root. Panel B: Posterior view of the canine heart showing 2 fat pads: the IVC-LA, located at the IVC-inferior LA junction, and the RPV, located at the RPV-atrial junction. SA = sinoatrial node; Rt and Lt = right and left; PA = pulmonary artery; PV = pulmonary vein; RV = right ventricle; and LV = left ventricle. (From Chiou CW. Efferent vagal innervation of the canine atria and sinus and atrioventricular nodes: the third fat pad. *Circulation* 1997; 95(11):2573–2584.)

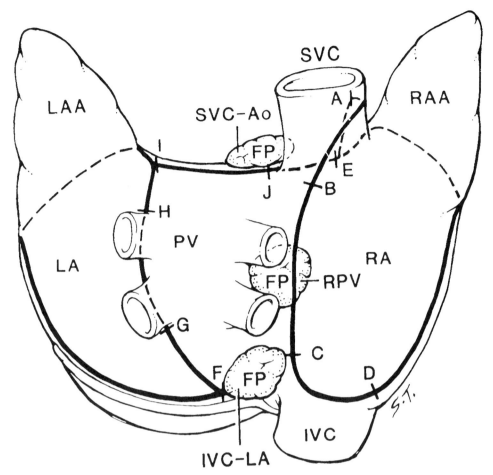

Figure 16. Locations of epicardial radiofequency lesions. Epicardial lesions were created in the RA connecting locations: E-A-B-C-D-E. Another set of lesions encircled the LA between F-G-H-I-J and from F to I. FP = fat pad; PV = pulmonary vein; A = anteriomedial SVC; B = lateral SVC at the superior RPV; C = lateral IVC at the inferior RPV; D = IVC-AV groove junction; E = medial SVC-sinus transversus junction; F = IVC-LA junction (IVC-LA fat pad was not included); G = at the inferior left pulmonary vein; H = at the superior left pulmonary vein; I = sinus transversus at the pulmonary trunk; and J = sinus transversus at aorta. (From Chiou CW. Efferent vagal innervation of the canine atria and sinus and atrioventricular nodes: the third fat pad. *Circulation* 1997;94(11):2573–2584.)

after using a custom-designed epicardial ablation plaque to create RF lesions in a pattern mimicking the Maze procedure. AF lasting from 7.3 to 20.1 minutes was observed in 5 pigs before ablation. After ablation, AF lasting no longer than 45 seconds could be induced in 4 of the 5 pigs. The remaining pig had a single episode lasting 4.5 minutes.

Elvan and associates[24] infused variable doses of methacholine to test the efficacy of epicardial lesion creation in reducing AF inducibility immediately after ablation (5 acute dogs) and 7–21 days postablation (4 chronic dogs). Epicardial lesions were created around the RAA, around the LAA, from the SVC to the IVC laterally, from the SVC medially to the RAA, and in the coronary sinus (see Fig-

Posterior View of the Atria

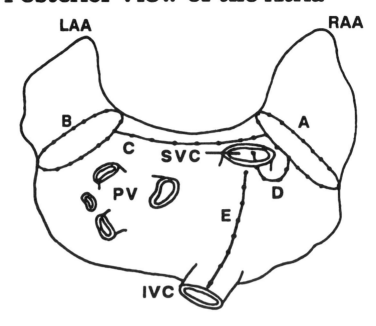

Superior View (Atria removed)

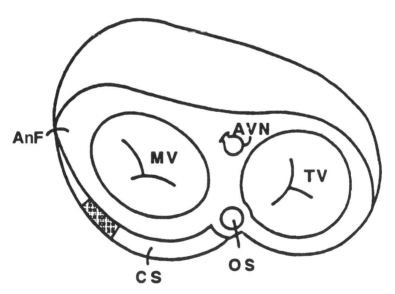

Figure 17. Locations of epicardial atrial ablations. The upper diagram shows localization of epicardial atrial RF catheter ablations. *A* shows a radiofrequency-induced lesion around the right atrial appendage (RAA); *B,* a lesion around the left atrial appendage (LAA); *C,* a lesion in the transverse sinus; *D,* a lesion extending from the medial superior vena cava (SVC) to lesion A; and *E,* a lesion extending from the lateral SVC to the lateral inferior vena cava (IVC). The lower diagram shows the endovascular ablation site in the coronary sinus (hatched area). PV = pulmonary veins; OS = ostium of the coronary sinus; AVN = AV node; TV = tricuspid valve; MV = mitral valve; and AnF = annular fibrosis. (From Elvan, et al. Radiofrequency catheter ablation of the atria reduces inducibility and duration of atrial fibrillation in dogs. *Circulation* 1995;91(8):2235–2244.)

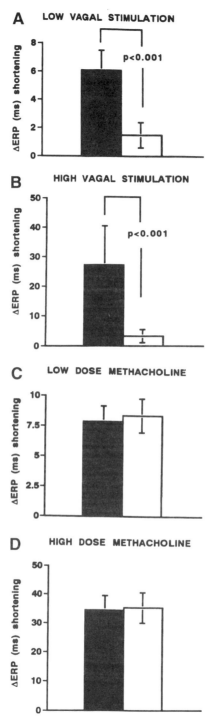

Figure 18. Effective refractory period shortening, before and after ablation. The bar graphs show the effects of radiofrequency catheter ablation (RFCA) on changes in atrial effective refractory period (ΔERP = mean ± standard deviation) induced by low-level (A) and high-level (B) cervical vagal stimulation and alterations in atrial ERPs induced by a low dose (C) and a high dose (D) of methacholine. Changes in ERP were measured at 5 left and right atrial sites before and after RFCA. Solid bar = before ablation; open bar = after ablation. (From Elvan, et al. Radiofrequency catheter ablation of the atria reduces inducibility and duration of atrial fibrillation in dogs. *Circulation* 1995;91(8):2235–2244.)

ure 17). Figure 19 shows the duration of AF induced in each of these sets of dogs before ablation, acutely postablation and chronically after ablation. Increasingly higher methacholine doses were required to generate AF postablation. Ablation had a more prominent effect on AF inducibility in the chronic set of dogs. The ability of low or high level vagal stimulation to shorten effective refractory period was not changed after ablation (See panels C and D in Figure 18).

In their study defining the vagal innervation of the atria, Chiou and colleagues[41] determined that sustained AF remained inducible after RF vagal denervation when either low doses (1.5 μg/kg/min) or high doses (3.6 μg/kg/min) of methacholine were infused. In 10 dogs, 3 RF lesions were created epicardially to ablate the SVC-Ao, the IVC-LA, and the RPV fat pads. Though the lesions eliminated the ability to induce AF via burst pacing during vagal stimulation, sustained AF was still inducible during methacholine infusion.

Mitral Regurgitation

Cox and associates used the mitral regurgitation model of AF to develop the surgical Maze procedure. Several versions of the technique have been used.

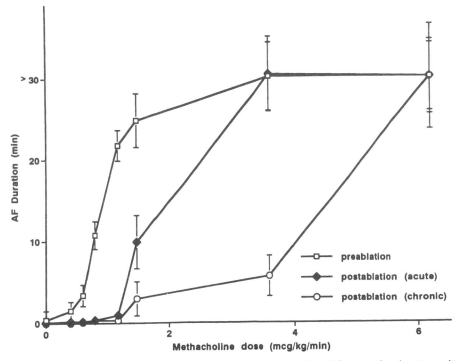

Figure 19. AF duration versus methacholine dose before and after ablation. The duration of induced AF during infusion of graded concentrations of methacholine was obtained in 5 dogs in an acute group and a chronic group before and after ablation. After ablation, larger doses of methacholine were required to induce runs of AF lasting >30 minutes. (From Elvan, et al. Radiofrequency catheter ablation of the atria reduces inducibility and duration of atrial fibrillation in dogs. *Circulation* 1995;91(8):2235–2244.)

They all involve the placement of multiple linear incisions in a very specific pattern that modifies conduction but does not result in electrical isolation of atrial tissues (Figure 20). Both the LA and RA appendages are removed, and the insertion site of the pulmonary veins into the LA is isolated. All the incisions are sutured closed, thus creating a maze-like pattern. This procedure divides atrial tissues into small separate territories that are smaller than the critical area that will support sustained AF. Various versions of the technique have been used to successfully cure AF in humans.[12] The long-term results have been encouraging, with a low risk of severe complications in selected patients. The atria appear to function well, with SA and AV nodal function preserved in most instances and low risk for embolization after the postoperative course. In general, these surgical procedures are technically very demanding and involve considerable intra- and perioperative morbidity. The development of minimally invasive transcatheter AF ablation technology is needed because many patients are not candidates for the Maze procedure due to the presence of contraindications to extensive surgery.

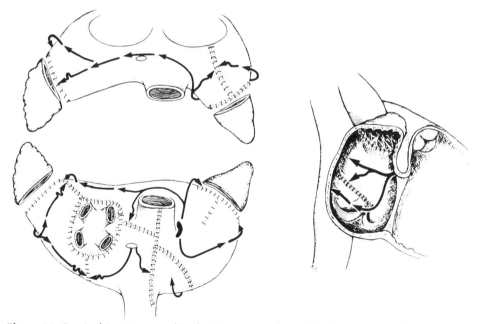

Figure 20. Surgical incisions used in the Maze procedure. This is a depiction of the locations of the incisions in the third version of Cox's Maze procedure. The pulmonary veins are totally isolated and both atrial appendages are removed. The remaining incisions are made to direct the atrial conduction so that significant atrial contraction is achieved while preventing the generation of AF. (From Cox JL. Evolving applications of the Maze procedure for atrial fibrillation. *Ann Thorac Surg* 1993:55; 578–580.)

Rapid Atrial Pacing

Epicardial Cryoablation

Morillo and associates[34] used cryotechnology to ablate sustained AF (> 15 minutes) after applying rapid RA pacing at 400 beats per minute for 6 weeks. Mapping of the atria revealed a region in the posterior left atrium with a consistently shorter AF cycle length. Figure 8 shows the locations of the mapping electrodes used and identifies the area where cryoablation was performed. In 9 of 11 dogs, AF was no longer inducible via burst-pacing or extrastimulus after cryoablation of this area. Nonsustained atrial flutter was induced in 7 of these 9 dogs postablation.

Epicardial RF Ablation

Elvan and associates[43] created atrial lesions in chronically paced dogs using a 6-pole catheter placed on the RA and LA epicardium as shown in Figure 21. RA lesions were created from the SVC to the IVC laterally, from the SVC to the RAA medially, around the RAA, and in the coronary sinus. After 10–14 weeks of chronic rapid atrial pacing, 9 out of 9 dogs had spontaneous sustained AF (> 24 hours) verified by Holter recordings. In 5 dogs, after creating right-sided lesions, conversion to sinus rhythm was achieved, and sustained AF (> 15 minutes) could not be induced via premature or burst pacing. However, AF lasting 9.3 ± 3.5 minutes could be induced. In the 4 remaining dogs, no conversion was noted after RA lesion generation. After a one-week recovery period, left-sided lesions were created around the LAA and in the coronary sinus. After an additional one-week recovery period, sustained AF (>15 minutes) was not inducible. In 2 dogs, atrial flutter was inducible but could be converted via burst pacing.

Adjustable Loop Catheter with 24 4-mm Ring Electrodes

Avitall and associates have used an adjustable loop catheter with 24 4-mm ring electrodes[44-48] to ablate chronic AF induced by dual-lead chronic rapid atrial pacing. This catheter system creates adjustable loops of various sizes (Figure 22). As the loop is expanded, the body of the catheter adapts to the curvature of the atrium forcing the electrodes to be in firm contact with the endocardium.

We have used this catheter to ablate chronic AF in 9 dogs. Rapid pacemakers were implanted and used to pace the RAA at 400 beats per minute and the RA free wall at 130 beats per minute. After development of chronic AF the pacemakers were turned off. Spontaneous chronic AF was still present after 24 hours.

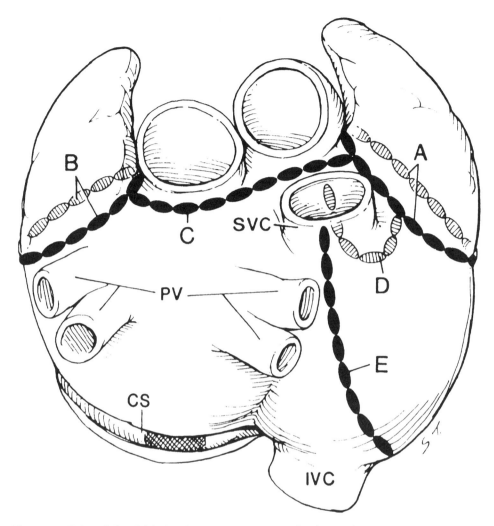

Figure 21. Epicardial atrial lesion locations: A = around right atrial appendage; B = around left atrial appendage; C = in transverse sinus; D = extending from medial SVC to lesion A; E = extending from lateral SVC to lateral IVC. The hatched area shows the endovascular ablation site in coronary sinus. IVC = inferior vena cava; SVC = superior vena cava; PV = pulmonary veins; CS = coronary sinus. (From Elvan, et al. Radiofrequency catheter ablation of the atria reduces inducibility and duration of atrial fibrillation in dogs. *Circulation* 1995;91(8):2235–2244.)

Various combinations of the following linear lesions were generated in a variety of sequences:

- *RA Loop:* A right atrial circular lesion extending from the anterior septal tricuspid valve to the RA appendage to the SVC and circling back to the IVC.
- *RAI:* A right atrial isthmus lesion where the catheter is looped into the RV with the ablation electrodes across the tricuspid valve ring extending into the IVC.

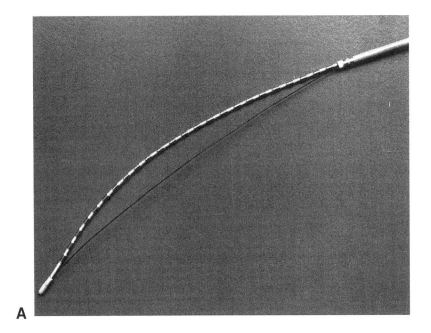

A

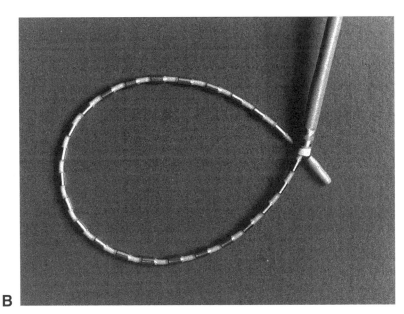

B

- *LAH:* A circular horizontal lesion placed under the pulmonary veins in the mid left atrium, above the mitral valve (as indicated by a coronary sinus catheter and the atrial and ventricular electrograms recorded from each of the electrodes on the 24-pole catheter).
- *LAV1:* A vertical lesion extending from the mitral valve annulus medial of the pulmonary veins.
- *LAV2:* A vertical linear lesion extending from the mitral valve to the LA appendage, lateral of the pulmonary veins.

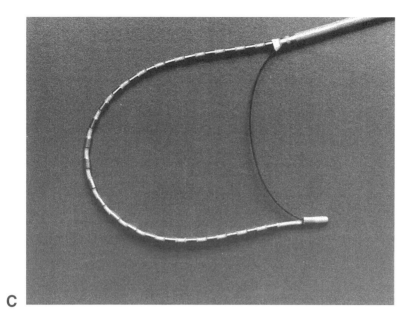

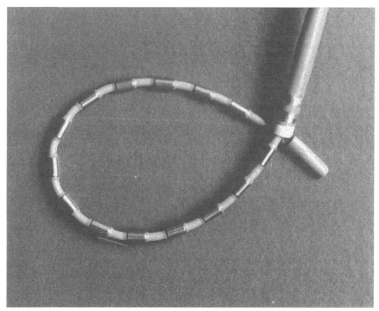

Figure 22. The loop catheter for AF ablation. Panel A shows the catheter extended; panel B shows it deflected to form a semicircular loop; in panel C it forms a large circular loop; and in panel D it forms a small circular loop.

Figure 23 depicts representative fluoroscopic images of the catheter positions for each of these lesions.

AF was converted to atrial flutter in 8 of 9 dogs, and sinus rhythm was achieved in 5 of these 8 dogs. Sinus rhythm occurred spontaneously in 1 dog and after overdrive burst pacing in 4 dogs. There was no specific lesion that

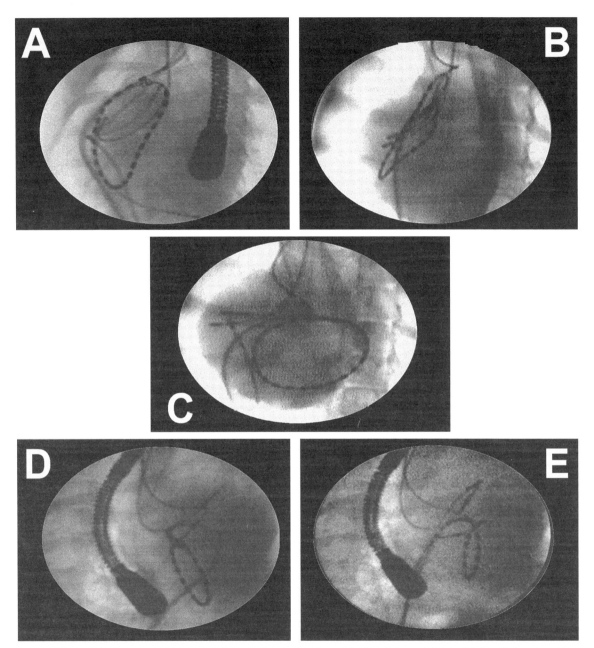

Figure 23. Fluoroscopic images of the catheter positioned in the right and left atria. Panel A: RA Loop. A right atrial circular lesion extending from the anterior septal tricuspid valve to the RA appendage to the SVC and circling back to the IVC. Panel B: RAI. A RA isthmus lesion where the catheter is looped into the RV with the ablation electrodes across the tricuspid valve ring and the IVC. Panel C: LAH. A circular horizontal lesion placed under the pulmonary veins in the mid left atrium, parallel to the mitral valve. Panel D: LAV1. A vertical lesion extending from the mitral valve annulus medial of the pulmonary veins. Panel E: LAV2. A vertical linear lesion extending from the mitral valve to the LA appendage, lateral of the pulmonary veins. Panels A, B, D, and E also show a transesophageal echocardiography probe. Standard catheters are shown including a coronary sinus catheter (Panels A and C) and a high right atrium catheter (Panels A, C, and E). The 2 endocardial pacing wires can be seen descending from the superior vena cava into the right atrium in panels A, D, and E.

caused the conversions from AF, although 6 of the 8 conversions occurred after creating a left atrial lesion. In 3 dogs, conversions were noted after ablating in a single atrium—the RA in 1 dog and the LA in 2 dogs. Five conversions occurred after both RA and LA lesions; 4 of these occurred while ablating in the LA. At the end of the procedure, 1 dog still maintained chronic AF.

Deflectable Catheter with Coil Electrodes

Haines and colleagues[49] used a deflectable catheter with 4 12.5-mm electrodes to ablate AF in a SLRAP/MR model. Lesions were created in 7 dogs in the following lines: lateral RA (intercaval), TV-IVC isthmus, SVC-TV anterior, LAA to posterior MV, and LAA to anterior MV. AF persisted after RA lesion generation. After LA lesion creation, AF could not be induced in 4 of 7 dogs acutely or 1–2 weeks postablation. Complications included death (n=2, tamponade and MI), heart block (n=2), and sinus arrest requiring permanent pacemaker insertion (n=1).

Kalman and associates[23] used a deflectable catheter with 3–6 12.5-mm coil electrodes to ablate AF in 8 dogs with chronic AF induced by atrial pacing at 400 beats per minute. Before ablation, 3 dogs had spontaneous AF for 24 hours, while the remaining 5 dogs had AF lasting >10 minutes post burst pacing. After creating RA lesions from the superior tricuspid annulus (TA) to the crista terminalis (CT), from the inferolateral TA to the CT, and from the SVC to the IVC, sustained AF could not be induced in 4 of 8 dogs. LA lesions were created from the lateral mitral annulus to the septum anteriorly and from the posterior mitral annulus to the roof of the LA. After RA and LA lesions, sustained AF could not be induced in 7 of 8 dogs. Sustained atrial flutter could be induced in 1 dog post RA lesions and in 1 dog post RA and LA lesions. One sudden death occurred during LA ablation due to myocardial infarction.

Additional Ablation Technology

A 4-mm Tip Electrode Deflectable Catheter Guided by Preshaped Sheaths

Haïssaguerre et al[15,16] and Swartz et al[17] have ablated paroxysmal AF in humans using a standard 4 mm, temperature-controlled, deflectable catheter along with multiple preshaped sheaths. They both created sequential lesions in the LA and the RA by dragging the catheter in predetermined paths similar to the Maze procedure. Although no clear pathological evidence has been presented as to the linearity and contiguity of the lesions, the users of this technique have reported success in ablating AF and paroxysmal AF in humans. Many of the patients require a second procedure to ablate recurrent AF and atrial flutter.

The major benefit of using 4-mm tip electrode catheters with preformed sheaths is its immediate availability. However, such an approach requires long procedure and radiation exposure times, since the catheter is dragged in small increments. In addition, moving the catheter over trabeculated tissues is unlikely to result in linear, contiguous lesions. This may lead to the formation of flutter circuits.[50] When dragging the catheter, it is possible that the tip will force free a clot that may result in a stroke. In order to create lesions using the drag technique, several different preshaped sheaths must be used. Multiple sheath replacements can increase the risk of creating air emboli.

Deflectable Catheter with 14 4-mm Electrodes

Haïssaguerre and associates[16] used a deflectable catheter with 14 4-mm electrodes spaced 3 mm apart in conjunction with the drag technique using a standard 4 mm tip electrode catheter to create lesions in the RA and LA (Figure 24) to ablate paroxysmal AF in humans. RA lesions ablated paroxysmal AF in 6 of 45

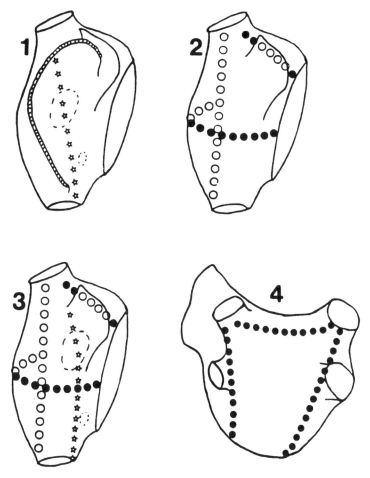

Figure 24. The ablation scheme used in the RA (1, 2, 3, anterior view) and LA (4, posterior view.) Group 1 (15 patients) underwent only a single septal right atrial line. Group 2 (15 patients) received a longitudinal and a transverse line in the right atrial free wall. Group 3 (15 patients) underwent an additional septal line. The fourth diagram shows the left atrial lines performed in 9 patients who failed attempts in one of the first 3 groups. From: Haïssaguerre M, et al. Right and left atrial radiofrequency catheter therapy of paroxysmal atrial fibrillation. *J Cardiovasc Electrophysiol* 1996; 7(12):1132–1144.

(13%) patients, while additional ablation of the LA increased the success rate to 40% (4 of 10). Stable sinus rhythm was restored during the procedure in 18 of 45 (40%) patients after RA ablation and 8 of 10 (80%) patients after additional LA lesions. Sustained AF could not be induced in 50% of patients after LA ablation, but in only 11% after RA ablation. RA or LA arrhythmogenic foci were demonstrated in 12 of 45 (27%) patients. Though some patients had decreased susceptibility to paroxysmal AF, most patients did not exhibit evidence of conduction block across the lines of ablation. No data regarding the character of the lesions was reported.

Saline Electrodes, Microwave Ablation, Laser Ablation

The infusion of saline during RF ablation is a technique that enables larger lesions to be created. The flow of cooled saline into the electrode-tissue interface allows for ablation at higher power levels, while preventing overheating and subsequent char formation. Nakagawa and associates[51] have used a deflectable catheter with 2 20 mm coil electrodes with saline infusion holes to create atrial lesions in dogs. They created lesions with the same catheter during saline infusion and without infusion. The lesions created with infusion were longer and more consistently transmural and the formation of coagulum on the electrodes was prevented. Wharton and colleagues[52] have described another saline infusion RF ablation catheter with 12 2-mm electrodes used to create atrial linear lesions. Though coagulum formation was avoided in this study, only 42% of the lesions were both contiguous and transmural.

Microwave and laser ablation do not require the high level of contact needed to generate large lesions with RF energy. Though no data has been published regarding their use in creating linear atrial lesions, their successful use in ventricular lesion generation suggests that in time these techniques may prove to be useful in atrial ablation.

Summary

In this chapter we have defined the safety and technological considerations for the development of catheter-based technology for the ablation of AF. Clearly, 2 major outcomes will define the future of this technology. The procedure will prove to be a failure if there is a high incidence of embolic stroke. In addition, the utility of this technology will be limited if it is only able to convert AF to an atrial flutter that is difficult to ablate and results in a rapid ventricular response that is difficult to control. Other troubling potential complications include sinus node dysfunction, AV nodal or His ablation necessitating pacemaker insertion, and perforations.

Goals

The primary goal of AF ablation is the restitution of normal sinus rhythm under autonomic control. With successful restoration of organized atrial activity, effective atrial mechanical contraction should be achieved. The resumption of atrial blood transport and the elimination of the need to anticoagulate the patient are crucial to the success of the procedure. AF can be ablated by simply burning all of the atrial tissues, but this will not result in significant hemodynamic benefit to the patient. Thus, the extent of the lesions must be minimized.

Models

To test the safety and efficacy of catheter-based technology to ablate AF, several experimental models are in use. Such models include acute-type AF induced in the pericarditis and vagal stimulation models, both of which can be ablated in the right atrium. These 2 models have few human analogs and do not represent the majority of human chronic AF. Chronic models include mitral regurgitation and single and dual lead variations of rapid atrial pacing. They create progressive electrical remodeling with decreasing atrial refractoriness, wavelength, and conduction velocity which, along with increased regional heterogeneity, results in the formation of reentrant circuits.[53] In both the acute and chronic models, investigators have noted electrical changes that are also present in humans with AF.

Lesions

In the acute burst pacing model, a single lesion in the RA along the medial intra-atrial septum eliminated the induction of AF in 10 of 11 dogs.[18] In the sterile pericarditis model, RA linear lesions were sufficient to eliminate the induction of AF.[22,25,39] In the vagal stimulation model, it has been shown that discrete lesions at the RA dome may eliminate the induction of AF during vagal stimulation.[21] Endocardial lesions at the SVC and base of the RA appendage may ablate the vagal insertion site included at the SVC aortic root space.[41]

In the chronic AF models of rapid pacing with or without mitral regurgitation, the location and the extent of lesions required to ablate AF is not uniformly established. From the limited experience in humans,[15–17] it appears that LA linear lesions involving the pulmonary veins and the territory around these veins are needed. The ablation of pacing induced chronic AF in the animal model appears to require the same type of lesions for successful conversion. The technology for the creation of such lesions is still evolving. In several investigations, multipolar electrodes placed on a deflectable shaft were able to create linear lesions 2.4 ± 0.7 cm in length.[49,54] However, such technology requires significant catheter manipulation and a variety of catheters of different sizes, deflection directions, and preformed shapes. In contrast, a loop catheter design may provide better catheter-tissue contact by creating an expandable loop within the atria. This technology also allows for the creation of lesions in a greater variety of locations. A nonfluoroscopic electromagnetic locating system may provide accurate guidance during anatomically-directed linear lesion formation using a tip ablation electrode that is dragged along the endocardial surface.[55] This system provides increased accuracy in creating lesions but does not resolve the limitation of procedure time and possible stroke complications. Clearly, minimizing LA catheter manipulation, total LA instrumentation time, and total procedure time may be crucial reducing complication risks.

It is hypothesized that mapping the atria for the maximal fractionated activity may provide further definition of the site of ablation. If the critical areas for ablation can be mapped, the extent of atrial ablation can be minimized. Therefore, more atrial tissue can be preserved to contribute to atrial mechanical contraction when AF is converted to normal sinus rhythm. Effective mapping capabilities also decrease the likelihood of ablating inappropriate areas such as the AV and SA nodes. The use of 4 mm ablation/recording electrodes allows for highly localized observation of atrial electrical activity and, therefore, catheter location. A catheter with 12 mm electrodes and 2 mm interelectrode spacing can efficiently generate linear lesions, but such a design has limited mapping resolution.

In summary, a catheter with multiple small electrodes that can be rapidly and accurately positioned with firm electrode-tissue contact will be able to create long contiguous transmural lesions, while avoiding excessive destruction and SA or AV nodal ablation. This desirable combination of capabilities can be achieved with a loop catheter design equipped with multiple 4-mm electrodes.

Though heightened focus has been placed on it in recent years, the evolution of catheter-based technology for the ablation of AF is a slow and ongoing process. Many initial investigations in animal models and in humans have shown great promise. However, several significant limitations remain to be overcome including procedure-related strokes, excessive radiation exposure, and the conversion of AF to atrial flutter with rapid ventricular response, which necessitates additional ablation procedures. With further technological development and methodology refinement, the ablation of AF may eventually offer a long-term solution for patients with this debilitating condition.

References

1. Olsson S, Alessie M, Campbell R. *Atrial Fibrillation: Mechanisms and Therapeutic Strategies.* Armonk, NY: Futura Publishing Co., Inc., 1994.
2. Boysen G, Nyboe J, Appleyard M, et al. Stroke incidence and risk factors for stroke in Copenhagen, Denmark. *Stroke* 1988;19:1345–1353.
3. Lake FR, Cullen KJ, de Klerk NH, et al. Atrial fibrillation and mortality in elderly population. *Aust NZ J Medication* 1989;19:321–326.
4. Alpert JS, Peterson P, Godtfredsen J. Atrial fibrillation: natural history, complications, and management. *Ann Rev Med* 1988;39:41–52.
5. Petersen P, Godtfredsen J. Atrial fibrillation: a review of course and prognosis. *Acta Med Scand* 1984;216:5–9.
6. Hankey GJ, Dennis MS, Slattery JM, et al. Why is the outcome of transient ischemic attacks different in different groups of patients. *Br Med J* 1993;306:1107–1111.
7. Crijns HJGM, Gosselink M. Prophylactic drug therapy after cardioversion of atrial fibrillation or flutter. *Cardiology* 1994;7:31–34.
8. Echt DS, Liebson PR, Mitchell LB, et al. Mortality and morbidity in pa-

tients receiving encainide, flecainide or placebo: the cardiac arrhythmia suppression trial. *N Engl J Med* 1991;324:781–788.

9. Gosselink ATM, Crijns HJGM, Van Gelder IC, et al. Low-dose amiodarone for maintenance of sinus rhythm after cardioversion of atrial fibrillation or flutter. *JAMA* 1992;267:3289–3293.

10. Cox JL, Boineau JP, Schussler RB, et al. Five-year experience with the Maze procedure for atrial fibrillation. *Ann Thorac Surg* 1993; 56:814–824.

11. Kuu-Gi S, Jun-Jack C, Jin-Jer C, et al. Recovery of atrial function after atrial compartment operation for chronic atrial fibrillation in mitral valve disease. *J Am Coll Cardiol* 1994;24(2):392–398.

12. Cox JL, Boineau JP, Schuessler RB, et al. Surgical interruption of atrial reentry as a cure for atrial fibrillation. In: Olsson SB, Allessie MA, Campbell RWF, eds. *Atrial Fibrillation: Mechanisms and Therapeutic Strategies.* Armonk, NY: Futura Publishing Co. Inc., 1994. pp 373–404.

13. Scheinman M. Catheter ablation: present role and projected impact on health care for patients with cardiac arrythmias. *Circulation* 1991;83:1489–1498.

14. Feld K. Radiofrequency catheter ablation versus modification of the AV node for control of rapid ventricular response in atrial fibrillation. *J Cardiovasc Electrophysiol* 1995;6(3):217–228.

15. Haïssaguerre M, Gencel L, Fischer B, et al. Successful catheter ablation of atrial fibrillation. *J Cardiovasc Electrophysiol* 1994;5(12):1045–1052.

16. Haïssaguerre M, Jaïs P, Shah D, et al. Right and left atrial radiofrequency catheter therapy of paroxysmal atrial fibrillation. *J Cardiovasc Electrophysiol* 1996; 7(12):1132–1144.

17. Swartz JF, Pellersels G, Silvers J, et al. A catheter-based curative approach to atrial fibrillation in humans [abstract]. *Circulation* 1994;90(4):I–335.

18. Tondo C, Otomo K, Antz M, et al. Successful radiofrequency catheter ablation of atrial fibrillation by a single lesion to the inter-atrial septum [abstract]. *Circulation* 1995:92(8); I–265.

19. Seifert M, Friedman M, Selike F, et al. Radiofrequency Maze ablation for atrial fibrillation [abstract]. *Circulation* 1994;90(4):I594.

20. Ortiz J, Miwano S, Abe H, et al. Mapping the conversion of atrial flutter to atrial fibrillation and atrial fibrillation to atrial flutter: insights into mechanism. *Circ Res* 1994;74(5):882–894.

21. Avitall B, Hare J, Helms R. Vagally mediated atrial fibrillation in a dog model can be ablated by placing linear radiofrequency lesions at the junction of the right atrial appendage and the superior vena cava [abstract]. *PACE* 1995;18(4):857.

22. Kumagai K, Khrestian C, Waldo A. Simultaneous multisite mapping studies during induced atrial fibrillation in the sterile pericarditis model: insights into the mechanism of maintenance. *Circulation* 1997;95(2):511–521.

23. Kalman J, Olgin J, Karch M, et al. Are linear lesions needed in both atria to prevent atrial fibrillation in a canine model? [abstract] *Circulation* 1996;94(8):I–555.

24. Elvan A, Pride H, Eble J, et al. Arrhythmias/radiofrequency ablation: radiofrequency catheter ablation of the atria reduces inducibility and duration of atrial fibrillation in dogs. *Circulation* 1995;91(8):2235–2244.

25. Nakagawa H, Kumagai K, Imai S, et al. Catheter ablation of Bachmann's bundle from the right atrium eliminates atrial fibrillation in a canine sterile pericarditis model [abstract]. *PACE* 1996;19(4):581.

26. Wijffels MC, Kirchhof C, Dorland R, et al. Atrial fibrillation begets atrial fibrillation: a study in awake chronically instrumented goats. *Circulation* 1995;92(7):1954–1968.

27. Cox JL, Canavan TE, Schuessler RB, et al. The surgical treatment of atrial fibrillation, II: intraoperative electrophysiologic mapping and description of the electrophysiologic basis of atrial flutter and fibrillation. *J Thorac Cardiovasc Surg* 1991;101:406–426.

28. Haines D, McRury I. Implementation of a modified canine model of chronic atrial fibrillation [abstract]. *Circulation* 1995;92(8):I–404.

29. Ortiz J, Igarashi M, Gonzalez X, et al. A new, reliable atrial fibrillation model with a clinical counterpart [abstract]. *J Am Coll Cardiol* 1993;21(2):183A.

30. Liu L, Nattel S. Differing sympathetic and vagal effects on atrial fibrillation in dogs: role of refractoriness heterogeneity. *Am J Physiol* 1997;273 (2Pt2):H805–816.

31. Geddes L, Hinds M, Babbs C, et al. Maintenance of atrial fibrillation in anesthetized and unanesthetized sheep using cholinergic drive. *PACE* 1996;19(2):165–175.

32. Wang Z, Page P, Nattel S. Mechanism of flecainide's antiarrhythmic action in experimental atrial fibrillation. *Circ Res* 1992;71:271–287.

33. Moriera D, Shepard R, Waldo A. Chronic rapid atrial pacing to maintain atrial fibrillation: use to permit control of ventricular rate in order to treat tachycardia induced cardiomyopathy. *PACE* 1989;12(5):761–775.

34. Rensma P, Allessie M, Lammers W, et al. The length of the excitation wave as an index for the susceptibility to reentrant atrial arrhythmias. *Circ Res* 1988;62:395–410.

35. Morillo C, Klein G, Jones D, et al. Chronic rapid atrial pacing: structural, functional, and electrophysiological characteristics of a new model of sustained atrial fibrillation. *Circulation* 1995;91(5):1588–1595.

36. Goette A, Honeycutt C, Langberg J. Arrhythmias/pacing: electrical remodeling in atrial fibrillation: time course and mechanisms. *Circulation* 1996; 94(11):2968–2974.

37. Elvan A, Wylie K, Zipes D. Arrhythmias/pacing: pacing-induced chronic atrial fibrillation impairs sinus node function in dogs: electrophysiological remodeling. *Circulation* 1996;94(11):2953–2960.

38. Avitall B, Bharati S, Kotov A, et al. Histopathologic similarities between the human mitral disease chronic atrial fibrillation and the canine rapid pacing model of chronic atrial fibrillation [abstract]. *PACE* 1997;20(4):1139.

39. Kotov A, Bharati S, Helms R, et al. The chronic atrial fibrillation canine model: a new approach to increase yield and efficiency [abstract]. *J Am Coll Cardiol* 1997;29(2):471A.

40. Avitall B, Hare J, Mughal K, et al. A catheter system to ablate atrial fibrillation in a sterile pericaditis dog model [abstract]. *PACE* 1994;17(2):774.

41. Avitall B, Hare J, Mughal K, et al. Right-sided driven atrial fibrillation in a sterile pericaditis dog model [abstract]. *PACE* 1994;17(2):774.

42. Chiou C-W, Eble J, Zipes D. Efferent vagal innervation of the canine atria and sinus and atrioventricular nodes: the third fat pad. *Circulation* 1997;95(11):2573–2584.

43. Avitall B, Helms R, Kotov A. A thoracoscopic approach to ablate atrial fibrillation via linear radiofrequency lesion generation on the epicardium of both atria [abstract]. *PACE* 1996;19(4):626.

44. Elvan A, Huang X, Pressler M, et al. Radiofrequency catheter ablation of the atria eliminates pacing-induced sustained atrial fibrillation and reduces connexin 43 in dogs. *Circulation* 1997;96(5):1675–1685.

45. Avitall B, Kotov A, Helms R. New monitoring criteria for transmural ablation of atrial tissues [abstract]. *Circulation* 1996;94(8):I-904.

46. Avitall B, Helms R, Kotov A, et al. The use of temperature versus local depolarization amplitude to monitor atrial lesion maturation during the creation of linear lesions in both atria [abstract]. *Circulation* 1996;94(8):I–904.

47. Avitall B, Helms R, Chiang W, et al. The impact of transcatheter generated atrial linear radiofrequency lesions on atrial function and contractility [abstract]. *PACE* 1996;19(4):698.

48. Avitall B, Kotov A, Bharati S, et al. Long-term remodeling of the atria after atrial fibrillation ablation with multiple long atrial linear lesions [abstract]. *PACE* 1997;20(4):1054.

49. Avitall B, Helms R, Kotov A, et al. Atrial fibrillation in the rapid pacing dog model: is there atrial dominance? Which atrium should be ablated? [abstract] *PACE* 1997;20(4):1139.

50. Haines D, McRury I. Primary atrial fibrillation ablation in a chronic atrial fibrillation model [abstract]. *Circulation* 1995;92(8):I–265.

51. Avitall B, Helms R, Chiang W, et al. Nonlinear atrial radiofrequency lesions are arrhythmogenic: a study of skipped lesions in the normal atria [abstract]. *Circulation* 1995;92(8):I–265.

52. Nakagawa H, Yamanashi W, Pitha J, et al. Creation of long linear transmural radiofrequency lesions in the atrium using a novel spiral ribbon-saline irrigated electrode catheter [abstract]. *J Am Coll Cardiol* 1996:27(2);188A.

53. Wharton M, Tomassoni G, Pomeranz M, et al. Saline perfused, balloon radiofrequency ablation catheter for creation of linear transmural atrial lesions [abstract]. *Circulation* 1996;94(8):I–493.

54. Gaspo R, Bosch R, Talajic M, et al. Functional mechanisms underlying tachycardia-induced sustained atrial fibrillation in a chronic dog model. *Circulation* 1997;96(11):4027–4035.

55. Whayne JG, Haines DE, Panescu D, et al. Catheter system designs to facilitate RF ablation of atrial fibrillation [abstract]. *PACE* 1996;19(4)II;I–339.

56. Shpun S, Gepstein L, Hayam G, et al. Accurate linear lesions guided by non-fluoroscopic electromagnetic mapping during sinus rhythm and atrial fibrillation [abstract]. *PACE* 1997;20(4):1099.

Chapter 19

New Catheter Technologies for the Ablation of Atrial Fibrillation

J. Michael Mangrum, M.D., David E. Haines, M.D.

Introduction

Atrial fibrillation is the most common sustained arrhythmia: it affects 0.2–0.6% of the general population, and 5–10% of those over 60 years old.[1–7] As the population ages, the number of patients who present with this arrhythmia will surely increase. Associated with this arrhythmia are hemodynamic changes due to atrioventricular asynchrony, increased risk of thromboembolic events, and symptoms of palpitations, dizziness, and angina in some patients. At the present time, conventional therapy is comprised of 2 dominant strategies: the restoration of sinus rhythm and maintenance using antiarrhythmic medications and the control of the ventricular response rate and anticoagulation. Neither of these approaches is uniformly effective. In addition there are side effects and drug interactions from the antiarrhythmics, and inconvenience and potential bleeding complications with anticoagulation therapy. Therefore, non-pharmacological therapies for prevention of atrial fibrillation are desirable.

An established non-pharmacological treatment for atrial fibrillation is atrioventricular (AV) nodal modification or complete AV junctional ablation with pacemaker insertion.[8,9] These procedures are designed to achieve rate control. However, because the atria continue to fibrillate, the risk of thromboembolism remains unchanged. Newer treatments such as atrial defibrillators have been implanted in highly selected individuals. Current devices are able to detect atrial fibrillation with near 100% specificity and very high sensitivity.[10] However, one major limitation of this therapy is that most patients experience pain with shocks at energy levels required for defibrillation. Finally, single- or dual-site atrial pacing has shown some promise in significantly reducing the

From Huang SKS, Wilber DJ (eds.): *Radiofrequency Catheter Ablation of Cardiac Arrhythmias: Basic Concepts and Clinical Applications,* 2nd ed. Armonk, NY: Futura Publishing Company, Inc. ©2000.

recurrences of atrial fibrillation in patients with paroxysmal atrial fibrillation and coexisting bradyarrhythmias.[11]

All of these management strategies are good treatment options but are not curative. Beginning in the 1980s, surgical techniques were developed to cure atrial fibrillation; success could be achieved but only at the cost of undergoing a major surgical procedure. In the 1990s, with the technical advances in catheter-based ablations using radiofrequency (RF) energy, it is possible to emulate surgical procedures without thoracotomy and cardiopulmonary bypass.

Background

The key to development of newer and improved therapies for atrial fibrillation is to understand its mechanisms. Despite the emergence of a new subset of atrial fibrillation that appears to have a focal mechanism, the accepted mechanism for the majority of cases of atrial fibrillation is reentry, consisting of multiple wavelets circulating around anatomic barriers and variable regions of functional conduction block. This theory was first proposed with a computer model in 1964 by Moe et al. They proposed that the refractory period, conduction velocity, and mass of tissue were the dominant factors that modulated the ability of the atria to sustain fibrillation.[12] In 1990, Allessie et al confirmed this hypothesis. They placed 2 mapping electrodes into the right and left atria of isolated blood-perfused canine hearts and initiated atrial fibrillation with programmed electrical stimulation during acetylcholine infusion. Simultaneous recordings were taken from 192 electrodes and sequence maps were constructed. Waves of activation were observed and noted to accelerate, decelerate, divide and/or change direction. It was noted that 4 to 6 wavelets were required in order to sustain continuous propagation of the atrial fibrillation.[13]

The self-perpetuation of atrial fibrillation has been of significant interest, and the electrophysiological changes have been termed electrical remodeling. The underlying mechanism of electrical remodeling is unknown, but one leading hypothesis holds the electrophysiological changes may be mediated through an increased level of intracellular calcium.[14,15] During electrophysiological studies in dogs, atrial fibrillation has been shown to prolong corrected sinus node recovery time and P-wave duration, decrease maximal and intrinsic heart rate, and shorten the atrial effective refractory period (ERP).[16] The significant decrease in ERP has been noted in several studies,[14,17–18] and recently it has been demonstrated that termination of sustained atrial fibrillation by RF ablation returns the ERP back to baseline.[19]

Therefore, with the understanding that fibrillatory wavelets require a critical amount of atrial tissue for propagation and electrical remodeling, the theory behind the surgical or catheter-based curative approach can be understood. That is, by forming lines of conduction block in the atrial wall with surgical incisions or RF ablation, the number of propagating wavelets will decrease and hence atrial fibrillation will be prevented (Figure 1).

During the 1980s, Cox et al developed a surgical technique referred to as the Maze procedure with its first clinical application in 1987.[20,21] Since its in-

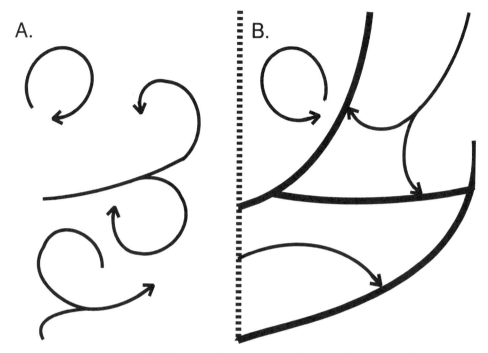

Figure 1. Cartoon of atrial fibrillation without and with linear atrial ablations. Panel A represents multiple atrial fibrillation wavelets propagating throughout the atria unimpeded by anatomic barriers. Panel B represents a similar region of atrial wall after the creation of lines of conduction block by surgical incisions or catheter ablation. Because the atrium is segmented, the wavelets are unable to propagate and atrial fibrillation cannot be sustained.

ception, the Maze procedure has been modified twice. All Maze procedures have included 1) excision of both atria appendages, and (2) isolation of the left atrial wall incorporating the 4 pulmonary vein ostia. The Maze-I procedure was modified because of a high prevalence of sinus node dysfunction and left atrial mechanical dysfunction.[22,23] The incision located anterior to the junction of the superior vena cava (SVC) in the right atrium was eliminated, and a counter incision on the anterior right atrium was added. In addition, there was modification of the incision located at the base of the heart across the atrial septum. Some of these modifications were technically challenging and time-consuming, and therefore further modifications were made to yield the Maze-III.[23] The main modification was to move the left atrial dome incision more posteriorly, thereby moving the atrial septotomy posterior to the SVC. Using these techniques, success rates ranging from 76–93% have been reported.[24,25] Thus, the concept that surgical linear atrial lesions can prevent recurrent atrial fibrillation has been proven.

More recently Suede et al reported success with a simple surgical procedure confined to the left atrium in patients with atrial fibrillation and mitral valve disease based on the hypothesis that the shorter fibrillatory cycle length in the left posterior atrial wall would act as a source of persisting reentrant wavelets for maintaining atrial fibrillation. The procedure consisted of excision of the left atrial appendage, isolation of the pulmonary veins, and cryoablation around the incision between the upper and lower left pulmonary veins and between incisions to the posterior mitral valvular annulus. In the Suede study of 51 patients, 86% who underwent this procedure had either elimination of atrial fibrillation or significant reduction in episodes.[26] This study indicated that more limited ablation than that performed in the Maze operation could be similarly successful in eliminating atrial fibrillation, but suggested that ablation site selection (in this case the pulmonary inflow region) was critical for success.

Catheter-Based Approaches to Atrial Fibrillation Ablation

The surgical approaches toward cure of atrial fibrillation all have the major limitations of thoracotomy and cardiopulmonary bypass with the accompanying morbidity, mortality, and cost.[27] Therefore, a less invasive approach to the cure of atrial fibrillation has been sought. Throughout this decade the feasibility of a catheter-based approach to create linear ablations has been demonstrated in a number of animal and human studies. However, the technical challenges of developing these catheter-based systems have been formidable. For instance, in the Maze procedure, it has been stated that the incisions/suture lines must be complete and continuous for procedure success; hence, it is likely that this will be a requirement for catheter-based approaches. This represents a significant challenge even in regions with smooth, thin atrial walls. The challenge increases as the catheter is manipulated along the varied topography of the atrial walls. The atrial wall thickens at the crista terminalis and at Bachman's bundle, necessitating much deeper radiofrequency ablative lesions. Around the pulmonary veins and the tricuspid and mitral annuli, high flow rates cause significant convective cooling which makes it difficult to achieve tissue temperatures high enough to result in irreversible tissue damage. Finally, tissue contact can be uneven where there is greater trabeculation, as around the atrial appendages and right atrium anterior to the crista terminalis. Thus, the catheter and electrode designs are very important. In order to achieve successful catheter ablation in these regions, the catheter not only must gain access to these sites, but also must then be positioned to assure stable wall contact. Finally, the use of aggressive catheter ablation maneuvers in order to achieve continuous transmural lesions may be associated with increased risks of catheter-induced trauma to the atrial wall, and thrombus or char formation in response to excessive delivery of RF energy. These can, in turn, result in embolic complications such as stroke. Thus, if a catheter-based cure of atrial fibrillation is to be developed, the benefits and risks of the procedure will need to be carefully considered.

Catheter and Electrode Design

In 1994, Swartz et al[28] reported the ability to produce long linear lesions using conventional ablation catheters and a series of long, shaped sheaths. This was achieved by selecting the appropriate sheath, ablating each line using continuous energy delivery with temperature monitoring, and moving the catheter 2–3 mm every 30 seconds. As might be expected, this procedure was very time-consuming and technically demanding as gaps in the ablation line necessitated repeated RF applications. The painstaking nature of linear drag techniques has prompted the development of catheters specifically designed to create lesions several centimeters in length without the need for repositioning (Figure 2). Initial attempts to improve ablation efficacy used long tip electrodes. Their deficiencies included nonuniform tissue heating and variability of tissue contact. Subsequently, catheters with multiple poles and specific electrode construction and spacing were developed. Multipolar ablation allows the creation of a line of lesions from a single fixed catheter position, but positioning the catheter to assure adequate tissue contact along its entire length can be challenging. New technologies including intracardiac echocardiography[29,30] and three-dimensional electroanatomic mapping[31,32] have been shown to aid in catheter positioning and improve adequate tissue contact. In addition, alternative catheter configurations

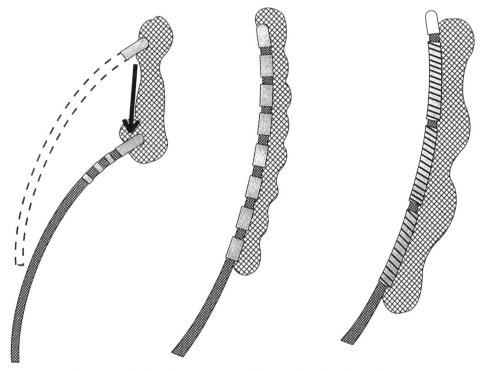

Figure 2. A schematic of a distal tip ablation catheter and multipolar catheters is presented. Areas of radiofrequency energy heating are represented by the cross-hatched regions. In order to create linear lesions with the distal tip of a standard ablation catheter, either a "drag" technique or "point-to-point" ablation technique must be used (left). These techniques are time-consuming and may result in lesion discontinuity. Therefore, catheters with multiple ablation poles have been created to avoid the need for catheter repositioning. These catheters are positioned parallel to the atrial wall targeted for ablation, and radiofrequency energy is delivered in sequence or simultaneously to multiple poles. The middle drawing represents a multipolar catheter with ring electrodes. The right drawing represents a multipolar catheter with a coil electrode.

such as expanding intracardiac loops have been used to optimize electrode-tissue contact. Specific components of new catheter ablation systems are discussed below.

Temperature Control

Temperature control is critical for the creation of continuous lesions and avoidance of char and coagulum (especially in the left atrium, because of the risk of systemic thromboembolism). Whayne et al[35] compared different multipolar linear ablation catheter systems in the canine atrium using 2 energy systems. The first system delivered energy to either coil or ring electrode in sequence, with each electrode having individual temperature control (70°C to 80°C). The second system (MECA, EP Technologies, San Jose, CA) delivered energy simultaneously to all electrodes. Each electrode segment consisted of a flexible coil with a pair of thermistors on either side of the coils and at each end. For temperature feedback power control, the higher of 2 measured temperatures was used.[36] In this comparison, 6% of the ablation lines using sequential energy to ring electrodes were correctly targeted, continuous and transmural, as compared to 36% with sequential coil electrodes and 76% with the MECA system and its coil electrodes that used simultaneous energy. The differences were likely due to the beneficial effects of heating adjacent electrodes simultaneously, improved temperature monitoring, long flexible electrodes with short interelectrode gaps, and bidirectional steering allowing improved tissue contact.

It is generally acknowledged that the avoidance of char and coagulum is extremely important, especially for ablations in the left atrium. McRury et al[37] described the "edge effect" phenomenon using long coil electrodes. This phenomenon, explained mathematically by the Laplace equation, states that from a radiating source of electrical potential there is higher current and power density at areas of high geometric gradients such as the edges of electrodes. Therefore, heating increases with power density and peak temperatures occur at the electrode edges (Figure 3). In the McRury study, 16 dogs underwent right and left atrial ablations using multicoil electrodes with either a single thermistor in the center of each coil, or a dual thermocouple design with each thermocouple located at opposing sides on each end of the coils. The results indicated that by monitoring the temperature at the electrode edges, the prevalence of a rise in electrical impedance could be lowered from 45% to 2%, and there was 74% less coagulum adherent to the catheter. The targeted temperature could be achieved with a mean power of 50.7 ± 32.3 watts versus 61.6 ± 38.0 watts using dual versus single temperature sensors. It was concluded that when using long RF electrodes for production of linear atrial lesions, monitoring temperatures at the electrode edge helped prevent the occurrence of potentially embolic thrombus and char on the catheter.

Novel Catheter Designs for Site Access

Avitall et al[38] proposed the use of a monorail sliding catheter system for the creation of linear lesions in the right atria of 7 dogs with atrial fibrillation.

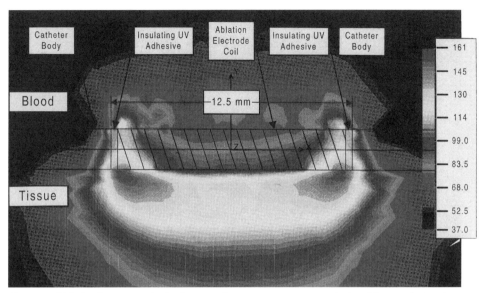

Figure 3. This isotherm graph depicts steady-state temperatures derived from a finite element analysis of radiofrequency ablation with a coil electrode 12 mm in length. The legend of temperatures is shown at right; the temperatures range from the physiological normal (violet = 37°C) to maximum tissue temperature (red = 161°C). In this example, the power is adjusted to maintain the temperature at the midpoint of the electrode at 70°C. In this case, tissue temperature may reach 161°C below the electrode edges, resulting in char and coagulum formation. (Reproduced with permission from *Circulation* 1997;96:4057–4064.) See color plate.

The ablation catheter was placed over a guidewire into the right atrium with deflection achieved by pushing the catheter shaft against a stopper located 10 cm from the guidewire tip. Examination of the heart revealed continuous and transmural lesions. This system was used to make left atrial lesions via a transseptal approach in 5 dogs.[34] In each dog 3 lesions were made: 1) from mitral ring to pulmonary veins and medially to the appendage, 2) mitral ring to pulmonary veins and laterally to the appendage, and 3) horizontally perpendicular to the first 2 lesions. As in their previous study, linear transmural lesions were created.

Using a similar concept, Haines et al created multiple lesions in both atria of 6 dogs.[33] The ablation catheter had an 8F shaft and 2 splines at its terminus that formed a loop. A central wire allowed the loop to straighten for venous entry and then to expand after atrial positioning. This technology has provided greater maneuverability around the heterogeneous geometry of the left atria. The Avitall catheter design has been merged with the coil electrode technology and is now comprised of 14 coil electrodes that are 12 mm in length and a distal pull wire (EP Technologies, San Jose, CA) (Figure 4). Manipulation of the catheter, pull wire, and introducer sheath can result in a variety of loop geometries deployed in the atrial chambers. Deploying more catheter length from the sheath while the wire is retracted produces a larger loop that conforms to the geometry of the atrial chamber, thus optimizing catheter-tissue contact.

Other experimental catheter designs are currently being investigated. One

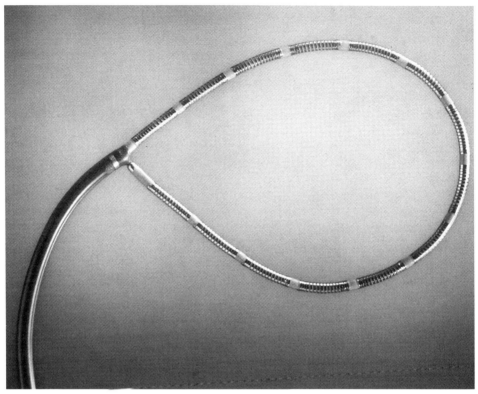

Figure 4. The loop ablation catheter consists of 14 coil electrodes, each 12 mm in length, and a distal tip pull-wire. The loop ablation catheter is seen placed through a long sheath with the pull-wire retracted. The retraction results in a large loop to conform to the geometry of the atria.

such device was recently reported by Liese et al. The investigators successfully created linear, contiguous, and transmural lesions using an expandable catheter with 12 7 mm coil electrodes with 1.5 mm spacing, a protective pigtail tip, and a novel steering system at the distal electrode to adjust the angle of contact.[39] Interestingly, creation of left atrial lesions appeared to be more successful than creation of right-sided lesions with this new tool. Another design proposed for atrial fibrillation ablation is a variation of the expandable loop, but instead of metal electrodes that contact the tissue, saline within perforated balloons is heated with RF energy and is perfused through the balloon perforations causing heating of contiguous tissue. It is proposed that this tool will reliably create transmural lesions with minimal risk of char, coagulum, or thrombus formation.[40]

Adjunctive Imaging for Guidance of Ablation Catheters

Intracardiac echocardiography (ICE) has been proposed as an adjunct to fluoroscopy for catheter guidance during RF ablation for a number of arrhythmias.[41] It has been useful in catheter site selection relative to anatomic structures, and with assessment of catheter-tissue contact, thereby resulting in improved energy coupling to tissue and greater lesion size.[42,43] Its greatest benefit may be in its use with ablations that are predominantly anatomically targeted, such as atrial flutter and primary ablation of atrial fibrillation. Olgin et al[44] used ICE as a guide to position a multiple coil (4 5 mm coils separated by 2 mm) array catheter (Medtronic-CardioRhythm, Minneapolis, MN). After good contact (defined as all 4 coils adjacent to the endocardium and lack of sliding on the endocardium) was assured, lesions were created in the right atria of 6 pigs. The results revealed accurate lesion targeting (within 0.3 mm), successful creation of long linear lesions with a single energy application without having to reposition the catheter, and reduced procedural and fluoroscopic times. Similar results have been demonstrated in a comparative study by Epstein et al.[30] In this study, 10 dogs underwent right atrial ablations with a multielement ablation catheter (MECA). Five canines underwent catheter ablation with blinded ICE acquisition by a second operator, and 5 canines had ablation useng both fluoroscopic and ICE guidance. Successful RF energy delivery (defined by achieving a temperature of 70°C with less than 0.9 amperes of RF current per electrode coil) was achieved in 61% of cases with ICE guidance versus 48% of ablations guided by fluoroscopy alone ($P = 0.02$) (Figure 5). Adequate lesion continuity (greater than 75%) was achieved in 100% of ICE-guided ablations compared to 56% of those performed with fluoroscopic guidance. Finally, the locations for ablation were inappropriately targeted with fluoroscopic guidance in 25% of cases compared to the assessment of catheter position by ICE. Thus, ICE guidance of linear atrial ablation allowed the operator to improve electrode-tissue contact and electrode targeting of the desired anatomic substrate.

An alternative technology to fluoroscopy and ICE that has been proposed as being potentially useful in the ablation of atrial fibrillation is three-dimensional anatomic mapping. The Carto system (Biosense, Inc., Orangeburg, New York) uses a catheter with a built-in sensor that allows its position to be determined within a three-dimensional magnetic field. Point-by-point acquisitions of electrical signals and precise anatomic positions allow for reconstruction of anatomic maps. It has been proposed that this may be a useful tool for guiding catheter ablation of arrhythmias with significant reduction of fluoroscopic time without increasing procedure times.[45] Since atrial fibrillation is not a stable rhythm, the value of electrogram mapping with this system is limited. However, any anatomically-based ablation procedure may benefit from this technology by assisting more precise and reproducible catheter placement. Kuck et al have reported the use of the electroanatomic mapping system for ablation of atrial fibrillation in humans. In their study, 27 patients with idiopathic atrial fibrillation were randomized to initial left atrial ablations (13 patients) or right atrial ablations only (14 patients). Nine of 13 patients within the left atrial group required additional right atrial lesions as there was no major change in their rhythm post left atrial ablation. The results revealed limited success with left-sided ablations, but demonstrated the feasibility of the electroanatomic mapping system for primary ablation of atrial fibrillation.[32]

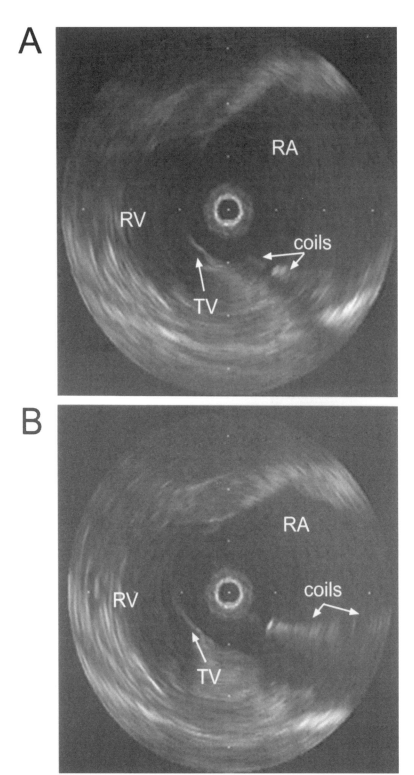

Figure 5. Intracardiac echocardiographic (ICE) image obtained during attempted positioning of a multi-electrode ablation catheter. The ICE catheter is placed in the right atrium with visualization of the right atrium (RA), right ventricle (RV), and tricuspid valve (TV). The multipolar catheter, consisting of multiple coils, is placed in the right atrium. Panel A demonstrates good electrode contact with the endocardium, compared to panel B which shows displacement of the electrode coils from the endocardial surface.

Lesion Location for Atrial Fibrillation Ablation

The ideal locations for radiofrequency catheter ablation are presently unknown. Various right-sided and biatrial ablations continue to be evaluated. Over the past few years, several studies have evaluated the success of right-sided ablations.[46-52] Although various endpoints for success have been used, it appears that there may be limited success (for no recurrence of atrial fibrillation) and improved response to pharmacological therapy.

A biatrial approach in humans was described by Swartz et al[28] in 1994. This ablation procedure used 8 lines of block and roughly followed the Maze procedure; however, linear and horizontal lines were used to separate the pulmonary veins and the atrial appendages were not separated from the remainder of the atria. Other investigators have preferred a staged approach, in which they attempted to perform more limited initial ablations with further ablation if the initial approach was unsuccessful. Studies that have used this staged approach have revealed an increased success rate with the additional left atrial lesions.[39,53,54]

Animal Studies

Animal models for atrial fibrillation have been developed in the goat, sheep, and dog. Because a variable for development of atrial fibrillation is atrial size, to maintain a critical number of wavelets, models in smaller animals have not been developed. Atrial fibrillation is usually produced by one of 4 techniques: 1) chronic rapid atrial pacing;[55,56] 2) chronic pericarditis;[57] 3) valvular disruption;[58] or 4) both rapid atrial pacing and valvular disruption.[59] The last technique has the advantage of producing chronic rather than sustained (self-terminating) atrial fibrillation.

Radiofrequency catheter ablation in the canine model was reported by Elvan et al.[60] In this study, 30 open-chest dogs received radiofrequency energy through the epicardium to the posterolateral right atrium, anteromedial side of the SVC, both the right and left atrial appendages, and the transverse sinus by use of 6F or 7F catheters with hexapolar or octapolar multielectrode steerable tips at A power output setting of 30 to 40 watts for 60 seconds. In addition, a 6F catheter with a hexapolar multielectrode tip was advanced through the external jugular vein to the distal coronary sinus with energy delivered at 10 to 20 watts for 30 seconds. The results indicated that atrial fibrillation induction by atrial pacing could be eliminated, as could the perpetuation of atrial fibrillation by low-level cervical vagal stimulation or infusion of low doses of methacholine. This study raises 2 interesting questions about the applicability of these findings to humans. First, the canine atrial dimensions are smaller than those of humans and the number of ablations required may be different. Second, the ablation in the canine model produces vagal denervation, which decreases the ERP shortening and thus may prevent atrial fibrillation induction; in contrast, paroxysmal atrial fibrillation induced by enhanced vagal tone in humans is rare.

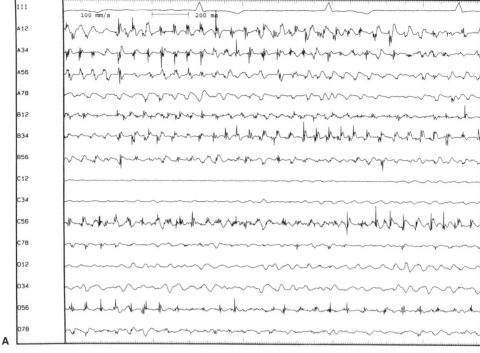

Figure 6. A basket catheter is used to record atrial electrograms during a linear atrial ablation procedure in an experimental model of chronic atrial fibrillation. Surface lead III and intra-atrial electrograms from 15 bipolar pairs from a 64-pole basket electrode are shown. Panel A shows the atrial fibrillation rhythm at baseline. The F-F intervals are irregular with very short cycle lengths. Early during linear atrial ablation (panel B), the rhythm organizes to a regular atrial tachycardia with a longer cycle length. This suggests the transition from a functional reentrant rhythm to an anatomically-based reentry. With further placement of linear ablative lesions, conversion of atrial tachycardia to sinus rhythm was observed. This persisted despite attempted atrial fibrillation induction with burst atrial pacing (panel C).

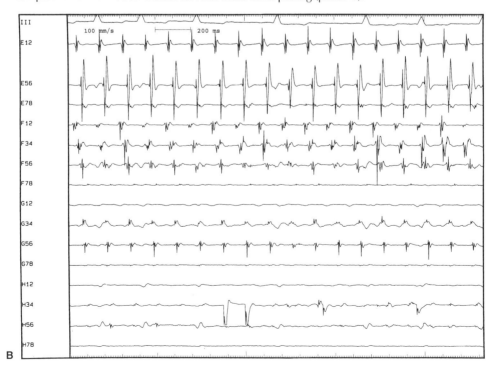

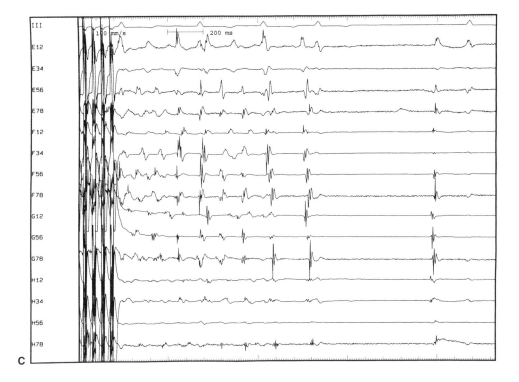

The atrial fibrillation model created with a combination of induced mitral regurgitation and high rate atrial pacing is associated with left atrial enlargement, probably as the consequence of chronic left atrial hypertension. The maintenance of atrial fibrillation does not appear to be dependent upon cholinergic stimulation, since it persists despite administration of atropine. Mitchell et al[59] reported their results of linear atrial ablation in this model using specially-designed radiofrequency ablation catheters that had 4–7 stainless steel coils, 8F in diameter, 12 mm in length, and one or 2 thermistors or thermocouples positioned at its midpoint or edge. The catheters were positioned along one of 3 targeted lines in the right atrium (between the superior and inferior vena cava, across the isthmus between the tricuspid annulus and inferior vena cava, and extending anteriorly from the crista terminalis across the pectinate muscles and intersecting the tricuspid annulus) and each of 5 targeted lines in the left atrium (transverse posterior and anterosuperior lines from the left atrial appendage base toward the septum, and lateral, posterior, and anterior vertical lines from the tricuspid annulus toward the appendage, pulmonary veins and anterior wall, respectively). At each catheter position, radiofrequency energy was delivered sequentially to selected electrodes via a MECA controller from a high power generator (150 watts RMS, EP Technologies, Inc., San Jose, CA). Power delivery was automatically controlled to maintain a present temperature of 70°C or 80°C. All ablations were initiated in the right atrium, then the left atrium. Ablation attempts were continued until all atrial reentrant arrhythmia had been terminated and could not be reinitiated with aggressive burst atrial pacing from both the left and right atria, or until the maximum procedure duration (10 hours) had been reached (Figure 6). The study evaluated

16 dogs: 11 in the ablation group and 5 in the control group. After the ablations, the dogs recovered and surviving animals underwent a follow-up electrophysiological study 13 ± 5 days later. The results of programmed atrial stimulation revealed sustained atrial fibrillation in 0 of 7 ablation dogs and 5 of 5 control dogs; and sustained atrial tachycardia in 2 of 7 ablation dogs and 1 of 5 control group. Of the 2 dogs with sustained atrial tachycardia, additional ablation was successful in one. Therefore, biatrial ablation was successful with no initiation of sustained atrial fibrillation or tachycardia in 6 of 7 surviving dogs. Of interest, at pathological examination discontinuity of the transmural lesions was often observed even in the setting of effective arrhythmia termination

Summary

The use of radiofrequency catheter ablation in treating atrial fibrillation is presently in its infancy but holds much promise. Several studies in both animal models and humans have demonstrated that this procedure can modify the arrhythmia in such a way that atrial fibrillation can be cured or significantly altered so that drug therapy is more effective. This technique provides AV synchrony and hemodynamic benefits and should lessen the risk of thromboembolism. It also has the advantage over the surgical Maze procedure in that it is less invasive and thereby can avert open-heart surgery.

However, before this technique can be widely applied many issues still remain: 1) Where are the ideal locations for ablation, and should different patient populations be treated differently (for instance, should mitral valve disease be treated primarily with left-sided ablations)? 2) Is the staged approach superior to an initial biatrial procedure? 3) Should intravascular ultrasound be routinely used to ensure location and tissue contact? 4) Should the lesions be based solely on anatomic positions or should there also be targeting based on an electrophysiological evaluation? 5) Will advancement in catheter and energy system design improve lesion continuity? 6) Will the safety issues such as prolonged procedural and fluoroscopy time and risk of thromboembolism from left atrial lesions be minimized as techniques and technology improve? 7) Ultimately, will there be a mortality benefit or cost from this procedure?

References

1. Ostrander LD Jr., Brandt RL, Kjelsberg MO, et al. Electrocardiographic findings among the adult population of a total natural community: Tecumseh, Michigan. *Circulation* 1965;31:888–898.
2. Brand FN, Abbott RD, Kannel WB, et al. Characteristics and prognosis of lone atrial fibrillation: 30-year follow-up in the Framingham Study. *JAMA* 1985;254:3449–3453.
3. Kopecky SL, Gersh BJ, McGoon MD, et al. The natural history of lone atrial fibrillation: a population-based study over 3 decades. *N Engl J Med* 1987;317:669–674.

4. Furberg CD, Psaty BM, Manolio TA, et al, for the CHS Collaborative Research Group. Prevalence of atrial fibrillation in elderly subjects (the Cardiovascular Health Study). *Am J Cardiol* 1994;74:236–241.

5. Prystowsky EN, Benson DW, Fuster V, et al. Management of patients with atrial fibrillation: a statement for healthcare professional from the Subcommittee on Electrocardiography and Electrophysiology, American Heart Association. *Circulation* 1996;93:1262–1277.

6. Cameron A, Schwartz MJ, Kronmal RA, et al. Prevalence and significance of atrial fibrillation in coronary artery disease (CASS registry). *Am J Cardiol* 1988;61:714–717.

7. Treseder AS, Sastry BSD, Thomas TPL, et al. Atrial fibrillation and stroke in elderly hospitalized patients. *Age Aging* 1986;15:89–92.

8. Homoud M, Foote CB, Estes NA III, et al. Atrioventricular junctional ablation and modification for atrial fibrillation. *Cardiol Clin* 1996;14:555–567.

9. Morady F, Hass C, Strickberger SA, et al. Long-term follow-up after radiofrequency modification of the artioventricular node in patients with atrial fibrillation. *J Am Coll Cardiol* 1997;29:113–121.

10. Lau CP, Tse HF, Lok NS, et al. Initial clinical experience with an implantable human atrial defibrillator. *PACE* 1997;20:220–225.

11. Saksena S, Prakash A, Hill M, et al. Prevention of recurrent atrial fibrillation with chronic dual-site right atrial pacing. *J Am Coll Cardiol* 1996;28: 687–694.

12. Moe GK, Rheinboldt WC, Abildshov JA. A computer model of atrial fibrillation. *Am Heart J* 1964;67:200–220.

13. Allessie MA, Rensma PL, Brugada J, et al. Pathophysiology of atrial fibrillation. In: Zipes DP, Jalife J, eds. *Cardiac Electrophysiology: From Cell to Bedside*. Philadelphia, PA: WB Saunders, 1990. pp 548–549.

14. Goette A, Honeycutt C, Langberg JJ. Electrical remodeling in atrial fibrillation: time course and mechanisms. *Circulation* 1996;94:2968–2974.

15. Tieleman RG, De Langen CDJ, Van Gelder IC, et al. Verapamil reduces tachycardia-induced electrical remodeling of the atria. *Circulation* 1997;95: 1945–1953.

16. Elvan A, Wylie K, Zipes DP. Pacing-induced chronic atrial fibrillation impairs sinus node function in dogs: electrophysiological remodeling. *Circulation* 1996;94:2953–2960.

17. Morillo CA, Klein GJ, Jones DL, et al. Chronic rapid atrial pacing: structural, functional, and electrophysiological characteristics of new model of sustained atrial fibrillation. *Circulation* 1995;91:1588–1595.

18. Wijffels MCEF, Kirchhof CJHJ, Dorland R, et al. Atrial fibrillation begets atrial fibrillation: a study in awake chronically instrumented goats. *Circulation* 1995;92:1954–1968.

19. Elvan A, Huang X, Pressler ML, et al. Radiofrequency catheter ablation of the atria eliminates pacing-induced sustained atrial fibrillation and reduces connexin 43 in dogs. *Circulation* 1997;1675–1685.

20. Cox JL, Schuessler RB, Cain ME, et al. Surgery for atrial fibrillation. *Sem Thorac Cardiovasc Surg* 1989;1:67–73.

21. Cox JL. The surgical treatment of atrial fibrillation IV: surgical technique. *J Thorac Cardiovasc Surg* 1991;101:584–592.

22. Cox JL, Boineau JP, Schuessler RB, et al. Modification of the Maze procedure for atrial flutter and atrial fibrillation I: rationale and surgical results. *J Thorac Cardiovasc Surg* 1995;110:473–484.

23. Cox JL, Jaquiss RDB, Schuessler RB, et al. Modification of the Maze procedure for atrial flutter and atrial fibrillation II: surgical technique of the Maze-III procedure. *J Thorac Cardiovasc Surg* 1995;110:485–495.

24. Kamata J, Kawazoe K, Izumoto H, et al. Predictors of sinus rhythm restoration after Cox-Maze procedure concomitant with other cardiac operations. *Ann Thorac Surg* 1997;64:394–398.

25. Cox JL, Schuessler RB, Lappas DG, et al. An 81/2 -year clinical experience with surgery for atrial fibrillation. *Ann Surg* 1996;224:267–273.

26. Sueda T, Nagata H, Orihashi K, et al. Efficacy of a simple left atrial procedure for chronic atrial fibrillation in mitral valve operations. *Ann Thorac Surg* 1997;63:1070–1075.

27. Kawaguchi AT, Kosakai Y, Sasako Y, et al. Risks and benefits of combined Maze procedure for atrial fibrillation associated with organic heart disease. *J Am Coll Cardiol* 1996;28:985–990.

28. Swartz JF, Pellersels G, Silvers J, et al. A catheter-based curative approach to atrial fibrillation in humans [abstract]. *Circulation* 1994;90:I-335.

29. Olgin J, Kalman J, Maguire M, et al. Electrophysiologic effects of long linear atrial lesions placed under intracardiac echo guidance. *PACE* 1996;19: 581.

30. Epstein LM, Mitchell MA, Smith TW, et al. A comparative study of fluoroscopy and intracardiac echocardiographic guidance for the creation of linear artial lesions. *Circulation* 1998;98(17):1796–1801.

31. Pappone C, Rillo M, Lamberti F, et al. New technique to create and verify continuity of long radiofrequency lesions in patients with atrial fibrillation [abstract]. *J Am Coll Cardiol* 1998:31;62A.

32. Kuck KH, Ernst S, Khanedani A, et al. Clinical follow-up after primary catheter ablation of atrial fibrillation using the CARTO system [abstract]. *PACE* 1998;21:868.

33. Haines DE, McRury ID, Whayne JG, et al. Atrial radiofrequency ablation: the use of a novel deploying loop catheter design to create long linear lesions [abstract]. *Circulation* 1994;90:I-335.

34. Avitall B, Helms RW, Chiang W, et al. Technology and method for the creation of left atrial endocardial linear lesions to ablate atrial fibrillation [abstract]. *J Am Coll Cardiol* 1996;27:400A.

35. Whayne JG, Haines DE, Panescu D, et al. Catheter system designs to facilitate RF ablation of atrial fibrillation [abstract]. *PACE* 1996;19:650.

36. Panescu D, Haines DE, Fleischman SD, et al. Atrial lesions by temperature-controlled radiofrequency ablation [abstract]. *Circulation* 1996;94:I-493.

37. McRury ID, Panescu D, Mitchell MA, et al. Nonuniform heating during radiofrequency catheter ablation with long electrodes: monitoring the edge effect. *Circulation* 1997;96:4057–4064.

38. Avitall B, Hare J, Mughal K, et al. A catheter system to ablate atrial fibrillation in a sterile pericarditis dog model [abstract]. *PACE* 1994;17(Part II):774.

39. Liese KS, Roithinger FX, Goseki Y, et al. Enhanced tissue contact using an expandable multi-electrode catheter for generating transmural biatrial RF lesions [abstract]. *PACE* 1998;(Part II):923.

40. Wharton M, Tommassoni G, Pomeranz M, et al. Saline perfused balloon radiofrequency ablation catheter for creation of linear transmural atrial lesions [abstract]. *Circulation* 1996;94:I493.

41. Kalman JM, Olgin JE, Karch MR, et al. Use of intracardiac echocardiography in interventional electrophysiology. *PACE* 1997;20(Part I):2248–2262.

42. Kalman JM, Fitzpatrick AP, Olgin JE, et al. Are linear lesions needed in both atria to prevent atrial fibrillation in a canine model? [abstract] *Circulation* 1996;94:I558.

43. Kalman JM, Fitzpatrick AP, Olgin JE, et al. Biophysical characteristics of radiofrequency lesion formation in vivo: dynamics of catheter tip-tissue contact evaluated by intracardiac echocardiography. *Am Heart J* 1997;133:8–18.

44. Olgin JE, Kalman JM, Chin M, et al. Electrophysiological effects of long, linear atrial lesions placed under intracardiac ultrasound guidance. *Circulation* 1997;96:2715–2721.

45. Khong A, Nademanee K, Kosar E, et al. Does nonfluoroscopic 3-D mapping aid arrhythmia ablation? [abstract] *PACE* 1998;21(Part II):923.

46. Man KC, Daoud E, Knight B, et al. Right atrial radiofrequency catheter ablation of paroxysmal atrial fibrillation [abstract]. *J Am Coll Cardiol* 1996; 27:188A.

47. Natale A, Tomassoni G, Kearney MM, et al. Catheter ablation approach on the right side only for paroxysmal atrial fibrillation therapy [abstract]. *Circulation* 1995;92:I266.

48. Riccardi R, Lamberti F, Scaglione M, et al. Vagal atrial fibrillation: atrial mapping and effectiveness of right atrial catheter ablation [abstract]. *Circulation* 1996;94:I675.

49. Haïssaguerre M, Jais P, Shah DC, et al. Right and left atrial radiofrequency catheter therapy in paroxysmal atrial fibrillation. *J Cardiovasc Electrophys* 1996;7:1132–1144.

50. Haines DE, Langberg JJ, Lesh MD, et al. Catheter ablation of atrial fibrillation using the multiple electrode catheter ablation (MECA) system: preliminary clinical trial results [abstract]. *PACE* 1998;21(Part II):832.

51. Gaita F, Riccardi R, Scaglione M, et al. Atrial mapping and effectiveness of a right atrial catheter ablation in patients with vagal atrial fibrillation [abstract]. *J Am Coll Cardiol* 1997;29:176A.

52. Feld G, Birgersdotter-Green U, Fijumura O, et al. Radiofrequency catheter ablation of the right atrium for control of atrial fibrillation refractory to antiarrhythmic drugs [abstract]. *J Am Coll Cardiol* 1997;29:176A.

53. Jais P, Haïssaguerre M, Shah D, et al. Catheter ablation for paroxysmal atrial fibrillation: high success rates with ablation in the left atrium [abstract]. *Circulation* 1996;94:I675.

54. Maloney JD, Chodimella, Sabe A, et al. Biatrial linear and focal ablation for restoring sinus rhythm in patients with refractory atrial fibrillation: initial experience with a two-stage procedure [abstract]. *J Am Coll Cardiol* 1997;29:176A.

55. Morillo CA, Klein GJ, Jones DL, et al. Chronic rapid atrial pacing: struc-

tural, functional, and electrophysiological characteristics of a new model of sustained atrial fibrillation. *Circulation* 1995;91:1588–1595.

56. Wijffels MCEF, Kirchlof CJHJ, Dorland R, et al. Atrial fibrillation begets atrial fibrillation: a study in awake chronically instrumented goats. *Circulation* 1995;92:1954–1968.

57. Page PL, Plumb VJ, Okumaur K, et al. A new model of atrial flutter. *J Am Coll Cardiol* 1986;8:872–879.

58. Cox JL, Canavan TE, Schuessler RB, et al. The surgical treatment of atrial fibrillation II: intraoperative electrophysiologic mapping and description of the electrophysiologic basis of atrial fibrillation. *J Thorac Cardiovasc Surg* 1991;101:406–426.

59. Mitchell MA, McRury ID, Haines DE. Linear atrial ablations in a canine model of chronic atrial fibrillation: morphologic and electrophysiologic observations. *Circulation* 1998;97:1176–1185.

60. Elvan A, Pride H, Eble J, et al. Radiofrequency catheter ablation of the atria reduces inducibility and duration of atrial fibrillation in dogs. *Circulation* 1995;91:2235–2244.

Part IV

Radiofrequency Catheter Ablation of Atrioventricular Nodal Reentrant Tachycardia

Chapter 20

Evolving Concepts of Atrioventricular Nodal Reentrant Tachycardia: Insights into the Anatomy and Physiology

Delon Wu, M.D., Yasuhiro Taniguchi, M.D., Ming-Shien Wen, M.D.

When Mines introduced the concept of reentry in 1913, he implied that reentry might be responsible for some cases of paroxysmal tachycardia in humans.[1] Reciprocal rhythm or circus contraction was considered to be the basis for auricular paroxysmal tachycardia in the 1920s.[2] In 1943, Barker et al first suggested that circus movement involving the atrioventricular (AV) node might be the mechanism of supraventricular tachycardia.[3] The first evidence that the AV node may dissociate functionally into 2 pathways was provided by Moe et al in animal studies including dogs, turtles, cats, and sheep in 1956.[4] In their study, the ventriculo-atrial (VA) propagation times were plotted against the coupling intervals of the premature ventricular stimulation, which showed that as the coupling interval of the premature impulse was shortened, the VA interval lengthened progressively until a critical coupling interval when a sudden prolongation of the VA interval was noted. The VA interval remained long as the coupling interval was shortened further. Reciprocating beats or echoes were noted when the premature stimulus was propagated with a long VA interval at short coupling intervals. They postulated a dual AV transmission system with a fast (β-pathway) and a slow (α-pathway) pathway. The fast pathway has a faster conduction time and a longer refractory period, while the slow pathway has a slower conduction time but recovers earlier than the fast pathway. Therefore, when a premature impulse arrives at a critical time, the fast pathway may be blocked and the impulse conducts through the slow pathway.

From Huang SKS, Wilber DJ (eds.): *Radiofrequency Catheter Ablation of Cardiac Arrhythmias: Basic Concepts and Clinical Applications,* 2nd ed. Armonk, NY: Futura Publishing Company, Inc. ©2000.

The impulse then returns in a retrograde fashion from the distal (relative to the origin of the impulse) fast pathway and echoes back to the chamber of origin. Subsequent macroelectrophysiological and microelectrophysiological studies in animals have provided evidence confirming the presence of a dual AV nodal conducting system that causes reciprocating responses.[5-12]

The first evidence of dual AV nodal pathways in humans was provided by Kistin in 1962.[13] Through analysis of electrocardiogram with simultaneous recording of the esophageal lead in 82 patients with ventricular premature beats, he noted that in many patients, the ventricular response following the interpolated premature ventricular beat was not from the sinus impulse but from the reciprocating impulse. He also noted 2 ranges of VA conduction time suggestive of dual AV nodal pathways in some patients. In addition, 2 ranges of PR interval in reciprocal ventricular beats, suggesting the presence of multiple AV nodal pathways, were noted in 2 patients. In 1968, Schuilenburg and Durrer delivered atrial extrastimulus to a patient with atrial septal defect and plotted ventricular responses against the atrial coupling intervals (A_1A_2, V_1V_2 curve). They found double discontinuities of the conduction curve with 3 types of atrial echoes, suggesting the presence of triple pathways.[14] One year later, they reported ventricular extrastimulus studies in 3 patients that showed a sudden prolongation of VA interval associated with the occurrence of reciprocating ventricular echo when V_1V_2 was propagated with a long VA interval.[15] Electrical induction and termination of supraventricular tachycardia were first described by Moe et al in 1963 in a dog.[16] In humans, Hunt et al[17] and Lister et al[18] reported successful termination of supraventricular tachycardia by rapid atrial pacing in the late 1960s. Gettes and Yoshonis observed spontaneous initiation of supraventricular tachycardia by a premature atrial beat that was associated with a long PR interval.[19] Bigger and Goldreyer induced supraventricular tachycardia by delivery of atrial premature stimulation in patients without Wolff-Parkinson-White syndrome in 1970.[20]

The above observations suggest that reentry is likely to be the mechanism of tachycardia. However, the site of reentry was not precisely localized. In 1971, Goldreyer and Bigger, using His bundle recording and atrial extrastimulus testing, localized the site of reentry in the AV node in several patients with supraventricular tachycardia.[21] Goldreyer and Damato further demonstrated that a critical delay (critical AH interval) is necessary for induction of AV nodal reentrant tachycardia (AVNRT).[22] The spectra of dual AV nodal pathway phenomena were subsequently described by Rosen, Denes, Wu, and their coworkers as well as other investigators in the 1970s and 1980s.[23-30] These phenomena include:

1) discontinuous anterograde or retrograde conduction curve (A_1A_2, A_2H_2 curve or V_1V_2, A_1A_2 curve);
2) 2 ranges of conduction intervals (2 ranges of nonoverlapping PR, AH intervals or VA intervals);
3) shift of atrial activation sequence with or without simultaneous shift in conduction time during incremental ventricular pacing or programmed stimulation;
4) double His bundle and ventricular responses to a single atrial impulse due to simultaneous conduction through the 2 pathways;
5) AVNRT

Anterograde Dual AV Nodal Pathways

In 1973, Denes et al demonstrated a discontinuous AV conduction curve in 2 patients with normal PR interval and paroxysmal supraventricular tachycardia.[23] Using His bundle recording and atrial extrastimulus testing techniques, they plotted A_2H_2 responses and H_1H_2 responses against A_1A_2 coupling intervals and found that at a critical A_1A_2 interval, a sudden jump of A_2H_2 and, thus, H_1H_2 response was noted. Further shortening of A_1A_2 interval resulted in a second A_1A_2, A_2H_2 or A_1A_2, H_1H_2 curve. The curve before the jump was defined as the fast pathway and that after the slow pathway (Figure 1). Induction

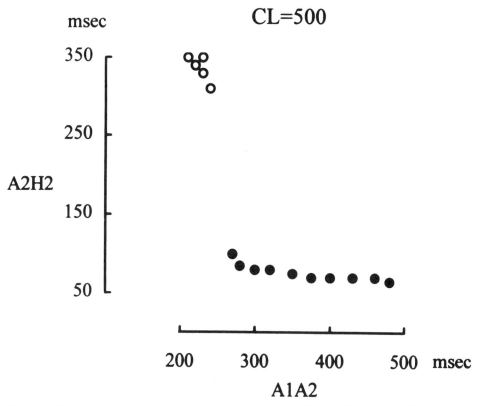

Figure 1. AV conduction curve of a patient showing dual AV nodal pathways. The A_2H_2 responses were plotted against the A_1A_2 coupling intervals at an atrial paced cycle length of 500 milliseconds. Note that as the A_1A_2 intervals were shortened from 480 to 250 milliseconds, A_2H_2 responses increased from 65 to 120 milliseconds. A sudden jump of the A_2H_2 from 120 to 310 milliseconds was noted as the A_1A_2 was shortened from 250 of 240 milliseconds. When the A_1A_2 was shortened further, the A_2H_2 remained prolonged. AV nodal reentrant echoes and tachycardia were induced when the A_2 was conducted with a long A_2H_2 response. The curve before the jump was defined as the fast pathway conduction curve, and that after the slow pathway conduction curve. The effective refractory period of the fast pathway was, therefore, 240 milliseconds, and the slow pathway 210 milliseconds. The echo zone was defined at A_1A_2 between 220 and 240 milliseconds, and was consistent with the whole slow pathway conduction curve. The critical AH interval for induction of AV nodal reentrant echoes or tachycardia was 310 milliseconds. CL = cycle length; close circles = responses without echoes or tachycardia; open circles = responses with echoes or tachycardia.

of echoes or tachycardia was noted when conduction shifted to the slow pathway (Figure 2). Subsequent studies have shown that an overlap of the fast pathway and the slow pathway curve is frequently noted, and 2 sets of conduction properties can be defined from the conduction curves.[29] The effective refractory period of the fast pathway is the longest A_1A_2 that is blocked in the fast pathway, and that of the slow pathway the longest A_1A_2 that is blocked in the slow pathway. The slow pathway effective refractory period is therefore equal to that of the AV node. AV nodal reentrant echo or tachycardia is induced when anterograde fast pathway conduction fails resulting in conduction through the slow pathway, that achieves a sufficient delay (a critical AH interval) to allow recovery of the blocked fast pathway for reexcitation.

The dual pathway conduction curve can be demonstrated in the majority of patients with AVNRT when careful study is performed.[29,30] The reported incidence of dual pathway AV conduction curve varies from 10–46% in patients with or without paroxysmal supraventricular tachycardia.[31–35] Demonstration of dual pathway conduction curve requires a longer effective refractory period of the fast pathway than that of the slow pathway and the atrial functional refractory period as well as a sufficient difference in conduction time between the 2 pathways. If the effective refractory period of the fast pathway is shorter than that of the slow pathway or the conduction time of the 2 pathways is not sufficiently different, a discontinuous A_1A_2, A_2H_2 curve will not be demonstrated. The effective refractory period and the conduction times of the 2 pathways are influenced by several physiological and pharmacological factors. Both the effective refractory period and the conduction time of the fast and the slow pathway increase with shortening of cycle length and thus demonstration of dual pathway curve may become possible with changes in driven cycle length.[28,31,36,37] In general, it is easier to demonstrate a discontinuous A_1A_2, A_2H_2 curve at a shorter driven cycle length, although it may require a delivery of 2 atrial extrastimuli in some patients. Atropine[24,37,38] and isoproterenol[39–41] shorten the conduction time and the effective refractory period of both pathways and may make demonstration of the dual pathway curve more difficult; β-blockers,[36] calcium blockers,[42–44] or digitalis[45–47] increase the conduction time and the effective refractory period of both pathways and, therefore, may unmask dual AV nodal pathways. Class I antiarrhythmic agents tend to shorten the conduction time and the effective refractory period of both pathways due to an indirect vagolytic effect.[48–50]

Dual AV nodal pathways can also be demonstrated during incremental atrial pacing by plotting the AA, AH curve.[28,29] The AH interval increases with shortening of atrial paced cycle length. At a critical paced cycle length, the atrial impulse may encounter the effective refractory period of the fast pathway and conducts through the slow pathway. If the slow pathway conduction delay is insufficient to allow the recovery of the blocked fast pathway for reexcitation and is capable of repetitive conduction, slow pathway conduction will sustain at this paced cycle length. Plotting of AA, AH curve will display a discontinuous curve. Otherwise, an atypical Wenckebach periodicity with or without induction of AVNRT will result. Atypical Wenckebach periodicity with a sudden increment of AH interval in the middle or terminal portion of the pacing induced Wenckebach period can be demonstrated in almost every patient with a discontinuous A_1A_2, A_2H_2 curve.[23,29,36]

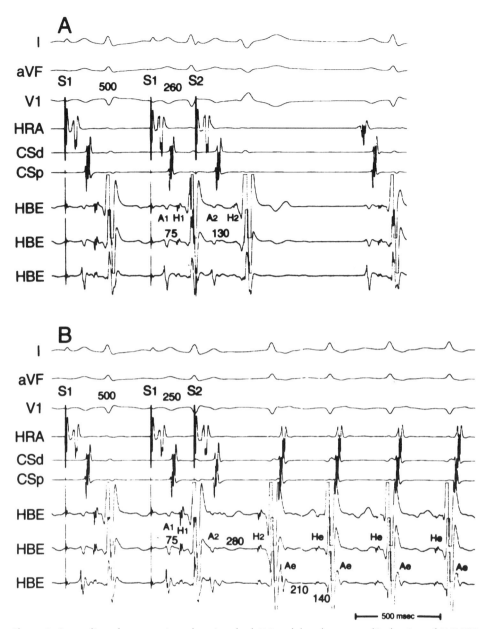

Figure 2. Recordings from a patient showing dual AV nodal pathways and induction of AVNRT. In both panels A and B, the atria were paced at a cycle length of 500 milliseconds with an AH of 75 milliseconds. In A, an atrial extrastimulus was delivered at a coupling interval of 260 milliseconds, and was conducted through the fast pathway with an AH of 130 milliseconds. In B, an atrial extrastimulus was delivered earlier at a coupling interval of 250 milliseconds, and was blocked in the fast pathway and conducted through the slow pathway with an AH of 280 milliseconds, resulting in induction of AVNRT. The tachycardia had a cycle length of 350 milliseconds, an AH of 210 milliseconds, and an HA of 140 milliseconds. The earliest atrial activation during tachycardia was registered from the ostium of the coronary sinus, and the P wave occurred slightly after the QRS complex. I, AVF & V$_1$ = surface ECG lead I, AVF & V$_1$; HRA, CSd, CSp & HBE = bipolar electrogram recorded from the high right atrium, the distal 2 electrodes of the coronary sinus catheter that was positioned inside of the coronary sinus, the proximal 2 electrodes of the coronary sinus catheter that was positioned at the ostium the coronary sinus, and the His bundle recording site. A$_1$ & H$_1$ = low septal right atrial and His bundle responses to the sinus or the basic paced beat; A$_2$ & H$_2$ = low septal right atrial and His bundle responses to the extrastimulus; Ae & He = low septal right atrial and His bundle responses during AV nodal reentrant echoes or tachycardia; S$_1$ & S$_2$ = stimulus artifact of the basic paced and the extrastimulus beat.

Less commonly, patients with dual AV nodal pathways may manifest with 2 ranges of nonoverlapping PR interval during sinus rhythm or 2 ranges of nonoverlapping AH interval during atrial pacing.[24,26,28,29,51] Manifestation of 2 PR intervals during sinus rhythm or 2 AH intervals at an identical cycle length during atrial pacing depends on a long effective refractory period of the fast pathway relative to the cycle length of sinus rhythm or atrial pacing, and a long retrograde effective refractory period of the fast pathway. Conduction with a short PR or AH interval reflects fast pathway conduction, while conduction with a long PR or AH interval reflects slow pathway conduction. Shift from short PR to long PR interval or vice versa is usually initiated by premature atrial or ventricular beats. When a premature atrial beat falls upon the effective refractory period of the fast pathway during sinus rhythm with fast pathway conduction and a short PR interval, the impulse will be blocked in the fast pathway and so conducts through the slow pathway resulting in a long PR interval. Repetitive retrograde concealed conduction to the blocked fast pathway will keep the anterograde fast pathway refractory and maintains the slow pathway conduction. Sustained slow pathway conduction with a long PR interval or a long AH interval also requires a long retrograde effective refractory period of the fast pathway; otherwise, AV nodal reentrant echoes or tachycardia will occur and a long PR or AH interval will not result. Resumption of fast pathway conduction during sustained slow pathway conduction can be initiated by a premature atrial or ventricular beat that produces a block in the anterograde slow pathway. Manifestation of 2 ranges of AH intervals is frequently demonstrated in patients with a discontinuous A_1A_2, A_2H_2 curve, when a special pacing technique is applied.[28] Thus, at a critical atrial paced cycle length, sustained slow pathway conduction may result when the first paced beat falls within the effective refractory period of the fast pathway. Sustenance of slow pathway conduction also requires an ability of the slow pathway for repetitive conduction otherwise fast pathway conduction will resume immediately.

Rarely, patients with dual AV nodal pathways may manifest with simultaneous fast and slow pathway conduction, resulting in double His bundle and ventricular responses to a single atrial impulse (Figure 3).[25,29,52,53] This phenomenon usually occurs during rapid atrial pacing. It was suggested that pacing induced Type I block in both pathways has put these 2 pathways out of phase so that the distal conduction system and the ventricles are able to respond to both the fast and the slow pathway impulses. Usually, the impulse from the slow pathway is sufficiently prolonged so that the retrograde fast pathway is capable of reexcitation and AV nodal reentrant echoes or tachycardia is the result. The occurrence of simultaneous fast and slow pathway conduction depends on a unidirectional block of the retrograde slow pathway, otherwise the anterograde fast pathway impulse will enter the distal slow pathway and collide with the oncoming slow pathway impulse. Intermittent second degree block in the 2 pathways associated with intermittent simultaneous fast and slow pathway conduction and aberrant conduction may produce a very complex tachyarrhythmia pattern clinically.[54,55] Nonetheless, it should be cautioned that pseudo-simultaneous fast and slow pathway conduction is a very common phenomenon during rapid atrial pacing.[56] Under such circumstances, the paced atrial impulses conduct through the slow pathway with a prolonged

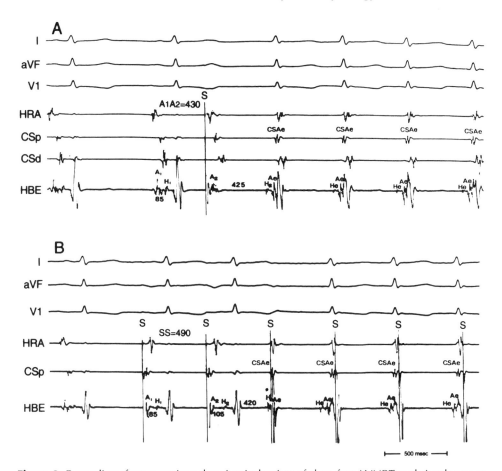

Figure 3. Recordings from a patient showing induction of slow-fast AVNRT and simultaneous fast and slow pathway conduction. In A, tachycardia was induced following delivery of an atrial extrastimulus at a coupling interval of 430 milliseconds during sinus rhythm. The AH interval of the sinus beat was 85 milliseconds. The atrial extrastimulus was blocked in the fast pathway and conducted through the slow pathway with an AH of 425 milliseconds, resulting in induction of the slow-fast AVNRT. In B, simultaneous fast and slow pathway conduction occurred at the beginning of atrial pacing with a cycle length of 490 milliseconds. The first paced beat was conducted through the fast pathway with an AH of 85 milliseconds, while the second paced beat was followed by 2 His bundle responses. The first His bundle response had an AH of 105 milliseconds, and the second 420 milliseconds. The second His bundle response was blocked in the His-Purkinje system and was not conducted to the ventricles, but was followed by initiation of a slow-fast AVNRT. Note that during tachycardia, the earliest atrial activation was registered from the His bundle recording site and was occurring slightly before the QRS complex. H_2* = second His bundle response to the second atrial paced beat; CSAe = atrial responses during tachycardia recorded at the ostium of the coronary sinus; S = stimulus artifact.

AH interval, so that the last paced atrial beat falls before the His bundle response of the preceding paced beat and is followed by 2 His bundle and ventricular responses. The last response is then followed by induction of AV nodal reentrant echoes or tachycardia, mimicking simultaneous fast and slow pathway conduction.

Retrograde Dual AV Nodal Pathways

In 1977, Wu et al demonstrated a discontinuous V_1V_2, A_1A_2 curve suggestive of retrograde dual pathways in 3 patients with paroxysmal supraventricular tachycardia.[27] Ventricular echoes were induced simultaneously when a sudden increment of VA interval occurred at a critical V_1V_2 interval (Figure 4 and Figure 5). These echoes have a reversed circuit using the slow pathway for retrograde and the fast pathway for anterograde conduction. As in patients

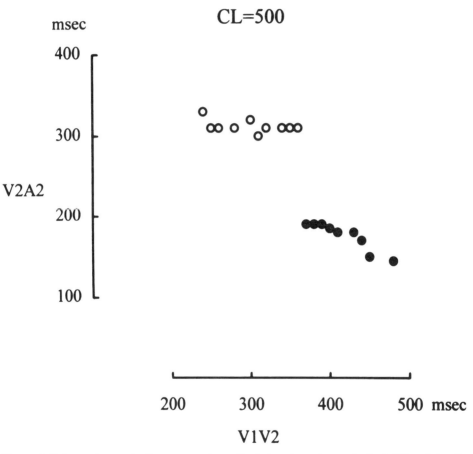

Figure 4. Retrograde conduction curve of a patient showing retrograde dual AV nodal pathways. The V_2A_2 responses were plotted against the V_1V_2 coupling intervals at a ventricular paced cycle length of 500 milliseconds. As the V_1V_2 intervals were shortened from 480 to 370 milliseconds, the V_2A_2 responses prolonged from 140 to 190 milliseconds; a sudden increment of V_2A_2 was noted at V_1V_2 of 360 milliseconds. When V_1V_2 was shortened further, V_2A_2 remained prolonged. AV nodal reentrant echoes and tachycardia were induced when V_1V_2 was responded with a long V_2A_2 interval. The curve before the sudden increment of V_2A_2 was the fast pathway conduction curve, and that after the slow pathway conduction curve. The effective refractory period of the fast pathway was 360 milliseconds, and the slow pathway 230 milliseconds.

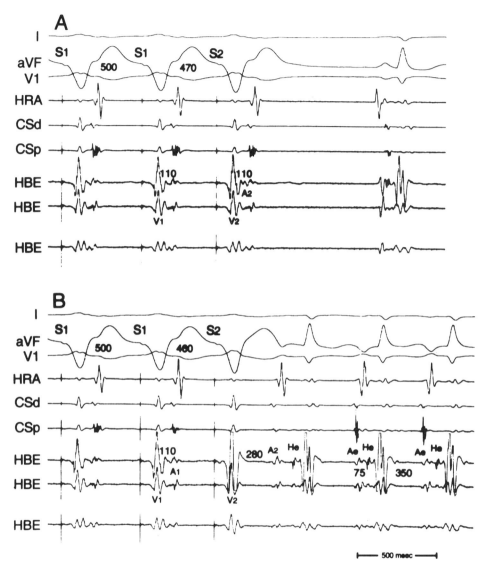

Figure 5. Recordings from a patient showing retrograde dual AV nodal pathways and the fast-slow form AVNRT. In both panels A and B, the ventricles were paced at a cycle length of 500 milliseconds with a VA of 110 milliseconds. In A, a ventricular extrastimulus was delivered at a coupling interval of 470 milliseconds, and was conducted to the atria through the fast pathway with a VA interval of 110 milliseconds; the earliest atrial activation was registered at the His bundle recording site. In B, a ventricular extrastimulus was delivered earlier at a coupling interval of 460 milliseconds, and was blocked in the fast pathway and conducted to the atria through the slow pathway with a VA interval of 280 milliseconds, resulting in induction of a reversed type of fast-slow AVNRT. The tachycardia had a cycle length of 425 milliseconds, an AH of 75 milliseconds, and an HA of 350 milliseconds. The earliest atrial activation during tachycardia was registered from the coronary sinus, and the P wave occurred in front of the QRS complex. V_1 & V_2 = ventricular responses to the basic paced beat and to the extrastimulus.

with anterograde dual AV nodal pathways, retrograde atypical Wenckebach periodicity was noted during rapid ventricular pacing. A discontinuous V_1V_2, A_1A_2 curve is frequently seen in patients with a clinical history of paroxysmal supraventricular tachycardia and a discontinuous A_1A_2, A_2H_2 curve, but without induction of AV nodal reentrant echo or tachycardia.[38,57] These patients have an increased retrograde fast pathway refractoriness and, therefore, induction of echoes or tachycardia may become possible after administration of atropine or isoproterenol, which improves the retrograde fast pathway conduction. Discontinuity of V_1V_2, A_1A_2 curves usually disappears after atropine or isoproterenol in these patients. A discontinuous V_1V_2, A_1A_2 curve may also be demonstrated in patients with dual pathway AVNRT following administration of a class I antiarrhythmic agent that depresses the retrograde fast pathway conduction.[48–50]

An important observation was made by Sung et al in 1981.[58] They noted a difference in retrograde atrial activation sequence depending on whether conduction utilizes the fast or the slow pathway. Retrograde fast pathway conduction is characterized by an earliest atrial activation occurring at the low right atrial septum at the His bundle recording site, while retrograde slow pathway conduction is characterized by the earliest atrial activation occurring at the ostium of the coronary sinus (see Figure 5).

Multiple AV Nodal Pathways

The possibility of multiple AV nodal pathways in humans was first suggested by Kistin in 1962.[13] He noted 2 ranges of PR intervals in reciprocating ventricular echo beats suggesting the presence of triple pathways. Schuilenburg and Durrer noted double discontinuities associated with 3 types of reciprocating atrial echoes suggesting the presence of triple AV nodal pathways in a patient with atrial septal defect.[14] Subsequently, triple or quadruple A_1A_2, A_2H_2 curves, suggestive of triple or multiple pathways, have been described from several laboratories.[59–63] However, the presence of multiple pathways in these patients was usually not supported by other evidence; therefore, whether or not multiple discontinuities in these patients indeed reflected conduction through different pathways cannot be ascertained. Spurrel et al[64] reported alternating AH intervals during tachycardia in a patient, suggesting 2 anterograde pathways and a common retrograde pathway. McGuire et al[65] noted differences in VA intervals, atrial activation sequence, and cycle length of tachycardia in 3 patients exhibiting 2 types of AVNRT. Wu et al[66] demonstrated 3 different types of retrograde pathways in 7 patients with multiple AVNRT. In these patients, the fast pathway had the earliest atrial activation at the His bundle area (Figure 6, panel A), the intermediate pathway had the earliest atrial activation at the ostium of the coronary sinus (Figure 7, panel B), and the slow pathway had the earliest atrial activation at the ostium of the coronary sinus (see Figure 6, panel B and Figure 7, panel A). These observations strongly support the existence of multiple AV nodal pathways.

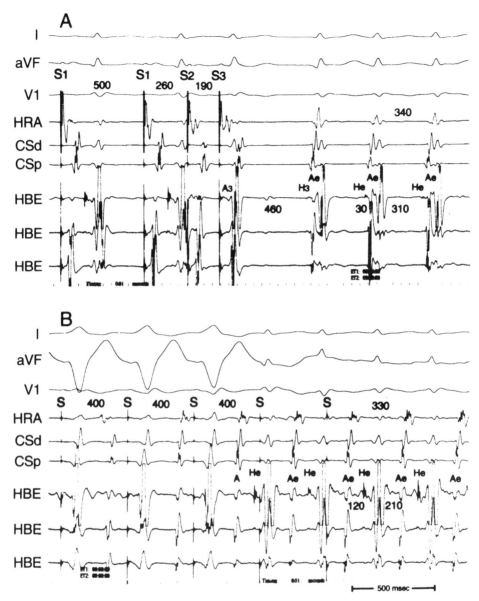

Figure 6. Recordings from a patient showing slow-fast and fast-slow AVNRTs. In A, slow-fast tachycardia was induced by delivery of 2 atrial extrastimuli to an atrial paced cycle length of 500 milliseconds. The coupling interval of the first extrastimulus was 260 milliseconds, and the second 190 milliseconds. The second extrastimulus was blocked in the fast pathway and conducted through the slow pathway with an AH of 460 milliseconds and induction of the slow-fast AVNRT. The tachycardia had a cycle length of 340 milliseconds, an AH of 310 milliseconds, and an HA of 30 milliseconds. The earliest atrial activation during tachycardia was registered simultaneously from the His bundle recording site and the ostium of the coronary sinus, and occurred slightly before the QRS complex. In B, a fast-slow AVNRT was induced by rapid ventricular pacing at a cycle length of 400 milliseconds. The ventricular paced stimulus was conducted to the atria through the slow pathway and the tachycardia was induced following cessation of the pacing. The tachycardia had a cycle length of 330 milliseconds, an AH of 120 milliseconds, and an HA of 210 milliseconds. The earliest atrial activation was recorded simultaneously from the His bundle catheter and the ostium of the coronary sinus. A_3 and H_3 = low septal right atrial and His bundle responses to the second extrastimulus; S_3 = stimulus artifact of the second extrastimulus.

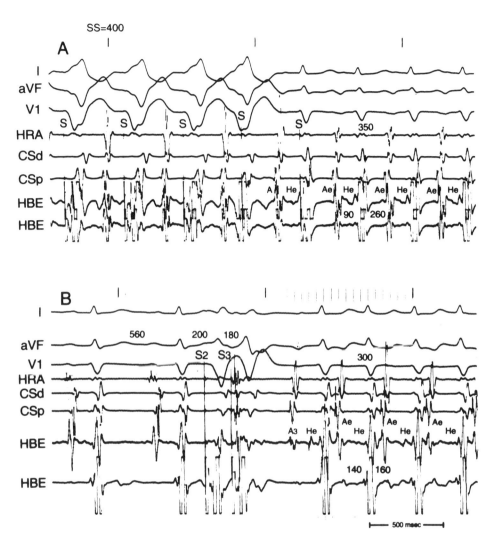

Figure 7. Recordings from a patient showing fast-slow and fast-intermediate AVNRTs. In A, a fast-slow tachycardia was induced following cessation of rapid ventricular pacing at a cycle length of 400 milliseconds; the last ventricular beat was a catheter induced premature beat. These ventricular beats were conducted to the atria through the slow pathway. The tachycardia had a cycle length of 350 milliseconds, an AH of 90 milliseconds, and an HA of 260 milliseconds. The earliest atrial activation during tachycardia was registered from the ostium of the coronary sinus. In B, a fast-intermediate tachycardia was induced by delivery of 2 ventricular extrastimuli during sinus rhythm. The sinus cycle length was 560 milliseconds, and the coupling interval of the first extrastimulus was 200 milliseconds and the second 180 milliseconds. The second ventricular extrastimulus was conducted to the atria through the slow pathway. The tachycardia had a cycle length of 300 milliseconds, an AH of 140 milliseconds, and an HA of 160 milliseconds. The earliest atrial activation during tachycardia was registered from the ostium of the coronary sinus.

Atrioventricular Nodal Reentrant Tachycardia

The most common form of AVNRT is the slow-fast form that utilizes a slow pathway for anterograde and a fast pathway for retrograde conduction.[23,29,30,32,33] The tachycardia is induced by delivery of atrial extrastimulus with a definable echo zone. It is also inducible with rapid atrial pacing during the atypical Wenckebach periodicity when anterograde block occurs in the fast pathway and conduction shifts to the slow pathway. Anterograde slow pathway conduction alone is not sufficient for induction of tachycardia. A critical delay in the slow pathway (reflected as the critical AH interval) is necessary to allow recovery of the blocked fast pathway for reexcitation.[22] The critical AH interval is not a fixed interval; it may change with changes in atrial driven cycle length, changes in sympathetic tone, or after drug administration. Slow-fast form of AVNRT may also be induced retrogradely by delivery of ventricular extrastimulus or with rapid ventricular pacing.[67] Retrograde induction of the slow-fast tachycardia is dependent on a block in the distal slow pathway and, therefore, is frequently limited by the refractoriness of the His-Purkinje system. It also requires a longer retrograde effective refractory period of the slow pathway than the fast pathway, as well as a sufficient delay in the circuit, which includes the retrograde fast pathway and the anterograde slow pathway conduction, otherwise the tachycardia cannot be induced.

The average heart rate during tachycardia is 169±28 beats per minute.[68] The atria are activated before, simultaneously with, or slightly after the QRS complex, depending on the conduction time from the distal link to the His bundle and to the atria (see Figure 2, Figure 3, and Figure 6, panel A). The ratio of AH/HA is less than one and remains fixed when the tachycardia is stable.[69] The earliest atrial activation is usually registered at the low septal right atrium from the His bundle recording site although there may be multiple sites of the earliest atrial activation, or the earliest atrial activation may be recorded in the coronary sinus or at the base of Koch's triangle.[70] The tachycardia can be entrained by atrial or ventricular overdrive pacing; it can be terminated by a faster overdrive pacing or programmed stimulation from either the atrium or the ventricle.[71,72] An excitable gap can be demonstrated by delivery of atrial or ventricular extrastimulus during tachycardia.[73–75] As the retrograde fast pathway conduction time is either fixed or prolonged very little, delivery of ventricular extrastimulus usually preexcites the atria during tachycardia. Rarely, an atrial extrastimulus delivered during tachycardia may engage the anterograde fast pathway and preempt the control of the His bundle and the ventricles; the impulse simultaneously enters the slow pathway, entrains the tachycardia, and results in double responses of the His bundle and the ventricles during tachycardia.[75]

A variant form of "slow-fast" AVNRT was described by Ross et al,[76] in that the earliest atrial activation was registered from the ostium of the coronary sinus during tachycardia. The electrophysiological and pharmacological characteristics of this tachycardia are similar to those of the slow-fast AVNRT. However, the HA interval is slightly longer and the atrial response usually occurs after the QRS complex during tachycardia (see Figure 2, panel B). The retrograde pathway of this tachycardia also has a limited decremental ability, but a minor prolongation of the HA interval is sometimes noted during incremental ventricular pacing or ventricular extrastimulus testing. This retrograde pathway was designated as the "intermediate or γ-pathway" and the tachycardia as "slow-intermediate" form by Wu et al.[66]

A reversed type of AVNRT using the fast pathway for anterograde conduction and the slow pathway for retrograde conduction was described by Wu et al[27] in 1977. This fast-slow form of AVNRT is characterized by a short AH and a long HA interval and the earliest atrial activation is registered from the ostium of the coronary sinus during tachycardia (see Figure 5, panel B).[27,77] It is induced by ventricular extrastimulus or with rapid ventricular pacing during retrograde atypical Wenckebach periodicity, when conduction shifts from the fast pathway to the slow pathway. The tachycardia can also be induced by programmed atrial stimulation. Anterograde induction of this tachycardia depends on a block in the slow pathway; therefore, a critical AH delay is not obvious.

With the presence of multiple pathways, multiple AVNRTs may occur in the same patient (see Figure 6 and Figure 7).[63,65,66,78] These include the slow-fast form, the slow-intermediate form, the fast-slow form, and the fast-intermediate form. The fast-intermediate form of tachycardia is an uncommon tachycardia characterized by a fast heart rate due to short anterograde and retrograde conduction time; the tachycardia may mimic atrial flutter clinically. In patients with multiple AVNRTs, shift of tachycardia from one type to the other may be initiated by premature atrial or ventricular beats due to a double loop figure-8 type of excitation wave among the pathways. The possibility of "intermediate-slow" form or "intermediate-fast" form of tachycardia may occur but has not been well substantiated so far.

The nature of the proximal and the distal link is unclear.[79–86] Block proximal to the His bundle potential recording site during tachycardia has been noted in a few patients with AVNRT, especially in those with the unusual form of tachycardia.[82-84] Therefore, a distal common pathway is likely to exist between the circuit and the His bundle. Although AV dissociation or second degree VA block has also been noted during tachycardia in a few case reports, the exact role of the atrium during reentry is unclear.[85,86] The reentrant circuit is likely to include some atrial tissue, but excitation of the whole atria is unnecessary.

Modification of the Reentrant Circuit by Physiological and Pharmacological Maneuvers

The reentrant circuit in the common slow-fast form tachycardia consists of an anterograde slow pathway, a retrograde fast pathway, a proximal link, and a distal link. The cycle length of tachycardia reflects the sum of conduction times within the circuit and is identical to the sum of the AH and HA intervals. Sustenance of tachycardia requires a tachycardia cycle length longer than the effective refractory period of all components of the circuit.[38,48,87] If anterograde block occurs in the slow pathway, the tachycardia will terminate with an atrial activation without a QRS complex. If retrograde block occurs in the fast pathway, tachycardia will terminate with a QRS complex without an atrial response. Physiological and pharmacological maneuvers may increase the anterograde slow pathway or retrograde fast pathway refractoriness and make the tachycardia nonsustainable. Vagal maneuvers,[88–93] digitalis,[45–47] β-blockers,[47] calcium-blockers,[42–44] and adenosine[94,95] increase the effective refractory period of the anterograde slow pathway and may terminate the tachycardia or prevent recurrence of the tachycardia. These agents may also increase the effective refractory period of the fast pathway, thus terminating the tachycardia in the retrograde direction. In contrast, class I antiarrhythmic agents selectively depress the retrograde fast pathway conduction and may prevent recurrence of the tachycardia.[48–50] Atropine and isoproterenol improve both the anterograde slow pathway and retrograde fast pathway conduction and thus facilitate induction of sustained tachycardia.[23,37–41] However, atropine and isoproterenol shorten the anterograde effective refractory period of the fast pathway and therefore may make induction of tachycardia more difficult.

Modification of the Reentrant Circuit by Surgery or Catheter Ablation

Surgical modification of the AV node with cure of the tachycardia and preservation of conduction was fortuitously accomplished in 1979 when Pritchett et al attempted to interrupt AV conduction by surgical dissection.[96] Subsequently, Ross et al[76] innovated surgical techniques for dissection of the perinodal tissue and Cox et al[97] developed cryocoagulation techniques for modification of the AV node. These techniques usually result in modification of the slow pathway conduction with preservation of anterograde AV conduction, although the retrograde fast pathway conduction is sometimes damaged. Selective modification of the slow pathway and the retrograde fast pathway using cryoablation may be achieved by careful application of ice-mapping technique to the discrete area of Koch's triangle.[98] The surgery requires thoracotomy and cardiopulmonary bypass, is associated with potential mortality and significant morbidity, and thus has limited value for a benign arrhythmia like AVNRT.

Catheter modification of the AV nodal reentrant circuit using direct current shocks was introduced by Haïssaguerre et al[99] and Epstein et al.[100] With this procedure, the current was delivered to the earliest atrial activation site during tachycardia at the anterior-superior region of Koch's triangle. It resulted in ablation or modification of either the fast or the slow pathway conduction. The innovation of radiofrequency current as the energy source for catheter ablation has revolutionized the therapy of AVNRT and has provided new insight to the understanding of dual pathway physiology. The radiofrequency current is capable of creating a small, dense, and well-defined lesion and is therefore more selective. There are 3 approaches: the anterior approach, the posterior approach, and the inferior approach. With the anterior approach, the current is applied to the anterior-superior region of Koch's triangle.[101,102] The anterior approach selectively ablates or modifies the retrograde fast pathway conduction, although it may also cause damage to the anterograde fast or slow pathway conduction and thus abolishes dual pathway physiology. As a consequence of selective retrograde fast pathway conduction, it may also reverse the reentrant circuit causing an induction of the fast-slow form of AVNRT. The posterior approach delivered the current to a strict posterior site between the ostium of the coronary sinus and the tricuspid annulus.[103,104] The posterior approach results in selective ablation of the slow pathway, although it also occasionally damages the retrograde fast pathway. The inferior approach delivers the current to the inferior-midseptal area of Koch's triangle and results in selective ablation or modification of the slow pathway, although it may also cause damage to the retrograde fast pathway.[41,105] A stepwise posterior-inferior approach with the initial current delivered to a posterior site near the ostium of the coronary sinus and the ablation site progressively moved anteriorly toward the apex of Koch's triangle along the tricuspid annulus has the same results.[106] Technical details of AV nodal modification by catheter techniques are described in other chapters.

The Anatomy and Physiology of the AV Node

Normal impulse transmission from the sinus node to the ventricles must pass through the AV junctional area. The AV rings insulate the atria from the ventricles and prevent direct impulse transmission from the atria to the ventricles. The AV junction is a complex anatomic structure located within an area called Koch's triangle.[107–109] Koch's triangle is bounded anteriorly and superiorly by the tendon of Todaro, posteriorly by the coronary sinus, and inferiorly by the annulus fibrosus of the tricuspid ring. The exact nature of the anatomic structure and the mode of impulse transmission within the AV junction has been a subject of controversy and remains unsettled. Basically, there are 2 theories concerning AV conduction. Some scholars proposed the existence of a sinoventricular conducting system and posited that the specialized conducting cells are different from the contractile myocardial cells.[110,111] They suggested that there are special internodal conduction pathways connecting the sinus node and the AV node and that there are special arrangements of the junctional area to accommodate these pathways before they converge to become the His bundle. Recently, Racker proposed a model for sinoventricular conduction in which 3 atrionodal bundles (superior, middle and lateral) converge to form a proximal AV bundle (Figure 8).[111,112] The proximal AV bundle is contiguous to the atrial end of the AV node (node of Tawara). The AV node is then connected to the distal AV bundle (the His bundle). Not only the AV node-distal AV bundle complex is encased within the fibrous tissue—the atrionodal bundles and the proximal AV bundles are also ensheathed heavily by the connective tissue. In contrast to these views, other scholars, represented by Anderson et al,[113–115] proposed that there are no special internodal pathways and that there are 4 special zones in the junctional area: a transitional cell zone (AN zone), the compact AV node (N zone), the penetrating AV bundle, and the branching AV bundle (Figure 9). With this proposal, the atria approach the compact AV node through the transitional cells, which can be further organized into 3 groups. The superficial anterior group of transitional cells approaches the compact node from the sinus septum and from the anterior limbs. The posterior group

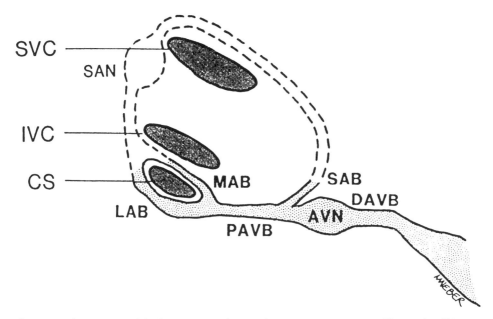

Figure 8. Schematic model of sinoventricular conducting system proposed by Racker.[112] AVN = AV node; CS = coronary sinus; DAVB = distal AV bundle; IVC = inferior vena cava; LAB = lateral atrionodal bundle; MAB = middle atrionodal bundle; PAVB = proximal AV bundle; SAB = superior atrionodal bundle; SAN = sinus node; SVC = superior vena cava. (Reproduced from Racker[112] with permission).

approaches the compact node from the sinus septum and also from a muscular tract extending beneath the coronary sinus into the posterior atrial wall. The deep middle group approaches the compact node from the left atrial septum. The superficial anterior group and the deep group of transitional cells is separated by the tendon of Todaro. The compact node bifurcates posteriorly into 2 limbs diverging toward the tricuspid and mitral side of the septal annulus fibrosus. The penetrating bundle is encased within the central fibrous body and courses distally to become the branching bundle. The methodology used by Racker differed from that of Anderson et al as well as that of other previous investigators. While Anderson et al performed transverse sections of the junctional area (with respect to the coronary sinus-His bundle axis) perpendicular to the annulus fibrosus of the tricuspid ring, Racker conducted studies with longitudinal sections. The AV node in Racker's model is encased within the central fibrous body and, therefore, is likely to be the proximal part of the penetrating bundle (or the nodo-Hisian junction, NH zone) in the model of Anderson et al. The compact node of Anderson et al probably includes most of the proximal AV bundle and the terminal part of the superior AV bundle in Racker's mode.

The transitional AN cells have a more negative resting membrane potential, fast upstroke velocity, higher amplitude with a phase I and plateau, and minimal cycle length-dependent changes.[116,117] In contrast, the compact nodal N cells have a more positive resting membrane potential, slow upstroke velocity, low amplitude, a round peak, and marked cycle length-dependent changes. The mode of impulse transmission through the AV junction in humans is less

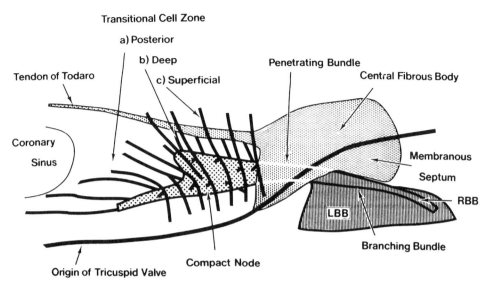

Figure 9. Schematic model of AV junction proposed by Becker AE and Anderson RH[115]. LBB = left bundle branch; RBB = right bundle branch. (Reproduced from Becker and Anderson[115] with permission).

clear. Animal mapping studies suggest that the normal anterograde impulse approaches the compact node simultaneously with 2 sources of inputs: an anterior input from the atrial septum as a broad wavefront descending via the superficial anterior and the deep middle transitional cell groups and a posterior input from the crista terminals.[117-120] The anterior input does not appear to bypass the proximal compact node, but curves posteriorly to join the posterior input. Disagreement exists concerning the major delay during normal impulse propagation. Some investigators suggested that the transitional cells (AN zone) account for most of the delay during normal conduction, while others contend that the compact node (N zone) is the site of major conduction delay. The cycle length dependent delay is less controversial: all evidence suggests that nodal cells are responsible for cycle length dependent delay, including the increment of conduction time and block during Wenckebach periodicity. Limited data during intra-operative mapping in humans suggest that the anterior input dominates the normal anterograde conduction.[121] The activation pattern of retrograde conduction is characterized by the earliest atrial exit being in the atrial septum anterior to the coronary sinus, which receives the impulse via the superficial anterior group of transitional cells; the crista terminalis receives the impulse from the posterior transitional cell group.

Hypothetical Model

The knowledge correlating the anatomic structure and impulse transmission of the junctional area was primarily obtained from studies of rabbit heart because the impulse transmission fails quickly in in vitro preparations of larger species, and because it is technically difficult or impossible to impale the compact node and the His bundle in larger species. The information obtained from in vivo mappings of the junctional area is limited to surface activation rather than the three-dimensional activation. Based on the terminology used by Anderson et al,[113–115] Wu[29] proposed a hypothesis in 1982 that the retrograde fast pathway conduction in AVNRT reflects the conduction over a portion of the anterior superficial transitional cells that insert to the distal compact node, while the anterograde slow pathway conduction reflects the conduction over the posterior transitional cells through the compact node (Figure 10, left panel). The anterograde fast pathway conduction is equivalent to the normal anterograde AV conduction in that the major impulse conducts through the anterior superficial transitional cells bypassing the proximal portion of the compact node. Anatomic studies of the AV junctional area in patients with clinical dual AV nodal pathways have shown no difference compared to persons without dual AV nodal pathways.[122] This hypothesis could explain almost all known dual AV nodal pathway phenomena, including the difference in atrial exit during retrograde fast pathway and slow pathway conduction. The retrograde fast pathway conduction is characterized by a lack of decremental conduction responsive to class I agents, and with the earliest atrial activation being registered from the His bundle recording catheter at the apical area of Koch's triangle. The slow pathway conduction is characterized by marked decremental conduction, responsive to vagal maneuvers, adenosine, calcium-blockers, β-blockers, and digitalis, and with the earliest atrial activation during retrograde slow pathway conduction registered near the ostium of the coronary sinus. This hypothesis also provides an expla-

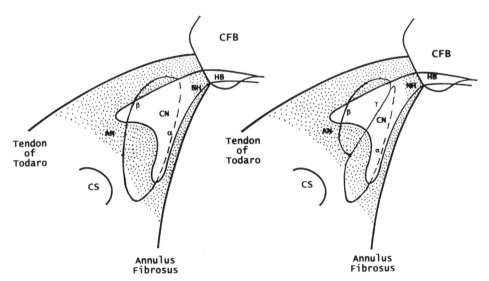

Figure 10. Schematic representation of Koch's triangle showing the hypothetical model of dual AV nodal pathways and the reentrant circuit (left panel) as well as the triple pathways and the double loop figure-of-8 reentrant circuit (right panel). Koch's triangle is bounded by the tendon of Todaro, the coronary sinus, and the annulus fibrosus of the tricuspid ring. The dotted area represents the transitional cell zone. AN = atrionodal transitional cell; CN = compact node; NH = nodo-Hisian transitional cell. α, β & γ = slow pathway, fast pathway, and intermediate pathway. CFB & CS = central fibrous body and coronary sinus.

nation for radiofrequency modification of the AVNRT in that selective ablation of the retrograde fast pathway can be achieved by delivery of the radiofrequency current to the anterio-superior portion of Koch's triangle while selective ablation of the slow pathway can be achieved by delivery of the radiofrequency current to the posterior-inferior portion of Koch's triangle along the tricuspid annulus.[123] Recently, Wu et al[66] further extended the hypothesis to include an intermediate pathway, where it reflects the conduction over a more proximal and inferior (as compared to the retrograde fast pathway) portion of the anterior superficial transitional cells (see right panel of Figure 10). Operating among these 3 AV nodal pathways could result in multiple AVNRTs. It also provides for an explanation that the multiple form of AVNRT can be effectively ablated by delivery of the radiofrequency current to a midseptal site similar to the site of inferior approach for ablation of the common slow-fast form of AVNRT.[78]

References

1. Mines GR. On dynamic equilibrium in the heart. *J Physiol* 1913;46: 349–382.
2. Iliescu CC, Sebastiani A. Notes on the effects of quinidine upon paroxysms of tachycardia *Heart* 1923;10:223–230.
3. Barker PS, Wilson FN, Johnston FD. The mechanism of auricular paroxysmal tachycardia with alternation of cycle length. *Am Heart J* 1943;26: 435–445.
4. Moe GK, Preston JB, Burlington H. Physiologic evidence for a dual A-V transmission system. *Circ Res* 1956;4:357–375.
5. Rosenblueth A, Rubio R. Ventricular echoes. *Am J Physiol* 1958;195;53–60.
6. Wallace AG, Daggett WM. Re-excitation of the atrium. "The echo phenomenon." *Am Heart J* 1964;68:661–666.
7. Mendez C, Han J, Garcia de Jalon PD, et al. Some characteristics of ventricular echoes. *Circ Res* 1965;16:562–581.
8. Moe GK, Mendez C, Han J. Some features of dual A-V conducting system. In: Dreifus LS, Likoff W, Moyer JH, eds. *Mechanisms and Therapy of Cardiac Arrhythmias.* New York, NY: Grune & Stratton, 1966. pp 361–372.
9. Watanabe Y, Dreifus LS. Inhomogeneous conduction in the A-V node. *Am Heart J* 1965;70:505–514.
10. Mendez C, Moe GK. Demonstration of a dual A-V nodal conduction system in the isolated rabbit heart. *Circ Res* 1966;19:378–393.
11. Janse MJ, Van Capelle FJL, Freud GE, et al. Circus movement within the A-V node as a basis for supraventricular tachycardia as shown by multiple microelectrode recording in the isolated rabbit heart. *Circ Res* 1971;28:403–414.
12. Wit AL, Goldreyer BN, Damato AN. An in vitro model of paroxysmal supraventricular tachycardia. *Circulation* 1971;43:862–875.
13. Kistin AD. Multiple pathways of conduction and reciprocal rhythm with interpolated ventricular premature systoles. *Am Heart J* 1963;65:162–179.
14. Schuilenburg RM, Durrer D. Atrial echo beats in the human heart elicited by induced atrial premature beats. *Circulation* 1968;37:680–693.

15. Schuilenburg RM, Durrer D. Ventricular echo beats in the human heart elicited by induced ventricular premature beats. *Circulation* 1969;40:337–3 47.
16. Moe GK, Cohen W, Vick RL. Experimentally induced paroxysmal A-V nodal tachycardia in the dog. *Am Heart J* 1963;65:87–92.
17. Hunt NC, Cobb FR, Waxman MB, et al. Conversion of supraventricular tachycardia with atrial stimulation. *Circulation* 1968;38:1060–1065.
18. Lister JW, Cohen LS, Bernstein WH, et al. Treatment of supraventricular tachycardias by rapid atrial stimulation. *Circulation* 1968;38:1044–1059.
19. Gettes LS, Yoshonis KF. Rapidly recurring supraventricular tachycardia. *Circulation* 1970;41:689–700.
20. Bigger JT Jr, Goldreyer BN. The mechanism of supraventricular tachycardia. *Circulation* 1970;42:673–687.
21. Goldreyer BN, Bigger JT Jr. Site of reentry in paroxysmal supraventricular tachycardia in man. *Circulation* 1971;43:15–26.
22. Goldreyer BN, Damato AN. Essential role of atrioventricular conduction delay in the initiation of paroxysmal supraventricular tachycardia. *Circulation* 1971;43:679–687.
23. Denes P, Wu D, Dhingra RC, et al. Demonstration of dual A-V nodal pathway in patients with paroxysmal supraventricular tachycardia. *Circulation* 1973;48:549–555.
24. Rosen KM, Metha A, Miller RA. Demonstration of dual atrioventricular nodal pathways in man. *Am J Cardiol* 1974;33:291–294.
25. Wu D, Denes P, Dhingra R, et al. New manifestations of dual A-V nodal pathways. *Eur J Cardiol* 1975;2:459–466.
26. Wu D, Denes P, Dhingra RC, et al. Determinants of fast and slow pathway conduction in patients with dual A-V nodal pathways. *Circ Res* 1975;36:782–790.
27. Wu D, Denes P, Amat-y-Leon F, et al. An unusual variety of atrioventricular nodal reentry due to retrograde dual atrioventricular nodal pathways. *Circulation* 1977;56:50–59.
28. Wu D, Hung JS, Kou CT. Determinants of sustained slow pathway conduction and relation to reentrant tachycardia in patients with dual atrioventricular nodal transmission. *Am Heart J* 1981;101:521–528.
29. Wu D. Dual atrioventricular nodal pathways: a reappraisal. *PACE* 1982;5:72–89.
30. Aktar M, Jazayeri MR, Sra J, et al. Atrioventricular nodal reentry: clinical, electrophysiological, and therapeutic considerations. *Circulation* 1993;88:282–295.
31. Denes P, Wu D, Dhingra R, et al. Dual A-V nodal pathways: a common electrophysiological response. *Br Heart J* 1975;37:1069–1976.
32. Bisset JK, de Soyza N, Kane JJ, et al. Atrioventricular conduction patterns in patients with paroxysmal supraventricular tachycardia. *Am Heart J* 1976;91:287–291.
33. Touboul P, Huerta F, Porte J, et al. Reciprocal rhythm in patients with normal electrocardiogram: evidence for dual conduction pathways. *Am Heart J* 1976;91:3–10.

34. Thapar MK, Gillette P. Dual atrioventricular nodal pathways: a common electrophysiologic response in children. *Circulation* 1979;60:1369–1374.
35. Casta A, Wolff GS, Mehta AV, et al. Dual atrioventricular nodal pathways: a benign finding in arrhythmia-free children with heart disease. *Am J Cardiol* 1980;46:1013–1018.
36. Wu D, Denes P, Dhingra RC, et al. Effect of propranolol on induction of A-V nodal reentrant tachycardia. *Circulation* 1974;50:665–677.
37. Neuss H, Schlepper M, Spies HF. Effects of heart rate and atropine on dual A-V conduction. *Br Heart J* 1975;37:1216–1227.
38. Wu D, Denes P, Bauernfeind R, et al. Effects of atropine on induction and maintenance of A-V nodal reentrant tachycardia. *Circulation* 1979;59: 779–788.
39. Hariman RJ, Gomes JAC, El-Sherif N. Catecholamine-dependent atrioventricular nodal reentrant tachycardia. *Circulation* 1983;67:681–686.
40. Niazi I, Naccarelli G, Dougherty A, et al. Treatment of atrioventricular node reentrant tachycardia with encainide: reversal of drug effect with isoproterenol. *J Am Coll Cardiol* 1989;13:904–916.
41. Wu D, Yeh SJ, Wang CC, et al. A simple technique for selective radiofrequency ablation of the slow pathway in atrioventricular node reentry tachycardia. *J Am Coll Cardiol* 1993;21:1612–1621.
42. Rinkenberger RL, Prystowsky EN, Heger JJ, et al. Effects of intravenous and chronic oral verapamil administration in patients with supraventricular tachyarrhythmias. *Circulation* 1980;62:996–1010.
43. Sung RJ, Elser B, McAllister RG Jr. Intravenous verapamil for termination of reentrant supraventricular tachycardias. Intracardiac studies correlated with plasma verapamil concentration. *Ann Intern Med* 1980;93:682–689.
44. Yeh SJ, Kou HC, Lin FC, et al. Effects of oral diltiazem in paroxysmal supraventricular tachycardia. *Am J Cardiol* 1983;52:271–278.
45. Wellens HJJ, Duren DR, Liem KL, et al. Effects of digitalis in patients with paroxysmal atrioventricular nodal tachycardia. *Circulation* 1975;52:779–788.
46. Wu D, Wyndham C, Amat-y-Leon F, et al. The effects of ouabain on induction of atrioventricular nodal reentrant paroxysmal supraventricular tachycardia. *Circulation* 1975;52:201–207.
47. Bauernfeind RA, Wyndham CR, Dhingra R, et al. Serial electrophysiologic testing of multiple drugs in patients with atrioventricular nodal reentrant paroxysmal tachycardia. *Circulation* 1980;62:1341–1349.
48. Wu D, Denes P, Bauernfeind R, et al. Effects of procainamide on A-V nodal reentrant paroxysmal tachycardia. *Circulation* 1983;57:1171–1179.
49. Wu D, Hung JS, Kou CT, et al. Effects of quinidine on atrioventricular nodal reentrant paroxysmal tachycardia. *Circulation* 1981;64:823–831.
50. Sethi KK, Jaishankar S, Gupta MP. Salutary effects of intravenous ajmaline in patients with paroxysmal supraventricular tachycardia mediated by dual atrioventricular nodal pathways; blockade of the retrograde fast pathway. *Circulation* 1984;70:876–883.
51. Fisch C, Mandrola JM, Rardon DP. Electrocardiographic manifestations of dual atrioventricular node conduction during sinus rhythm. *J Am Coll Cardiol* 1997;29:1015–1022.

52. Lin FC, Yeh SJ, Wu D. Determinants of simultaneous fast and slow pathway conduction in patients with dual atrioventricular nodal pathways. *Am Heart J* 1985;109:963–970.

53. Gomes JAC, Kang PS, Kelen G, et al. Simultaneous anterograde fast-slow atrioventricular nodal pathway conduction after procainamide. *Am J Cardiol* 1980;46:677–684.

54. Csapo G. Paroxysmal non-reentrant tachycardia due to simultaneous conduction in dual atrioventricular nodal pathways. *Am J Cardiol* 1979;43: 1033–1045.

55. Sutton FJ, Lee YC. Supraventricular non-reentrant tachycardia due to simultaneous conduction through dual atrioventricular nodal pathways. *Am J Cardiol* 1983;51:897–900

56. Yeh SJ, Wu YC, Lin FC, et al. Pseudosimultaneous fast and slow pathway conduction: a common electrophysiologic finding in patients with dual atrioventricular nodal pathways. *J Am Coll Cardiol* 1985;6:927–932.

57. Brugada P, Heddle B, Green M, et al. Initiation of atrioventricular nodal reentrant tachycardia in patients with discontinuous anterograde atrioventricular nodal conduction curves with and without documented supraventricular tachycardia: observations on the role of a discontinuous retrograde conduction curve. *Am Heart J* 1984;107:685–697.

58. Sung RJ, Waxman HL, Saksena S, et al. Sequence of retrograde atrial activation in patients with dual atrioventricular nodal pathways. *Circulation* 1981;64:1059–1067.

59. Dopirak MR, Schaal SF, Leier CV. Triple A-V nodal pathways in man? *J Electrocardiol* 1980;13:185–188.

60. Swiryn S, Bauernfeind RA, Palileo FA, et al. Electrophysiologic study demonstrating triple antegrade AV nodal pathways in patients with spontaneous and/or induced supraventricular tachycardia. *Am Heart J* 1982; 103:168–176.

61. Kuck KH, Kuch B, Bleifeld W. Multiple antegrade and retrograde AV nodal pathways: demonstration by multiple discontinuities in the AV nodal conduction curves and echo time intervals. *PACE* 1984;7:656–662.

62. Sebag C, Chevalier P, Davy JM, et al. Triple antegrade nodal pathway in a patient with supraventricular paroxysmal tachycardia. *J Electrocardiol* 1986;19(1):85–90.

63. Tai CT, Chen SA, Chiang CE, et al. Multiple antegrade atrioventricular nodal pathways in patients with atrioventricular node reentrant tachycardia. *J Am Coll Cardiol* 1996;28:725–731.

64. Spurrell RAJ, Krikler D, Sowton E. Two or more intra A-V nodal pathways in association with either a James or Kent extranodal bypass in 3 patients with paroxysmal supraventricular tachycardia. *Br Heart J* 1973;35:113–122.

65. McGuire MA, Lau KC, Johnson DC, et al. Patients with two types of atrioventricular junctional (AV nodal) reentrant tachycardia: evidence that a common pathway of nodal tissue is not present above the reentrant circuit. *Circulation* 1991;83:1232–1246.

66. Wu D, Yeh SJ, Wang CC, et al. Double loop figure-of-8 reentry as the mechanism of multiple atrioventricular node reentry tachycardias. *Am Heart J* 1994;127:83–95.

67. Wu D, Kou HC, Yeh SJ, et al. Determinants of tachycardia induction using ventricular stimulation in dual pathway atrioventricular nodal reentrant tachycardia. *Am Heart J* 1984;108:44–55.

68. Denes P, Amat-y-Leon F, et al. Clinical electrocardiographic and electrophysiologic observations in patients with paroxysmal supraventricular tachycardia. *Am J Cardiol* 1978;41:1045–1051.

69. Akhtar M, Damato AN, Ruskin JN, et al. Antegrade and retrograde conduction characteristics in 3 patterns of paroxysmal atrioventricular junctional reentrant tachycardia. *Am Heart J* 1978;95:22–42.

70. Anselme F, Hook B, Monahan K, et al. Heterogeneity of retrograde fast-pathway conduction pattern in patients with atrioventricular nodal reentry tachycardia. Observations by use of simultaneous multiple catheter mapping of Koch's triangle. *Circulation* 1996;93:960–968.

71. Portillo B, Mejias J, Leon-Portillo N, et al. Entrainment of atrioventricular nodal reentrant tachycardias during overdrive pacing from high right atrium and coronary sinus. With special reference to atrioventricular dissociation and 2:1 retrograde block during tachycardias. *Am J Cardiol* 1984;53:1570–1576.

72. Brugada P, Waldo AL, Wellens HJJ. Transient entrainment and interruption of atrioventricular nodal tachycardia. *J Am Coll Cardiol* 1987;9:767–775.

73. Wu D, Denes P, Wyndham C, et al. Demonstration of dual atrioventricular nodal pathways utilizing a ventricular extrastimulus in patients with atrioventricular nodal reentrant paroxysmal supraventricular tachycardia. *Circulation* 1975;52:789–798.

74. Schuger CD, Steinman RT, Lehmann MH. The excitable gap in atrioventricular nodal reentrant tachycardia: characterization with ventricular extrastimuli and pharmacologic intervention. *Circulation* 1989;80:324–334.

75. Lai WT, Lee CS, Sheu SH, et al. Electrophysiologic manifestations of the excitable gap of slow-fast AV nodal reentrant tachycardia demonstrated by single extrastimulation. *Circulation* 1995;92:66–76.

76. Ross DL, Johnson DC, Denniss AR, et al. Curative surgery for atrioventricular junctional ("AV nodal") reentrant tachycardia. *J Am Coll Cardiol* 1985;6:1383–1392.

77. Sung RJ, Styperek JL, Myerburg RJ, et al. Initiation of 2 distinct forms of atrioventricular nodal reentrant tachycardia during programmed ventricular stimulation in man. *Am J Cardiol* 1978;42:404–415.

78. Yeh SJ, Wang CC, Wen MS, et al. Radiofrequency ablation therapy in atypical or multiple atrioventricular node reentry tachycardia. *Am Heart J* 1994;128:742–758.

79. Josephson ME, Kastor JA. Paroxysmal supraventricular tachycardia: is the atrium a necessary link? *Circulation* 1976;54:430–435.

80. Miller JM, Rosenthal ME, Vassallo JA, et al. Atrioventricular nodal reentrant tachycardia: studies on upper and lower "common pathways." *Circulation* 1987;75:930–940.

81. Josephson M, Miller J. Atrioventricular node reentry tachycardia: is the atrium a necessary link? In: Touboul P, Waldo A, eds. *Atrial Arrhythmias: Current Concepts and Management.* St Louis, MO: Mosby Year Book, 1990. pp 311–329.

82. Wellens HJJ. Unusual examples of supraventricular reentrant tachycardias. *Circulation* 1975;51:997–1002.
83. Hamer AWF, Zahen CA, Peter T, et al. Verapamil effects in AV node reentry tachycardia with intermittent supra-Hisian AV block. *Am Heart J* 1984;107:431–439.
84. Yeh SJ, Yamamoto T, Lin FC, et al. Atrioventricular block in atypical form of junctional reciprocating tachycardia; evidence supporting the atrioventricular node as the site of reentry. *J Am Coll Cardiol* 1990;15:385–392.
85. Bauernfeind RA, Wu D, Denes P, et al. Retrograde block during dual pathway atrioventricular nodal reentrant paroxysmal tachycardia. *Am J Cardiol* 1978;42:499–505.
86. Wang CC, Yeh SJ, Lin FC, et al. Spontaneous atrioventricular dissociation in atrioventricular nodal reentrant tachycardia. *Am Heart J* 1990;119:1426–1429.
87. Denes P, Wu D, Amat-y-Leon F, et al. The determinants of AV nodal reentrance in patients with dual AV nodal pathways. *Circulation* 1977;56:253–259.
88. Klein HO, Hoffman BF. Cessation of paroxysmal supraventricular tachycardias by parasympathomimetic interventions. *Ann Intern Med* 1974;81:48–50.
89. Josephson ME, Seides SE, Batsford WB, et al. The effects of carotid sinus pressure in reentrant paroxysmal supraventricular tachycardia. *Am Heart J* 1974;88:694–697.
90. Curry PVL, Rowland E, Fox KM, et al. The relationship between posture, blood pressure and electrophysiological properties in patients with paroxysmal supraventricular tachycardia. *Arch Mal Coeur* 1977;71:293–299.
91. Waxman MB, Bonet JF, Finley JP, et al. Effects of respiration and posture on paroxysmal supraventricular tachycardia. *Circulation* 1980;62:1011–1020.
92. Waxman MB, Wald RW, Sharma AD, et al. Vagal techniques for termination of paroxysmal supraventricular tachycardia. *Am J Cardiol* 1980;46:655–664.
93. Metha D, Wafa S, Ward DE, et al. Relative efficacy of various physical manoeuvres in the termination of junctional tachycardia. *Lancet* 1988;331:1181–1185.
94. Lai WT, Wu JC, Wu SN, et al. Differential effect of adenosine on antegrade fast, antegrade slow, and retrograde fast pathways in patients with atrioventricular nodal reentrant tachycardia [abstract]. *Circulation* 1996;94:I284.
95. DiMarco JP, Sellers TD, Berne RM, et al. Adenosine: electrophysiologic effects and therapeutic use for terminating paroxysmal supraventricular tachycardia. *Circulation* 1983;68:1254–1263.
96. Pritchett ELC, Anderson RW, Benditt DG, et al. Reentry within the atrioventricular node: surgical cure with preservation of atrioventricular conduction. *Circulation* 1979;60:440–450.
97. Cox JL, Holman WL, Cain ME. Cryosurgical treatment of atrioventricular node reentrant tachycardia. *Circulation* 1987;76:1829–1836.
98. Keim S, Werner P, Jazayeri M, et al. Localization of the fast and slow pathways in atrioventricular nodal reentrant tachycardia by intraoperative ice mapping. *Circulation* 1992;86:919–925.

99. Haïssaguerre M, Warin JF, Lemetayer P, et al. Closed-chest ablation of retrograde conduction in patients with atrioventricular nodal reentrant tachycardia. *N Engl J Med* 1989;320:426–433.

100. Epstein LM, Scheinman MM, Langberg JJ, et al. Percutaneous catheter modification of the atrioventricular nodal reentrant tachycardia. *Circulation* 1989;80:757–768.

101. Goy JJ, Fromer M, Schlaepfer J, et al. Clinical efficacy of radiofrequency current in the treatment of patients with atrioventricular node reentrant tachycardia. *J Am Coll Cardiol* 1990;16:418–423.

102. Lee MA, Morady F, Kadish A, et al. Catheter modification of the atrioventricular junction with radiofrequency energy for control of atrioventricular nodal reentry tachycardia. *Circulation* 1991;83:827–835.

103. Jackman WM, Beckman KJ, McClelland JH, et al. Treatment of supraventricular tachycardia due to atrioventricular nodal reentry by radiofrequency ablation of slow-pathway conduction. *N Engl J Med* 1992;327:313–318.

104. Kay GN, Epstein AE, Dailey SM, et al. Selective radiofrequency ablation of the slow pathway for the treatment of atrioventricular nodal reentrant tachycardia: evidence for involvement of perinodal myocardium within the reentrant circuit. *Circulation* 1992;85:1675–1688.

105. Haïssaguerre M, Gaita F, Fischer B, et al. Elimination of atrioventricular nodal reentrant tachycardia using discrete slow potentials to guide application of radiofrequency energy. *Circulation* 1992;85:2162–2175.

106. Jazayeri M, Hempe SL, Sra J, et al. Selective transcatheter ablation of fast and slow pathways using radiofrequency energy in patients with atrioventricular nodal reentrant tachycardia. *Circulation* 1992;85:1318–1328.

107. James TN. Morphology of the human atrioventricular node, with remarks pertinent to its electrophysiology. *Am Heart J* 1961;62:756–771.

108. Truex RC, Smythe MQ. Reconstruction of the human atrioventricular node. *Anat Rec* 1967;101:17–57.

109. Dean JW, Ho SY, Rowland E, et al. Clinical anatomy of the atrioventricular junctions. *J Am Coll Cardiol* 1994;24:1725–1731.

110. James TN. The connecting pathways between the sinus node and A-V node and between the right and the left atrium in the human heart. *Am Heart J* 1963;66:498–508.

111. Racker DK. Atrioventricular node and input pathways: a correlated gross anatomical and historical study of the canine atrioventricular junctional region. *Anat Rec* 1989;224:336–354.

112. Racker DK. Sinoventricular transmission in 10 mM K+ by canine atrioventricular nodal inputs. Superior atrionodal bundle and proximal atrioventricular bundle. *Circulation* 1991;83:1738–1753.

113. Anderson RH, Janse MJ, van Cavelle FJ, et al. A combined morphological and electrophysiological study of the atrioventricular node of the rabbit heart. *Circ Res* 1974;35:909–922.

114. Anderson RH, Becker AE, Brechenmacher C, et al. The human atrioventricular junctional area: a morphologic study of the AV node and bundle. *Eur J Cardiol* 1975;3:11–25.

115. Becker AE, Anderson RH. Morphology of the human atrioventricular junc-

tional area. In: Wellens HJJ, Lie KI, Janse MJ, eds. *The Conduction System of the Heart*. Leiden, the Netherlands: HE Stenfert Kroese BV, 1976. pp 263–286.

116. Paes de Carvalho A, de Almeida DF. Spread of activity through the atrioventricular node. *Circ Res* 1960;8:801–809.

117. Meijler FL, Janse MJ. Morphology and electrophysiology of the mammalian atrioventricular node. *Physiol Rev* 1988;62:608–647.

118. Janse MJ. Influence of the direction of the atrial wave front on A-V nodal transmission in isolated hearts of rabbits. *Circ Res* 1969;25:439–449.

119. Van Cappelle FJL, Janse MJ, Varghese PJ, et al. Spread of excitation in the atrioventricular node of isolated rabbit hearts studied by multiple microelectrode recording. *Circ Res* 1972;31:602–616.

120. Zipes DP, Mendez C, Moe GK. Evidence for summation and voltage dependency in rabbit atrioventricular nodal fibers. *Circ Res* 1973;32:170–177.

121. McGuire MA, Bourke JP, Robotin MC, et al. High resolution mapping of Koch's triangle using sixty electrodes in humans with atrioventricular junctional (AV nodal) reentrant tachycardia. *Circulation* 1993;88:2315–2328.

122. Ho SY, McComb JM, Scott CD, et al. Morphology of the cardiac conduction system in patients with electrophysiologically poven dual atrioventricular nodal pathways. *J Cardiovasc Electrophysiol* 1993;4:504–512.

123. Wu D, Yeh SJ, Wang CC, et al. Nature of dual atrioventricular nodal pathways and the tachycardia circuit as defined by radiofrequency ablation technique. *J Am Coll Cardiol* 1992;20:889–895.

Chapter 21

Ablation of Atrioventricular Nodal Reentrant Tachycardia with the Anterior Approach: Is It Obsolete in the Year 2000?

Ling-Ping Lai, M.D., Jiunn-Lee Lin, M.D., Shoei K. Stephen Huang, M.D.

Atrioventricular (AV) nodal reentrant tachycardia (AVNRT) is the most common form of paroxysmal supraventricular tachycardia in adults.[1] Some patients can develop incapacitating recurrent tachycardia that is resistant to drug therapy; others who are responsive to medications frequently develop intolerable adverse effects or are not compliant with the treatment. Nowadays, radiofrequency (RF) catheter ablation has proven to be a safe and effective treatment modality for AVNRT. Historically, the initial approach to the RF catheter ablation for AVNRT was modification of AV conduction by lesions created near the anterosuperior aspect of the triangle of Koch (the anterior approach method).[2-4] Lately, selective ablation of the slow pathway of AV nodal reentry has been introduced by lesions created near the posteroinferior base of the triangle of Koch (the posterior approach method) between the ostium of the coronary sinus and the tricuspid annulus.[5-7] Though both techniques can achieve a high success rate, the latter technique has gained overwhelming popularity over the former because of a lower incidence of complete AV block. In this chapter, we will review the data published in the literature regarding the anterior approach and address the possible value of this technique in the year 2000.

From Huang SKS, Wilber DJ (eds.): *Radiofrequency Catheter Ablation of Cardiac Arrhythmias: Basic Concepts and Clinical Applications,* 2nd ed. Armonk, NY: Futura Publishing Company, Inc. ©2000.

Techniques of the Anterior Approach

The development of the anterior approach method for RF treatment of AVNRT was based on earlier experience with animal experiments in which the investigators were interested in creating partial or incomplete AV block by RF catheter ablation to avoid implantation of a permanent pacemaker.[8,9] Huang and coworkers demonstrated that persistent incomplete (first- and second-degree) AV block was achieved in 13 of 20 dogs 2 to 3 months after RF ablation of the AV junction by titration of the RF output and regulation of the ablation end points.[8] Marcus et al[9] also produced chronic first-degree AV block in 4 of 6 dogs. On the basis of these data in animal experiments, it is quite clear that chronic incomplete AV block could be induced by careful titration of RF output applied to the AV junction where the His bundle potential was small or barely visible and the ratio of atrial to ventricular amplitudes was ≥1.0 after the His bundle catheter was withdrawn from the site where the maximum His bundle potential was recorded.[8] However, inadvertent induction of complete AV block can occur even with a 2 mm-tipped catheter electrode. The major lesions in animals with incomplete AV block were confined in the approaches to and in the AV node with varying degrees of damage to the His bundle.[8,9]

The technique of the anterior approach method presented here was developed and modified from the initial animal experiments described above.[8] There

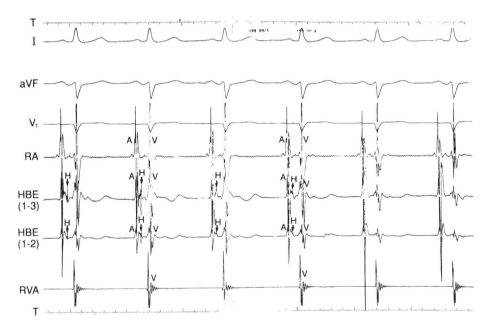

Figure 1. Demonstration of withdrawing the His-bundle ablation catheter (from left to right tracings) to the point where a small or barely visible His bundle potential with a relatively large atrial amplitude was recorded from the distal pair of the ablation catheter. Tracings were recorded at a paper speed of 100 mm/second. A = atrial potentials; HBE = His bundle electrograms; H = His bundle potential (indicated by an arrow); RA = right atrium electrograms; RVA = right ventricular apex electrograms; V = ventricular potentials; T = time line.

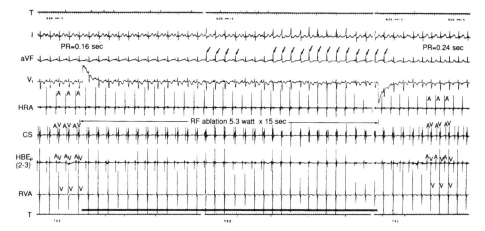

Figure 2. Simultaneous recordings of the surface electrogram (lead I, aVF, and V1) and intra-cardiac electrograms during radiofrequency (RF) catheter modification of the atrioventricular node in a patient with atrioventricular nodal reentrant tachycardia. Note that accelerated junctional beats (arrows) occurred during RF energy delivery. The PR interval increased from a baseline of 0.16 second to 0.24 second (increased by 50%) immediately after RF application. The paper speed was 25 mm/second. HRA = high right atrium electrograms; CS = coronary sinus electrograms; HBE = His bundle electrograms; RVA = right ventricular apex electrograms; T = time line.

may be minor differences among various reports with regard to the technique. The following is usually a typical practice.

The ablation catheter at the AV junction is initially positioned to record the maximum amplitude of the bipolar His bundle potential recorded from the distal pair of the electrodes. The catheter is then carefully withdrawn, while a firm clockwise torque is maintained, until the His bundle potential becomes small or barely visible or disappearing and a relatively large atrial amplitude (A/V ratio, ≥1.0) is recorded (Figure 1). At this point, the ablation catheter is held steadily and energy is applied until one of the following events occurs: 1) PR prolongation ≥30% to 50% (Figure 2); 2) impedance rise; or 3) transient high grade AV block. The end point of ablation is 1) noninducibility of AVNRT with isoproterenol, or 2) complete AV block. Although the anterior approach is very effective in eliminating AVNRT, the risk of inadvertent complete AV block remains high.

Risk of Complete AV Block with the Anterior Approach

When compared with the posterior approach, the target site for the anterior approach is located more approximately to the compact AV node and the bundle of His. Therefore, the anterior approach has a smaller safety margin and is theoretically associated with a higher risk of inadvertent complete AV block. The incidence of inadvertent complete AV block in the literature ranged from 0% to 22% (Table 1). The wide variation in the incidence of complete AV block might be attributed to the operator's experience and the so-called learning curve effect.

Table 1
Incidence of Inadvertent Complete AV Block Produced by
RF Ablation of AVNRT Using the Anterior Approach

Study group	Incidence of AV block		Ref	RF energy titration
Lee et al, 1991	3/39	(7.7%)	3	No
Langberg et al, 1993	9/127	(7.1%)	4	Titration in the last 37
Jazayeri et al, 1992	4/19	(21%)	10	Yes
Mitrani et al, 1993	3/13	(23%)	11	No
Chen et al, 1993	2/32	(6.3%)	12	No
Huang et al, 1996	3/56	(5.4%)	13	Yes
Mehta et al, 1995	0/31	(0%)	14	Yes
Kottkamp et al, 1995	0/53	(0%)	15	No

There are several reports in which a comparison between the 2 techniques was made.[10–14,16,17] All except one showed a higher incidence of complete AV block with the anterior approach when compared to with the posterior approach. In the Multicenter European Radiofrequency Survey (MERFS), the incidence of complete AV block in 880 patients with AVNRT who underwent RF ablation was 5.3% with the anterior approach and 2.0% with the posterior approach.[17] In the "Guidelines for Clinical Intracardiac Electrophysiological and Catheter Ablation Procedures" the ACC/AHA Task Force Report stated that slow pathway ablation is preferred because of a lower incidence of producing AV block, a greater likelihood of maintaining a normal PR interval during sinus rhythm, and its efficacy in the atypical forms of AVNRT.[18]

Can Inadvertent AV Block Be Avoided When Performing the Anterior Approach?

Inadvertent complete AV block is a very depressing outcome for the treatment of AVNRT. Since the anterior approach is associated with a higher risk of AV block, how to avoid the AV block has been the focus of several reports.

Titrating the energy application has been stressed in early reports with regard to the anterior approach. The rationale for titrated energy applications is that the RF lesion is created by gradual desiccation along the current flow. Physicians can stop energy delivery before a disastrous outcome occurs should any warning signs appear. However, the incidence of complete AV block was still high in several reports although titrated energy applications were performed.[10,13]

On the other hand, Kottkamp et al reported no incidence of permanent complete AV block in 53 patients with AVNRT using the anterior approach without titrating the energy output.[15] They clearly showed that in experienced hands, the anterior approach could be performed with a very low risk of complete AV block. In our experiences, careful monitoring of the AV conduction during RF energy application and prompt discontinuation of the energy output upon transient AV block are the keys to minimize the incidence of permanent complete AV block. We also suggest that overdrive atrial pacing be used to monitor the AV conduction should junctional ectopies occur during RF energy application. These precautions should apply to all sessions when the ablation site is near the AV junction, such as in the ablation procedure for AVNRT with the posterior approach, for midseptal accessory pathway, or for atrial tachycardia from the triangle of Koch.[19,20] Recently, Lin et al reported that the distal end of the AV nodal artery could be used as a landmark for predicting the occurrence of complete AV block during RF slow-pathway ablation of AVNRT.[21] They proved that the distal end of the AV nodal artery identified by selective coronary angiography can be a fluoroscopic marker for the compact AV node, and energy application at or near this location may result in AV block.

Conclusions

Ablation of AVNRT with the anterior approach is effective but is associated with a higher risk of inadvertent AV block when compared with the posterior approach. Although inadvertent complete AV block can be avoided with several precautions in the experienced hands, and some reports did show that the anterior approach could be performed with a very low risk of AV block, the posterior approach should still be considered as the preferred method. The anterior approach may be appropriate for patients in whom the posterior approach is ineffective. However, in experienced hands, the success rate of the posterior approach is approaching 100% and a back-up anterior approach is hardly needed. On the other hand, for those who are on the start of a learning curve, the anterior approach is associated with a fairly high incidence of complete AV block and is not worth a trial. Therefore, ablation of AVNRT with the anterior approach will be hardly useful, if not obsolete, in the year 2000.

References

1. Manolis AS, Estes NAM III. Supraventricular tachycardia: mechanism and therapy. *Arch Intern Med* 1987:147:1706–1716.
2. Goy J-J, Fromer M, Schlaepfer J, et al. Clinical efficacy of radiofrequency current in the treatment of patients with atrioventricular node reentrant tachycardia. *J Am Coll Cardiol* 1990;16:418–423.
3. Lee MA, Morady F, Kadish A, et al. Catheter modification of the atrioventricular junction with radiofrequency energy for control of atrioventricular nodal reentry tachycardia. *Circulation* 1991;83:827–835.
4. Langberg JJ, Harvey M, Calkins H, et al. Titration of power output during radiofrequency catheter ablation of atrioventricular nodal reentrant tachycardia. *PACE* 1993;16:465–470.
5. Jackman WM, Beckman KJ, McClelland JM, et al. Treatment of supraventricular tachycardia due to atrioventricular nodal reentry by radiofrequency catheter ablation of the slow-pathway conduction. *N Engl J Med* 1992;327:313–318.
6. Kay GN, Epstein AE, Dailey SM, et al. Selective radiofrequency ablation of

the slow pathway for the treatment of atrioventricular nodal reentrant tachycardia. *Circulation* 1992;85:1675–1688.

7. Haïssaguerre M, Gaita F, Fischer B, et al. Elimination of atrioventricular nodal reentrant tachycardia using discrete slow potentials to guide application of radiofrequency energy. *Circulation* 1992;85:2162–2175.

8. Huang SKS, Bharati S, Graham AR, et al. Chronic incomplete atrioventricular block induced by radiofrequency catheter ablation. *Circulation* 1989;80:951–961.

9. Marcus FI, Blouin LT, Bharati S, et al. Production of chronic first degree atrioventricular block in dogs using closed-chest electrode catheter with radiofrequency energy. *J Electrophysiol* 1988;2:315–326.

10. Jazayeri MR, Hempe SL, Sra JS, et al. Selective transcatheter ablation of the fast and slow pathways using radiofrequency energy in patients with atrioventricular nodal reentrant tachycardia. *Circulation* 1992;85:1318–1328.

11. Mitrani RD, Klein LS, Hackett FK, et al. Radiofrequency ablation for atrioventricular node reentrant tachycardia: comparison between fast (anterior) and slow (posterior) pathway ablation. *J Am Coll Cardiol* 1993;21: 432–441.

12. Chen SA, Chiang CE, Tsang WP, et al. Selective radiofrequency catheter ablation of fast and slow pathways in 100 patients with atrioventricular nodal reentrant tachycardia. *Am Heart J* 1993;125:1–10.

13. Pires LA, Huang SKS, Mazzola F, et al. Long-term outcome after radiofrequency catheter ablation of atrioventricular nodal reentrant tachycardia with the anterior-approach method. *Am Heart J* 1996;132:125–129.

14. Mehta D, Gomes JA. Long-term results of fast pathway ablation in atrioventricular nodal reentry tachycardia using a modified technique. *Br Heart J* 1995;74:671–675.

15. Kottkamp H, Hindricks G, Willems S, et al. An anatomically and electrogram-guided stepwise approach for effective and safe catheter ablation of the fast pathway for elimination of atrioventricular node reentrant tachycardia. *J Am Coll Cardiol* 1995;25:974–981.

16. Langberg JJ, Leon A, Borganelli M, et al. A randomized, prospective comparison of anterior and posterior approaches to radiofrequency catheter ablation of atrioventricular nodal reentry tachycardia. *Circulation* 1993;87: 1551–1556.

17. Hindricks G, on behalf of the Multicenter European Radiofrequency Survey (MERFS) Investigators of the Working Group on Arrhythmias of the European Society of Cardiology: incidence of complete atrioventricular block following attempted radiofrequency catheter modification of the atrioventricular node in 880 patients. *Eur Heart J* 1996;17:82–88.

18. ACC/AHA Task Force report: guidelines for clinical intracardiac electrophysiological and catheter ablation procedure. *J Am Coll Cardiol* 1995;26: 555–573.

19. Lin JL, Huang SKS, Lai LP, et al. Radiofrequency catheter ablation of septal accessory pathways within the triangle of Koch: importance of energy titration testing other than the local electrogram characteristics for identifying the successful target site. *PACE* 1998;21:1909–1917.

20. Lai LP, Lin JL, Chen TF, et al. Clinical electrophysiological characteristics

and radiofrequency catheter ablation of atrial tachycardia near the apex of Koch's triangle. *PACE* 1998;21:367–374.

21. Lin JL, Lai LP, Lin LJ, et al. The distal end of the atrioventricular nodal artery serves as a landmark identifying the risk of complete heart block during radiofrequency catheter ablation of the slow pathway in atrioventricular nodal reentrant tachycardia [abstract]. *J Am Coll Cardiol* 1998;31(suppl A);202A.

Chapter 22

Selective Slow Pathway Ablation for Treatment of AV Nodal Reentrant Tachycardia

Gregg W. Taylor, M.D., G. Neal Kay, M.D.

Clinical Features and Traditional Concepts of Atrioventricular Nodal Reentry

The most common cause of paroxysmal supraventricular tachycardia is atrioventricular nodal reentry. Atrioventricular nodal reentrant tachycardia (AVNRT) is more common in females than males, is relatively uncommon in infants and young children, and is characterized by the onset of recurrent episodes of rapid palpitations in young adulthood or middle age. Electrocardiographically, the P waves are either absent or can be seen distorting the terminal portion of the QRS, suggesting to early investigators that the atria and ventricles are activated simultaneously. Esophageal and intracardiac electrograms in patients with this arrhythmia later confirmed these findings and demonstrated that a long atrio-His (AH) interval and a short His-to-atrial (HA) interval were typical of AVNRT. Strong evidence supporting a reentrant mechanism in AVNRT was provided by Denes and associates who demonstrated that inititiation of tachycardia was dependent upon attainment of a critical delay in the AH interval, and by observing that dual conduction pathways were typical of patients with AVNRT.[1] Additional support for the presence of dual conduction pathways through the AV node was presented by Rosen and colleagues who demonstrated the presence of 2 distinct sets of PR intervals on the surface electrocardiogram of a patient with AVNRT.[2] Based on these observations, typical AVNRT has traditionally been thought to involve reentrant activation within

From Huang SKS, Wilber DJ (eds.): *Radiofrequency Catheter Ablation of Cardiac Arrhythmias: Basic Concepts and Clinical Applications,* 2nd ed. Armonk, NY: Futura Publishing Company, Inc. ©2000.

the AV node, with antegrade conduction via a slowly conducting (slow) pathway and retrograde conduction over a more rapidly conducting (fast) pathway.

Animal Models of the AV Junction

Functional Division of the AV Junction

Based on the velocity of action potential propagation and the upstroke velocity of the action potential, the region of the AV junction can be divided into 3 functional areas[3,4] which are diagrammatically displayed in Figure 1. The AN region is composed of transitional cells that join the atrium to the atrioventricular node. This region is characterized by slowing of the upstroke velocity of the action potential and reduction in the velocity of propagation of the wavefront of excitation. The N region, corresponding to the compact AV node, consists of cells with the slowest rate of rise of the action potential upstroke and conduction velocity. Located between the compact AV node and the penetrating bundle of His are cells in the NH region, with action potentials and conduction velocities that are more rapid than the N region (similar to the AN region). The cells at the atrial border of the AV node are generally oriented with their long axis parallel to that of the node.[3,4] In the N region, however, the cells are more densely packed with greater diameter and a more rounded appearance than in

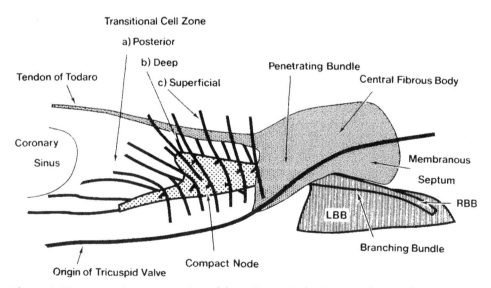

Figure 1. Diagrammatic representation of the atrioventricular junctional area. The AN region is composed of 3 groups of transitional cells that join the compact node. The NH region connects the compact node and the His bundle. LBB = left bundle branch; RBB = right bundle branch. (Reproduced by permission from Becker AE, Anderson RH. Morphology of the human atrioventricular junctional area. In: Wellens HJJ, Lie KI, Janse MJ, eds. *The Conduction System of the Heart.* Philadelphia, PA: Lea and Febiger, 1976. p 276.)

the transitional zones. Conduction through the compact AV node is associated with gradually decaying amplitude and rising velocity of the action potential (decremental conduction).

Atrial Inputs to the AV Junction

Much of the available anatomic information concerning the atrial inputs to the AV junction is derived from animal models, particularly the rabbit and canine heart. In the rabbit model, as shown schematically in Figure 2, the compact atrio-

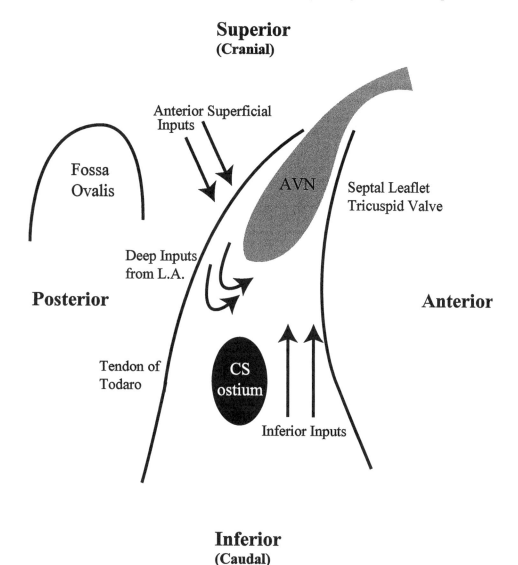

Figure 2. Schematic representation of the atrial inputs to the AV node. See text for details. CS = coronary sinus; AVN = atrioventricular node.

ventricular node receives atrial input from superficial (relative to the right atrial endocardium) transitional cells approaching superiorly from the region of the limbus of the fossa ovalis, and from a deep group of transitional cells that approach the node from the left atrial side of the interatrial septum.[5,6] Inferior input is via transitional cells that extend from the crista terminalis and approach the AV node from the region of the coronary sinus ostium.[5] During normal sinus rhythm, the superior superficial cells in the interatrial septum and the deep left-sided group of transitional cells provide preferential input to the compact AV node. In the case of block in these approaches, antegrade conduction occurs via the inferior transitional cells approaching the AV node from the crista terminalis.[5,6] In the rabbit model, retrograde AV nodal conduction is associated with earliest atrial activation in the region of the superior superficial cells.[3,4]

AV Node Echo Beats

Atrioventricular node echo beats have been demonstrated to involve antegrade conduction over the inferior group of cells approaching from the crista terminalis with retrograde atrial activation via the superior superficial fibers.[7,8] The safety margin for conduction over the slower, inferior input to the node has been shown to be greater than that of the more rapidly conducting, superior input from the interatrial septum.[7] With programmed atrial stimulation, unidirectional block in either the region of the crista terminalis or the interatrial septal input to the AV node could result in AV nodal echo beats.[9,10] Antegrade conduction block along the interatrial septal input to the AV node has been shown to result in conduction over the posterior input to the node at the insertion of the crista terminalis, subsequently producing reentrant echo beats.[8] By placing a surgical incision in the perinodal tissue, reentrant echo beats could be abolished.[8] These experiments suggest a critical role of the perinodal atrium in atrioventricular nodal reentry.

Anatomic and Functional Concepts of Human AVNRT

Unlike other reentrant arrhythmias which have been well characterized by intracardiac mapping, the precise anatomic circuit maintaining AVNRT remains undefined. Incomplete understanding of the anatomic and functional characteristics of the reentrant circuit in AVNRT stems from its location in the center of the heart, and from the complex three-dimensional structure of the AV node. Debate over the presence of an upper and lower common pathway, and whether the reentrant circuit is purely intranodal or contains extranodal atrial inputs, is still unsettled.[11–18] The arguments surrounding these controversies come from anatomic and functional observations made at the time of intracardiac mapping, either in the electrophysiological laboratory or in the operating room, and are described in the following paragraphs.

Anatomic Separation of Fast and Slow Pathways

Sung and colleagues first described an abrupt shift in the site of earliest retrograde atrial activation during ventricular pacing from the His bundle electrogram to the region near the ostium of the coronary sinus coincident with a sudden prolongation of the HA interval in patients with dual AV nodal pathways.[19] This observation has been confirmed by several investigators and interpreted as evidence that the atrial insertion of the slow pathway may be located more inferior to the fast pathway. In a study by Keim and colleagues, reversible cooling (ice mapping) was performed to localize the functional fast and slow pathways during surgical ablation of AV nodal reentrant tachycardia (AVNRT).[15] In 4 of 6 patients studied, conduction over the slow pathway was blocked during reversible cooling of atrial myocardium along the tricuspid annulus inferior to the AV node (extending from the coronary sinus). In the additional patients, antegrade slow pathway conduction was interrupted by reversible cooling along the tricuspid annulus superior to the AV node (1 patient) or in the interatrial septum as it approached the AV node from the limbus of the fossa ovalis (1 patient). Retrograde fast pathway conduction was interrupted by ice mapping along the tendon of Todaro. Importantly, AV nodal reentry could not be interrupted by reversible cooling at sites intermediate to the functional fast and slow pathways, suggesting no obligate linking of these fibers by a specialized anatomic structure in the perinodal atrium. Additional direct evidence in support of an anatomic separation of the slow and fast pathway has been provided by patients undergoing operative dissection of the perinodal atrial myocardium for long-term cure of AVNRT.[15,20–25] In these studies, surgical dissection eliminated either the fast or slow pathway, leaving the alternate conduction pathway intact. These data suggest that the fast conducting fibers are located superiorly, extending from the AV node towards the tendon of Todaro and foramen ovale. The slowly conducting fibers were shown to be located inferiorly, extending toward the compact AV node, along the tricuspid annulus, from the direction of the coronary sinus ostium.

Changes in Fast and Slow Pathway Conduction with Pacing Location

In addition to these anatomic observations, the site of pacing within the atria affects the AV nodal conduction interval.[17] Thus, the AH interval is typically shorter with pacing from the coronary sinus ostium than during pacing from the right atrium. This may suggest that the "fast pathway" fibers approaching the AV node from the left side of the interatrial septum have a shorter conduction time than fibers entering from the right side of the septum.[5] The slow pathway, representing fibers approaching the AV node inferiorly, is also activated with a shorter AH interval during pacing from the coronary sinus than from the right atrium. An alternative explanation for this finding may be that the AH interval measured with a standard electrode catheter may not reflect the true AV nodal conduction time. Rather, this increase may include intraatrial but extranodal conduction.

Evidence For and Against an Upper Common Pathway

Evidence for the existence of an upper common pathway proximal to fast and slow fibers located within the AV node has been suggested by the finding of AV Wenckebach block during atrial pacing at a pacing rate slower than that of AVNRT.[11] This difference in AV Wenckebach rates has been reported in a minority of patients with AV nodal reentry.[11] In addition, the AH interval during atrial pacing (measured from the end of the atrial deflection to the onset of the His deflection) may exceed the AH interval during AVNRT (measured from the onset of the atrial deflection to the onset of the His deflection) in some patients (less than 10%). Retrograde VA block in the fast pathway during atrioventricular nodal reentry has also been observed[12,13] suggesting that the atrium may not be a necessary portion of the reentry circuit. The observation of retrograde VA block, however occurs in a rare minority of patients with AVNRT.[12]

In contrast to these observations, premature atrial extrastimuli introduced from the inferior interatrial septum near the coronary sinus during AVNRT just before the expected time of retrograde fast pathway conduction can activate the slow pathway and advance the tachycardia (activate the His bundle early).[14] This point strongly suggests that there is an extranodal gap between the fast and slow pathway. Additionally, in 9 patients, Satoh and colleagues[26] paced the coronary sinus and high right atrium, attempting to entrain AVNRT. In 5 of 9 patients, orthodromic capture of the atrial electrogram recording at the His bundle potential was observed leading the investigators to conclude that an upper common pathway was absent. Further observations from intraoperative ice mapping[15] and high-resolution electrical mapping of Koch's triangle at the time of surgical dissection[16,25] in patients with AVNRT demonstrated no evidence of a proximal common pathway in the reentrant circuit (see below). In addition to these observations, the widespread recognition that ablation of the inferior inputs to the AV node in patients with AVNRT may prevent inducibility of this arrhythmia without affecting slow pathway conduction further supports the absence of a proximal common pathway. The sum of the available evidence calls into question the existence of a proximal common pathway[14–16,25,26]

Evidence for a Distal Common Pathway

Perhaps less controversial is the evidence that supports the existence of a distal common pathway, located proximal to the His bundle, in the lower region of the AV node. Miller and colleagues studied the HA interval during AVNRT and during ventricular pacing in 28 patients with this arrhythmia.[11] The HA interval during pacing exceeded the HA interval during AVNRT in 19 of 28 patients (68%) by a mean of 25 milliseconds, suggesting the presence of AV nodal tissue between the His bundle and the distal turnaround of the fast and slow pathways.[11] In addition, VA Wenckebach block occurred at a ventricular pacing rate slower than that of AVNRT in 2 patients. The spontaneous occurrence of 2:1 AV block proximal to the His bundle during AVNRT, as shown in Figure 3, also strongly supports the existence of a distal common pathway.[12,61]

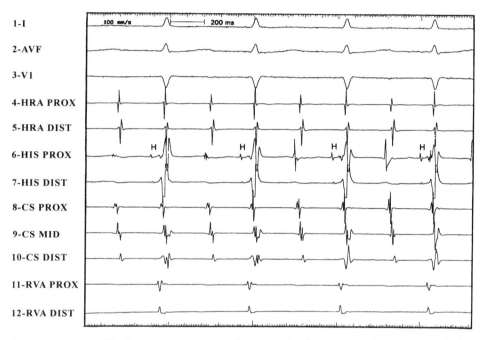

Figure 3A. 2:1 AV block during AVNRT. Surface ECG leads 1, aVF, and V₁ are recorded simultaneously with bipolar intracardiac electrograms recorded from the high right atrium proximal (HRA PROX) and distal (HRA DIST) electrode pairs, His bundle proximal (HIS PROX) and distal (HIS DIST) pairs, coronary sinus proximal (CS PROX), mid (CS MID), and distal (CS DIST) pairs, and right ventricular apex proximal (RVA PROX) and distal (RVA DIST). Note that block is proximal to the His bundle as indicated by an absence of a His bundle deflection during beats not conducted to the ventricle.

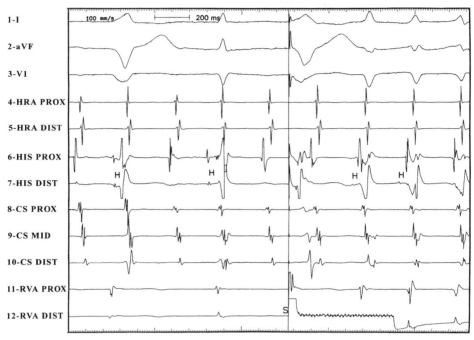

Figure 3B. A premature ventricular extrastimulus (S) delivered during AVNRT results in 1:1 AV conduction, without a change in the atrial cycle length. This finding suggests the presence of a lower common pathway that is proximal to the bundle of His.

Evidence For and Against the Necessity of the Atrium in the Reentrant Circuit

The concept that AVNRT involves a reentrant circuit that is confined to the AV node (atria unnecessary) was supported by the observation of several investigators that spontaneous retrograde block in the HA interval may occur without interruption of the tachycardia.[12,13] Others demonstrated that premature atrial stimuli delivered during AVNRT could render the atrium refractory to retrograde atrial activation without interrupting the tachycardia.[18] Also, the delivery of premature atrial stimuli during AVNRT has been shown to advance the tachycardia (shorten the HA) without affecting the tachycardia cycle length. Finally, the presence of atrial fibrillation during AVNRT would suggest that the atria do not form part of the reentrant circuit, although this phenomenon is exceedingly rare.[27]

The experimental evidence suggesting that the atria are required to maintain the reentrant circuit in human AVNRT comes from multiple mapping studies at the time of surgery. As previously noted,[15,20–25] these studies show that cure of AVNRT can be produced by placing ablative lesions in the perinodal atrial myocardium, as much as 10 millimeters or more from the compact AV node. Pathological studies at the time of autopsy[28] or heart transplantation[29] in patients previously cured of AVNRT with RF catheter ablation reveal an absence of necrosis in the compact AV node. In the case described by Olgin and colleagues,[28] there was no evidence of any gross or histological damage to the AV node or to the transitional cells approaching the compact AV node in a patient dying 5 months after successful slow pathway ablation of typical AVNRT. Experimental evidence provided by surgical and histological examination strongly supports the requirement of atrial tissue in the reentrant circuit in some patients.

Electrophysiological Properties of Fast and Slow Pathways in Humans

There are several important functional differences in the fast and slow AV nodal pathways. First, the effective refractrory period (ERP) of the antegrade fast pathway is usually longer than that of the slow pathway.[2,30] There are many exceptions to this observation, a factor with great practical importance for the demonstration of slow pathway conduction. Second, the fast and slow pathways may have quantitatively differing responses to autonomic and pharmacological manipulations. For example, adrenergic stimulation tends to shorten the ERP of the fast pathway (both antegrade and retrograde) to a greater extent than that of the slow pathway.[31,32] This finding can be exploited by administration of isoproterenol to stimulate antegrade and retrograde fast pathway conduction when slow pathway conduction predominates at rest. Conversely, for patients with high catecholamine states, slow pathway conduction may not be demonstrable if the ERP of the fast pathway is less than that of the slow pathway. In these individuals, the use of a b- adrenergic blocking agent such as propranolol[32] or esmolol[31] tends to prolong the ERP of the antegrade fast pathway to a greater extent than it does for the slow pathway, thereby allowing demonstration of slow pathway conduction. Although retrograde fast pathway conduction tends to result in earliest retrograde atrial activation at the apex of Koch's triangle while retrograde slow pathway conduction activates the base of the triangle near the coronary sinus ostium, there are exceptions to this rule.[19,33] The retrograde fast pathway has been reported by several authors to be associated with nondecremental conduction properties in the HA interval, suggesting to some investigators that the retrograde fast pathway may be an accessory bypass tract.[34–37] The surgical cure of AVNRT may be accomplished without influencing the nondecremental nature of the retrograde fast pathway.[34] Studies of patients with AVNRT and controls have shown that retrograde VA conduction is almost uniformly depressed by Type 1 antiarrhythmic drugs such as procainamide,[38] constituting evidence against the notion that the retrograde fast pathway is an accessory bypass tract.

Catheter Ablation Techniques for AV Nodal Modification

Armed with these important clues to the anatomic substrate of AV nodal reentry, several investigators have used catheter ablation techniques to modify AV nodal conduction and eliminate AVNRT in cases of patients who have been refractory to medical therapy.[36,39-47] Haïssaguerre and colleagues reported that DC shocks applied to the region of the superior margin of the tricuspid annulus near the apex of Koch's triangle were effective in ablating retrograde fast pathway conduction in patients with AVNRT.[45] Lee and associates demonstrated that the application of radiofrequency (RF) current in the same region was capable of eliminating retrograde fast pathway conduction with prolongation of the PR and AH intervals, suggesting that the antegrade fast pathway had been eliminated or significantly modified.[41] More recently, several investigators have shown that antegrade slow pathway conduction can be selectively eliminated by the application of RF current along the tricuspid annulus near the ostium of the coronary sinus.[36,42,43,46,47] Based on these observations, a revised concept of AVNRT has been proposed that suggests the fast pathway is usually located superiorly in Koch's triangle with the slow pathway located more inferiorly and using perinodal atrial myocardium.[36,42,47] Although this revised concept implies that the fast and slow pathways are anatomically distinct, it remains uncertain whether either of these pathways are composed of normal AV nodal transitional cells, specialized atrial myocardium, or ordinary working atrial myocardium with conduction properties analogous to an accessory AV pathway. However, several pathological examinations of hearts in patients who have undergone catheter ablation for AVNRT have been published. In none of these cases can a discrete structure composed of specialized conduction tissue be identified in the region ablated.

Technique of Selective Slow Pathway Ablation

The standard technique for slow pathway ablation is to perform the diagnostic electrophysiological study during the same session as the therapeutic procedure. Therefore, after sedation with an intravenous narcotic (fentanyl) and a benzodiazepine (midazolam or diazepam) and local anesthesia with 1% mepivacaine, a 6F hexapolar or octapolar catheter is inserted into the right internal jugular vein and positioned in the coronary sinus. Quadripolar catheters are then advanced from the femoral vein to the high right atrium, right ventricular apex and across the tricuspid valve for recording of His bundle activation. Heparin 2500–5000 IU (depending on body surface area) is administered intravenously following catheter insertion, followed by an additional 1000 IU each subsequent hour of the procedure.

Programmed atrial stimulation is performed from the high right atrium for construction of an AV nodal function curve. Rapid atrial pacing is performed starting at a rate slightly faster than that of the sinus node and increased gradually until AV Wenckebach block is observed. The development of a PR interval that is greater than the atrial pacing cycle length is a strong indicator of antegrade slow pathway conduction.[70] In order for this sign to be meaningful, the PR interval should exceed the RR interval with rapid atrial pacing during stable 1:1 AV conduction. Programmed ventricular stimulation is also performed to construct a retrograde AV conduction system function curve with careful attention to the site of earliest atrial activation. In addition, incremental ventricular pacing is performed to evaluate the sequence of retrograde atrial activation and the VA and HA intervals. Isoproterenol is routinely infused to allow assessment of antegrade and retrograde conduction during adrenergic stimulation and to facilitate the induction of AVNRT (if necessary).

In patients in whom a discontinuous AV nodal function curve cannot be demonstrated during programmed atrial stimulation, it is important to determine the reason. If the fast pathway conduction is suppressed in the baseline state, as evidenced by a long AH interval at all atrial pacing rates or VA block during ventricular pacing, isoproterenol is infused. Isoproterenol usually facilitates fast pathway conduction in such cases, often allowing recognition of dual AV nodal pathways and induction of AVNRT. Occasionally atropine must also be administered in such patients. In contrast, if the baseline ERP of the fast pathway is very short, conduction over the slow pathway may be difficult to document. In this situation, increasing the degree of sedation or infusing esmolol may prolong the fast pathway refractory period and allow recognition of slow pathway conduction.[31]

Perhaps before discussing the typical location of the slow and fast AV nodal pathways, the terminology used to discuss the anatomy of this region should be clarified. As noted in Figure 2, the septal leaflet of the tricuspid valve is actually the *anterior* boundary of Koch's triangle. The superior boundary of this region is the membranous interventricular septum. The posterior border of the triangle is the tendon of Todaro, and the inferior boundary is the ostium of the coronary sinus. Therefore, the slow pathway is inferior (caudal) to the compact AV node. RF ablation of the slow pathway is usually directed *anterior* to the coronary sinus ostium in the rim of myocardium between the tricuspid valve and the ostium of the coronary sinus. In contrast, the fast pathway fibers actually approach the compact AV node from a posterior and superior direction. Therefore, the true anatomy is somewhat different than that commonly used by electrophysiologists to discuss ablation in this region.

Once slow pathway conduction can be reproducibly demonstrated, the ablation catheter is positioned along the tricuspid annulus immediately anterior to the coronary sinus ostium. The right anterior oblique view is especially useful for positioning of catheters as it best displays Koch's triangle in profile. The target zone is the isthmus of tissue between the tricuspid valve annulus and os of the coronary sinus (Figure 4). Positioning of the catheters is best performed during sinus rhythm as the atrial and ventricular deflections in the tricuspid annulus electrogram are more easily discerned. The ablation catheter should have a distal electrode of at least 4 mm in length and should have a deflectable distal segment. The length of the deflecting segment of the ablation catheter that has proven most effective has ranged from 2.0 to 3.0 inches. The number of electrodes on the ablation catheter is largely a matter of operator preference. A quadripolar catheter with an interelectrode distance of 2 mm and a spacing of 5 mm between the proximal and distal pairs has been most commonly used. The ablation catheter is advanced into the right ventricle, moved inferiorly so that it lies anterior to the ostium of the coronary sinus, and then withdrawn towards the tricuspid annulus until the distal pair of electrodes records a small atrial deflection and a large ventricular deflection. Although there are many exceptions, the proximal electrode pair typically records a larger atrial than ventricular deflection. The AV ratio recorded from the distal electrode pair in sinus rhythm may range from approximately 0.7:1 to 1:3.

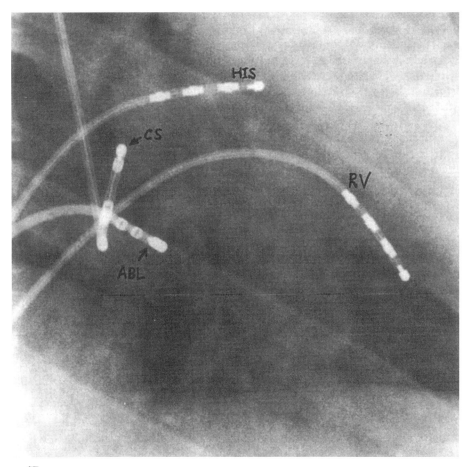

Figure 4. Fluoroscopic images of typical catheter position used for RF ablation of the slow AV nodal pathway. Panel A (right anterior oblique view). Note that this view demonstrates Koch's triangle in profile. The ablation catheter is positioned anterior to the coronary sinus ostium along the tricuspid annulus. The His bundle catheter marks the apex of the triangle. (*continued*)

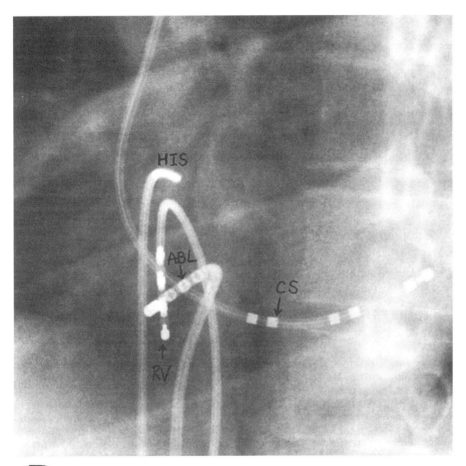

B

Figure 4. (*continued*) Panel B (left anterior oblique view). Note that the left anterior oblique view allows recognition of the catheter positions relative to the interatrial septum.

Our convention for describing the position of the ablation catheter in the region of Koch's triangle is to divide the length of the tricuspid annulus into 12 segments, with site 1 located at the apex of the triangle near the central fibrous body, site 10 located at the most inferior extent (floor) of the coronary sinus os- tium, and site 12 located more caudally as the tricuspid annulus begins to curve toward the free wall of the right atrium (Figure 5). The most common site for effective ablation of slow pathway conduction is along the tricuspid annulus im- mediately anterior to the coronary sinus ostium (sites 8–10). The slow pathway is successfully ablated at these sites in approximately 95% of patients with AVNRT. Elimination of slow pathway conduction may sometimes require that the catheter be repositioned along the tricuspid annulus inferior to the coro- nary sinus ostium (sites 11 and 12). If ablation of the slow pathway is not suc-

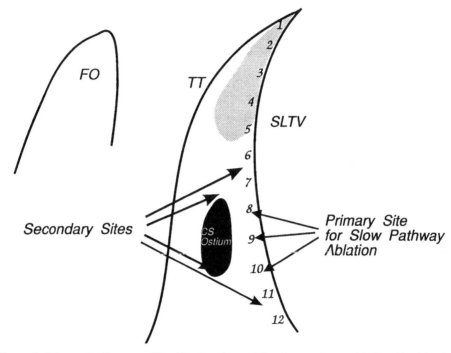

Figure 5. Schematic diagram of Koch's triangle used for slow pathway ablation. Koch's triangle is bounded anteriorly by the septal leaflet of the tricuspid valve (SLTV), posteriorly by the tendon of Todaro (TT), superiorly by the central fibrous body, and inferiorly by the coronary sinus ostium. The tricuspid annulus is divided into 12 sites, with site 1 being located at the apex of the triangle and site 10 located at the level of the inferior extent of the coronary sinus ostium. Sites 11 and 12 are located inferior to the level of the coronary sinus ostium. The most common site for ablation of the slow AV nodal pathway (Primary site) is along the tricuspid annulus immediately anterior to the coronary sinus ostium (sites 8–10). Less commonly, application of RF current may be effective in ablating slow pathway conduction at other sites (Secondary sites) immediately superior or inferior to the coronary sinus ostium, or along the tricuspid annulus at sites 7–8 or 11–12.

cessful at these locations, the ablation catheter is then moved more superiorly along the tricuspid annulus (site 7). In a very small percentage of patients, elimination of slow pathway conduction may require application of RF energy at other sites, such as those more cephalad along the tricuspid annulus (sites 5 or 6), in the ostium of the coronary sinus, or against the interatrial septum immediately superior to the coronary sinus ostium.

Application of RF Current

Several investigators have examined the role of temperature and impedance monitoring, and the effect of power output titration on initial success and tachycardia recurrence. Using fixed power output in 35 patients with AVNRT, Strickberger and colleagues[48] showed that the steady state electrode-tissue interface temperature during successful applications of energy was $48.5\pm3.3°C$ versus $46.8\pm5.5°C$ for unsuccessful applications. The change in mean impedance did not differ between successful and unsuccessful applications of RF energy. In this study there were no recurrences of AVNRT during 114 ± 21 days of follow-up. Calkins and colleagues[49] examined the relationship of electrode temperature and recurrent tachycardia in 201 patients undergoing AVNRT ablation. In this group of patients, there was no relation found between the likelihood of tachycardia recurrence and peak electrode temperature during RF ablation. Finally, Epstein and colleagues[50] used a closed-loop, temperature-feedback energy source in a series of 39 patients with AVNRT and retrospectively compared their results with 43 patients undergoing RF ablation of AVNRT with a nontemperature guided energy source. Procedural success was the same in both groups as was the number of RF applications and procedure duration. There was a significant difference in fluoroscopic duration and the formation of coagulum, in favor of temperature control.

In our laboratory, RF current is delivered in a unipolar configuration from the distal electrode of the ablation catheter toward a pair of dispersive electrode pads placed over the posterior thorax. RF current is delivered with an initial power of 30–40 watts for 30 seconds. Impedance is carefully monitored and RF energy is halted with any sudden rise in impedance. The electrocardiogram is continuously monitored for the presence of an accelerated junctional rhythm which typically occurs at the effective slow pathway ablation site. It should be stressed that an accelerated junctional rhythm is not specific to slow pathway ablation as it is routinely observed during intentional ablation of the AV node as well as in many instances of intentional fast pathway ablation.

After each RF current application, programmed atrial stimulation and/or rapid atrial pacing are performed to determine the presence or absence of slow pathway conduction, AV nodal echoes, or inducible AVNRT (Figure 6). If any of these characteristics remain, the catheter is repositioned and RF current is applied at a slightly different position. The sequence of ablation sites chosen for delivery of RF energy is related to the probability of successful slow pathway ablation at each site and the risk of impairing AV conduction. Thus, RF energy applications are initially delivered at Koch's triangle sites 8–10, then at site

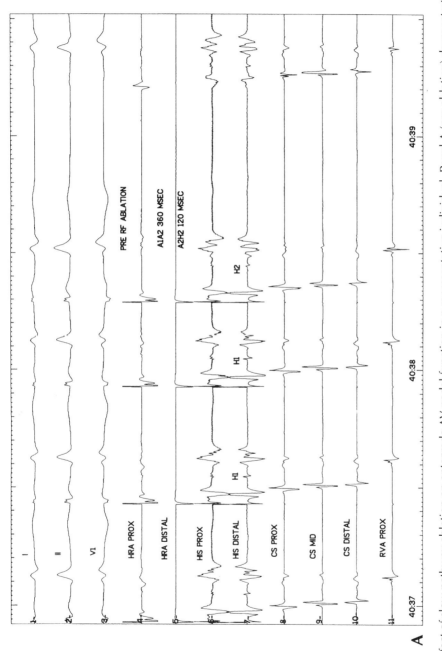

Figure 6. Effect of slow pathway ablation on antegrade AV nodal function in a representative individual. Panel A (pre-ablation) demonstrates surface electrocardiographic leads I, II, and V_1 recorded simultaneously with bipolar intracardiac electrograms recorded from the high right atrium proximal (HRA PROX) and distal (HRA DISTAL) electrode pairs, His bundle proximal (HIS PROX) and distal (HIS DISTAL) pairs, coronary sinus proximal (CS PROX), mid (CS MID), and distal (CS DISTAL) pairs, and right ventricular apex (RVA PROX). During programmed atrial stimulation from the HRA at a basic drive cycle length of 500 milliseconds, a premature extrastimulus with A1A2 coupling interval of 360 milliseconds is introduced. Note that the A2H2 interval measures 120 milliseconds. (*continued*)

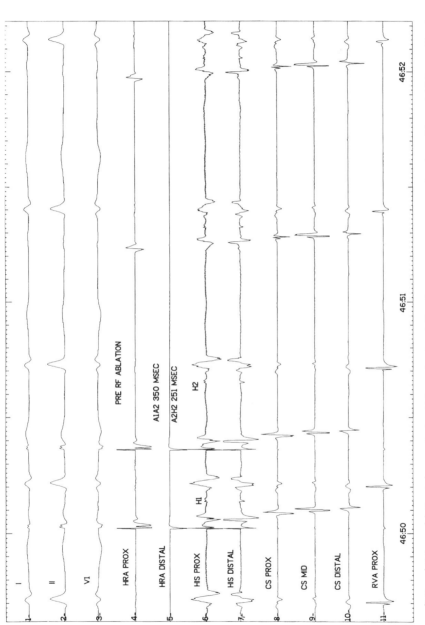

Figure 6. (*continued*) Panel B (pre-ablation) demonstrates AV conduction following a premature extrastimulus with an A1A2 coupling interval of 350 milliseconds. Note that the A2H2 interval prolongs to 251 milliseconds, consistent with block of conduction in the fast AV nodal pathway with antegrade conduction via the slow pathway. (*continued*)

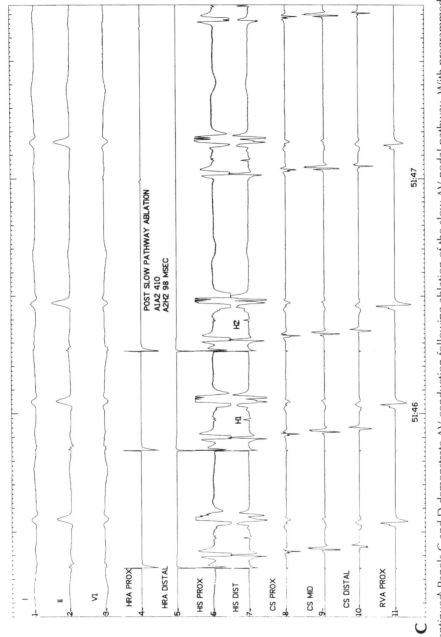

Figure 6. (*continued*) Panels C and D demonstrate AV conduction following ablation of the slow AV nodal pathway. With programmed stimulation at a basic drive cycle length of 500 milliseconds, a premature extrastimulus with A1A2 coupling interval of 410 milliseconds is associated with an A2H2 interval of 98 milliseconds (Panel C). (*continued*)

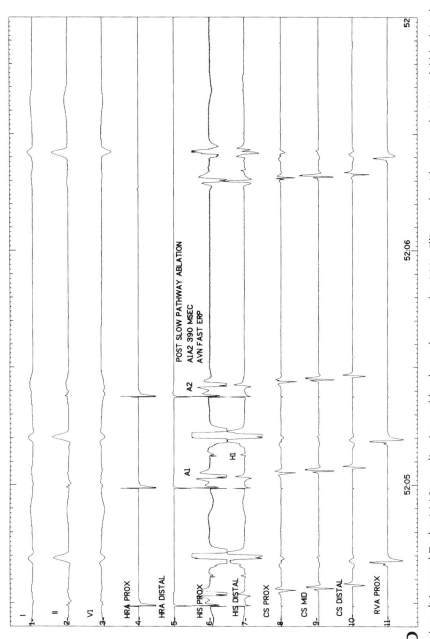

Figure 6. (*continued*) In panel D, the A1A2 coupling interval has been decreased to 390 milliseconds with antegrade AV nodal block in the fast pathway and no further evidence of slow pathway conduction.

6–7, and finally at Koch's triangle site 5, only if the risk of complete AV block can be justified by the severity of the clinical symptoms.

In our experience, the number of RF applications necessary to initially render AVNRT noninducible was 5.1 ± 6.1 lesions. The total number of RF lesions delivered (including "bonus applications") was 6.8 ± 6.4 RF applications. The mean RF energy delivered at the effective site was 41 ± 20 watts.

Study Population

Between June 10, 1990, and July 31, 1997, 1055 patients with AVNRT were referred to the clinical electrophysiology laboratory at the University of Alabama at Birmingham for catheter ablation. The ablation procedure was performed in accordance with an experimental protocol approved by the Institutional Review Board for Research Involving Human Subjects and all patients gave written, informed consent. Antiarrhythmic drugs had been discontinued for at least 4 half-lives in all subjects. There were 717 females (68%) and 338 males (32%) ranging in age from 7 to 93 years (mean 47.8 ± 17.1 years). The clinical arrhythmia was typical AVNRT (slow antegrade-fast retrograde) in 97% of patients, atypical AVNRT (fast antegrade-slow retrograde) in 1% patients, and both typical and atypical forms of AVNRT in 1% patients. The mean cycle length of AVNRT was 345 ± 92 milliseconds. The demonstration of dual AV nodal pathways required the administration of isoproterenol, isoproterenol plus atropine, or esmolol in 19% of patients. The intent of AV nodal modification was to selectively ablate the slow AV nodal pathway in 1051 patients. In 4 patients the fast pathway was chosen for selective ablation because of inability to reliably demonstrate slow pathway conduction in 2 patients, recurrence of AVNRT following a previous slow pathway ablation procedure in 1 patient, and concerns regarding the functional status of the antegrade fast pathway in 1 patient.

Efficacy of AV Nodal Modification

The slow pathway was selectively ablated in 1043 of 1051 patients (99%) in whom the procedure was attempted, with 8 patients developing some impairment of antegrade fast pathway conduction. The fast pathway was intentionally ablated in 4 of 4 patients attempted. AVNRT was rendered noninducible in 1054 of 1055 patients (99.9%). The one primary failure in our experience occurred in a patient with both the typical and atypical forms of AVNRT. Although selective slow pathway ablation did not prevent inducibility of a slow form of atypical AVNRT in this individual, AVNRT of the typical form was rendered noninducible following the procedure. This patient has had no recurrence of palpitations in over 7 years of follow-up. Complete AV block occurred in 6 patients (0.5%), following a single ablation session in 5 patients and 2 sessions in one. AV block was observed when the application of RF current was confined to Koch's triangle site 7 or more inferiorly in 3 cases. In our entire series of 1055 patients, the mean fluoroscopic exposure has been 13.8 minutes.

Follow-up

AVNRT recurred in 36 of 1055 patients (3.4%) who had an initially successful procedure, including 35 patients after selective slow pathway ablation and 1 patient after inadvertent fast pathway ablation. A second, successful ablation procedure was performed in 34 of 35 patients with tachycardia recurrence. One patient declined a repeat ablation procedure as her case has been well controlled with medical therapy that had been previously ineffective. Overall, 1052 of 1055 patients (99.7%) have had long-term elimination of AVNRT without antiarrhythmic medications. Several patients have complained of rapid palpitations that have been documented to be sinus rhythm or premature atrial and ventricular depolarizations. The cases of these patients have been managed with reassurance.

The Effect of Slow Pathway Ablation on Residual AV Nodal Conduction

The effect of slow pathway ablation on residual AV nodal conduction is shown in Table 1. As our data and others' demonstrate, selective ablation of the slow pathway by application of RF current along the tricuspid annulus caudal to the expected location of the compact AV node eliminates the typical discontinuous AV conduction curve without impairing fast pathway function.[36,42,46,47] In many cases the ERP of the fast pathway actually shortens following slow pathway ablation.[36,51] The mechanism of shortening was investigated by Natale and colleagues[51] who compared changes in the fast pathway ERP with and without autonomic blockade both before and after RF ablation of the slow pathway. Before ablation, autonomic blockade did not alter the ERP of the fast pathway. After ablation, the fast pathway ERP was shortened in both groups of patients but there was no difference in the degreee of shortening between patients with and without autonomic blockade. In another study designed to look at changes in fast pathway ERP after slow pathway ablation, Strickberger and colleagues[52] found that the fast pathway ERP was shortened only after complete loss of slow pathway conduction (loss of dual AV nodal physiology and the absence of echo beats). These observations led the authors to suggest that changes in fast path-

Table 1
Effect of Slow Pathway Ablation on AV Conduction

Parameter	Preablation	Postablation	P
Sinus CL (msec)	769±172	688±170	0.10
AH Interval (msec)	69.3±18.5	71.7±27	NS
Antegrade ERP Fast (msec)	360.9±100.2	342.2±90	0.09
Retrograde ERP Fast (msec)	296.3±118	290.0±79.2	NS
AV Wenckebach Rate (bpm)	179.2±65.5	175.4±73.4	NS
VA Wenckebach Rate (bpm)	188.3±47.2	194.1±45.4	NS

Table 2
Complications

Complication	n	%
Complete AV Block	6	.6
Pulmonary Edema	1	0.1
Hematoma	2	0.2
Femoral Artery Pseudoaneurysm	1	0.1
Deep Vein Thrombosis	1	0.1
Pericardial Tamponade	2	0.2
Total	13/1055	1.2

way ERP after RF ablation of the slow pathway were secondary to a withdrawal of electrotonic inhibition of the fast pathway by the slow pathway. In general, retrograde fast pathway conduction is not influenced by slow pathway ablation.[36,42] However, if the ablation site is moved more superiorly (closer to the AV node), several authors have found that antegrade slow pathway ablation may be associated with elimination of retrograde fast pathway conduction.[36,47] If the ablation site is in the usual inferior location (at the level of the coronary sinus ostium), retrograde conduction remains intact in the fast pathway and continues to be associated with a nondecremental HA interval.[36]

Complications

Complications observed during the course of our experience are shown in Table 2. Six patients have developed complete AV block, with 3 cases occurring in our initial 50 patients. Pericardial tamponade occurred in 2 patients; in both, it was managed with percutaneous drainage without long-term sequelae. Two patients developed groin hematomas, and one developed a femoral artery pseudoaneurysm, requiring surgical repair. One patient developed a deep vein thrombosis that was treated with long-term anticoagulation. Thus the total complication rate has been 1.2%.

Importance of Accelerated Junctional
Rhythm During Slow Pathway Ablation

Our data[53] and that of others[54,55] suggest that an accelerated junctional rhythm is to be expected with successful ablation of slow pathway conduction. Indeed, among 127 patients in whom this phenomenon was carefully studied[53] the RF current application that was effective in eliminating slow pathway conduction was associated with an accelerated junctional rhythm (Figure 7) in 120 patients (94%). In another study designed to characterize the difference between junctional ectopy associated with successful and unsuccessful RF abla-

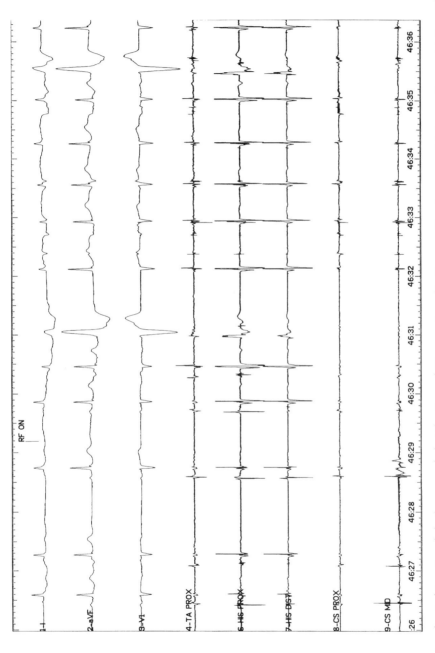

Figure 7. Accelerated junctional rhythm recorded at the time of RF current application resulting in successful slow pathway ablation. The ablation catheter was positioned along the tricuspid annulus inferior to the coronary sinus ostium. Note that following the initiation of RF current delivery (RF ON), premature atrial and ventricular beats and junctional extrasystoles are produced. The development of an accelerated junctional rhythm during application of RF current is typical of successful slow pathway ablation.

tion of AVNRT, junctional ectopy was seen more frequently (100% versus 65%), and for a longer duration (7.1±7.1 versus 5.0±7.0 seconds) during successful versus unsuccessful RF applications.[55] Because the absence of junctional ectopy during RF ablation corresponds to an ineffective ablation site, it is our practice to terminate the application of RF current at a given site if an accelerated junctional rhythm is not observed within 10–15 seconds. It should be emphasized that observation of an accelerated junctional rhythm is not specific to ablation of the slow pathway, as it is routinely induced during intentional AV nodal ablation, and is thought to be a response to thermal injury of the compact AV node or perinodal inputs of the slow and fast pathway.

Importance of Recording Slow Pathway Potentials

Several investigators have reported that activation of the slow pathway is associated with the inscription of discrete electrical potentials (Figure 8), often referred to as "slow pathway potentials" or "slow potentials."[42,56] In these studies, the presence of a slow potential was used to locate the slow pathway, serving as a site to target RF energy. The origin of these potentials is uncertain, though McGuire and colleagues[57] concluded that they were produced by asynchronous activation of muscle bundles at various sites in Koch's triangle in blood-perfused porcine and canine hearts. The electrogram morphology has been variously described as either sharp and rapid or slow and broad with a low amplitude, and the timing of slow pathway potentials during the cardiac cycle has been reported either to closely follow local atrial activation near the coronary sinus ostium[42] or to span the AH interval.[56] Such potentials are neither specific to Koch's triangle nor to patients with AVNRT.[58] Niebauer and colleagues investigated the prevalence of slow pathway potentials at various sites in the atrium in patients with and without AVNRT.[58] In their study, there was no difference in the number or morphology of "slow potentials" in the posteroseptal area in patients with and without AVNRT. In addition, slow pathway potentials were found at locations outside Koch's triangle, at the anterior, posterior, and lateral aspects of the tricuspid valve annulus in a minority of patients with and without AVNRT.[58] These data support the notion that slow pathway potentials are not specific to individuals with AVNRT and may occur in regions of the right atrium where transitional cells are not thought to be found.

Despite these observations, the probability of recording putative slow pathway potentials at the site of effective slow pathway ablation is quite high, probably in excess of 90% of cases.[42,56]

The specificity of these deflections to predict an effective ablation site is likely to be much lower, however. In our experience, the recording of electrograms compatible with slow pathway potentials at a site along the tricuspid annulus does not necessarily predict successful RF ablation of the slow pathway. In addition, slow pathway conduction can also be eliminated by the delivery of RF current at sites that do not record putative slow pathway potentials. Nevertheless, fractionated atrial electrograms are usually recorded at sites along the tricuspid annulus that have other characteristics predictive of successful

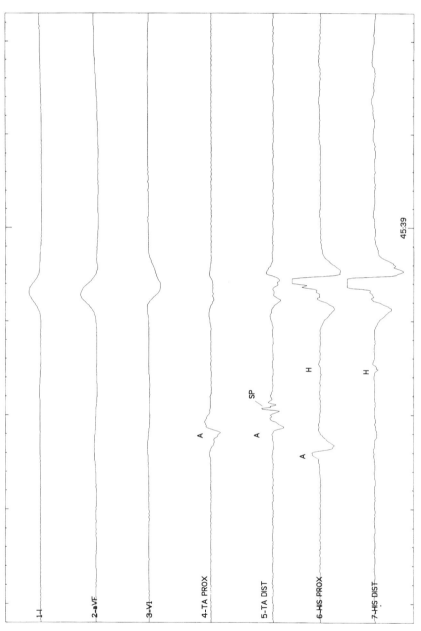

Figure 8. A representative example of bipolar electrograms recorded along the tricuspid annulus proximal (TA PROX) and distal (TA DISTAL) electrode pairs immediately anterior to the ostium of the coronary sinus in a patient with AVNRT. Note that the atrial and ventricular deflections have approximately equal amplitude in the distal electrode pair. In the distal (but not the proximal) tricuspid annulus electrogram, a discrete deflection with relatively rapid upstroke is recorded (SP). Application of RF current at the TA Distal site resulted in successful slow pathway ablation. (Paper speed 400 mm/sec).

slow pathway ablation. Thus, we prefer to refer to these characteristic signals as "fractionated atrial electrograms" rather than imply a discrete specialized conduction pathway.

Potential Advantages of Slow Pathway Ablation as Compared to Fast Pathway Ablation

There are 2 overriding advantages of the slow pathway ablation technique that favor its use as compared to fast pathway ablation. First, the risk of complete AV block is significantly lower with slow pathway ablation than with fast pathway ablation. For example, rates of complete heart block ranging from 8% have been reported with fast pathway ablation.[41] In contrast, the risk of AV block has been less than 1% in our experience with selective slow pathway ablation. The second major advantage of slow pathway ablation is the avoidance of a prolonged PR interval following the procedure. Fast pathway ablation can be associated with a very long PR interval (related to residual AV conduction over the slow pathway). If the RP interval is less than the PR interval during slow pathway conduction, patients may complain of symptoms similar to those encountered with VVI pacing (pacemaker syndrome).[59] These symptoms are avoided with selective slow pathway ablation.

Potential Disadvantages of Slow Pathway Ablation as Compared to Fast Pathway Ablation

Slow pathway ablation can be technically challenging in several clinical situations. If dual AV nodal pathways cannot be demonstrated with programmed stimulation, the end point for defining successful ablation of the slow pathway can be difficult to determine. For example, if the antegrade fast pathway ERP is shorter than the slow pathway ERP, an antegrade discontinuous AV nodal function curve often cannot be demonstrated. In this situation, pharmacological manipulations such as increasing the degree of sedation or administration of a β-blocking agent (esmolol) may lengthen the ERP of the fast pathway to a greater extent than that of the slow pathway, allowing reliable recognition of slow pathway conduction. Despite these techniques, a discontinuous AV nodal function curve may not be demonstrable in some patients. Another marker of slow pathway conduction is the consistent occurrence of a very long AH interval during incremental atrial pacing (Figure 9). The slow pathway can be assumed to be responsible for AV conduction if the PR interval during rapid atrial pacing exceeds the pacing cycle length during consistent 1:1 AV conduction. Thus, a steady state can usually be reached during slow pathway conduction in which the PR interval exceeds the RR interval without the development of Wenckebach block. This marker provides a rapid and easily reproducible means to assess whether the slow pathway remains

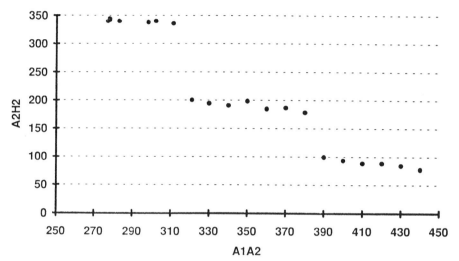

Figure 9. AV conduction intervals during rapid atrial pacing are illustrated for an individual before (Panel A) and after (Panel B) RF ablation of the slow AV nodal pathway. Note that before slow pathway ablation rapid atrial pacing from the high right atrium at a constant cycle length of 373 milliseconds is associated with a stimulus-to-QRS interval (402 seconds) that is consistently greater than the pacing cycle length. Note the very long AH inteval (357 milliseconds). The PR interval that consistently exceeds the pacing cycle length (PR>RR) is evidence of slow pathway conduction. Following slow ablation (Panel B), atrial pacing at a cycle length of 388 milliseconds results in AV Wenckebach conduction with a maximum AH interval of 126 milliseconds. Following ablation the PR interval never exceeded the RR interval in this individual, indicating no evidence of slow pathway conduction. This is an easily reproducible test of the presence or absence of antegrade conduction over the slow AV nodal pathway.

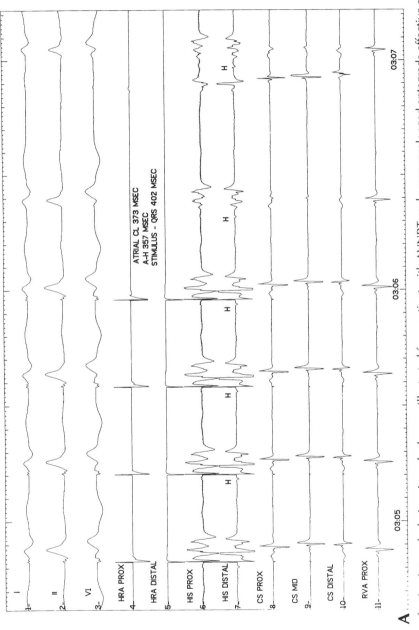

Figure 10. Conduction intervals during sinus rhythm are illustrated for a patient with AVNRT and a very prolonged antegrade effective refractory period of the fast AV nodal pathway. This elderly woman suffered from very frequent episodes of AVNRT at rates ranging from 110 to 140 bpm. Tracings were made with the patient heavily sedated with intravenous meperidine and midazolam. During sinus rhythm with a cycle length of 882 milliseconds, the AH interval measured 110 milliseconds with antegrade conduction over the fast AV nodal pathway (Panel A). *(continued)*

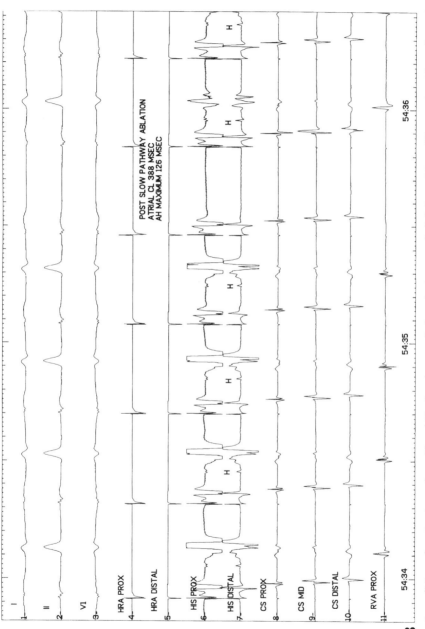

Figure 10. (*continued*) Less than 1 minute later (Panel B), the sinus cycle length decreased slightly to 866 milliseconds with prolongation of the AH interval to 367 milliseconds, indicating antegrade block in the fast AV nodal pathway and resultant slow pathway conduction. Despite the very prolonged antegrade effective refractory period of the fast AV nodal pathway, it was elected to ablate the slow AV nodal pathway. Following slow pathway ablation, the AH interval during sinus rhythm with a cycle length of 948 milliseconds measured 104 milliseconds. This patient has developed occasional episodes of asymptomatic AV Wenckebach block during sleep but has maintained normal AV conduction with a normal PR interval while awake during follow-up.

intact following RF applications. Following successful slow pathway ablation, incremental atrial pacing results in prolongation of the AH interval with Wenckebach block without evidence of a PR interval that is consistently longer than the RR interval.

Another potential disadvantage of slow pathway ablation involves the patient with evidence of impaired fast pathway conduction (Figure 10). These patients are usually elderly with relatively slow AVNRT (typically 100–150 bpm). In these individuals, ablation of the slow pathway results in mandatory AV conduction via the fast pathway and may result in AV Wenckebach block during rest. Although the development of AV Wenckebach block during sleep or rest has not been symptomatic in our experience, the potential for evidence of impaired residual AV conduction should be suspected in these individuals following successful slow pathway ablation. In addition, we have observed one elderly individual with AVNRT who had no evidence of antegrade fast pathway conduction at rest or during isoproterenol infusion. Since all antegrade AV conduction occurred via the slow pathway in this individual, the retrograde fast pathway was targeted for ablation.

A more difficult clinical situation involves the patient who has previously had an unsuccessful attempt at fast pathway ablation with persistent AVNRT. In these individuals, slow pathway ablation may result in high degree AV block because of impairment of fast pathway conduction related to the previous fast pathway ablation attempt. Indeed, in our experience, 3 episodes of AV block occurred in patients with previous ablation attempts. Therefore, for patients who have had recurrence of conduction or primary failure of an ablation attempt involving either the slow or fast pathways, it is probably wise to confine further ablation efforts to the pathway originally targeted for ablation.

Slow Pathway Ablation of Multiple Anterograde AV Nodal Pathways

The presence of multiple "slow" anterograde AV nodal pathways, as demonstrated by the discontinuous AV nodal function curve (Figure 11) may represent up to 5% of patients with AVNRT.[60] Whether these pathways represent discrete anatomically distinct circuits or are functionally present because of nonuniform anisotrophy is unclear. Frequently, multiple slow pathways (whether functional or anatomic) are in close proximity within Koch's triangle. Tai and colleagues found that 42% of a series of 26 patients with multiple slow pathways had elimination of multiple slow pathways with RF ablation at one site. In this series and others, it was noted that slow pathways with longer conduction times have a more inferior location in Koch's triangle when compared with locations producing a shorter AH interval. In patients with multiple slow pathways, RF ablation of the fast pathway may be associated with persistently inducible AVNRT with anterograde conduction over a second slowly conducting pathway. Thus, the presence of a discontinuous AV nodal function curve suggestive of multiple slow pathways should be considered an indication for catheter ablation of the slow pathway.

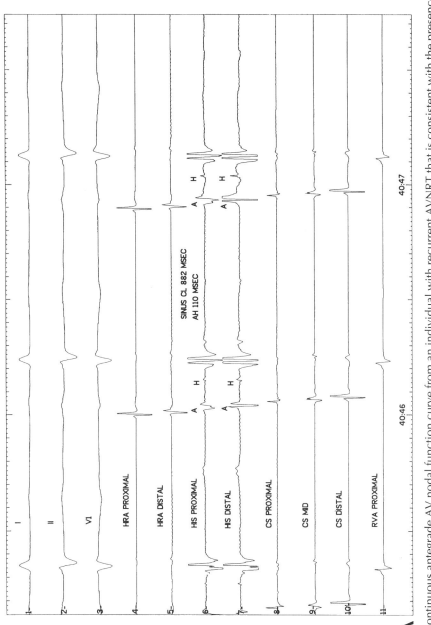

Figure 11. Discontinuous antegrade AV nodal function curve from an individual with recurrent AVNRT that is consistent with the presence of 2 slow AV nodal pathways. Note that the A2H2 interval markedly prolongs at an A1A2 coupling interval of 380 milliseconds in this individual. At an A1A2 coupling interval of 308 milliseconds, there was further prolongation of the A2H2 conduction interval. In this patient, inducible AVNRT was eliminated following ablation of the pathway associated with intermediate A2H2 intervals. The catheter was then positioned more inferiorly along the tricuspid annulus with ablation of the pathway supporting the longest A2H2 intervals. This pattern has been observed in several patients, suggesting that the slowest of the slow pathways is consistently located more inferiorly. *(continued)*

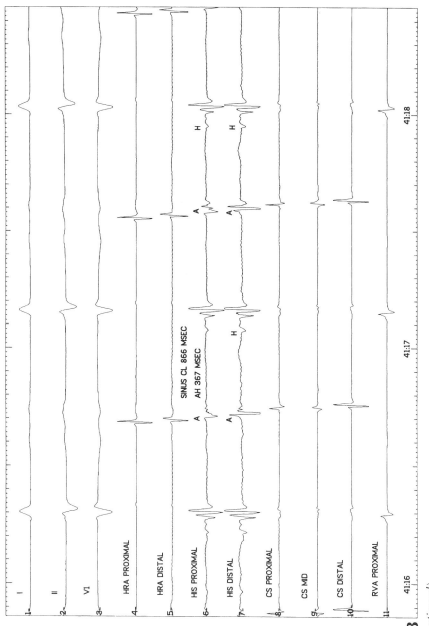

Figure 11. (*continued*)

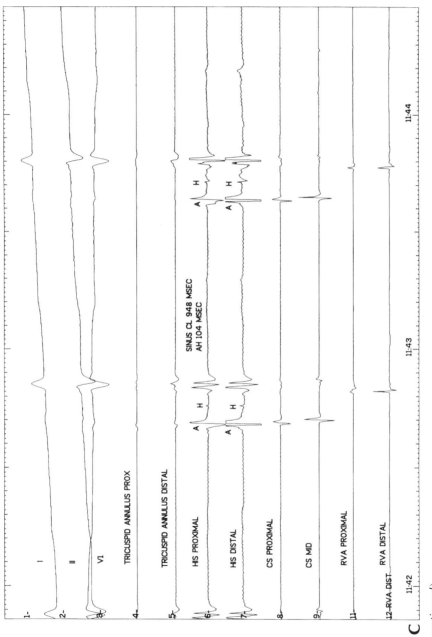

Figure 11. (*continued*)

Slow Pathway Ablation in Patients with Continuous AV Node Function Curves

Although typical of patients with AVNRT, discontinuous AV nodal physiology can be initially demonstrated with programmed atrial stimulation (Figure 12) in only 60–85% of patients in whom this arrhythmia is inducible.[56,51] Anterograde slow and retrograde fast pathway conduction is the usual arrhythmic substrate in these patients although Silka and colleagues,[62] in a study of younger patients, commonly observed the unusual form of AVNRT in patients with smooth AV nodal function curves. Several investigators have attempted to unmask, in patients with a continuous AV nodal function curve, evidence of dual AV nodal pathways by using aggressive extrastimulation protocols including double extrastimuli[63] autonomic maneuvers[64,65] and the administration of pharmacological agents.[32,66] Nevertheless, some patients do not demonstrate discontinuous AV nodal function. During rapid atrial pacing, the PR interval often exceeds the pacing cycle length when there is anterograde conduction over the slow pathway and AVNRT is induced. The prognostic value of the PR/RR ratio was examined by Baker and colleagues[67] in patients known to have AVNRT and in controls. In patients with AVNRT and smooth AV nodal function curve, 96% had a PR/RR ratio greater than one during rapid atrial pacing at the maximum rate with consistent 1:1 AV conduction. In controls, the

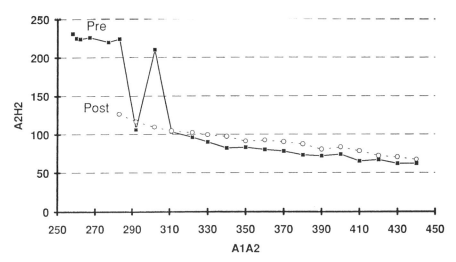

Figure 12. Antegrade AV nodal function curves for a representative individual pre and post RF ablation of the slow AV nodal pathway. The A2H2 conduction intervals are plotted on the ordinate versus the A1A2 extrastimulus coupling interval on the abscissa. Before slow pathway ablation (solid symbols), there is smooth and gradual prolongation of the A2H2 interval and A1A2 coupling intervals of 440 to 312 milliseconds. At an A1A2 coupling interval of 305 milliseconds, there is marked prolongation of the A2H2 interval compatible with antegrade block in the fast pathway with conduction over the slow AV nodal pathway. Following slow pathway ablation (open circles), the A2H2 interval gradually prolongs at all coupling intervals (440–283 milliseconds), suggesting that conduction over the slow pathway has been eliminated without adversely influencing fast pathway conduction.

PR/RR ratio greater than one was demonstrated in 11%, leading the authors to conclude that a PR/RR ratio greater than one at the maximum atrial pacing rate with 1:1 AV conduction was a particularly useful method for demonstrating slow AV nodal pathway conduction in patients with inducible AVNRT and continuous AV nodal function curves.

End Point for Slow AV Nodal Pathway Ablation

It is clear that delivery of RF current at the sites along the tricuspid annulus discussed above may eliminate inducible AVNRT in some patients without eliminating all evidence of slow pathway conduction.[42,53,68–70] In most patients who no longer have inducible AVNRT following application of RF current in the slow pathway region but who demonstrate a residual discontinuous AV nodal function curve and AV nodal echo beats, AVNRT does not recur during a follow-up of several years. Thus, elimination of all evidence of slow pathway conduction is not a necessary requirement for a successful slow pathway ablation procedure. Despite one series[68] which did not show a correlation, our data[53] and others[69,70] have demonstrated that residual evidence of slow AV nodal pathway conduction is the strongest predictor of recurrent AVNRT following an apparently successful slow pathway ablation procedure. Additionally, the absence of junctional tachycardia during RF application[70] also predicts an increased risk of recurrent tachycardia.

Conclusions

To date, the available evidence suggests that, for patients with AVNRT, the slow AV nodal pathway is located inferior to the compact AV node and utilizes perinodal atrial myocardium anterior to the coronary sinus ostium along the tricuspid annulus. In the vast majority of individuals, the application of RF current in this location selectively abolishes slow pathway conduction and AVNRT without impairing residual AV nodal function. Slow pathway ablation appears to be associated with a lower risk of AV block than reported for fast pathway ablation and should be considered the procedure of choice for patients with recurrent AVNRT.

References

1. Denes P, Wu D, Dhingra RC, et al. Demonstration of dual AV nodal pathways in patients with paroxysmal supraventricular tachycardia. *Circulation* 1973;48:549–555.
2. Rosen KM, Mehta A, Miller RA. Demonstration of dual atrioventricular nodal pathways in man. *Am J Cardiol* 1974;33:291–294
3. Paes de Carvalho AF, de Almeida D. Spread of activity through the atrioventricular node. *Circ Res* 1960;8:801–809.

4. Anderson RH, Janse MJ, van Capelle FJL, et al. A combined morphological and electrophysiological study of the atrioventricular node of the rabbit heart. *Circ Res* 1974;35:909–922.

5. van Capelle FJL, Janse MJ, Varghese PJ, et al. Spread of excitation in the atrioventricular node of isolated rabbit hearts studied by multiple micro-electrode recording. *Circ Res* 1972;31:602–616.

6. Janse MJ. Influence of the direction wave front on A-V nodal in isolated hearts of rabbit. *Circ Res* 1969;25:439–449.

7. Mendez C, Moe GK. Demonstration of a dual A-V nodal conduction system in the isolated rabbit heart. *Circ Res* 1966;19:378–393.

8. Inuma H, Dreifus LS, Mazgalev T, et al. Role of perinodal region in atrio-ventricular nodal reentry: evidence in an isolated rabbit heart preparation. *Am J Cardiol* 1983;2:465–473.

9. Mazgalev T, Dreifus LS, Bianchi J, et al. The mechanism of AV junctional reentry: role of atrio-nodal junction. *Anat Rec* 1981;201:179–188.

10. Watanabe Y, Dreifus LS. Inhomogeneous conduction in the AV node: a model for reentry. *Am Heart J* 1965;70:505–512.

11. Miller JM, Rosenthal ME, Vassallo JA, et al. Atrioventricular nodal reentrant tachycardia: studies on upper and lower "common pathways". *Circulation* 1987;75:930–940.

12. Wellens HJJ, Wesdorp JC, Duren DR. Second degree block during reciprocal atrioventricular nodal tachycardia. *Circulation* 1976;53:595–599.

13. Bauernfeind RA, Wu D, Denes P, et al. Retrograde block during dual pathway atrioventricular nodal reentant paroxysmal tachycardia. *Am J Cardiol* 1978;42:499–505.

14. Jackman WM, Beckman KJ, McClelland JH, et al. Participation of atrial myocardium (posterior septum) in AV nodal reentrant tachycardia: evidence for resetting by atrial extrastimuli [abstract]. *PACE* 1991;14:646.

15. Keim S, Werner P, Jazayeri M, et al. Localization of the fast and slow pathways in atrioventricular nodal reentrant tachycardia by intraoperative ice mapping. *Circulation* 1992;86:919–924.

16. McGuire MA, Lau KC, Johnson DC, et al. Patients with 2 types of atrioventricular junctional (AV nodal) reentrant tachycardia. *Circulation* 1991; 83:1232–1246.

17. Kay GN, Epstein AE, Plumb VJ. Evidence for posterior input of both fast and slow AV nodal pathways in patients with AV nodal reentrant tachycardia [abstract]. *Circulation* 1992;85:1675–1688.

18. Josephson ME, Kastor JA. Paroxysmal supraventricular tachycardia: is the atrium a necessary link? *Circulation* 1976;54:430–435.

19. Sung RJ, Waxman HL, Saksena S, et al. Sequence of retrograde atrial activation in patients with dual atrioventricular nodal pathways. *Circulation* 1981;64:1059–1067.

20. Holman WL, Ikeshita M, Lease JG, et al. Alteration of antegrade atrioventricular conduction by cryoablation of periatrioventricular nodal tissue. *J Thorac Cardiovasc Surg* 1984;88:67–80.

21. Cox JL, Holman WL, Cain ME. Cryosurgical treatment of atrioventricular node reentrant tachycardia. *Circulation* 1987;76:1329–1336.

22. Ross DL, Johnson DC, Dennis R, et al. Curative surgery for atrioventricu-

lar junctional ("AV nodal") reentrant tachycardia. *J Am Coll Cardiol* 1985; 6:1383–1392.

23. Pritchett ELC, Anderson RW, Benditt DG, et al. Reentry within the atrioventricular node: surgical cure with preservation of atrioventricular conduction. *Circulation* 1979;60:440–446.

24. Fujimuar O, Guiraudon GM, Yee R, et al. Operative therapy of atrioventricular node reentry and results of an anatomically guided procedure. *Am J Cardiol* 1989;64:1327–1332.

25. McGuire MA, Bourke JP, Robotin MC, et al. High resolution mapping of Koch's triangle using sixty electrodes in humans with atrioventricular junctional (AV Nodal) reentrant tachycardia. *Circulation* 1993;88(part 1): 2315–2328.

26. Satoh M, Miyajima S, Koyama S, et al. Orthodromic capture of the atrial electrogram during transient entrainment of atrioventricular nodal reentrant tachycardia. *Circulation* 1993;88(part 1):2329–2236.

27. Surawicz Z, Reddy C, Prystowsky E, eds. *Tachycardias*. Boston, MA: Martinus Nijhoff, 1984.

28. Olgin JE, Ursell P, Kao AK, et al. Pathological findings following slow pathway ablation for AV nodal reentrant tachycardia. *J Cardiovasc Electrophysiol* 1996;7:625–631.

29. Gamache MC, Bharati S, Lev M, et al. Histopathological study following catheter guided radiofrequency current ablation of the slow pathway in a patient with atrioventricular nodal reentrant tachycardia. *PACE* 1994;17: 247–251.

30. Wu D, Denes P, Dhingra R, et al. Determinants of fast- and slow-pathway conduction in patients with dual atrioventricular nodal pathways. *Circ Res* 1975;36:782–790.

31. Philippon F, Plumb VJ, Kay GN. Differential effect of esmolol on fast and slow AV nodal pathways in patients with AV nodal reentrant tachycardia. *J Cardiovasc Electrophysiol* 1994;5:810–817.

32. Wu D, Denes P, Dhingra R, et al. The effects of propranolol on induction of A-V nodal reentrant paroxysmal tachycardia. *Circulation* 1974;50:665–677.

33. Engelstein ED, Stein KM, Markowitz SM, et al. Posterior fast atrioventricular node pathways: implications for radiofrequency catheter ablation of atrioventricular node reentrant tachycardia. *J Am Coll Cardiol* 1996; 27:1098–1105.

34. Ruder MA, Mead RH, Smith NA, et al. Comparison of pre-and postoperative conduction patterns in patients surgically cured of atrioventricular node reentrant tachycardia. *J Am Coll Cardiol* 1991;17(2):397- 402.

35. Gomes JAC, Dhatt MS, Damato AN, et al. Incidence, determinants and significance of fixed retrograde conduction in the region of the atrioventricular node. *Am J Cardiol* 1979;44:1089–1098.

36. Kay GN, Epstein AE, Dailey SM, et al. Selective radiofrequency ablation of the slow pathway for the treatment of atrioventricular nodal reentrant tachycardia. *Circulation* 1992;85:1675–1687.

37. Gomes JAC, Dhatt MS, Rubenson DS, et al. Electrophysiologic evidence for selective retrograde utilization of a specialized conduction system in atrioventricular nodal reentrant tachycardia. *Am J Cardiol* 1979;43:687–698.

38. Shenasa M, Gilbert CJ, Schmidt DH, et al. Procainamide and retrograde atrioventricular nodal conduction in man. *Circulation* 1982;65:355–362.

39. Goy JJ, Fromer M, Schlaepfer J, et al. Clinical efficacy of radiofrequency current in the treatment of patients with atrioventricular node reentrant tachycardia. *J Am Coll Cardiol* 1990;16:418–423.

40. Epstein LM, Scheinman MM, Langberg JJ, et al. Percutaneous catheter modification of the atrioventricular node. A potential cure for atrioventricular nodal reentrant cardia. *Circulation* 1989;80:757–768.

41. Lee MA, Morady F, Kadish A, et al. Catheter modification of the atrioventricular junction with radiofrequency energy for control of atrioventricular nodal reentry tachycardia. *Circulation* 1991;83:827- 835.

42. Jackman WM, Beckman KJ, McClelland JH, et al. Treatment of supraventricular tachycardia due to atrioventricular nodal reentry by radiofrequency catheter ablation of slow-pathway conduction. *N Engl J Med* 1992;327:313–318.

43. Jazayeri MR, Hempe SL, Sra JS, et al. Selective transcatheter ablation of the fast and slow pathways using radiofrequency energy in patients with atrioventricular nodal reentrant tachycardia. *Circulation* 1992;85:1318–1328.

44. Calkins H, Sousa J, El-Atassi R, et al. Diagnosis and cure of the Wolff-Parkinson-White syndrome or paroxysmal supraventricular tachycardia during a single electrophysiologic test. *N Engl J Med* 1991;324:1612–1618.

45. Haïssaguerre M, Warin JF, Lemetayer P, et al. Closed-chest ablation of retrograde conduction in patients with atrioventricular nodal reentrant tachycardia. *N Engl J Med* 1989;320:426–433.

46. Wathen M, Natale A, Wolfe K, et al. An anatomically guided approach to atrioventricular node slow pathway ablation. *Am J Cardiol* 1992;70:886–889.

47. Wu D, Yeh SJ, Wang CC, et al. Nature of dual atrioventricular node pathways and the tachycardia circuit as defined by radiofrequency ablation technique. *J Am Coll Cardiol* 1992;20:884–894.

48. Strickberger SA, Zivin A, Daoud EG, et al. Temperature and impedance monitoring during slow pathway ablation in patients with AV nodal reentrant tachycardia. *J Cardiovasc Electrophysiol* 1996;7:295–300.

49. Calkins H, Prystowsky E, Berger RD, et al, and the ATAKR Multicenter Investigators Group. Recurrence of conduction following radiofrequency catheter ablation procedures: relationship to ablation target and electrode temperature. *J Cardiovasc Electrophysiol* 1996;7:704–712.

50. Epstein LM, Jung S, Lee RJ, et al. Slow AV nodal pathway ablation utilizing a unique temperature controlled radiofrequency energy system. *PACE* 1997;20(part I):664–670.

51. Natale A, Klein G, Yee R, et al. Shortening of fast pathway refractoriness after slow pathway ablation. *Circulation* 1994;89:1103–1108.

52. Strickberger SA, Daoud E, Niebauer M, et al. Effects of Partial and complete ablation of the slow pathway on fast pathway properties in patients with atrioventricular nodal reentrant tachycardia. *J Cardiovasc Electrophysiol* 1994;5:645–649.

53. Baker JH II, Plumb VJ, Epstein AE, et al. Predictors of recurrent atrioventricular nodal reentry after selective slow pathway ablation. *Am J Cardiol* 1994;73:765–769.

54. Wang X, McClelland JH, Beckman KJ, et al. Accelerated junctional rhythm during slow pathway ablation. *Circulation* 1991;84(suppl);II-582.

55. Jentzer JH, Goyal R, Williamson BD, et al. Analysis of junctional ectopy during radiofrequency ablation of the slow pathway in patients with atrioventricular nodal reentrant tachycardia. *Circulation* 1994;90:2820–2826.

56. Haïssaguerre M, Gaita F, Fischer B, et al. Elimination of atrioventricular nodal reentrant tachycardia using discrete slow potentials to guide application of radiofrequency energy. *Circulation* 1992;85:2162–2175.

57. McGuire MA, de Bakker JMT, Vermeulen JT, et al. Origin and significance of double potentials near the atrioventricular node. *Circulation* 1994;89:2351–2360.

58. Niebauer MJ, Daoud E, Williamson B, et al. Atrial electrogram characteristics in patients with and without atrioventricular nodal reentrant tachycardia. *Circulation* 1995;92:77–81.

59. Zornoza JP, Crossley GH, Haisty WK, et al. Pseudopacemaker syndrome: a complication of radiofrequency ablation of the AV junction [abstract]. *PACE* 1992;15:590.

60. Tai CT, Chen SA, Chiang CE, et al. Multiple anterograde atrioventricular node pathways in patients with atrioventricular node reentrant tachycardia. *J Am Coll Cardiol* 1996;28:725–731.

61. Wu D, Denes P, Dhingra R, et al. Clinical electrocardiographic and electrophysiological observations in patients with paroxysmal supraventricular tachycardia. *Am J Cardiol* 1978;41:1045–1051.

62. Silka MJ, Kron J, Halperin BD, et al. Mechanisms of AV node reentrant tachycardia in young patients with and without dual AV node physiology. *PACE* 1994;17(part II):2129–2133.

63. Brooks R, Goldberger J, Kadish A. Extended protocol for demonstration of dual AV nodal physiology. *PACE* 1993;16:277–284.

64. Mann D, Reiter M. Effects of upright posture on atrio-ventricular nodal reentry and dual atrioventricular nodal pathways. *Am J Cardiol* 1988;62:408–412.

65. Paparella N, Alboni P, Pirani R, et al. Effects of autonomic blockade on dual atrioventricular nodal pathways pattern. *J Electrocardiol* 1986;19:269–274.

66. Wu D, Denes P, Bauernfeind R, et al. Effects of atropine on induction and maintenance of atrioventricular nodal reentrant tachycardia. *Circulation* 1979;59:779–788.

67. Baker JH II, Plumb VJ, Epstein AE, et al. PR/RR interval ratio during rapid atrial pacing: a simple method for confirming the presence of slow AV nodal pathway conduction. *J Cardiovasc Electrophysiol* 1996;7:287–294.

68. Manolis AS, Wang PJ, Estes NAM III. Radiofrequency ablation of slow pathway in patients with atrioventricular nodal reentrant tachycardia. *Circulation* 1994;90:2815–2819.

69. Huagui GL, Klein GJ, Stites HW, et al. Elimination of slow pathway conduction: an accurate indicator of clinical success after radiofrequency atrioventricular node modification. *J Am Coll Cardiol* 1993;22:1849–1853.

70. Tebbenjohanns J, Pfeiffer D, Schumacher B, et al. Impact of the local atrial electrogram in AV nodal reentrant tachycardia: ablation versus modification of the slow pathway. *J Cardiovasc Electrophysiol* 1995;6:245–251.

Part V

Radiofrequency Catheter Ablation of Accessory Pathways

Chapter 23

Ablation of Right Free Wall Accessory Pathways

William M. Miles, M.D.

Right free wall accessory pathways include those that bridge the tricuspid annulus along its posterior, lateral and anterior aspects. They comprise approximately 12% of all accessory pathways.[1–5] Right sided accessory pathways that involve the complex posteroseptal space, those in the right midseptal region, and those that involve the anteroseptal region in proximity to the His bundle are not addressed in this chapter. However, it may be difficult to distinguish right posteroseptal and anteroseptal accessory pathways from right posterior or anterior free wall pathways, respectively, prior to detailed intracardiac mapping.

Ablation of right free wall accessory pathways is based on the same principles as ablation of accessory pathways at other sites. On first thought, one might anticipate that ablation of right free wall pathways would be relatively easy because of the catheter accessibility of the tricuspid annulus. However, due to unique anatomic features of the tricuspid annulus, one may encounter difficulty in maintaining catheter stability, mapping difficulties, increased cooling of the ablation tip by the blood pool, and the possibility of multiple or unusual accessory pathways (such as atriofascicular fibers). Thus, ablation of right free wall pathways is often more challenging than that of left free wall pathways, and the recurrence rate after apparent successful ablation is higher. However, the complication rate is low and the vast majority of right free wall pathways can be successfully ablated with routine radiofrequency ablation techniques.

From Huang SKS, Wilber DJ (eds.): *Radiofrequency Catheter Ablation of Cardiac Arrhythmias: Basic Concepts and Clinical Applications,* 2nd ed. Armonk, NY: Futura Publishing Company, Inc. ©2000.

Electrocardiographic Localization of Right Free wall Accessory Pathways

Patients with right free wall accessory pathways usually have marked pre-excitation during sinus rhythm if anterograde conduction exists. This is because the sinus impulse travels through the right atrial tissue and reaches the atrial insertion of the accessory pathway at approximately the same time as it enters the atrioventricular (AV) node. If the accessory pathway has typical rapid anterograde conduction characteristics, then maximal or near maximal preexcitation may occur before the impulse has a chance to travel through the AV node and His-Purkinje system. On occasion, anterograde necessary pathway conduction may be slow enough that anterograde preexcitation is minimal or absent despite the ability of the accessory pathway to conduct anterogradely if given enough time; an example of this would be a right free wall accessory AV pathway with decremental (AV node-like) conduction properties or an atriofascicular (Mahaim) fiber.[6–9] If the QRS complex in sinus rhythm is not maximally or near-maximally preexcited, atrial pacing should be used to maximize preexcitation and help determine delta wave orientation. Adenosine may also be used to maximize preexcitation but may block accessory pathways with decremen-

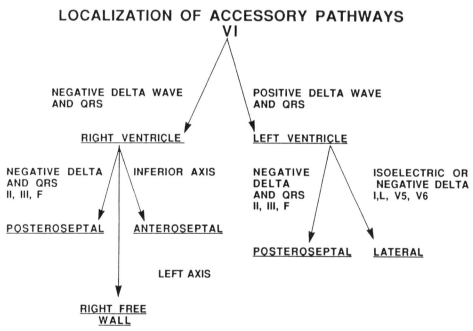

Figure 1. Algorithm for localization of accessory pathways using delta wave orientation. Analysis of lead V_1 helps determine whether the accessory pathway bridges the mitral or tricuspid annulus. The frontal plane axis is then used to determine whether the pathway is anterior, posterior, or lateral. (Reprinted with permission from Zipes DP. Specific arrhythmias: diagnosis and treatment. In Braunwald E, ed: *Heart Disease. A Textbook of Cardiovascular Medicine*, Philadelphia, PA: WB Saunders, 1992. p 695.)

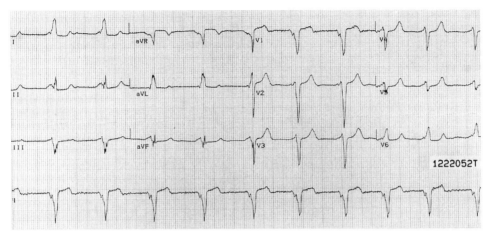

Figure 2. 12-lead electrocardiogram during sinus rhythm in a patient with a right free wall accessory pathway. Note the short PR interval and marked preexcitation with a left bundle branch block QRS morphology in lead V_1.

tal conduction properties.[9] Obviously, a concealed (retrogradely-conducting only) right free wall accessory pathway would not generate a delta wave.

In patients with right free wall pathways, the delta wave in lead V_1 is either totally negative or may have an initial isoelectric portion or positive R wave followed by a wide, deep preexcited S wave; thus the resultant delta wave is predominantly negative, representing ventricular activation from right to left (Figures 1 and 2).[10–14] The delta wave axis in the limb leads helps to determine the right free wall accessory pathway location along the tricuspid annulus. If the delta wave axis is superiorly oriented with negative delta waves in leads 2, 3, and AVF (pseudo-inferior infarct pattern), the accessory pathway is located in the right posterior region. If the delta wave axis is oriented inferiorly with positive delta waves in leads 2, 3, and AVF, the accessory pathway is located in the anterior region. Detailed mapping is necessary to make sure that the accessory pathway is not located posteroseptally or anteroseptally, and to determine its proximity to the His bundle. Accessory pathways located along the anterolateral, lateral, and posterolateral tricuspid annulus have a delta wave with a left axis in the limb leads. It should be noted that right midseptal accessory pathways may have a delta wave axis very similar to that of right lateral pathways and may be difficult to distinguish on surface ECG. It has been suggested that body surface mapping can distinguish these 2 locations prior to electrophysiological study.[15,16] This may be helpful in preablation patient counseling since there is risk of AV block during ablation of a right midseptal pathway.

Electrophysiological Localization of Right Free wall Accessory Pathways

Right free wall accessory pathways, like all AV connections, are mapped by utilizing both their anterograde and retrograde conduction to identify ventricular and atrial insertion sites, respectively. Because accessory pathways may have an oblique orientation across the AV groove, the earliest site of retrograde atrial activation and earliest site of anterograde ventricular activation may not be directly across the AV groove from each other, and may be as much as 2 centimeters apart in some patients.[17,18] If one anticipates ablating the accessory pathway from the atrial aspect of the tricuspid annulus (the most common approach), the site of earliest atrial activation, preferably with an accessory pathway potential present, would be the optimal site for ablation. On the other hand, if the ventricular aspect of the tricuspid annulus is the ablation target, the site of earliest ventricular activation (again, preferably with an accessory pathway potential present) would be the optimal site. When an accessory pathway is concealed (retrograde but no anterograde conduction), the ventricular insertion site cannot be determined by ventricular activation mapping. In the more unusual situation where an accessory pathway conducts anterogradely but not retrogradely, the atrial insertion site cannot be determined by atrial activation mapping. Therefore, the appropriate site of energy delivery along the triscupid annulus is more difficult to determine. In this situation, the recording of an accessory pathway potential may be particularly useful to guide the ablation procedure. Proving that a potential represents accessory pathway activation is tedious and often impossible; therefore, potentials suspected of originating from an accessory pathway have been classified as "probable" or "possible" accessory pathway potentials.[19]

Identification of the earliest site of atrial activation is usually performed during orthodromic AV reciprocating tachycardia; the anterograde limb of tachycardia is the normal AV node/His-Purkinje system and the retrograde limb is the accessory pathway. The earliest obtainable atrial activation along the AV groove (using the roving ablation catheter, a tricuspid annular multielectrode catheter such as a "halo" catheter {Figure 3}[20] or a right coronary artery mapping electrode[16, 21]) defines the atrial insertion site of the accessory pathway (Figure 4). Similar mapping can be performed during ventricular pacing. However, retrograde conduction via the normal VA conduction system (AV node and His bundle) may contribute to atrial activation and interfere with localization of the accessory pathway. Pacing from the right ventricular base rather than the apex may accentuate accessory pathway activation of the atrium.[22]

The ventricular insertion site of the accessory pathway is determined during sinus rhythm, atrial pacing (to accentuate the delta wave)—see Figure 4—or any arrhythmia resulting in activation of the ventricle via the accessory pathway, such as atrial fibrillation, atrial flutter, or antidromic AV reciprocating tachycardia. Again, if there is difficulty locating exactly where along the tricuspid annulus activation is earliest, a tricuspid annular multipolar mapping catheter such as a "halo" catheter or in rare instances a right coronary artery mapping electrode may be used. Our experience is that right sided accessory pathways can usually be ablated without using multipolar electrode catheter mapping along the tricuspid annulus, but if multiple accessory pathways are suspected or the anatomy is distorted (for example in Ebstein's anomaly), or if there is difficulty effecting adequate ablation, these mapping techniques may be used.

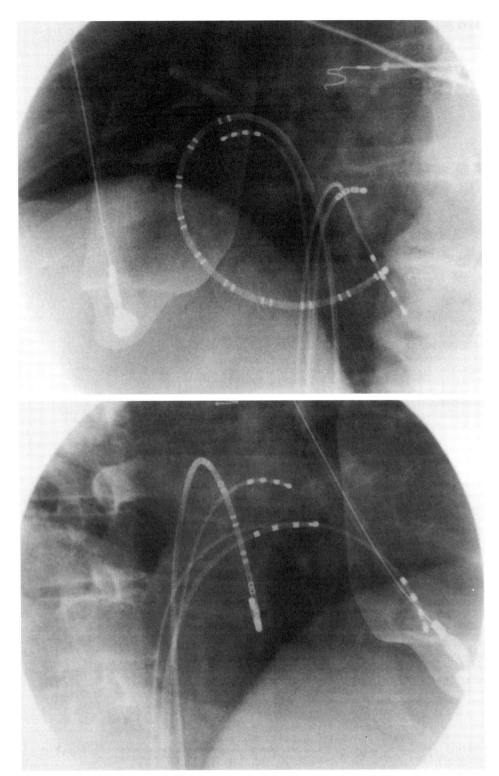

Figure 3. Fluoroscopic image of a 20-pole deflectable catheter positioned along the tricuspid annulus. Panel A is left anterior oblique, panel B is right anterior oblique projection. High right atrial, His bundle, and right ventricular apical catheters are also present.

A

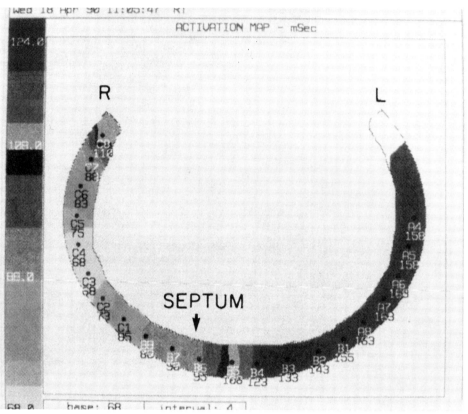

Figure 4. Intraoperative maps before (panels A and B) and after (panel C) surgical ablation of a right free wall accessory pathway. Maps are obtained by placing a multielectrode strip on the epicardium along the atrial or ventricular side of the mitral and tricuspid annulus intraoperatively. The strip simultaneously records electrograms extending from the left anterior region (L), the posterior septum and the right anterior region (R). Earliest activation is represented by yellow followed by orange, green, and blue as illustrated in the color scale on the left. In panel A, atrial activation is recorded during orthodromic reciprocating tachycardia. The earliest site of activation is on the right free wall. (*continued*)

B

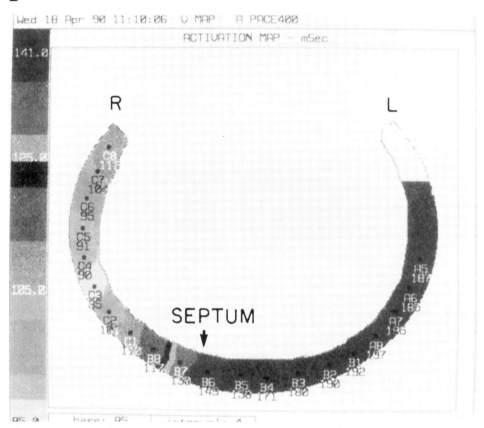

Figure 4. (*continued*) In panel B, ventricular activation is recorded during atrial pacing, showing earliest anterograde activation in the right free wall region just across the annulus from that in panel A. (*continued*)

C

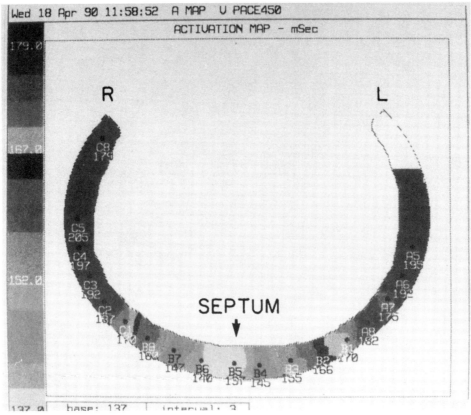

Figure 4. (*continued*) In panel C, post ablation, reciprocating tachycardia is no longer inducible. During ventricular pacing, earliest atrial activation is at the posterior septum. See color plate.

Right free wall accessory pathways that exhibit "decremental" or AV nodal-like conduction properties are most often atriofascicular pathways, the mapping and ablation of which are discussed elsewhere. However, a minority of right free wall necessary pathways with decremental conduction properties are true AV connections.[8,9] The distinction can usually be made very quickly during maximal preexcitation (either atrial pacing or antidromic tachycardia); in atriofascicular pathways earliest ventricular activation occurs near the right ventricular apex, and in AV connections it is near the right ventricular base along the tricuspid annulus.

Characteristics of Successful Ablation Sites

Successful ablation sites exhibit stable fluoroscopic and electrical characteristics. Experienced operators become familiar with the appearance of a catheter moving with the cardiac cycle yet stable against the endocardium as opposed to a catheter moving freely with each heartbeat without stable contact. Fluoroscopic stability is confirmed by also observing a stable electrogram, one of the most important predictors of catheter ablation success.[19] Whether one is ablating on the atrial or ventricular side of the tricuspid annulus, both atrial and ventricular electrogram components should be recorded from the ablating electrode. When ablating from the atrial aspect of the tricuspid annulus, the atrial potential is usually larger than or equal to the ventricular potential. Sometimes the 2 can merge and it may be difficult to determine whether both components are present. A probable accessory pathway potential is desirable but not always present at successful sites. During sinus rhythm with anterograde conduction over an accessory pathway, the local ventricular electrogram on the ablation catheter should precede the onset of the delta wave on the surface electrocardiogram by at least 10 milliseconds, and preferably preceded even earlier by an electrogram representing accessory pathway activation (Figure 5). In addition, the activation time between local atrial and ventricular electrograms recorded from the ablation catheter is usually short,

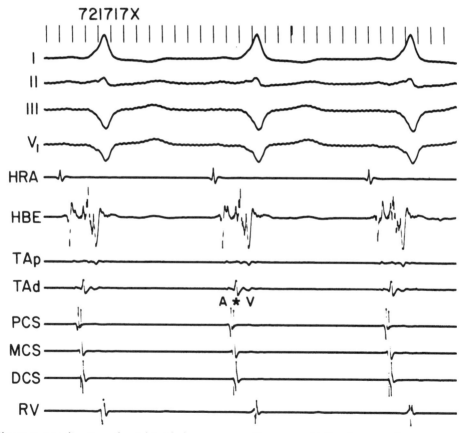

Figure 5. Localization of a right-sided accessory pathway preablation by recording accessory pathway potentials. TAp and TAd represent proximal and distal electrograms recorded from an ablation catheter positioned along the posterior tricuspid annulus. Panel A illustrates sinus rhythm with a delta wave consistent with a right posterior accessory pathway. On the distal tricuspid annulus electrodes, an accessory pathway potential (asterisk) is recorded between the atrial potential (A) and the ventricular potential (V). (*continued*)

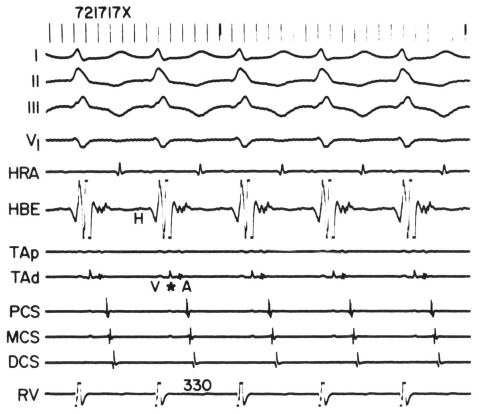

Figure 5. (*continued*) In panel B, orthodromic AVRT uses the right posterior accessory pathway as the retrograde limb. An accessory pathway potential (asterisk) is now recorded between ventricular activation (V) and atrial activation (A). (*continued*)

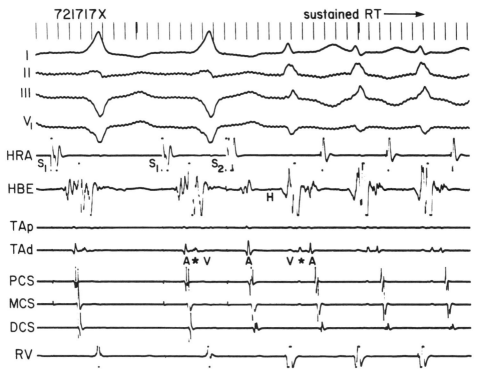

Figure 5. (*continued*) Panel C illustrates induction of orthodromic AVRT. During atrial pacing (S₁), the right posterior tricuspid annulus electrodes (TAd) record an accessory pathway potential (asterisk) between atrial activation (A) and ventricular activation (V). After introduction of an atrial extrastimulus (S₂) there is anterograde block in the accessory pathway and the accessory pathway potential is not recorded after atrial activation. The impulse reaches the ventricle via the normal AV node/His-Purkinje system (H) and AVRT is induced. The TAd electrodes now record a reversal of activation with the ventricular electrogram followed by accessory pathway and then atrial activation. The accessory pathway potential could be dissociated from the atrial potential with atrial pacing techniques, proving that it was not part of the atrial potential. (*continued*)

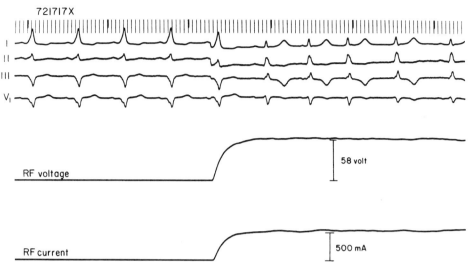

Figure 5. (*continued*) Panel D: ablation of the accessory pathway when radiofrequency energy is delivered through the electrode labeled TAd in the previous panels. (Reprinted with permission from Miles WM, et al. Atrioventricular reentry and variants: mechanisms, clinical features, and management. In: Zipes DP, Jalife J, eds. *Cardiac Electrophysiology: From Cell to Bedside.* Philadelphia: WB Saunders, 1995. p 649.)

approximately 40 milliseconds; however, exceptions occur when the antero-grade conduction time over an accessory pathway is prolonged. Prolonged accessory pathway conduction time may occur due to damage from previous radiofrequency ablation energy deliveries or due to inherently slow accessory pathway conduction. In addition, short activation times between local atrial and ventricular potentials may occur at sites other than the accessory pathway insertion site; both atrial and ventricular activation may proceed circumferentially along the tricuspid annulus and timing of local atrial and ventricular activation may be close to one another at multiple sites along the annulus. Thus, early ventricular activation prior to the delta wave is the most important timing criterion.

During orthodromic reciprocating tachycardia, the VA interval (that is, the interval between the onset of ventricular activation recorded from any surface or intracardiac lead and local atrial activation recorded from the roving ablation catheter) is usually between 70 and 90 milliseconds at the eventual successful site.[23] Again, this may be longer in an occasional patient with prolonged accessory pathway conduction. The time between the local ventricular and atrial electrograms during AVRT (both recorded simultaneously from the ablation catheter) is again approximately 40 milliseconds at the eventual successful site unless prolonged accessory pathway conduction time is present. Note that the criteria to define early activation using anterograde mapping with a delta wave are not dependent on accessory pathway conduction time, whereas retrograde timing criteria (VA intervals) are. Thus if the accessory pathway conducts anterogradely and especially if one plans to ablate on the ventricular side of the annulus, mapping during sinus rhythm or atrial pacing may be most effective.[19,24]

Ablation energy may be delivered during sinus rhythm, atrial pacing, ventricular pacing, or AV reentrant tachycardia. Energy delivery during AV reentrant tachycardia may result in termination of tachycardia and may dislodge the catheter, resulting in an inadequate burn. Therefore, if retrograde mapping during AV reentrant tachycardia is used to determine the optimal atrial ablation site (especially if the accessory pathway is concealed and no delta wave is available for mapping), we prefer to entrain the AV reentrant tachycardia by pacing the ventricle at a slightly shorter cycle length than the tachycardia just before the ablation energy is delivered. Thus, when the accessory pathway conduction is eliminated by the ablation pulse, the paced rhythm of the heart is uninterrupted and the likelihood of catheter movement during continued energy delivery is minimized. If one uses ventricular pacing for mapping the atrial insertion site of right free wall accessory pathways, one must be sure that earliest atrial activation is via the accessory pathway and not via the AV node. If ventricular pacing must be used for mapping, a tricuspid annulus mapping catheter may be useful to ensure that retrograde activation is all or in part via the accessory pathway.

When ablation catheters with temperature monitoring capabilities are used, a stabile catheter tip temperature is a helpful adjunct to ensure catheter stability and adequate catheter-tissue contact.[25–27] In general, when the tip temperature of the catheter rises to greater than 50°C, adequate catheter tissue contact is verified.[28] If the accessory pathway does not disappear despite a good temperature rise, the catheter is probably located in an incorrect position and a slightly different catheter location should be sought. Catheter tip temperature monitoring is also useful in determining whether the catheter moves during the energy delivery and in preventing an impedance rise due to coagulum formation when the tip temperature exceeds 100°C. Inadequate heating due to catheter instability and blood-pool cooling is a common problem when ablating along the tricuspid annulus.

New mapping technologies may be useful in helping to direct the ablation catheter to the atrial or ventricular accessory pathway insertion sites. For example, two-dimensional, nonfluoroscopic imaging (Carto System, Biosense, Orangeburg, New York) may be used to construct electroanatomic activation maps along the tricuspid annulus, either on the atrial side during AV reciprocating tachycardia or ventricular pacing or along the ventricular side during anterograde preexcitation.[29] This map is displayed as a color-coded activation map superimposed on a three-dimensional anatomic reconstruction of the tricuspid annulus (Figure 6). In addition, the ablation catheter tip can be returned to any site along the tricuspid annulus using electromagnetic nonfluoroscopic electroanatomic localization, and sites of ablation can be tagged on the map for further reference. This system has the advantage of providing immediate electroanatomic mapping information that may be especially useful if complicated anatomy or multiple accessory pathways are present. It also gives information during radiofrequency energy delivery with regard to catheter stability and movement.

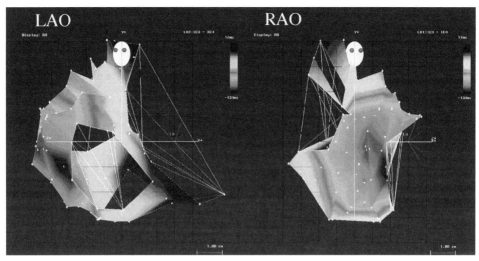

Figure 6. Electroanatomic mapping of the right atrium in a patient with a right free wall accessory pathway. Left anterior oblique (LAO) and right anterior oblique (RAO) projections of the right atrium are displayed during ventricular pacing. Earliest atrial activation is indicated by red, followed by yellow, green, blue, and lastly purple. In the LAO view, one can see the entirety of the tricuspid annulus, whereas in the RAO view the annulus is on the right of the image. Note that earliest atrial activation (red) during ventricular pacing is at the lateral aspect of the annulus, consistent with retrograde conduction via a right free wall accessory pathway. (Courtesy of Jeffrey E. Olgin, M.D., Indianapolis, IN.) See color plate.

Special Anatomic Features of the Tricuspid Annulus

There are differences between the anatomic structure of the tricuspid and mitral annuli that influence accessory pathway ablation.[30,31] The tricuspid annulus is larger in circumference than the mitral annulus. In addition, there is a portion of the mitral annulus (the region of continuity between the aortic and mitral valves) where accessory pathways do not occur. Therefore, a larger region must be mapped to ablate right free wall versus left free wall accessory pathways. The mitral valve attaches to its fibrous annulus at a right angle whereas the attachment of the tricuspid valve is more of an acute angle oriented toward the right ventricle, making it more difficult to wedge an ablation catheter underneath the tricuspid than the mitral valve. Whereas the mitral valve has a well-formed fibrous annulus, the tricuspid annulus may not be a complete fibrous ring and may have regions of discontinuity. On the right side, the atrium and ventricle fold over one another instead of terminating at a distinct fibrous ring as on the left (Figure 7). These anatomic differences may make it more difficult to position a catheter along the tricuspid annulus, and accessory pathways that run within this area may be more difficult to heat with radiofrequency energy. Accessory pathways may bridge the annulus at any point between its epicardial and subendocardial aspect.[32] In addition, pathways may have atrial or ventricular insertion sites displaced a few millimeters above or below the AV groove, respectively, further complicating mapping.

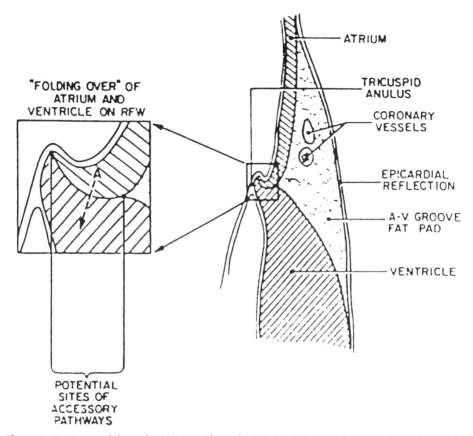

Figure 7. Anatomy of the right AV ring. The right AV ring is incomplete and the atrium "folds over" the ventricle at the AV groove. In contrast, the annulus along the left AV ring is continuous, the atrial and ventricular myocardium meet at the ring and do not fold over. (Reprinted with permission from Ferguson TB Jr, Cox JL. Surgical treatment for the Wolff-Parkinson-White Syndrome: the endocardial approach. In: Zipes DP, Jalife J, eds. *Cardiac Electrophysiology: From Cell to Bedside.* Philadelphia, PA: WB Saunders, 1990. pp 897–907.)

In Ebstein's anomaly, the posterior leaflet of the tricuspid valve is displaced a variable distance into the right ventricle away from the anatomic tricuspid annulus.[33] Right posteroseptal, posterior, and posterolateral accessory pathways occur commonly and may be manifest or concealed. An echocardiogram should be performed to exclude Ebstein's anomaly in patients with ECGs suggestive of accessory pathways in this region. As many as one-quarter of patients with Ebstein's anomaly and Wolff-Parkinson-White syndrome have more than one accessory pathway. The accessory pathways bridge the anatomic tricuspid annulus regardless of where the valve is located. Identification of the true anatomic annulus may be difficult especially because the electrical signals recorded from the endocardium near the annulus in patients with Ebstein's anomaly are often prolonged and fractionated. Ablation is usually accomplished at the true annulus, above the displaced tricuspid leaflet, although some patients may undergo successful ablation from the ventricular side of the annulus (but still above the valve leaflet). If more than one accessory pathway is suspected, differential atrial pacing from both the right atrial appendage and the coronary sinus may be helpful for mapping ventricular activation; pacing from the right atrial appendage tends to activate the posterolateral accessory pathway earlier than the septal pathway, and pacing from the coronary sinus tends to activate the septal pathway prior to the posterolateral pathway. Induction of atrial fibrillation may also help identify 2 distinct delta wave morphologies.

Ablation of right free wall pathways with decremental conduction properties are discussed in detail elsewhere. Most of these fibers are atriofascicular but a minority are atrioventricular.[8,9] They are rare and probably represent duplicate AV node/His-Purkinje systems.[6,7,9] Ablation techniques for the true atrioventricular variety are similar to those for any other right free wall AV connection. It is especially useful to record pathway potentials to ablate the atriofascicular variety. The pathways can be easily traumatized transiently with catheter movement, and this feature can be used for mapping.[34]

Whereas the coronary sinus provides an easily accessible structure for mapping along the mitral annulus, no such easily accessible structure exists along the tricuspid annulus. However, in rare cases it may be useful to introduce a tiny electrode catheter into the right coronary artery for localization of right free wall accessory pathways analogous to mapping using the coronary sinus on the left.[16,21]

Closely adjacent but anatomically discrete sites of catheter ablation may be necessary to eliminate both anterograde and retrograde accessory pathway conduction in up to 10% of patients;[18] the incidence of this phenomenon appears to be highest in patients with right free wall pathways (18.6% of cases). The explanation for this phenomenon is not clear but probably relates to complexity of fiber orientation, possibly branching over 1–2 centimeters along the annulus. This factor again emphasizes the importance of identifying atrial and ventricular insertion sites.

Mapping Considerations for Right Freewall Accessory Pathways

Right free wall accessory pathways are located in the right posterior, right posterolateral, right lateral, right anterolateral, or right anterior free wall positions (Figure 8). In the left anterior oblique fluoroscopic projection of the tricuspid annulus, the His is located at approximately 1 o'clock and the coronary sinus at 5 o'clock; right free wall pathways span from approximately 6 o'clock to 12 o'clock. Right anterior accessory pathways are at the most superior aspect of the tricuspid valve; right anteroseptal pathways, which are very close to the normal AV conduction system, are located near the catheter recording His bundle activation. Likewise, right posterior free wall accessory pathways are located at the most posterior aspect of the tricuspid valve, whereas posteroseptal accessory pathways are located closer to the coronary sinus ostium. During AV reciprocating tachycardia, right free wall accessory pathways demonstrate VA prolongation of 30 milliseconds or more during functional right bundle branch block,[35] whereas right anteroseptal and posteroseptal pathways are

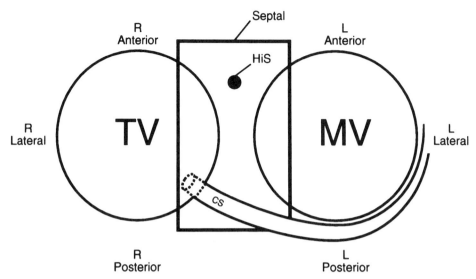

Figure 8. Schematic of free wall accessory pathway locations around the mitral and tricuspid annuli as visualized in the left anterior oblique projection. TV = tricuspid valve, MV = mitral valve, CS = coronary sinus, and His = His bundle. (Reprinted with permission from Zipes DP, ed. *Catheter Ablation of Arrhythmias.* Futura Publishing Co., 1994.)

characterized by less than 30 milliseconds increase in the VA interval with functional right bundle branch block. There should be no risk of damage to the normal AV conduction system if energy is delivered in the appropriate location for right free wall accessory pathways.

When routine diagnostic catheters are used to record high right atrial, His bundle, and coronary sinus atrial electrograms during AV reciprocating tachycardia using a right free wall accessory pathway, an apparent "high-to-low" atrial activation sequence may mimic that of an atrial tachycardia originating from the high right atrium (Figure 9). This pattern occurs because there is no right lateral recording to reveal the true earliest atrial activation.

The criteria for successful ablation sites have been described above. Mapping is performed in anterograde and retrograde directions. If mapping or positioning of the ablating catheter along the tricuspid annulus is particularly difficult, a small wire or electrode catheter can be introduced into the right coronary artery (after angiography and heparinization) for electrical mapping and as a target for the ablating catheter.[16,21] This is not necessary in routine cases but some investigators have found it to be useful in highly selected patients with multiple accessory pathways or in Ebstein's anomaly where the anatomy of the AV groove may be distorted. It has been reported to be safe, but complications of right coronary artery spasm, thrombosis, or endocardial injury are potentially severe. More commonly, a circular duodecapolar "halo" catheter may facilitate endocardial mapping of the tricuspid annulus.[20]

Transient interruption of accessory pathway conduction during radiofrequency energy delivery (with subsequent reappearance of conduction seconds to minutes after the energy delivery is completed) is more common with right

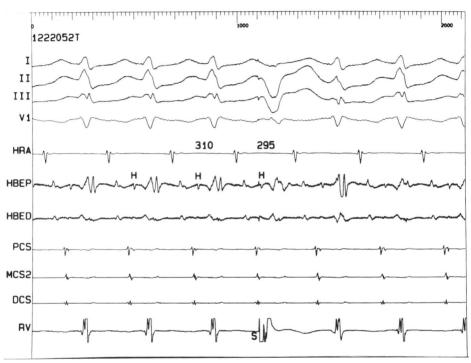

Figure 9. Intracardiac electrograms during orthodromic reciprocating tachycardia in the same patient as shown in Figure 1. Surface leads I, II, III, and V₁ are displayed along with high right atrial (HRA), proximal and distal His bundle (HBEP, HBED), proximal, middle and distal coronary sinus (PCS, MCS2, DCS), and right ventricular (RV) electrograms. Panel A: in this patient with a right lateral accessory pathway, there is an apparent "high to low" right atrial activation sequence during reciprocating tachycardia. This is a clue that the pathway is right free wall, and even earlier atrial activation will be found when the tricuspid annulus is mapped. The "high to low" atrial activation sequence must represent atrial activation via the accessory pathway because the atrial activation is advanced with identical sequence after the PVC (S) when the His (H) is refractory. (*continued*)

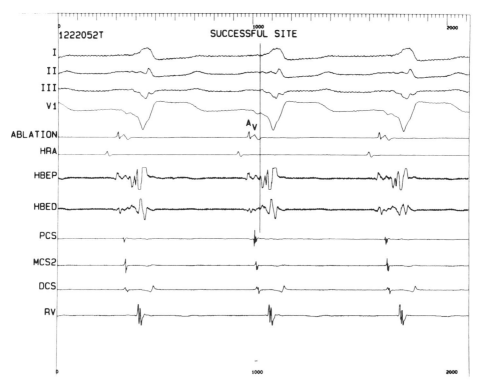

Figure 9. (*continued*) In panel B, the ablation electrograms at the successful site are displayed. Both atrial and ventricular components are present, and the ventricular electrogram precedes the onset of the delta wave in the surface tracings. In this example, no distinct accessory pathway potential is recorded. (*continued*)

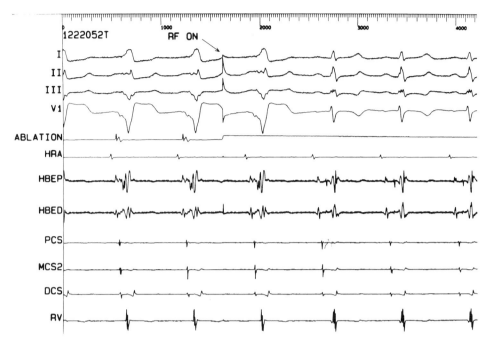

Figure 9. (*continued*) Panel C illustrates almost immediate disappearance of the delta wave upon onset of radiofrequency energy delivery.

free wall than left free wall pathways. This may be due to poor catheter-tissue contact and less heating, or possibly to the fact that some right free wall pathways do not travel as close to the endocardium as do left free wall pathways. The recurrence rate over the first few weeks after right free wall accessory pathways exceeds that of left free wall pathways (see below).[1,3,4,36–39]

Techniques of Right Free wall Ablation

Right free wall accessory pathways are usually approached by advancing the tip of the mapping/ablating deflectable catheter directly to the tricuspid annulus (Figure 10). Both atrial and ventricular potentials should be recorded from the distal electrodes. The tricuspid annulus is usually mapped in the left anterior oblique projection (see Figure 8). With experience, the operator can obtain recordings from any location around the tricuspid annulus, although good catheter tissue contact is more difficult to obtain than on the left. In our experience, the right posterior, posterior lateral, and lateral regions are usually best mapped and ablated from the femoral venous approach. The right anterolateral and anterior regions can also often be successfully ablated using the femoral venous approach, but alternatively a catheter introduced from the subclavian or internal jugular vein may obtain better contact in these areas (Figure 11). The catheter may be prolapsed across the tricuspid valve to help sta-

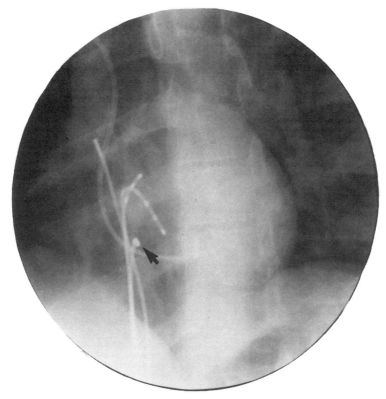

Figure 10. Fluoroscopic appearance of an ablation catheter (arrow) position for ablation of a right posterior accessory pathway (left anterior oblique projection). The catheter is at the most posterior aspect of the tricuspid annulus just off the septum. (Reprinted with permission from Zipes DP, ed. *Catheter Ablation of Arrhythmias.* Futura Publishing Co., 1994.)

bilize the tip on the tricuspid annulus. Most right free wall accessory pathways can be ablated by positioning the ablation catheter on the atrial side of the tricuspid annulus. Occasionally, however, a right free wall accessory pathway may be better approached by placing the catheter underneath the tricuspid apparatus, analogous to the technique used for left free wall accessory pathways (Figure 12). To do this, a catheter is introduced across the tricuspid valve and looped back upon itself in the right ventricle underneath the tricuspid apparatus until a small atrial potential as well as a larger ventricular potential is recorded, confirming adequate proximity to the tricuspid annulus. Several catheters with different degrees of stiffness, radius of curvature, or deflectability may be tried to achieve adequate contact. In addition, a set of sheaths has been developed that direct the catheter along the tricuspid annulus to the anterior, anterolateral, lateral, posterior lateral, and posterior regions (Figure 13). Once the location of the accessory pathway has been determined grossly, then the appropriate sheath is selected to direct the catheter along the annulus to that location. In addition, a simple long sheath with a slight bend at the tip can also be used to direct the catheter to several different locations along

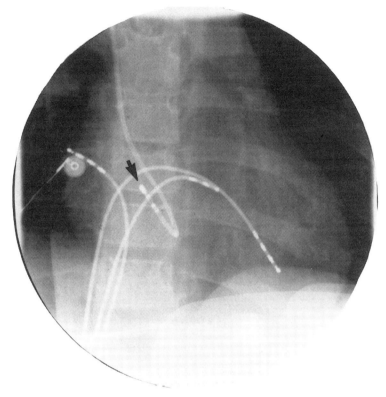

Figure 11. Fluoroscopic appearance of an ablation catheter (arrow) advanced to the tricuspid annulus from the right subclavian vein to ablate a right anterior accessory pathway (right anterior oblique projection). Adequate catheter contact could not be obtained from the femoral venous approach. (Reprinted with permission from Zipes DP, ed. *Catheter Ablation of Arrhythmias.* Futura Publishing Co., 1994.)

Figure 12. Fluoroscopic appearance of an ablation catheter (arrow) advanced into the right ventricle and underneath the tricuspid annulus to ablate the ventricular insertion of a right lateral accessory pathway. Upper panel is the right anterior oblique projection and lower panel is the left anterior oblique projection. Adequate tissue contact could not be obtained on the atrial side of the tricuspid annulus.

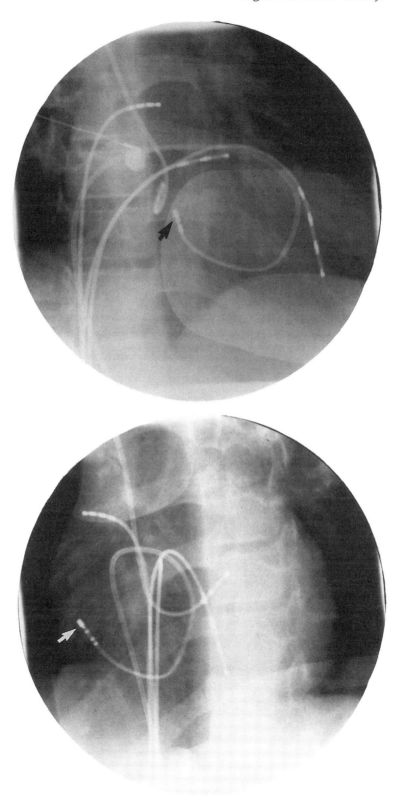

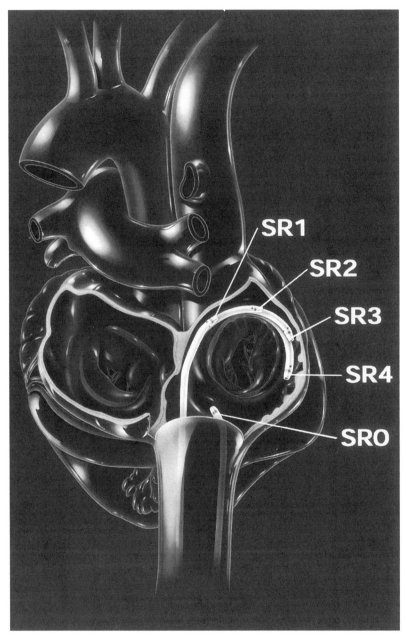

Figure 13. Preformed long atrial sheaths designed to facilitate placement of a mapping/ablation catheter along the atrial aspect of the tricuspid annulus. One selects a sheath with an appropriate curve and length (SRO–SR4) depending on the estimated location of the accessory pathway along the annulus. (Courtesy of Daige Corporation/St. Jude Medical, Inc.)

the tricuspid annulus. The advantage of the sheath is not only that it may help direct the catheter along the annulus, but also that it can stabilize the body of the catheter and improve the ability to obtain good catheter-tissue contact. A catheter with a groove in the distal electrode may also be used to stabilize the ablating electrode on the annulus. Transesophageal or intracardiac echocardiography may aid in identifying catheter position with respect to the tricuspid annulus or coronary sinus.[40]

Results of Right Freewall Accessory Pathway Ablation

The success rates for catheter ablation of right free wall accessory pathways is somewhat lower than that for accessory pathways at other locations: 88% versus 97% for left free wall, 96% for anteroseptal, and 91% for posteroseptal.[1-5,38,41] The recurrence rate (approximately 21% in earlier studies) after an apparently successful ablation is also higher than that at other sites: 8% for left free wall, 15% for anteroseptal and posteroseptal).[1,3,4,36-39,41] Indeed, in our experience, it is not uncommon for right free wall pathway conduction to repetitively disappear with energy delivery and reappear within the 30 minute waiting period after energy delivery. Again, this phenomenon is probably due to a combination of inadequate heating (catheter instability), difficult mapping, and possibly epicardial or complex accessory pathway anatomy.

Complications

Serious complications from ablation of right free wall accessory pathways are rare and less common than at any other accessory pathway site.[1-5,38,41] Complications are usually related to catheter introduction and manipulation; for example, complications of subclavian or internal jugular venous puncture (pneumothorax) or venous thromboembolism. Cardiac perforation may rarely occur, related to manipulation of either the diagnostic catheters or the ablation catheter. There is a small risk of pulmonary embolism due to clot or coagulum at the ablation site or due to thrombosis in the femoral venous system. Complications typical of left-sided accessory pathway ablation (arterial access complications, transseptal complications, systemic emboli) or septal pathway ablation (AV block) are very unusual.

Follow-up

In uncomplicated right free wall accessory pathway ablations, the patient can often be discharged on the same day as the procedure. Recurrent accessory pathway conduction is usually manifest as a delta wave on follow-up electrocardiogram or recurrent symptoms of tachycardia. Routine follow-up electrophysiological study in asymptomatic patients without delta waves is not indicated. However, follow-up electrophysiological study may be indicated in selected asymptomatic patients without delta waves who had highly symptomatic AV reciprocating tachycardiac as their presenting arrhythmia, or in patients with occupations in which definitive knowledge of accessory pathway absence is important (for example, airline pilots or professional athletes). Patients with a recurrent delta wave or symptoms of tachycardia should undergo repeat electrophysiology study because the vast majority can undergo successful reablation. Patients who had a delta wave prior to ablation may occasionally have recurrent orthodromic tachycardia without reappearance of the delta wave postablation due to recurrence of only retrograde accessory pathway conduction. The need for antithrombotic therapy post ablation is unknown; our practice is to give the patient aspirin 325 mg a day for 6 weeks after the procedure to prevent platelet deposition at the site of ablation.

Acknowledgement

The author appreciates the expert secretarial assistance of Kathy Orchin in the preparation of this manuscript and the help of M. Erick Burton, M.D. in the review of the manuscript.

References

1. Jackman WM, Xunzhang W, Friday KJ, et al. Catheter ablation of accessory atrioventricular pathways (Wolff-Parkinson-White Syndrome) by radiofrequency current. *N Engl J Med* 1991;324:1605–1611.
2. Calkins H, Langberg J, Sousa J, et al. Radiofrequency catheter ablation of accessory atrioventricular connections in 250 patients. *Circulation* 1992; 85:1337–1346.
3. Lesh MD, Van Hare GF, Schamp DJ, et al. Curative percutaneous catheter ablation using radiofrequency energy for accessory pathways in all locations: results in 100 consecutive patients. *J Am Coll Cardiol* 1992;19: 1303–1309.
4. Swartz JF, Tracy CM, Fletcher RD. Radiofrequency endocardial catheter ablation of accessory atrioventricular pathway atrial insertion sites. *Circulation* 1993;87:487–499.
5. Haïssaguerre M, Gaita F, Marcus FI, et al. Radiofrequency catheter ablation of accessory pathways. *J Cardiovasc Electrophysiol* 1994;5:532–552.
6. Tchou P, Lehmann MH, Jazayeri M, et al. Atriofascicular connection or a nodoventricular Mahaim fiber? Electrophysiological elucidation of the pathway and associated reentrant circuit. *Circulation* 1988;77:837.
7. Leitch J, Klein GJ, Yee R, et al. New concepts on nodoventricular accessory pathways. *J Cardiovasc Electrophysiol* 1990;1:220.
8. Klein LS, Hackett FK, Zipes DP, et al. Radiofrequency catheter ablation of Mahaim fibers at the tricuspid annulus. *Circulation* 1993;87:738.
9. McClelland JH, Xunzhang W, Beckman KJ, et al. Radiofrequency catheter ablation of right atriofascicular (Mahaim) accessory pathways guided by acessory pathway activation potentials. *Circulation* 1994;89:2655.

10. Gallagher J, Pritchett E, Sealy W, et al. The preexcitation syndromes. *Prog Cardiovasc Dis* 1978;20:285–327.

11. Milstein S, Sharma AD, Guiraudon GM, et al. An algorithm for the electrocardiographic localization of accessory pathways in the Wolff-Parkinson-White Syndrome. *PACE* 1987;10:555–563.

12. Fitzpatrick AP, Gonzales RP, Lesh MD, et al. New algorithm for the localization of accessory atrioventricular connections using a baseline electrocardiogram. *J Am Coll Cardiol* 1994;23:107–116.

13. Scheinman M, Wang Y, Van Hare G, et al. Electrocardiographic and electrophysiologic characteristics of anterior, mid-septal and right free-wall accessory pathways. *J Am Coll Cardiol* 1992;20:1220–1229.

14. Rodriguez LM, Smeets JLMR, Chillou C, et al. The 12-lead electrocardiogram in midseptal, anteroseptal, posteroseptal, and right free wall accessory pathways. *Am J Cardiol* 1993;72:1274–1280.

15. Liebman J, Zeno J, Olshansky B, et al. Electrocardiographic body surface potential mapping in the Wolff-Parkinson-White Syndrome: noninvasive determination of the ventricular insertion sites of accessory atrioventricular connections. *Circulation* 1991;83:886–899.

16. Lesh MD. Techniques for localization and radiofrequency catheter ablation of right free wall accessory pathways. In: Zipes DP, Jalife J, eds. *Cardiac Electrophysiology: From Cell to Bedside*. Philadelphia: WB Saunders, 1995. pp 1078–1092.

17. Jackman WM, Friday KJ, Yeung-Lai-Wah JA, et al. New catheter technique for recording left free-wall accessory atrioventricular pathway activation: identification of pathway fiber orientation. *Circulation* 1988;78:598–610.

18. Chen SA, Tai CT, Lee SH, et al. Electrophysiologic characteristics and anatomical complexities of accessory atrioventricular pathways with successful ablation of anterograde and retrograde conduction at different sites. *J Cardiovasc Electrophysiol* 1996;7:907–915.

19. Calkins H, Kim YN, Schmaltz S, et al. Electrogram criteria for identification of appropriate target sites for radiofrequency catheter ablation of accessory atrioventricular connections. *Circulation* 1992;85:565–573.

20. Olgin JE, Miles WM. Ablation of atrial tachycardias. In: Singer I, Barold S, Camm A, eds. *Nonpharmacologic Therapy of Arrhythmias for the 21st Century: The State of the Art*. Armonk, NY: Futura Publishing Co., 1998. pp 197–217.

21. Swartz JF, Cohen AI, Fletcher RD, et al. Right coronary epicardial mapping improves accessory pathway catheter ablation success [abstract]. *Circulation* 1989;80(suppl II):II–431.

22. Martinez-Alday JD, Almendral J, Arenal A, et al. Identification of concealed posteroseptal Kent pathways by comparison of ventriculoatrial intervals from apical and posterobasal right ventricular sites. *Circulation* 1994;89:1060–1067.

23. Benditt DG, Pritchett ELC, Smith WM, et al. Ventriculoatrial intervals: diagnostic use in paroxysmal supraventricular tachycardia. *Ann Int Med* 1979;91:161–166.

24. Chen X, Borggrefe M, Shenasa M, et al. Characteristics of local electrogram

predicting successful transcatheter radiofrequency ablation of left-sided accessory pathways. *J Am Coll Cardiol* 1992;20:656–665.

25. Langberg JJ, Calkins H, El-Atassi R, et al. Temperature monitoring during radiofrequency catheter ablation of accessory pathways. *Circulation* 1992; 86:1469–1474.

26. Calkins H, Prystowsky E, Carlson M, et al. Temperature monitoring during RF catheter ablation procedures using closed loop control. *Circulation* 1994;90:1279–1286.

27. Calkins H, Prystowsky E, Berger RD, et al. Recurrence of conduction following radiofrequency catheter ablation procedures: relationship to ablation target and electrode temperature. *J Cardiovasc Electrophysiol* 1996;7: 704–712.

28. Haines DE, Watson DD. Tissue heating during radiofrequency catheter ablation: a thermodynamic model and observations in isolated perfused and superfused canine right ventricular free wall. *PACE* 1989;12:962–976.

29. Shpun S, Gepstein L, Hayam G, et al. Guidance of radiofrequency endocardial ablation with real-time three-dimensional magnetic navigation system. *Circulation* 1997;96:2016–2021.

30. Ferguson TB Jr, Cox JL. Surgical treatment for the Wolff-Parkinson-White Syndrome: the endocardial approach. In: Zipes DP, Jalife J, eds. *Cardiac Electrophysiology: From Cell to Bedside*. Philadelphia, PA: WB Saunders, 1990. pp 897–907.

31. Guiraudon GM, Klein GJ, Yee R, et al. Surgery for the Wolff-Parkinson-White syndrome. In: Zipes DP, Jalife J, eds. *Cardiac Electrophysiology: From Cell to Bedside*. 2nd edition. Philadelphia, PA: WB Saunders, 1995. pp 1553–1562.

32. Becker AG, Anderson RW, Durrer D, et al. The anatomical substrates of Wolff-Parkinson-White syndrome: a clinicopathological condition seen in patients. *Circulation* 1978;57:870.

33. Giuliani ER, Fuster V, Brandenburg RO, et al. Ebstein's anomaly: the clinical features and natural history of Ebstein's anomaly of the tricuspid valve. *Mayo Clin Proc* 1979;54:163–173.

34. Cappato R, Schlüter M, Weiss C, et al. Catheter-induced mechanical conduction block of right-sided accessory fibers with Mahaim-type preexcitation to guide radiofrequency ablation. *Circulation* 1994;90:282–290.

35. Kerr CR, Gallagher JJ, German LD. Changes in ventriculoatrial intervals with bundle branch block aberration during reciprocating tachycardia in patients with accessory atrioventricular pathways. *Circulation* 1982;66: 196–201.

36. Twidale N, Wang X, Beckman KJ, et al. Factors associated with recurrence of accessory pathway conduction after radiofrequency catheter ablation. *PACE* 1991;14:2042–2048.

37. Langberg JJ, Calkins H, Kim YN, et al. Recurrence of conduction in accessory atrioventricular connections after initially successful radiofrequency catheter ablation. *J Am Coll Cardiol* 1992;19:1588–1592.

38. Leather RA, Leitch JW, Klein GJ, et al. Radiofrequency catheter ablation of accessory pathways: a learning experience. *Am J Cardiol* 1991;68:1651–1655.

39. Chen X, Kottkamp H, Hindricks G, et al. Recurrence and late block of accessory pathway conduction following radiofrequency catheter ablation. *J Cardiovasc Electrophysiol* 1994;5:650–658.

40. Olgin JE, Kalman JM, Fitzpatrick AP, et al. Role of right atrial endocardial structures as barriers to conduction during human type I atrial flutter: activation and entrainment mapping guided by intracardiac echocardiography. *Circulation* 1995;92:1839–1848.

41. Rosenthal LS, Calkins H. Catheter ablation of right free wall accessory pathways and Mahaim fibers. In: Singer I, ed. *Interventional Electrophysiology*. Baltimore, MD: Williams & Wilkins, 1997. pp 207–229.

Chapter 24

Radiofrequency Catheter Ablation of Posteroseptal Accessory Atrioventricular Pathways

Shih-Ann Chen, M.D., Chern-En Chiang, M.D., Ching-Tai Tai, M.D., Mau-Song Chang, M.D.

Anatomic Considerations

The posteroseptal area is a complex anatomic entity.[1-5] It corresponds to a region where the 4 cardiac chambers reach their maximal proximity posteriorly. In this area, the interatrial sulcus is to the far left of the interventricular sulcus, while the mitral annulus usually inserts into the right fibrous trigone as much as 5 mm superior to the insertion of the tricuspid annulus. Between the mitral annulus and the tricuspid annulus lies the right atrio-left ventricular sulcus, which was the junction between the inferomedial right atrium and the posterior superior process of the left ventricle. The undersurface of the coronary sinus abuts the superior margin of the right atrio-left ventricular sulcus.

To know the true dimensions of the posterior septum is important because it may provide a basis for consensus among electrophysiologists and facilitate more accurate comparison of the outcome and risks of catheter ablation techniques in relation to the anatomic sites of the accessory pathways (APs). Davis et al studied the dimensions of the posterior septum in 48 adult cadaver hearts.[6] They found that the mean distance from the coronary sinus ostium to the left margin of the posterior septal space was 2.3±0.4 cm and that the junction of the posterior septum and the left free wall lies > 1.75 cm to the left of

From Huang SKS, Wilber DJ (eds.): *Radiofrequency Catheter Ablation of Cardiac Arrhythmias: Basic Concepts and Clinical Applications,* 2nd ed. Armonk, NY: Futura Publishing Company, Inc. ©2000.

the coronary sinus ostium in more than 75 % of all but the smallest adults. Sealy and Mikat demonstrated that the distance from the central fibrous body to the left free wall ranged from 15 to 28 mm in 20 adult cadaver hearts by intraoperative measurement.[2] From the surgical findings, most posteroseptal APs consist of "right atrio-left ventricular" fibers with the ventricular insertion attaching onto the posterior superior process of the left ventricle, but some posteroseptal APs were considered to be left posteroseptal and a left atrial approach was needed for successful dissection.[1–4]

Jackman et al have shown that the AP activation potential could be recorded as far as 18 mm from the coronary sinus ostium distally for left posteroseptal APs.[7] Dhala et al defined posteroseptal APs as that in which the earliest atrial or ventricular activation was recorded less than 1 cm from the coronary sinus ostium, much narrower than the actual dimension.[8] Thus, some of the posteroseptal APs might have been classified by Dhala et al as left posterior free wall pathways for which left-sided ablation was indeed necessary.

In this laboratory, we defined the margin of the left posteroseptal space as 2 cm from the coronary sinus ostium, which was reasonable and compatible with the previous reports.[9] The earliest atrial activity recorded at the posteroseptal mitral annulus was always earlier than that recorded from the right posteroseptal area, suggesting that the atrial end might insert into the posteroseptal mitral annulus. Besides, these APs could be ablated successfully by radiofrequency energy delivered at the ventricular aspect of the posteroseptal mitral annulus, which implies that ventricular insertion was on the left ventricle. The above findings provided evidence that the APs were composed of "left atrio-left ventricular" fibers and comprised a subgroup of posteroseptal APs (Figure 1).

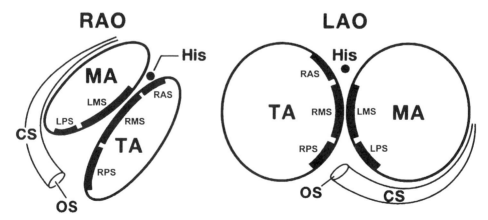

Figure 1. Schematic definition of septal accessory atrioventricular pathways in both right anterior oblique (RAO) and left anterior oblique (LAO) views. CS indicates coronary sinus; LMS = left midseptal; LPS = left posteroseptal; MA = mitral annulus; OS = ostium of the coronary sinus; RAS = right anteroseptal; RMS = right midseptal; RPS = right posteroseptal; TA = tricuspid annulus.

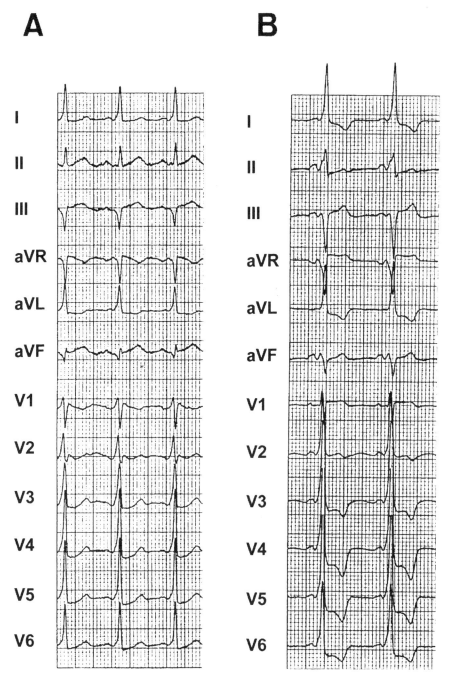

Figure 2A-C. VA interval and ΔVA of orthodromic tachycardia obtained during baseline electrophysiology study from patients who had a successful ablation site at the left posteroseptal area (B). The VA interval is defined as the interval from the initiation of QRS complex on the surface ECG to the local and middle atrial activation of intracardiac recording of the proximal (VA$_P$) and middle (VA$_M$) circumferential groups of electrodes of the coronary sinus catheter as well as the His bundle catheter (VA$_H$). The ΔVA is defined as the difference in VA interval between that recorded at the His bundle catheter (VA$_H$) and that at one of the electrode groups of the coronary sinus catheter that recorded the earliest atrial activation (VA$_P$ or VA$_M$). Tracings from top to bottom are ECG leads (I, II, and V$_1$), and high right atrium (HRA) electrograms. His bundle electrograms (HBE), and coronary sinus electrograms for proximal (CS$_P$), middle (CS$_V$), and distal (CS$_D$) electrode groups of the orthogonal catheter. (From Chiang et al, *Circulation* 1996;93:982–991.) (*continued*)

C

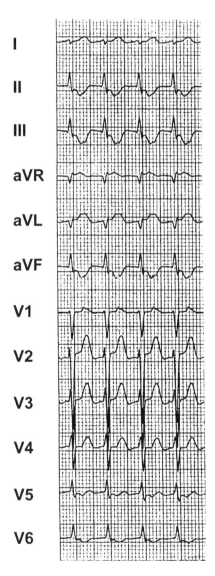

Figure 2A-C. (*continued*)

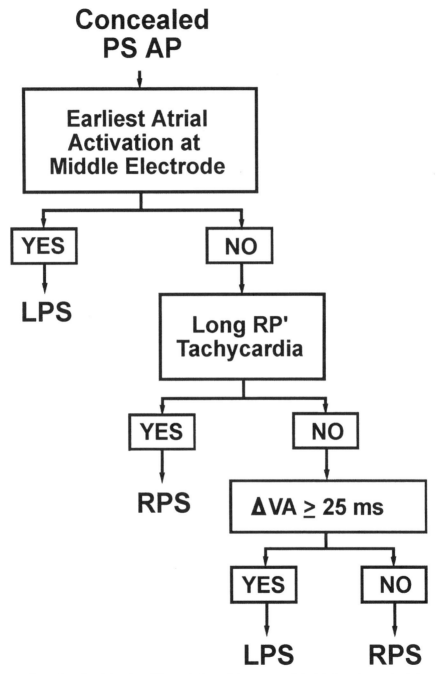

Figure 3. Stepwise algorithm for differentiation of the successful ablation site at the left posteroseptal area (LPS) from that at the right posteroseptal area (RPS). PS AP indicates posteroseptal accessory pathway. (From Chiang et al, *Circulation* 1996;93:982–991.)

Electrocardiographic Features

The most constant features on the 12-lead electrocardiograph that indicate a presence of a posteroseptal accessory pathway are the abrupt development of an R wave between leads V_1 and V_2 and a predominantly negative QRS in lead III. Arruda et al developed an ECG algorithm using the initial forces of preexcitation (initial 20 milliseconds) after the earliest delta wave onset in any of the limb leads as well as the precordial leads to predict accessory pathway location.[10] They demonstrated that a negative or isoelectric delta wave in lead V_1 indicated a septal pathway, and a positive delta wave indicated a right free wall pathway after excluding patients with a left free wall pathway. They also found that a negative delta wave in lead II identifies the subepicardial posteroseptal pathway with a sensitivity of 100%, a specificity of 100%, and a positive predictive value of 100%. Chiang et al from this laboratory reported that the polarity of the initial 40 millisecond segment of the most preexcited QRS complex in each of the frontal leads, and the polarity of the initial 60 millisecond segment of the most preexcited QRS complex in each of the precordial leads proved to be the best representatives of delta wave polarity in the respective leads; we also showed in the ECG algorithm that right septal pathways did not have the ECG manifestation of positive delta waves in lead V_1.[11] Thus, the posteroseptal accessory pathway was recognized by the following ECG features of preexcitation: 1) R/S ratio > 1 in lead V_2; 2) negative delta wave in lead III; and 3) R/S ratio < 1 in lead III (see below, Figure 4, panel A, for details).[12,17] Left posteroseptal pathways may be differentiated from right posteroseptal pathways by positive delta waves in lead V_1, and from left posterior or posterolateral pathways by R/S ratio < 1 in lead V_1.[10–13]

Furthermore, the characteristics of the retrograde P waves in posterior-type atrioventricular (AV) nodal reentrant tachycardia (AVNRT) are similar to those in AV reciprocating tachycardia using a posteroseptal pathway.[14] The report from this laboratory showed that with the difference of RP' intervals in leads V_1 and V_3 > 20 milliseconds, the posterior-type AV node reentrant tachycardia could be differentiated from AV reciprocating tachycardia using a posteroseptal pathway with a sensitivity of 71%, a specificity of 87% and a positive predictive value of 75%.[14] Ng et al also reported that in their patients with a long RP' tachycardia and negative P waves in the inferior leads, a positive or isoelectric P wave in lead I strongly supports a diagnosis of atypical AV node reentrant tachycardia, whereas a negative or biphasic P wave in lead I favors a diagnosis of permanent junctional reciprocating tachycardia or low right atrial tachycardia (Figures 2 and 3).[15]

Electrophysiological Characteristics and Radiofrequency Ablation

Accessory pathways located in this area pose a relatively difficult task for cardiac surgeons and electrophysiologists. Initial results from surgical ablation of APs in this area were associated with high success rate but also a high incidence of complete AV block because of the close proximity of the AV node to this area.[1–4] With the use of epicardial techniques, surgical results have been much improved. Catheter ablation has replaced surgical intervention in the treatment of patients with drug-refractory supraventricular tachycardia in recent years. Initially, direct current delivered through an electrode catheter at the coronary sinus ostium achieved a high success rate in eliminating these APs but carried a potential risk of cardiac tamponade and complete AV block.[16] Radiofrequency energy, with a more homogeneous lesion and devoid of barotrauma, has recently become a more favored energy source.

In some studies, radiofrequency catheter ablation of the posteroseptal accessory pathways has been identified as being more difficult than for pathways located in other areas.[17–19] Schluter et al reported that more radiofrequency pulses, longer procedure time, and longer radiation exposure were needed to achieve successful results.[17] In addition to the complex anatomic structure involved, difficulty in the discrimination of the successful ablation site on the right versus left posteroseptal area before the ablation procedure was a major reason. Arruda et al reported that approximately 40% of patients referred after at least one unsuccessful ablation attempt for a posteroseptal accessory pathway required ablation from coronary veins or anomalies of the coronary sinus.[10] They found that a posteroseptal accessory pathway associated with a negative delta wave in lead II requires subepicardial approach from the coronary venous system. Dhala et al also showed that among 11 patients with a positive or biphasic delta wave in lead II, 9 (82%) were ablated in the posteroseptal region of the tricuspid annulus; and of 25 patients with a negative delta wave in lead II, 13 (52%) were successfully ablated within the terminal coronary sinus including the ostium.[8] However, Wen et al showed that of the 146 posteroseptal accessory pathways, 94 (64%) were successfully ablated from the left posteroseptal region, 45 (31%) from the right posteroseptal region, and only 3 (2%) from the proximal coronary sinus.[18] They concluded that delivery of current to the coronary sinus or middle cardiac vein is unnecessary in most patients with posteroseptal pathways.[18] When ablation is unsuccessful from either right-side or left-side approach, Bashir et al have reported favorable results with the application of current using a bipolar configuration between the distal poles of a left- and right-sided catheter.[20]

The usual approach method in most of the above reports was that after baseline electrophysiological study, the posteroseptal tricuspid annulus including the coronary sinus ostium and its most proximal parts and the inferomedial right atrium were carefully mapped. If ablation at these areas failed or no appropriate ablation site could be obtained, the left posteroseptal area was then mapped with the use of a transaortic or transseptal approach. In the case that the appropriate electrogram was again unavailable at the left posteroseptal area, switch of the mapping procedure back to the right posteroseptal area was not uncommon. More radiofrequency pulses, prolonged procedure time, and radiation exposure were inevitable by these approaches.

In this laboratory, we developed a stepwise algorithm for differentiating left posteroseptal from right posteroseptal concealed accessory pathways; the presence of long RP' tachycardia suggested a right endocardial approach, while the ΔVA (defined as the difference in the VA intervals between that recorded at the His bundle catheter and that at one of the electrode groups recording the earliest atrial activation) ≥ 25 milliseconds during tachycardia suggested a left endocardial approach.[9] The position of the coronary sinus ostium was verified by angiography, and the coronary sinus catheter was fixed on the vascular sheath with the proximal electrode straddling the ostium. The "left atrio-left ventricular" fibers could be predicted by the algorithm from the baseline electrophysiological study without the inducement of functional bundle-branch block or the search for AP activation potential. In other words, if the earliest atrial activation could be recorded on the middle electrode for a "left atrio-left ventricular" AP, there was hardly a chance for a right endocardial approach to be effective in ablation except by applying radiofrequency energy deep into the coronary sinus, an approach not undertaken in this laboratory. The radiofrequency energy pulses, ablation time, and fluoroscopic time were therefore markedly reduced, as proven in the prospective study. Almost all APs (98.9%) could be successfully ablated on the endocardial surface without complications. The cut value, ΔVA≥25 milliseconds, could not be explained fully because throughout the literature, no previous reports have been found that study the intra-atrial conduction time from the posteroseptal tricuspid annulus to the His bundle area versus that from the posteroseptal mitral annulus. More electrophysiological studies may be needed to answer this (Figure 4, 5).

Posteroseptal pathways with decremental conduction properties are not unusual.[21,22] The presence of long RP' tachycardia predicts a right endocardial ablation site. Chien et al reported 6 patients with concealed posteroseptal APs with decremental properties presented as a permanent form of junctional reciprocating tachycardia.[23] All the APs could be treated successfully by DC shock via a catheter positioned just outside the coronary sinus ostium. Haïssaguerre et al also reported successful ablation with DC shock, using a right endocardial approach, in all 8 patients with long RP' tachycardia.[24] Gaita et al recently reported 32 patients with permanent junctional reciprocating tachycardia.[25] Twenty-five of them had concealed posteroseptal APs, and all the APs could be ablated with radiofrequency current delivered at the right posteroseptal area; this is in accordance with our previous study that all 11 patients with long RP' tachycardia including 3 patients with permanent junctional reciprocating tachycardia could have successful ablation on the right endocardial surface.[9] As far as is known, no one has ever reported a left endocardial approach achieving successful ablation of posteroseptal APs presenting as long RP' tachycardia. These findings suggested that in patients with posteroseptal APs presenting with long RP' tachycardia, the right endocardial approach should be tried first.

Coronary sinus venography or the venous phase of left coronary arteriography can clearly delineate the coronary sinus morphology and its ostium, and this information is very important for guiding the ablation procedure.[10,26,27] The importance of the stability of the electrode catheter in the vascular sheath should be addressed. In this laboratory, the catheter was locked to the vascular sheath, which was then sutured to the skin. Any dislodgment or displacement of the proximal electrode group away from the coronary sinus ostium might compromise the accuracy of the intracardiac electrode and the algorithm for determining the ablation site.

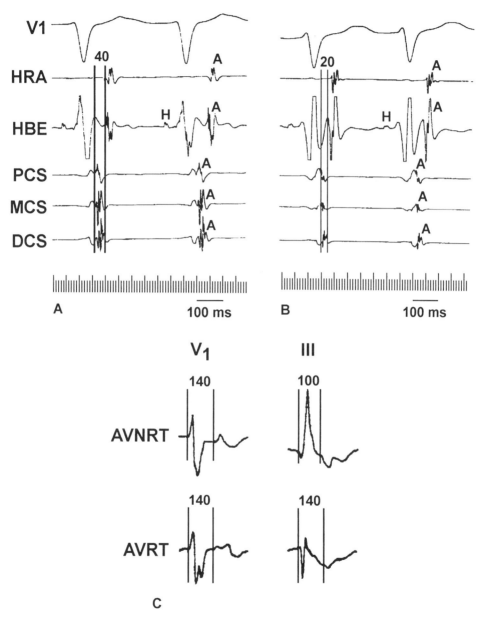

Figure 4. Twelve-lead ECGs show ventricular preexcitation. Panel A: right posteroseptal pathway. Panel B: left posteroseptal pathway. The delta wave is negative in leads II, III, aVF and positive in leads I and aVL. The precordial R/S ratio becomes more than 1 in lead V_2. The retrograde P wave is negative in lead II and positive in lead V_1.

A

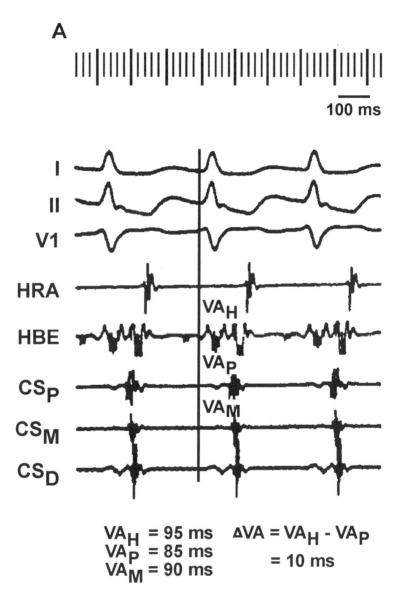

100 ms

VA_H = 95 ms
VA_P = 85 ms
VA_M = 90 ms

$\Delta VA = VA_H - VA_P$
= 10 ms

Figure 5. Panel A: The conduction time between atrial electrograms (A) recorded at the proximal coronary sinus (PCS) and His bundle area (HBE) during posterior type atrioventricular nodal reentry tachycardia (AVNRT) is 40 milliseconds. (*continued*)

B

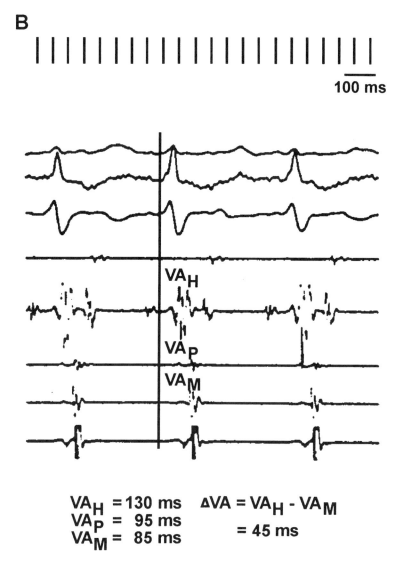

100 ms

$$VA_H = 130 \text{ ms} \quad \Delta VA = VA_H - VA_M$$
$$VA_P = 95 \text{ ms}$$
$$VA_M = 85 \text{ ms} \quad = 45 \text{ ms}$$

Figure 5. (*continued*) Panel B: The conduction time between atrial electrograms recorded at PCS and HBE during atrioventricular reciprocating tachycardia (AVRT) using a posteroseptal pathway is 20 milliseconds. HRA = high right atrium; H = His potential; MCS = middle coronary sinus; DCS = distal coronary sinus. (From Tai et al, *J Am Coll Cardiol* 1997;29:394–402.)

Conclusion

Catheter ablation of posteroseptal accessory pathways is technically challenging. Further understanding of the anatomy, electrocardiogrophy, and electrophysiology of accessory pathways in the septal area would improve the results of catheter ablation in the postersoseptal space.

References

1. Sealy WC, Gallagher JJ. The surgical approach to the septal area of the heart based on the experiences with forty-five patients with Kent bundles. J Thorac Cardiovasc Surg 1980;79:542–551.
2. Sealy WC, Mikat EM. Anatomical problems with identification and interruption of posterior septal Kent bundles. *Ann Thorac Surg* 1983;36:584–595.
3. Cox JL, Gallagher JJ, Cain ME. Experience with 118 consecutive patients undergoing surgery for Wolff-Parkinson-White syndrome. *J Thorac Cardiovasc Surg* 1985;90:490–501.
4. Guiraudon GM, Klein GJ, Sharma AD, et al. Surgical ablation of posterior septal accessory pathways in the Wolff-Parkinson-White syndrome by a closed heart technique. *J Throac Cardiovasc Surg* 1986;92:406–413.
5. Dean JW, Ho SY, Rowland E, et al. Clinical anatomy of the atrioventricular junctions. *J Am Coll Cardiol* 1994;24:1725–1731.
6. Davis LM, Byth K, Ellis P, et al. Dimensions of the human posterior septal space and coronary sinus. *Am J Cardiol* 1991;68:621–625.
7. Jackman WM, Friday KJ, Fitzgerald DM, et al. Localization of left free-wall and posteroseptal accessory atrioventricular pathways by direct recording of accessory pathway activation. *PACE* 1989;12:201–214.
8. Dhala AA, Deshpnde SS, Bremner S, et al. Transcatheter ablation of posteroseptal accessory pathways using a venous approach and radiofrequency energy. *Circulation* 1994;90:1799–1810.
9. Chiang CE, Chen SA, Tai CT, et al. Prediction of successful ablation site of concealed posteroseptal accessory pathways by a novel algorithm using baseline electrophysiological parameters: implication for an abbreviated ablation procedure. *Circulation* 1996;93:982–991.
10. Arruda MS, McClelland JH, Wang X, et al. Development and validation of an ECG algorithm for identifying accessory pathway ablation site in Wolff-Parkinson-White syndrome. *J Cardiovasc Electrophysiol* 1998;9:2–12.
11. Chiang CE, Chen SA, Teo WS, et al. An accurate stepwise electrocardiographic algorithm for localization of accessory pathways in patients with Wolff-Parkinson-White syndrome from a comprehensive analysis of delta waves and R/S ratio during sinus rhythm. *Am J Cardiol* 1995;76:40–46.
12. Fitzpatric AP, Gonzales RP, Lesh MD, et al. New algorithm for the localization of accessory atrioventricular connections using a baseline electrocardiogram. *J Am Coll Cardiol* 1994:23:107–116.
13. Tai CT, Chen SA, Chiang CE, et al. Electrocardiographic and electrophysi-

ologic characteristics of anteroseptal, midseptal, and para-Hisian accessory pathways: implication for radiofrequency catheter ablation. *Chest* 1996; 109:730–740.

14. Tai CT, Chen SA, Chiang CE, et al. A new electrocardiographic algorithm using retrograde P waves for differentiating atrioventricular node reentrant tachycardia from atrioventricular reciprocating tachycardia mediated by concealed accessory pathway. *J Am Coll Cardiol* 1996;29:394–402.

15. Ng KS, Lauer MR, Young C, et al. Correlation of p-wave polarity with underlying electrophysiologic mechanisms of long RP' tachycardia. *Am J Cardiol* 1996;77:1129–1132.

16. Morady F, Scheinman MM, Kou WH, et al. Long-term results of catheter ablation of a posteroseptal accessory atrioventricular connection in 48 patients. *Circulation* 1989;79:1160–1170.

17. Schluter M, Geiger M, Siebels J, et al. Catheter ablation using radiofrequency current to cure symptomatic patients with tachyarrhythmias related to an accessory pathway. *Circulation* 1991;84:1644–1661.

18. Wen MS, Yeh SJ, Wang CC, et al. Radiofrequency ablation therapy of the posteroseptal accessory pathway. *Am Heart J* 1996;132:612–620.

19. Lesh MD, Van Hare GF, Schamp DJ, et al. Curative percutaneous catheter ablation using radiofrequency energy for accessory pathways in all locations: results in 100 consecutive patients. *J Am Coll Cardiol* 1992;19: 1303–1309.

20. Bashir Y, Heald SC, O'Nunain S, et al. Radiofrequency current delivery by way of a bipolar tricuspid annulus-mitral annulus electrode configuration for ablation of posteroseptal accessory pathways. *J Am Coll Cardiol* 1993;22:550–556.

21. Coumel P, Cabrol C, Fabbiato A, et al. Tachycardie permanente par rhythm reciprozue. I-Preuves du diagnostic par stimulation auriculaire et ventriculaire. *Arch Mal Coeur* 1967;60:1830–1864.

22. Gallagher JJ, Sealy WC. The permanent form of junctional reciprocating tachycardia: further elucidation of the underlying mechanism. *Eur J Cardiol* 1978;8:413–430.

23. Chien WW, Cohen TJ, Lee MA, et al. Electrophysiological findings and long-term follow-up of patients with the permanent form of junctional reciprocating tachycardia treated by catheter ablation. *Circulation* 1992;85: 1329–1336.

24. Haïssaguerre M, Montserrat P, Warin JF, et al. Catheter ablation of left posteroseptal accessory pathways and of long RP' tachycardias with an endocardial approach. *Eur Heart J* 1991;12:845–859.

25. Gaita F, Haïssaguerre M, Giusetto C, et al. Catheter ablation of permanent junctional reciprocating tachycardia with radiofrequency current. *J Am Coll Cardiol* 1995;25:648–654.

26. Chiang CE, Chen SA, Yang CR, et al. Major coronary sinus abnormalities: identification of occurrence and significance in radiofrequency ablation of supraventricular tachycardia. *Am Heart J* 1994;127:1279–1289.

27. Weiss C, Cappato R, Schluter M, et al. Anomalies of the coronary venous system in patients with and without accessory pathways [abstract]. *J Am Coll Cardiol* 1995;25:18A.

Chapter 25

Catheter Ablation of Left Free Wall Accessory Pathways

Mark A. Wood, M.D.
John F. Swartz, M.D.

Introduction

Understanding the approach to left sided accessory pathways is important to the interventional electrophysiologist for many reasons. First, 40–70% of all accessory pathways presenting for ablation are located along the left free wall.[1–4] Left free wall pathways are therefore the most commonly encountered accessory pathway locations in clinical practice. Second, much of the clinical data on radiofrequency ablation of accessory pathways is derived from pathways in this location.[1–10] Third, the technical skills required to ablate these pathways are more demanding than for other locations and the risk for complications may be higher.[11–13]

Anatomy of Left Free Wall Accessory Pathways

A knowledge of the anatomy of left free wall accessory pathways is essential to understanding the mapping and ablation procedure. Left free wall pathways are typically thin strands of myocardial tissue crossing the adipose tissue on the epicardial aspect of the A-V annulus (Figure 1).[14] The annulus is typically normal in structure. The pathway may cross in close proximity to the annulus but may cross at some distance from the annulus within the fat pad nearer to the epicardium.[14,15] The atrial insertion of left free wall pathways is typically discrete (<1–3 mm in size) and close to the annulus.[14] The ventricu-

From Huang SKS, Wilber DJ (eds.): *Radiofrequency Catheter Ablation of Cardiac Arrhythmias: Basic Concepts and Clinical Applications,* 2nd ed. Armonk, NY: Futura Publishing Company, Inc. ©2000.

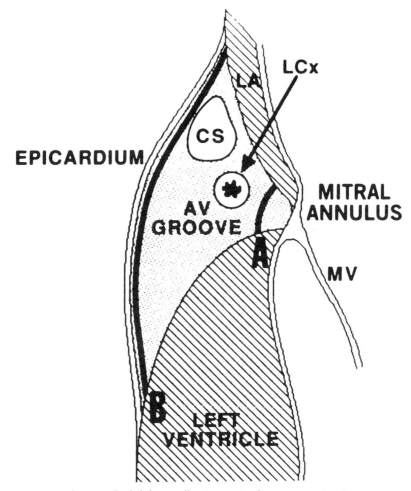

Figure 1. Diagram showing the left free wall atrioventricular (AV) junction in cross section. Left free wall accessory pathways may cross the AV junction close to the annulus (A) or at a distance within the fat pad. "Epicardial pathways" (B) course nearer to the epicardial reflection than to the mitral annulus. These pathways may not be successfully ablated from endocardial catheter positions due to atrial and/or ventricular insertions distant from the annulus, but may be ablated from within the coronary sinus.

lar insertion site is more variable and may be displaced away from the annulus toward the ventricular apex.[14] The ventricular insertion also tends to ramify over a region of tissue. These factors can influence the success of annular and subannular ablation attempts. Finally, most left free wall pathways cross the annulus obliquely. The atrial insertions are typically 4–30 mm proximal (posterior) to the more distal (anterior) ventricular insertion as mapped from within the coronary sinus.[16] The pathways tend to course less obliquely in the left paraseptal locations.[16]

The Transaortic Approach

Since its introduction in 1986 the transaortic or retrograde approach has been the most widely used technique for the ablation of left sided accessory pathways.[17] The advantages of the technique include ready access via the femoral artery, familiarity by most electrophysiologists, no need for specialized sheaths or equipment, and feasibility following full anticoagulation.

Catheter Manipulation

Arterial access is most commonly obtained via the right femoral artery although the brachial artery can also be used. Long vascular sheaths may be needed to cross tortuous femoral or iliac anatomy and may provide added catheter stability. The patient is fully heparinized and the ablation catheter is then passed into the descending aorta. In this position a tight curve is formed with the catheter tip before passage to the aortic root to minimize catheter manipulation in the arch and ascending aorta. The ablation catheter should be capable of forming a tight "J" curve, possess a 4 mm temperature monitoring tip electrode, and readily transmit applied torque. "Peanut" electrodes should be avoided due to risk of entrapment within the mitral apparatus.[18] In the RAO 30° projection the curved catheter most easily crosses the aortic valve when the curve is parallel to the fluoroscopic image plane with the "J" opening to the right. With this technique the curved catheter passes into the left ventricle oriented anterolaterally. In the aortic root, a straightened catheter tip may perforate aortic valve leaflets or enter the coronary artery system.[2,19] For these reasons the straightened catheter tip must *never* be used to cross the aortic valve. By maintaining a tight curve the catheter can be rotated counterclockwise and withdrawn into the left atrium as the tip turns posteriorly. By opening the catheter curve slightly the tip can easily map the annulus; clockwise torque moves the tip distally (anteriorly) along the coronary sinus and counterclockwise torque returns the catheter posteriorly (proximally along the coronary sinus). When the ablation site is approximated along the annulus the catheter tip is simultaneously withdrawn and straightened slightly to slip under the annulus for fine manipulation. Catheter positions beneath the annulus between the ventricular myocardium and mitral leaflet are most stable and target the ventricular accessory pathway insertion for ablation. In the authors' opinion catheter positions above or along the annulus are frequently too unstable for successful energy delivery using the retrograde approach. Others have successfully targeted the atrial insertions with the technique, however.[20]

Alternatively, after crossing the aortic valve the catheter can be straightened and steered directly under the annulus to the pathway location or withdrawn into the outflow tract, rotated posteriorly with a slight curve, and then advanced under the posterior mitral valve annulus for left paraseptal or posterior pathways.[6] For far left lateral and anterior pathways, extended reach catheters may be required. The use of long vascular sheaths into the ascending aorta or left ventricle has been described to improve catheter handling.[6] For manifest left free wall pathways a single catheter technique has been developed to minimize procedure time.[21,22] This approach has not gained widespread use due to selective patient criteria, requirement for extensive operator experience, difficulty in mapping retrograde pathway conduction, and the eventual need for additional catheter placement for postablation testing.

Mapping

The general pathway location is defined by a mapping atrial and ventricular activation using a diagnostic multipole coronary sinus catheter. The coronary sinus catheter also provides a visual target for placement of the ablation catheter. The pathway location defined by coronary sinus mapping is, however, only an approximation of the subannular ablation site due to the oblique course of left free wall pathways, displacement of the coronary sinus above the mitral annulus, variable basilar-apical ventricular insertion of the pathway or pathway location distal to reach of the coronary sinus catheter. Coronary sinus mapping may be enhanced by use of orthogonal electrode catheters to more specifically identify the electrogram components and accessory pathway potentials.[16]

Mapping with the ablation catheter should utilize both a close bipolar (2 mm spacing) and the unipolar configuration.[23] The unipolar electrogram is useful to initially localize the ablation site and to accurately reflect local ventricular activation. The bipolar electrogram more clearly displays the electrogram components and accessory pathway potentials.[8–10] Low amplifier gains should be used to reduce overlap of atrial and ventricular electrograms and to facilitate recognition of accessory pathway potentials.

During preexcitation the ablation site is first approximated by recording a QS potential on the unipolar electrogram. For retrograde activation mapping, the earliest atrial activation time is sought. As described above, initial mapping can be performed with the ablation catheter on the annulus. From this general area, the catheter is next positioned beneath the annulus for more precise mapping. Catheter tip positions beneath the mitral annulus are suggested by proximity to coronary sinus catheter, motion concomitant with the coronary sinus catheter and an atrial to ventricular electrogram ratio <1.0 (Figures 2 and 3). Once beneath the mitral annulus, specific electrogram criteria are applied to identify ablation sites.

Mapping Antegrade Activation

Because the transaortic approach targets the ventricular accessory pathway insertion site, this technique is best suited to map antegrade pathway activation. In mapping antegrade preexcitation from beneath the mitral annulus 5 electrogram characteristics serve as independent predictors of successful ablation sites.[8,9,24–27] These characteristics are presence of an accessory pathway (AP) potential, local atrial to ventricular conduction time (local A-V interval),

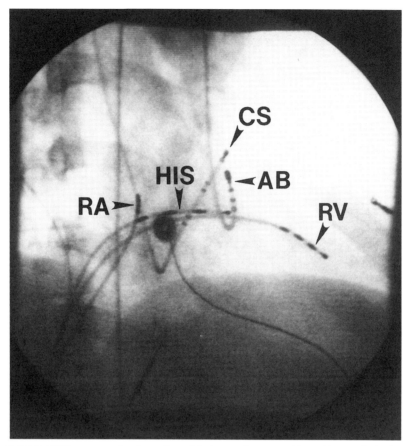

Figure 2. RAO 30° fluoroscopic view of an ablation catheter positioned beneath the lateral mitral annulus from the transaortic approach. The catheter positions are labeled as follows: RA = right atrium, CS = coronary sinus, HIS = His bundle, AB = ablation, RV = right ventricle. The tip of the ablation catheter is positioned beneath the mitral annulus just below the distal electrodes of the coronary sinus catheter.

delta (Δ) wave onset to local ventricular electrogram time (Δ-V interval), atrial electrogram amplitude and electrogram stability (Figures 4 and 5).

AP Potentials

The validation of AP potentials by the extrastimulus technique is not practical in clinical settings.[16,28,29] Instead, the presence of an AP potential can be presumed for discrete high frequency potentials occurring between the atrial and ventricular electrograms during antegrade accessory pathway conduction and occurring ≥ 10 milliseconds before Δ wave onset (see Figures 4 and 5).[4,9,19,24,26,27] The AP potential amplitude averages 0.5–1 mV at successful

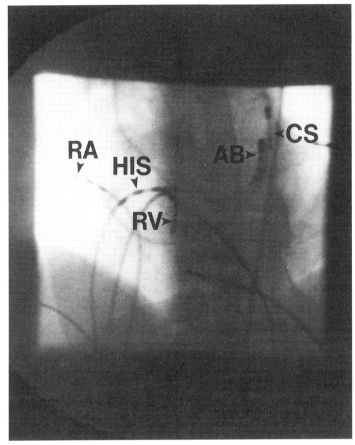

Figure 3. LAO 30° fluoroscopic view of catheter positions shown in Figure 2. Abbreviations per Figure 2.

sites.[27] Validated or presumed AP potentials are identified at 35–94% of successful left free wall ablation sites but are also noted at up to 72% of unsuccessful sites.[4,9,10,26–28]

Local A-V Interval

For left sided accessory pathways the time from the local atrial to ventricular electrograms at successful ablation sites averaged 25–50 milliseconds (see Figure 4).[10,25,26] Intervals ≤ 40 milliseconds should be sought.[10] Notably, the A-V intervals for left free wall pathways are longer than those for right sided pathways.[30] A wide overlap in the A-V intervals between successful and unsuccessful sites limits its specificity in some studies.[23,27]

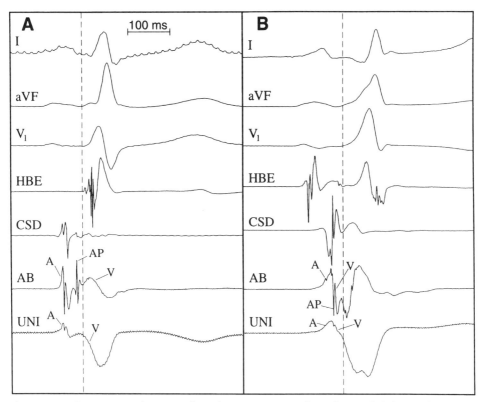

Figure 4. Surface ECG and intracardiac electrogram recordings from 2 left free wall ablation sites using the transaortic approach in different patients. I, aVF, and V_1, are surface ECG leads. HBE = His bundle electrogram, CSD = distal coronary sinus, AB = bipolar ablation electrogram, UNI = unipolar ablation electrogram, A = atrial electrogram, AP = accessory pathway potential, V = ventricular electrogram. The label pointers indicate the points of electrogram timing for interval measurements. The broken vertical lines delineate Δ wave onset in each panel. Panel A: Despite recording a large presumed AP potential from the ablation catheter, the electrogram represents an unfavorable ablation site. The bipolar ablation electrogram shows local V onset 20 milliseconds after Δ onset, and the A/V amplitude ratio is >2. The atrial electrogram amplitude is 0.97 mV. The unipolar electrogram shows a 25 milliseconds isoelectric interval between A and V, and ventricular activation is 15 milliseconds after Δ onset. This electrogram was recorded overlying the mitral annulus as evidenced by the low ventricular electrogram amplitude; A/V ratio >1.0. Panel B: Successful ablation site showing highly favorable electrogram characteristics in another patient. The bipolar ablation recording shows a presumed AP potential, ventricular activation 15 milliseconds before Δ onset and A/V ratio of 0.33. The atrial electrogram amplitude is 0.25 mV. The unipolar electrogram shows continuous electrical activity between A and V. Ventricular activation precedes Δ onset by 15 milliseconds. This electrogram was recorded from beneath the lateral mitral annulus.

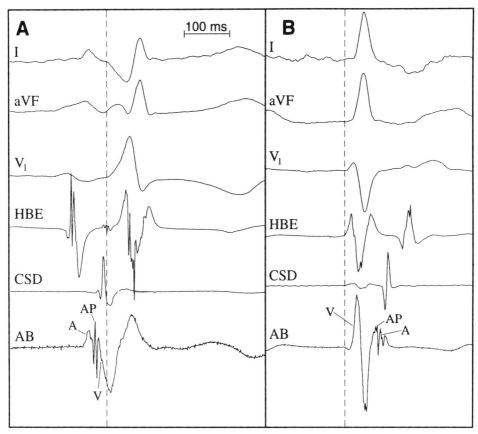

Figure 5. Successful ablation site shown during sinus rhythm and orthodromic reciprocating tachycardia from the same patient with a left lateral accessory pathway. Abbreviations and annotations per Figure 4. Panel A: During sinus rhythm with preexcitation there is continuous electrical activity between A and V with an interposed presumed AP potential. The local A-V interval is 25 milliseconds and local V precedes Δ onset by 15 milliseconds. The A/V ratio is 0.1. Panel B: During orthodromic tachycardia, the A electrogram fuses with the terminal portion of the V electrogram. The QRS onset (dotted line) to local A is 70 milliseconds. The local V-A interval is 55 milliseconds. A small presumed AP potential is noted.

Atrial Electrogram Amplitude

Successful subannular ablation sites demonstrate a minimal atrial electrogram amplitude as evidence of proximity to the annulus. Generally, an atrial electrogram amplitude greater than 0.4–1 mV or A/V ratios greater than 0.1 are necessary for success.[1,10,26,27]

Δ -V interval

For bipolar electrograms local ventricular activation should be measured at the peak of the major electrogram deflection or at the intrinsicoid deflection (see Figures 4 and 5).[9,23,27] The maximal negative dV/dt on the unipolar electrogram most accurately reflects local ventricular activation, however.[23,30] At successful sites the local ventricular activation precedes Δ wave onset by an average of only 2–10 milliseconds for left sided pathways compared to 15–20 milliseconds for right sided pathways.[8,27,31] A Δ-V interval ≤ 0 is typically necessary for successful ablation.

Stability

Electrogram stability is usually assessed by a <10% change in the amplitude of the atrial and ventricular electrograms (or the ratio of these electrograms) over 5–10 beats.[4,8,25,27] No major changes in the electrogram morphologies should occur at stable positions. Because catheter stability is typically good for subannular sites "wedged" between the left ventricle and mitral valve, this parameter frequently carries only negative predictive value.[24]

The sensitivity, specificities, and predictive values of these characteristics during antegrade mapping are shown in Table 1. Other predictors of success-

Table 1
Antegrade Activation Mapping by the Transaortic Approach

Electrogram Feature	Successful Sites (n=36)	Transiently Effective Sites (n=48)	Failed Sites (n=229)	Sensi-tivity	Speci ficity	+ PV	− PV	Accuracy
AP Potential	81%	63%	42%*	81%	51%	27%	92%	56%
Δ-V ≤0 ms	84%	54%*	62%*	75%	43%	23%	88%	49%
AEGM ≥ 1mV	81%	58%*	47%*	84%	49%	25%	92%	44%
Stability	94%	63%*	61%*	96%	35%	25%	97%	62%

Comparison of electrogram characteristics at successful and unsuccessful left-sided ablation sites by mapping antegrade activation using the transaortic approach in 50 patients.

n = number of electrograms analyzed in each category; AP = accessory pathway; Δ-V = time interval from Δ wave onset to local ventricular electrogram; AEGM = atrial electrogram amplitude; +PV = positive predictive valve; −PV = negative predictive value; * indicates $P <0.05$ compared to successful sites. Reproduced with permission from Chen X, et al. *J Am Coll Cardiol* 1992;20:656–665.

ful ablation sites may include continuous electrical activity and characteristic "Z" shaped bipolar electrogram morphologies.[26,27,31]

Mapping Retrograde Activation

Data specific to retrograde activation mapping of left free wall accessory pathways by the transaortic approach is relatively limited.[24,25,27] Mapping retrograde atrial activation from the subannular position is more difficult than for antegrade activation due to obfuscation of the low amplitude atrial electrograms following the large ventricular signal.[24] Multivariate predictors of successful ablation sites during retrograde activation mapping of left sided pathways include presence of an AP potential and the local ventricle to atrial (V-A) interval.[24]

AP Potential

AP potentials are noted in only 37–67% of successful ablation sites during retrograde AP conduction and are presumed to be frequently obscured by the ventricular electrogram (see Figure 5).[24,25,27]

Local V-A Interval

The local V-A interval during retrograde activation of left sided accessory pathways is typically 25–50 milliseconds at successful sites (see Figure 5).[8,10,24] At successful sites the short V-A interval often results in the inscription of the atrial electrogram on the ascending portion of the terminal ventricular electrogram. The "pseudo-disappearance" of the atrial electrogram within the terminal portion of the ventricular electrogram during orthodromic tachycardia is a manifestation of extremely short V-A intervals which correlates with successful sites.[24]

Other electrogram features serving as univariate predictors of successful ablation sites include stability, surface QRS-local atrial activation interval ≤ 70 milliseconds and continuous electrical activity defined as an isoelectric interval ≤ 5 milliseconds between the ventricular and atrial electrograms.[24,27] The sensitivity, specificity and predictive values of these electrogram features for mapping retrograde activation are shown in Table 2.

Tables 1 and 2 demonstrate the limited sensitivity, specificity, and predictive value of any single electrogram criteria to identify successful ablation sites. In fact, single criteria rarely exceed a 30% positive predictive value.[4,8] By meeting 3 or 4 criteria, however, electrograms with 62–87% positive predictive value for successful ablation can be identified (Table 3). In general, recording an AP potential, Δ-V interval ≤ 0, local A-V interval ≤ 40 milliseconds, or local V-A interval ≤ 50 milliseconds are most important.

Table 2
Retrograde Activation Mapping by the Transaortic Approach

Electrogram Feature	Sensitivity	Specificity	+ PV	− PV
Stability	100%	3%	15%	100%
AP Potential	27%	91%	45%	82%
CEA	85%	19%	22%	82%
V-A Interval	39%	93%	59%	85%

Electrogram predictors of successful ablation sites for concealed left free wall pathways by the transaortic approach in 33 patients. One hundred fifty-seven electrograms were analyzed.

CEA = continuous electrical activity; V-A Interval = local ventricular atrial electrogram interval manifest as the "pseudo-disappearance" phenomenon. (See text for details.) Other abbreviations per Table 1.

Reproduced with permission from Villacastin J, et al. *J Am Coll Cardiol* 1996;27:853–859.

Radiofrequency Delivery

The use of a temperature monitoring ablation system is highly recommended to insure adequate tissue heating and to prevent coagulum formation. At the target site, energy is delivered from catheter tip to a skin patch (or patches to reduce impedance) on the left chest. Temperatures of 60°C to 65°C should be sought.[5] Favorable ablation sites should not be abandoned until temperatures above 55°C are achieved.[5] Conversely, repeated energy deliveries at the same location after achieving ≥ 60°C are unlikely to succeed.[5] Adequate temperatures are readily achieved from beneath the mitral annulus compared to other locations due to better tissue contact and minimal convective heat loss.[5] Loss of pathway function is expected within 1–6 seconds for most successful lesions.[32] If antegrade preexcitation is present, radiofrequency energy should be delivered during sinus rhythm or continuous atrial pacing. For concealed pathways, energy delivery during ventricular pacing usually allows for detection of an altered retrograde activation sequence. Energy delivery during reciprocating tachycardia should be avoided due to the potential for catheter

Table 3
Multivariate Predictors of Successful Left Free-Wall Ablation Sites by the Transaortic Approach

Author	AP Potential	Δ-V Interval	A/V Ratio	Local A-V Interval	Local V-A Interval	Best + PV
Hindricks [9]	+		−			70%
Bashir [8]	+	+				20%
Chen [27]	+	+	+	+		62%
Cappota [26]	+	+	+	+		87%
Xie [25]	+	+		+		67%
Villacastin [24]	+				+	59%

Multivariate electrogram predictors of successful ablation of left sided accessory pathways by the transaortic approach from 6 published studies. Abbreviations per Tables 1 and 2. Best + PV is the optimal predictive value obtained by combination of the multivariate predictors. All studies include only antegrade mapping data except for Villacastin et al, which is exclusively retrograde mapping.

dislodgement with termination of the tachycardia. For incessant tachycardia, energy should be delivered during ventricular pacing at rates to entrain the tachycardia. This will permit termination of the tachycardia without abrupt changes in heart rate that may dislodge the catheter. Also, ventricular pacing at rates of 100–150 beats per minute can enhance catheter stability by reducing otherwise vigorous cardiac motion during sinus rhythm.

Following successful radiofrequency energy delivery, thorough electrophysiological testing is essential to confirm complete pathway ablation and to exclude other inducible arrhythmias. Rarely, retrograde accessory pathway function may persist despite ablation of antegrade conduction. This may result from modification of the ventricular pathway insertion or from the presence of a second pathway in close proximity to one that is ablated.[14,28]

Clinical Results

Immediate success rates for left lateral accessory pathway function by the transaortic approach are 86–100% in clinical studies.[1,2,9,26,27,33] The success rates are highest when antegrade accessory pathway activation can be mapped. Success rates for retrograde-only mapping of concealed pathways are frequently lower, but range from 64–100%.[24,27] Success rates should exceed 90% for experienced centers. The recurrence rates for left free wall accessory pathway function is approximately 2–5% and is less frequent than for pathways in other locations.[32–34] Recurrence is more likely in ablations involving concealed pathways, delivery of transiently effective energy pulses, or which require more than 5 energy deliveries for initial success.[1,32–34] Ablation of left free wall pathways by transaortic approach can be performed on an outpatient basis with complication rates similar to those of inpatient procedures.[35] In a study of outpatient procedures, 2 out of 100 patients developed femoral artery pseudoaneurysms after discharge; one after an overnight stay.[35] In the author's opinion, overnight stay is usually warranted to allow for recovery from sedation, observation for complications, and to limit early ambulation after femoral arterial access.

Troubleshooting the Failed Retrograde Approach

Difficulty with catheter manipulation is the most common cause of ablation failure.[36] Changing to catheters with different curvatures, different distal reaches, or enhanced torque transmission early into difficult cases may limit ineffective efforts. The use of long vascular sheaths may facilitate catheter manipulation. The use of unipolar electrograms enhances precise ventricular activation mapping. Attention must be given to catheter stability and to achieving appropriate temperatures before abandoning favorable sites. Coronary sinus pacing may enhance preexcitation to facilitate antegrade mapping. If early ventricular activation (Δ -V $\leq$ 0 milliseconds) is not recorded from beneath the mitral annulus, mapping the atrial insertion should be attempted.

Changing to the transseptal technique frequently achieves success when the transaortic approach fails.[20,37–39] The transseptal approach particularly enhances mapping of retrograde atrial activation.[13] Failure of both endocardial approaches to left free wall pathway ablation may be due to an epicardial pathway location.[15] These pathways usually require an epicardial approach to ablation either surgically or through the coronary sinus (see below).

Complications

Because of catheter manipulation in the aorta and left ventricle, the transaortic technique predisposes to vascular, embolic, and valvular complications. Vascular problems account for up to 50% of all complications with ablation procedures.[40,41] Complications of femoral artery access include groin hematomas, arterial thrombosis, aortic dissection, pseudoaneurysm, and arterio-venous fistula formation.[2,7,12,33,40,41] During catheter manipulation in the aortic root, extreme caution must be taken to avoid cannulation and especially energy delivery within the coronary artery system.[2] Left main coronary artery dissection and left anterior descending artery thrombosis resulting from direct catheter trauma have been reported.[42] The left circumflex coronary artery can rarely sustain thermal injury or spasm from subannular energy delivery.[2,34,36,43,44] Embolic complications are reported in 2% of left sided ablations.[11,45] Sources of emboli include thrombus formation on the catheter or at the site of lesion generation beneath the mitral annulus.[44,45] Catheter motion in the ascending aorta or frequent crossing of a calcified aortic valve may also mobilize atherosclerotic debris.

Valvular damage is a unique complication of the transaortic approach. In a pediatric population mild aortic or mitral insufficiency are reported in 30% and 12% of patients, respectively, after transaortic ablation.[46] New valvular regurgitation is not routinely noted in adults; however, perforation of the aortic valve is reported.[2,47] Entanglement of the ablation catheter within the mitral valve apparatus may result in acute mitral regurgitation and entrapment of the catheter.[18] The catheter can usually be extracted by straightening and countering the entangling maneuver. Removal of the coronary sinus catheter may be useful to relax the annulus and chordae tendonae. Transesophageal echocardiography can be helpful to direct extrication of the catheter.[18]

Life-threatening complications of tamponade, pericardial effusion, cardiac perforation, and stroke total 1.5% in a large series of ablations in all locations.[48] Complications are more frequent in patients older than 65 years of age.[12]

Radiofrequency Ablation Within the Coronary Sinus

When no effective sites result from endocardial mapping of a left free wall pathway the presence of an epicardial pathway should be considered.[15] Epicardial pathways are reported in 4% of left lateral ablation cases and 10% of failed ablation attempts.[15,36,49] These pathways have atrial and ventricular insertions distant from the mitral annulus and therefore may not be ablated from endocardial catheter positions (see Figure 1). The closer proximity of these pathways to the coronary sinus than to the mitral annulus results in large coronary sinus AP potentials and susceptibility to ablation from within the coronary sinus. The large coronary sinus AP potentials recorded from epicardial pathways exceed the local atrial and/or ventricular electrogram amplitudes in virtually all cases.[15,50] Coronary sinus angiography may be useful to delineate the venous anatomy before ablation. Unipolar radiofrequency energy of 20–30 watts for 30–60 seconds has been delivered at these sites with the ablation catheter tip positioned toward the ventricle within the coronary sinus.[15,49,50] Guidelines for target catheter tip temperatures within the coronary sinus are not reported, but use of temperature monitoring to limit temperatures to 55°C to 60°C is advisable.[35,36] Published data on ablation of left free wall accessory pathways is limited to small series (Table 4). The success rate for ablation within the coronary sinus is 62–100%.[15,49,51] Postablation coronary artery and coronary sinus angiograms reveal only localized coronary sinus thrombus formation in the minority of cases.[49] Of concern is coagulum formation "welding" the catheter tip to the thin wall of the coronary sinus. Pericarditis and venous branch occlusion have been reported.[52]

Radiofrequency energy delivery within the coronary sinus in "bipolar" configuration to a catheter beneath the mitral annulus has been described for endocardial accessory pathway ablation as well.[3,53] The success rate for endocardial pathway ablation from the coronary sinus is limited.[50] While no complications of bipolar ablation are reported in these very small series, coronary artery occlusion and extensive lesion formation involving the left atrium, ventricle, and coronary artery are described in animal models of this technique.[54] Given the limited experience with coronary sinus radiofrequency delivery for left free wall pathways, this technique should be attempted only for epicardial pathways and the potential for serious complications must be recognized.

Table 4
Radiofrequency Ablation of Left Free-Wall Pathways from within the Coronary Sinus

Author	# Patients	Success	# RF	Power	Complications	AP > A or V
Wang [51]	5	5/5 (100%)	—	—	—	—
Haïssaguerre [49]	7	6/7 (85%)	5±4	28±2.4	mural thrombus 2 patients	—
Giorgberidze [50]	5	3/5 (60%)	—	—	0	66%
Langberg [15]	2	2/2 (100%)	1.2±0.04	28±9	—	100%
Cappota [52]	6	6/6 (100%)	—	—	0	—

Summary of data on radiofrequency ablation of left free wall accessory pathways from within the coronary sinus. # RF = average number of radiofrequency lesions delivered; Power = average power delivered; AP>A or V = percent of patients with the coronary sinus accessory pathway potential of greater amplitude than the local atrial or ventricular electrogram.

Adapted from Giorgberidze I et al. *Interventional Electrophysiology: A Textbook.* Saksena S, Luderitz B eds. Armonk, NY: Futura Publishing Co., 1996. pp 409–421.

The Transseptal Approach

The transseptal approach to left free wall accessory pathway ablation was first reported in a large series in 1993 by Swartz et al.[13] This technique was developed to eliminate the prolonged intra-arterial catheter manipulation and potential for vascular complications attending the transaortic approach. Despite its potential benefits, the fact that most electrophysiologists are unfamiliar with the transseptal technique has slowed its widespread adoption. Nevertheless, transseptal catheterization is becoming increasingly important for the ablation of accessory pathways and other arrhythmias.

Transseptal Access

The technique of transseptal catheterization has recently been modified to facilitate its use in the electrophysiology laboratory.[55] Nevertheless, transseptal catheterization remains an exacting procedure that demands vigilance and operator experience. A brief overview of the procedure is given here. The reader is referred to detailed sources for a complete description.[56,57]

In addition to standard electrophysiological catheters, transseptal catheterization requires a 0.028–0.032 inch 145 cm guidewire, a transseptal sheath/dilator assembly and a Brockenbrough needle. Suitable transseptal sheaths include the standard single plane 180° curve Mullins sheath (USCI/C. R. Bard, Inc., Billerica, MA) or compound curve sheaths to direct and stabilize the ablation catheter in different locations (Daige Corp., Minnetonka, MN).[58] (Figure 6.) Before introducing the standard Mullins sheath, curvature may be modified according to the pathway location (see Figure 6). The curve is left intact for left posterior pathways, but curvature is progressively removed for more lateral positions. The curve is almost entirely removed for anterior pathways. The preformed transseptal sheaths are designed to direct and stabilize the catheter in different locations, thus obviating the need for sheath modification.

Transseptal left atrial catheterization is performed by passing the sheath/dilator assembly over the guidewire in the right femoral vein into the superior vena cava. The guidewire is withdrawn, the dilator flushed, and the Brockenbrough needle advanced to 1 cm from the dilator tip. Care must be taken to maintain the needle tip within the dilator at all times except during transseptal puncture. The sheath, dilator, and needle assembly are then oriented leftward and posterior orienting the needle hub arrow to approximately the 4 o'clock position. By withdrawing the assembly over the atrial septum in the LAO view (≈30°) the dilator tip moves slightly leftward on entering the right atrium, then leftward again while descending below the aortic root. A third abrupt leftward movement below the aortic root indicates passage over the limbus into the fossa ovalis (Figure 7). Once this position is obtained, the sheath position is documented in the RAO view (30–40°) to confirm a proper anterior-posterior position. The posterior extent of the aortic root is marked by a pigtail catheter in the noncoronary cusp or in the absence of aortic root dilation, by the His bundle catheter which lies at the level of the fibrous trigone opposite and

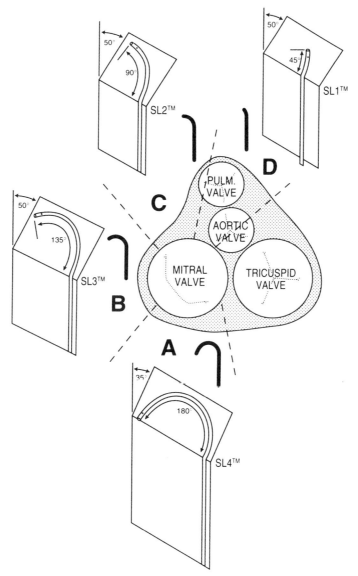

Figure 6. Preformed sheaths and method of Brockenbrough transseptal sheath modification for left-sided accessory pathways. The Brockenbrough sheath (solid figures) is modified before left atrial catheterization according to the targeted pathway location. Left posterior paraseptal and left posterolateral locations (A) require little, if any, modification of the 180° sheath curvature. Left free wall locations (B) are best approached with approximately 130–140° of the sheath curvature remaining. Left anterolateral ablations (C) require that only 90°of the sheath curve remain. For left anterior paraseptal locations (D) nearly all of the sheath curve is removed to permit access to the left fibrous trigone area. The preformed sheaths for each location are shown. The compound curvatures of these 4 different sheaths (SL1–SL4, Daige Corporation, Minnetonka, MN) facilitate stable positioning on the annulus.

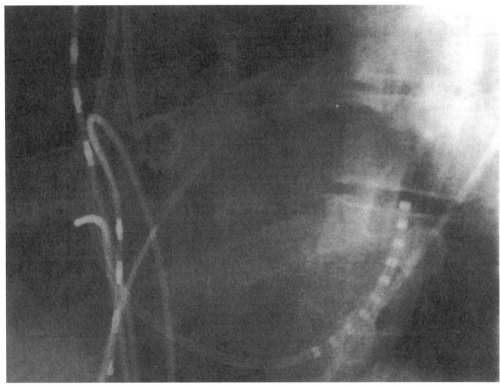

Figure 7. Fluoroscopic view of proper transseptal needle placement. Panel A: In this 40° LAO projection, the tip of the transseptal needle and sheath assembly is well seated below the limbus of the fossa ovalis. A pigtail catheter is positioned in the noncoronary cusp of the aortic valve. When properly positioned, the transseptal assembly is always below the level of the noncoronary cusp in this view. Higher placement may result in perforation of the right atrial roof or aortic root. (*continued*)

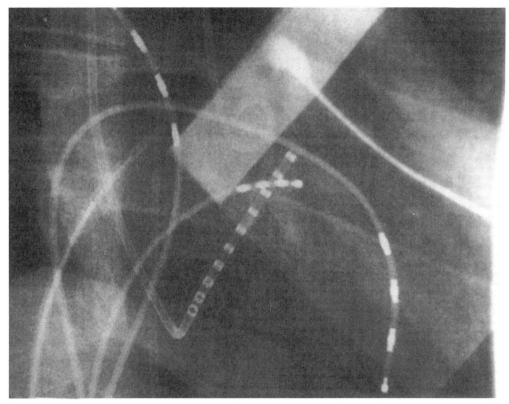

Figure 7. (*continued*) Panel B: In this 35° RAO view, the tip of the transseptal assembly is properly positioned approximately midway between the coronary sinus and pigtail catheters. Note the position of the His bundle catheter defining the caudal limit of the aortic root. In this view the posterior aspect of the true interatrial septum is demarcated by the coronary sinus catheter as it courses inferiorly from the superior vena cava to the coronary sinus os. The anterior border of the true interatrial septum is defined by the pigtail catheter in the noncoronary aortic cusp.

caudal to the noncoronary cusp.[55] In the RAO view the dilator tip should be anterior to the descending portion of the CS catheter and posterior to the His catheter or pigtail (see Figure 7). The sheath assembly should be oriented parallel to the distal portion of the coronary sinus catheter. The foramen should be probed with the dilator assembly for a patent foramen ovale which is present in 15–20% of adult patients. If the foramen is not patent the needle is advanced outside the dilator during continous pressure monitoring in the LAO view. The use of transesophageal or intracardiac echocardiography can confirm the dilator position against the foramen ovale. After passage through the foramen, a left atrial waveform should be recorded from the needle tip. Contrast injection through the needle can be performed to confirm the intra-atrial needle position before advancing the sheath across the septum. The dilator and needle are removed slowly and the sheath is flushed before introduction of the ablation catheter. Preformed sheaths should be positioned along the annulus at this time. The catheter is flexed as it extends out of the sheath to lie along the atrial aspect of the mitral annulus (Figure 8). The patient is fully heparinized after successful transseptal puncture.

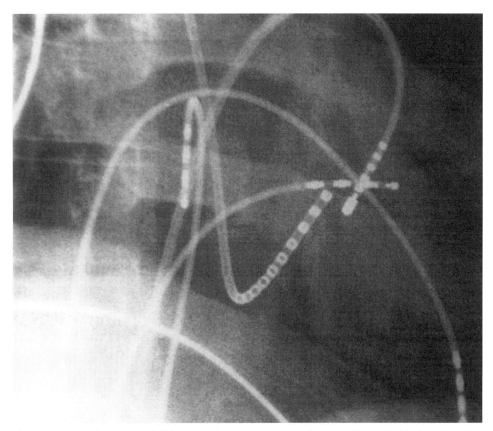

Figure 8. Typical transseptal ablation catheter appearance for mapping and ablation. Panel A: This 35° RAO view emphasizes the parallel orientation of the transseptal endocardial ablation catheter with the mitral annulus (outlined by the the decapolar coronary sinus catheter). Although the ablation catheter appears slightly below the coronary sinus catheter in this example, the position of the ablation catheter with respect to the coronary sinus catheter is variable. (*continued*)

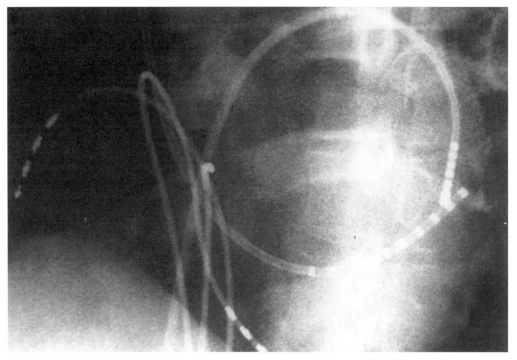

Figure 8. (*continued*) Panel B: Accurate incremental movement of the ablation catheter is greatly assisted by the regularly spaced electrodes of the coronary sinus catheter which serve as fluoroscopic reference points. In this 45° LAO view the ablation catheter is positioned in close proximity to the second coronary sinus electrode.

Catheter Manipulation

Once the catheter is positioned on the mitral annulus in the RAO view, mapping is performed in the LAO orientation. In the absence of preformed transseptal sheaths, gentle clockwise torque is needed to maintain the catheter on the posterior annulus; no torque is needed for lateral positions. As the catheter is moved more anteriorly, counterclockwise torque is necessary to keep the catheter tip on the annulus. In anterior positions the catheter tip may dislodge into the left atrial appendage or left ventricle. Attention to the intracardiac electrograms is necessary when mapping anterior regions as the coronary sinus catheter rarely provides an accurate fluoroscopic reference in this area. The goal is to maintain the catheter tip on the atrial aspect of the mitral annulus such that the annulus can be easily mapped by advancing and withdrawing the catheter. The ventricular aspect of the annulus can be mapped by passing the catheter tip across the mitral valve and deflecting the tip toward the annulus.

Mapping

The transseptal approach was developed to facilitate mapping of the atrial aspect of the mitral annulus. With proper catheter position this can be rapidly accomplished by advancing and withdrawing the catheter tip, causing it to slide along the annulus freely in parallel to the coronary sinus catheter.[13,59] Advancing the catheter moves the tip posteriorly; withdrawing it moves the tip anteriorly. Use of a closely spaced (2 mm) steerable bipolar catheter (4 mm tip) recording bipolar (30–500 Hz filter) and distal unipolar electrograms (.01–500 Hz filter) is recommended for mapping and ablation.[13,59]

Catheter position on the atrial aspect of the annulus is documented by recording a bipolar A:V electrogram amplitude ratio ≥ 1 and a unipolar electrogram P-R segment displacement from the baseline without ST segment displacement.[13] The stability of the catheter position is assessed by the P-R segment elevation (confirming good atrial tissue contact), consistent local electrogram amplitudes and by concordant motion of the coronary sinus and ablation catheters.[13] Mapping may begin at the site of pathway localization by the coronary sinus catheter or by moving the ablation catheter in 5 mm increments along the extent of the annulus. Target sites for ablation of the atrial insertion site are the shortest local atrial activation time (local V-A interval) or QRS to atrial electrogram interval during orthodromic tachycardia or ventricular pacing. Data on electrogram characteristics of successful ablation sites are much more limited than for the transaortic approach.[13,20,37,59] Most studies have utilized mapping criteria derived from the transaortic approach.[20,37] The differing catheter orientation, electrogram ratios, and oblique course of left free wall pathways may lead to discrepancies between mapping techniques for the 2 approaches, however.

Mapping Retrograde Activation

V-A Intervals

In a series of 76 patients with left sided accessory pathways, the local V-A interval at successful atrial ablation sites was 40 ± 15 milliseconds during orthodromic reentry and 38 ± 16 milliseconds during ventricular pacing.[13] The endocardial atrial activation precedes the earliest coronary sinus atrial activation during orthodromic tachycardia by an average of 10 milliseconds (Figure 9).[13,20]

In the series by Swartz et al, the QRS-atrial electrogram interval was 79 ± 17 milliseconds during orthodromic tachycardia and 141 ± 27 milliseconds during right ventricular pacing.[13] Fisher et al reported the local V-A of 33 ± 12 milliseconds and QRS-atrial of 69 ± 16 milliseconds during orthodromic tachycardia in 31 patients undergoing left lateral pathway ablation.[59] Manolis et al reported on the use of morphological electrogram characteristics to identify the shortest local V-A intervals.[60] A "W-sign" formed by the merging of local atrial and ventricular electrograms was found to have 100% sensitivity, 94% speci-

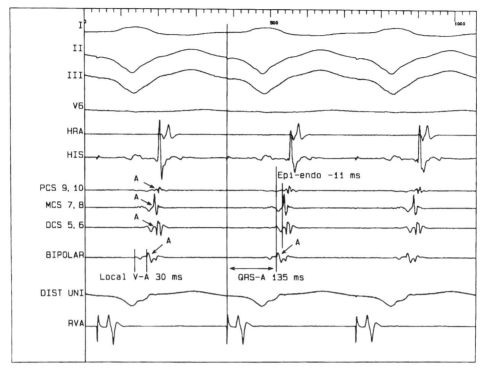

Figure 9. Typical left sided accessory pathway map recordings. Surface electrocardiogram I, II, III, and V₆ recordings are shown at the top of the figure. Intracardiac recordings from the high right atrium (HRA), bundle of His (HIS), proximal (PCS), middle (MCS), and distal (DCS), coronary sinus follow. The bipolar (BIPOLAR) and unipolar (DIST UNI) electrograms from the endocardial left atrial mapping catheter reveal a right ventricular pacing spike to local atrial electrogram interval (QRS-A) of 135 milliseconds and a local ventriculoatrial interval (Local V-A) of 30 milliseconds. The local A:V electrogram ratio is 3.6. The earliest atrial activation is recorded by the ablation catheter 11 milliseconds before the earliest atrial activation in the coronary sinus (Epi-endo). RVA indicates right ventricular apex recording.

ficity, and 73% positive predictive value in identifying successful ablation sites in 31 patients. This electrogram morphology was associated with A-V or V-A intervals of 58±17 milliseconds with an isoelectric interval less than 20 milliseconds between electrogram components.

A:V Electrogram Ratio

Swartz et al found the local A:V electrogram ratio to be 2.3±2.2 during sinus rhythm and 1.1±0.8 during orthodromic tachycardia at successful ablation sites.[13] Ratios of 0.6 have been reported by others, but the rhythms during which the ratio was determined were not given.[20,37]

AP Potentials

AP potentials have not been specifically sought in most large series of transseptal ablation.[13,20,37] Swartz reported presumed AP potentials to be present at only 30% of successful ablation sites.[13] This low incidence may be due to obfuscation of the AP potential by the large ventricular electrogram during retrograde activation mapping. In addition, the perpendicular orientation of the bipolar electrodes relative to the AP orientation may impede recording of AP potentials.[13]

Stability

Swartz et al assessed atrial electrogram stability by measuring the ratio of the smallest and largest atrial electrograms at the target site during the respiratory cycle.[13] The ratio was 0.8 ± 0.2 for successful sites. As an indicator of atrial contact, 0.45 ± 0.29 mV of PR segment deviation from baseline was recorded at the distal unipolar electrode.[13]

Mapping Antegrade Activation

Because the transseptal is used primarily for atrial mapping, limited data is available on antegrade mapping with this technique. Swartz, et al measured antegrade activation parameters at the atrial insertion site of 39 patients finding a Δ-V interval of -18 ± 13 milliseconds and a local A-V interval of 38 ± 10 milliseconds.[13] A Δ-V interval of 20 ± 6 milliseconds is reported by Deshpande, et al.[20] The "W sign" as described for retrograde mapping can be used for antegrade mapping as well.[60]

Mapping Atrial Electrogram Polarity Reversal

Because of the mobility of the ablation catheter and the electrode orientation parallel with atrial activation along the annulus, a unique vectorial mapping technique is possible with the transseptal approach.[13,59] This technique obviates the need to measure activation times during retrograde activation mapping. Using wide bandpass bipolar recordings (1–2500 Hz), the ablation catheter is moved incrementally along the annulus during orthodromic tachycardia (or ventricular pacing) while noting the amplitude and polarity of the atrial electrogram (Figure 10). Because the atrial insertion site is usually discrete, atrial electrical activation proceeds radially from this source immediately adjacent to the annulus. Thus, along the annulus, atrial activation proceeds anteriorly and posteriorly from the insertion. As the bipole approaches and then passes directly over the atrial insertion site the atrial electrogram becomes diminished in amplitude, isoelectric and fractionated. As the catheter

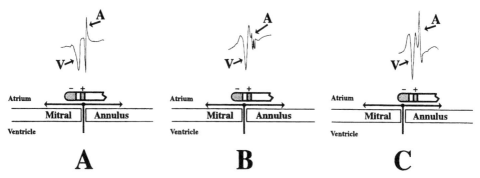

Figure 10. Localization of accessory pathway insertion site with electrogram polarity reversal. In these illustrations, the atrial insertion of an accessory pathway is modeled as a discrete point from which retrograde atrial activation spreads both anteriorly and posteriorly in a simultaneous fashion. Three different ablation/mapping catheter positions and their corresponding recordings during orthodromic atrioventricular reentrant tachycardia are shown in panels A-C. Note that the polarity of the recording electrodes has the distal pole as negative by convention. Panel A: When a mapping catheter is resting on the mitral annulus just posterior to the atrial insertion, the atrial electrogram (A) is recorded as a negative deflection. Panel B: As the catheter is pulled anteriorly so that the recording bipole straddles the accessory pathway insertion site, the atrial electrogram becomes smaller in amplitude and fractionated. Panel C: With further anterior catheter movement, the atrial electrogram increases in amplitude and becomes positive. At this point the distal ablation electrode is directly over the accessory pathway insertion site and successful ablation can be accomplished.

moves past the insertion site, reversal of the atrial electrogram polarity is observed. With the tip electrode negative and the catheter lying in the annulus from anterior to posterior, an upright atrial electrogram indicates a catheter position anterior to the insertion while negative electrograms indicate positions posterior to the atrial insertion.

The sensitivity, specificity, and positive predictive value of electrogram reversal were 97%, 46% and 75%, respectively, in 72 patients studied by Swartz et al.[13] Fisher et al combined this atrial electrogram vectoral data with electrogram timing and amplitude information into a computerized 3-dimensional mapping system to improve on the low accuracy of conventional electrogram timing variables in predicting successful ablation sites.[59] This sophisticated analysis decreased the procedure time, fluoroscopy time, number of lesions, and duration of radiofrequency energy for successful ablation compared to conventional mapping techniques.[59]

Radiofrequency Delivery

Guidelines for radiofrequency energy delivery by the transseptal approach have generally followed those for the transaortic approach.[20,37,58] Swartz et al, however, used abbreviated energy deliveries of 25 watts for only 20–30 seconds if pathway block occurred within 5 seconds of energy application.[13] Most studies have used 30–60 second energy deliveries. Little data is available on the guidelines for transseptal temperature controlled energy delivery.[58] The authors use target temperatures of 60°C to 65°C. There are no studies comparing the energy requirements or temperatures achieved between the transseptal and transaortic approaches. It is conceivable that the higher blood flow and less forceful tissue contact with transseptal atrial positions may require higher energies to achieve target temperatures.

Clinical Results

In the largest series of 388 patients with transseptal approach to left free wall pathways, 371 (96%) were successfully ablated.[55] Swartz reported 97% success in 76 patients.[13] Success rates range from 85–100% in series of pediatric and adult patients.[20,37] Recurrence rates of 3–6.6% are reported.[13,60] A summary of the clinical outcomes of transseptal ablation of left free wall pathways is provided in Table 5.

Complications

The incidence of complications related to transseptal ablation is 0–6% in series of adult patients.[13,37,38] The risk of complications in pediatric series of transseptal ablation varies from 3–25%.[61,62] Complications may result from

Table 5
Results of Transseptal Ablation for Left Free Wall Accessory Pathways

Author	# Pt	Success	Compli-cation	Recur-rence	X-over	Fluoro Time (min)	Procedure Time (hr)	Comments
DePonti [55]	388	96%	1.2%	1.2%	2%	—	—	complication rate includes ablation of atrial tachycardias
Swartz [13]	76	97%	2%	2%	0%	63±47	4.9±2.2	complication rate includes other pathway locations
Fisher [59]	26	100%	0%	0%	0%	25±10.5	2.8±0.9	vectorial 3-D mapping
Yip [58]	49	92%	4%	4%	4%	22.5±15.2	1.7±0.05	preformed transseptal sheaths
Manolis [60]	31	100%	0%	3%	0%	76±48	5.4±1.9	"W sign" used for mapping

Summary of results from transseptal ablation of left free wall accessory pathways. X-over = cross over to transaortic approach; Fluoro time = fluoroscopy time.

catheter manipulation, radiofrequency energy delivery or from the transseptal access. Reported complications include coronary spasm[37] and pericardial effusion with tamponade[20] due to left atrial perforation. Because arterial access is not required, peripheral vascular complications are rare. Coronary artery air embolism from the transseptal sheath has also beem reported.[37]

The transseptal approach may be complicated by cardiac perforation of the right atrium, aortic root, or left atrium. Usually, "needle only" punctures with the tip of the Brockenbrough needle are uncomplicated in the unanticoagulated patient. After errant needle puncture, however, the procedure should be discontinued and the patient closely monitored. Hemopericardium requiring pericardiocentesis has been reported with transseptal access for ablation.[20] Perforation with the dilator or sheath is usually catastrophic and requires emergent cardiac surgery to repair. In a series of 1279 transseptal procedures in the cardiac catherization laboratory, the incidence of major complications was 1.3%.[63] This series included 1.2% risk of tamponade, 0.08% risk of systemic embolization and 0.08% risk of death.

Comparison of Transaortic and Transseptal Approaches

Of the numerous studies comparing the transaortic and transseptal approaches, most authors report similar success rates for the 2 techniques (Table 6). The ability to utilize both techniques enhances the overall procedural success compared to either technique used separately.[20,37–39] Direct comparisons demonstrate total procedure times, fluoroscopy times, and incidence of crossovers similar to the other approach in most studies.[20,37,38,64] Most comparisons also report similar complication rates, although the small patient numbers and low overall complication rates make formal statistical analysis difficult.[20,37,64] Trends toward more complications and recurrences with the transaortic approach are noted in some reports.[38,39] Lesh found no electrophysiological factors useful to guide selection of ablation approach in 123 patients.[37] In this study the 2 approaches were equally effective for concealed and manifest pathways and no difference in success rate by pathway location was found. It should be noted, however, that most of these comparisons trials are not truly randomized for approach to ablation.[20,37,38]

Despite the similar outcomes in these studies, important differences exist between the 2 techniques. Complications, especially vascular complications, may be less frequent with the transseptal approach. In the author's opinion, far left lateral and anterior pathways are more accessible using the transseptal approach, while left posterior and posterolateral positions are readily achieved by both the transaortic and transseptal techniques. In general, the transseptal approach should be favored in the presence of a patent foramen ovale, aortic valve disease, significant peripheral arterial or aortic atherosclerotic disease, or hypertrophic or small left ventricles. The enhanced atrial recordings from the transseptal approach favors mapping of concealed pathways as well. The transseptal approach should be used in children weighing less than 30 kg to limit peripheral arterial complications, trauma to the left heart valve, and

Table 6
Comparison of Transaortic and Transseptal Ablation Procedures

Author	Approach	Patients	Success	Recurrence	Complication	X-over	Procedure Time (min)	Fluoro Time (min)	Comments
Deshpande [20]	TA	42	95%	—	4.7%	4.7%	244±82	51±22	
	TS	58	75%	—	3.4%	24%	268±88	53±22	
Lesh [37]	TA	89	85%	—	6.7%	12%	220±13	44±4	
	TS	33	85%		6.1%	12%	205±13	45±5	
Natale [38]	TA	49	88%	4%	4%	6%	—	42±29	
	TS	31	100%	0%	0%	0%	—	34±18	
Saul [6]	TA	50	40%	—	—	14%	3.3(2–9.5)hr*	52(18–259)	pediatric patients
	TS	13	100%	—	—	0%	4.3(2–6) hr*	58(14–197)	
Manolis [39]	TA	50	87%	11%	8%	10%	7.1±2.4 hr*	121±81*	
	TS	23	96%	4%	0%	7%	5.5±2.1 hr*	81±57	
Vora [61]	TA	13	100%	16%	8%	0%	—	38±30*	non-randomized pediatric patients
	TS	36	100%	0%	3%	0%	—	61±45	
Ma [64]	TA	50	100%	0%	0%	4%	77±20	12±7	
	TS	50	96%	0%	0%	0%	81±19	13±8	
Montenero [65]	TA	10	100%	—	—	—	—	45±10	pediatric patients
	TS	18	100%	—	—	—	—	23±1	

Summary of studies comparing the transaortic and transseptal approaches to ablation of left free wall pathways. TA = transaortic; TS = transseptal. Other abbreviations per Table 5. * P <0.05 TA vs. TS approaches.

the potential for growth-related expansion of ventricular radiofrequency lesions.[46,66,67] The transseptal approach is also recommended in elderly patients with the potential for complications due to arteriosclerotic disease. The transseptal approach may be contraindicated in the presence of distorted cardiac anatomy, such as from severe kyphoscoliosis, pneumonectomy, congenital heart disease, aortic root dilation or severely dilated right atrium. The transaortic approach is also preferred in anticoagulated patients and for operators lacking the considerable experience required for the transseptal approach. In general the operator should use the technique with which he or she is most familiar.

References

1. Lesh MD, Van Hare GF, Schamp DJ, et al. Curative percutaneous catheter ablation using radiofrequency energy for accessory pathways in all locations: results in 100 consecutive patients. *J Am Coll Cardiol* 1992;19: 1303–1309.
2. Calkins H, Langberg J, Sousa J, et al. Radiofrequency catheter ablation of accessory atrioventricular connections in 250 patients: abbreviated therapeutic approach to Wolff-Parkinson-White Syndrome. *Circulation* 1992;85: 1337–1349.
3. Jackman WM, Wang X, Friday KJ, et al. Catheter ablation of accessory atrioventricular pathways (Wolff-Parkinson-White syndrome) by radiofrequency current. *N Engl J Med* 1991;324:1605–1611.
4. Calkins H, Kim Y-N, Schmaltz S, et al. Electrogram criteria for identification of appropriate target sites for radiofrequency catheter ablation of accessory atrioventricular connections. *Circulation* 1992;85:565–573.
5. Langberg JJ, Calkins H, El-Atassi R, et al. Temperature monitoring during radiofrequency ablation of accessory pathways. *Circulation* 1992;86:1469–1474.
6. Saul JP, Hulse JE, De W, et al. Catheter ablation of accessory atrioventricular pathways in young patients: use of long vascular sheaths, the transseptal approach and a retrograde left posterior parallel approach. *J Am Coll Cardiol* 1993;21:571–583.
7. Schlüter M, Geiger M, Siebels J, et al. Catheter ablation using radiofrequency current to cure symptomatic patients with tachyarrhythmias related to an accessory atrioventricular pathway. *Circulation* 1991;84:1644–1661.
8. Bashir Y, Heald SC, Katritsis D, et al. Radiofrequency ablation of accessory atrioventricular pathways: predictive value of local electrogram characteristics for the identification of successful target sites. *Br Heart J* 1993;69: 315–321.
9. Hindricks G, Kottkamp H, Chen X, et al. Localization and radiofrequency catheter ablation of left-sided accessory pathways during atrial fibrillation. *J Am Coll Cardiol* 1955;25:444–451.
10. Silka J, Kron J, Halperin BD, et al. Analysis of local electrogram characteristics correlated with successful radiofrequency catheter ablation of accessory atrioventricular pathways. *PACE* 1992;15:1000–1007.

11. Epstein MR, Knapp LD, Martindill M, et al. Embolic complications associated with radiofrequency catheter ablation. *Am J Cardiol* 1996;77:655–658.

12. Chen S-A, Chiang C-E, Yang C-J, et al. Accessory pathway and atrioventricular node reentrant tachycardia in elderly patients: clinical features, electrophysiologic characteristics and results of radiofrequency ablation. *J Am Coll Cardiol* 1994;23:7002–7008.

13. Swartz JF, Tracy CM, Fletcher RD. Radiofrequency endocardial catheter ablation of accessory pathway atrial insertion sites. *Circulation* 1993;87:487–499.

14. Becker AE, Anderson RH. The Wolff-Parkinson-White syndrome and its anatomical substrates. *Anat Rec* 1981;201:169–177.

15. Langberg JJ, Man KC, Vorperian VR, et al. Recognition and catheter ablation of subepicardial accessory pathways. *J Am Coll Cardiol* 1993;22:1100–1104.

16. Jackman WM, Friday KJ, Yeung-Lai-Wah JA, et al. New catheter technique for recording left free wall accessory atrioventricular pathway activation. *Circulation* 1988;70:598–610.

17. Kuck KH, Jackman W, Pitha J, et al. Percutaneous catheter ablation at mitral annulus using a bipolar epicardial-endocardial electrode configuration. *PACE* 1986;9:287.

18. Conti JB, Geiser E, Curtis AB. Catheter entrapment in the mitral valve apparatus during radiofrequency ablation. *PACE* 1994;17:1681–1685.

19. Kosinski DJ, Grubb BP, Burket MW, et al. Occlusion of the left main coronary artery during radiofrequency ablation for the Wolff-Parkinson-White syndrome. *Eur J Cardiac Pacing Electrophysiol* 1993;1:63–66.

20. Deshpande SS, Bremmer S, Sra JS, et al. Ablation of left free wall accessory pathways using radiofrequency energy at the atrial insertion site: transseptal versus transaortic approach. *J Cardiovasc Electrophysiol* 1994;5:219–231.

21. Kuck K-H, Schlüter M. Single catheter approach to radiofrequency current ablation of left-sided accessory pathways in patients with Wolff-Parkinson-White syndrome. *Circulation* 1991;84:2366–2375.

22. Brugada J, Garcia-Bolao I, Figueiredo M, et al. Radiofrequency ablation of concealed left free wall accessory pathways without coronary sinus catheterization: results in 100 consecutive patients. *J Cardiovasc Electrophysiol* 1997;8:249–253.

23. Simmers TA, Hauer RNW, Wever EFD, et al. Unipolar electrogram models for prediction of outcome in radiofrequency ablation of accessory pathways. *PACE* 1994;17:186–198.

24. Villacastin J, Almendral J, Medina O, et al. "Pseudodisappearance" of atrial electrogram during orthodromic tachycardia: new criteria for successful ablation of concealed left-sided accessory pathways. *J Am Coll Cardiol* 1996;27:853–859.

25. Xie B, Heald SC, Camm AJ, et al. Successful radiofrequency ablation of accessory pathways with the first energy delivery: the anatomic and electrical characteristics. *Eur Heart J* 1996;17:1072–1079.

26. Cappato R, Schlüter M, Mont L, et al. Anatomic, electrical, and mechanical

factors affecting bipolar endocardial electrogram: impact on catheter ablation of manifest left free wall accessory pathways. *Circulation* 1994;90: 884–894.

27. Chen X, Borggrefe M, Shenasa M, et al. Characteristics of local electrogram predicting successful transcatheter radiofrequency ablation of left-sided accessory pathways. *J Am Coll Cardiol* 1992;20:656–665.

28. Jackman WM, Friday KJ, Fitzgerald DM, et al. Localization of left free wall and posteroseptal accessory atrioventricular pathways by direct recordings of accessory pathway activation. *PACE* 1989;12:204–214.

29. Niebauer MJ, Daoud E, Goyal R, et al. Assessment of pacing maneuvers used to validate anterograde accessory pathway potentials. *J Cardiovasc Electrophysiol* 1995;6:350–356.

30. Pieper CF, Blue R, Pacifica A. Simultaneously collected monopolar and discrete bipolar electrograms: comparison of activation time detection algorithm. *PACE* 1993;16:426–433.

31. Haïssaguerre M, Fischer B, Warin J-F, et al. Electrogram patterns predictive of successful radiofrequency catheter ablation of accessory pathways. *PACE* 1992;15:2138–2145.

32. Twidale N, Wang Z, Beckman KJ, et al. Factors associated with recurrences of accessory pathway conduction after radiofrequency catheter ablation. *PACE* 1991;14:2042–2048.

33. Chen X, Kotthemp H, Hendricks G, et al. Recurrence and late block of accessory pathway conduction following radiofrequency catheter ablation. *J Cardiovasc Electrophysiol* 1994;5:650–658.

34. Langberg JJ, Calkins H, Kim Y-N, et al. Recurrence of conduction in accessory atrioventricular connections after initially successful radiofrequency catheter ablation. *J Am Coll Cardiol* 1992;19:1588–1592.

35. Kalbfleisch SJ, El-Atassi R, Calkins H, et al. Safety, feasibility and cost of outpatient radiofrequency catheter ablation of accessory atrioventricular connections. *J Am Coll Cardiol* 1993;21:567–570.

36. Morady F, Strickberger SA, Man KC, et al. Reasons for prolonged or failed attempts at radiofrequency catheter ablation of accessory pathways. *J Am Coll Cardiol* 1996;27:683–689.

37. Lesh MD, Van Hare GF, Scheinman MM, et al. Comparison of the retrograde and transseptal methods for ablation of left free wall accessory pathways. *J Am Coll Cardiol* 1993;22:542–549.

38. Natale A, Wathen M, Yee R, et al. Atrial and ventricular approaches for radiofrequency catheter ablation of left-sided accessory pathways. *Am J Cardiol* 1992;70:114–116.

39. Manolis AS, Wang PJ, Estes NAM III. Radiofrequency ablation of left-sided accessory pathways: Transaortic versus transseptal approach. *Am Heart J* 1994;128:896–902.

40. Greene TO, Huang SKS, Wagshal AB, et al. Cardiovascular complications after radiofrequency catheter ablation of supraventricular tachyarrhythmias. *Am J Cardiol* 1994;74:615–617.

41. Chen S-A, Chiang C-E, Tai C-T, et al. Complications of diagnostic electrophysiologic studies and radiofrequency catheter ablation in patients with

tachyarrhythmias: an eight-year survey of 3966 consecutive procedures in a tertiary referral center. *Am J Cardiol* 1996;77:41–46.

42. Kosinski DJ, Grubb BP, Burket MW, et al. Occlusion of the left main coronary artery during radiofrequency ablation for the Wolff-Parkinson-White syndrome. *Eur J Cardiac Pacing Electrophysiol* 1993;1:63–66.

43. Solomon AJ, Tracy CM, Swartz JF, et al. Effect on coronary artery anatomy of radiofrequency catheter ablation of atrial insertion sites of accessory pathways. *J Am Coll Cardiol* 1993;21:1440–1444.

44. Metzger JT, Cheriex EC, Smeets JLRM, et al. Safety of radiofrequency catheter ablation of accessory atrioventricular pathways. *Am Heart J* 1994;127:1533–1538.

45. Thakur RK, Klein GJ, Yee R, et al. Embolic complications after radiofrequency catheter ablation. *Am J Cardiol* 1994;74:278–279.

46. Minich LL, Snider AR, Dick M. Doppler detection of valvular regurgitation after radiofrequency ablation of accessory connections. *Am J Cardiol* 1992;70:116–117.

47. Seifert MJ, Morady F, Calkins H, et al. Aortic leaflet perforation during radiofrequency ablation. *PACE* 1991;14:1582–1585.

48. Hindricks G. The Multicentre European Radiofrequency Survey (MERFS): complications of radiofrequency catheter ablation of arrhythmias. *Eur Heart J* 1993;14:1644–1653.

49. Haïssaguerre M, Gaita F, Fischer B, et al. Radiofrequency catheter ablation of left lateral accessory pathways via the coronary sinus. *Circulation* 1992;86:1464–1468.

50. Giorgberidze I, Saksena S, Krol RB, et al. Efficacy and safety of radiofrequency catheter ablation of left-sided accessory pathways through the coronary sinus. *Am J Cardiol* 1995;76:359–365.

51. Wang X, McClelland J, Beckman K, et al. Left free wall accessory pathway ablation from the coronary sinus: unique coronary sinus electrogram pattern. *Circulation* 1992;86:I586.

52. Cappota R, Weiss C, Brown E, et al. Catheter ablation of manifest accessory pathways related to the coronary sinus. *N Trends Arrhythmias* 1993;9:421.

53. Kuck K-H, Kunze K-P, Schlüter M, et al. Modification of a left-sided accessory atrioventricular pathway by radiofrequency current using a bipolar epicardial-endocardial configuration. *Eur Heart J* 1988;9:927–932.

54. Huang SKS, Graham AR, Bharati S, et al. Short and long term effects of transcatheter ablation of the coronary sinus by radiofrequency energy. *Circulation* 1988;78:416–427.

55. De Ponti R, Zardini M, Storti C, et al. Trans-septal catheterization for radiofrequency catheter ablaton of cardiac arrhythmias. *Eur Heart J* 1998;19:943–950.

56. Clugston R, Lau FYK, Ruiz C. Transseptal catheterization update 1992. *Cathet Cardiovasc Diagn* 1992;26:266–274.

57. Croft CH, Lipscomb K. Modified technique of transseptal left heart catheterization. *J Am Coll Cardiol* 1985;5:904–910.

58. Yip ASB, Chow W-H, Yung T-C, et al. Radiofrequency catheter ablation of

left-sided accessory pathways using a transseptal technique and specialized long intravascular sheaths. *Jpn Heart J* 1997;38:643–650.

59. Fisher WG, Swartz JF. Three dimensional electrogram mapping improves ablation of left-sided accessory pathways. *PACE* 1992;15:2344–2356.
60. Manolis AS, Wang PJ, Estes NAM III. Radiofrequency ablation of atrial insertion of left-sided accessory pathways guided by the "W sign." *J Cardiovasc Electrophysiol* 1995;6:1068–1076.
61. Vora AM, McMahon S, Jazayeri MR, et al. Ablation of atrial insertion sites of left-sided accessory pathways in children: efficacy and safety of transseptal versus transoartic approach. *Pediatr Cardiol* 1997;18:332–338.
62. Benito F, Sanchez C. Radiofrequency catheter ablation of accessory pathways in infants. *Heart* 1997;78:160–162.
63. Roelke M, Smith AJC, Palacios IF. The technique and safety of transseptal left heart catheterization: the Massachusetts General Hospital experience with 1279 procedures. *Cathet Cardiovasc Diagn* 1994;32:332–339.
64. Ma C, Dong J, Yang X, et al. A randomized comparison between retrograde and transseptal approach for radiofrequency ablation of left-sided accessory pathways. *PACE* 1995;18:479.
65. Montenero AS, Drago F, Crea F, et al. Ablazione transcatetere con radiofrequenza delle tachicardie sopraventricolari in eta pediatricia: risultati immediati e di un follow-up a medio termine. *G Ital Cardiol* 1996;26:31–40.
66. Hulse, JE, Papagionnis J, Van Proagh R, et al. Late assessment of radiofrequency lesions in infant sheep: Increased lesion size and myocardial tissue loss with growth. *Circulation* 1992;86:1239.
67. Dick M, O'Conner BK, Serwer GA, et al. Use of radiofrequency current to ablate accessory connections in children. *Circulation* 1991;84:2318–2324.

Chapter 26

Ablation of Anteroseptal and Midseptal Accessory Pathways

Michael Schlüter, Ph.D., Riccardo Cappato, M.D., Feifan Ouyang, M.D., Karl-Heinz Kuck, M.D.

An accessory atrioventricular (AV) pathway has been recognized as a strand of (usually) working myocardial cells connecting atrial and ventricular myocardium across the electrically insulating fibro-fatty tissues of the AV junction at anatomic sites not intended by nature (that is, remote from the locus of the bundle of His). In the days before catheter ablation, curative treatment of tachyarrhythmias mediated by such connections has been the exclusive domain of the cardiac surgeon. To describe their anatomic location, the cardiac surgeons have distinguished parietal accessory AV connections, located along the right and left free walls, from accessory connections confined to the areas anterior and posterior to the septum. Those accessory pathways (APs) were loosely labeled "anteroseptal" and "posteroseptal," respectively.[1–3] The latter terms, along with that of "intermediate septal," have also been used by electrocardiographers for accessory connections giving rise to specific patterns of delta wave polarity in the preexcited 12-lead electrocardiogram.[4,5] Finally, electrophysiologists performing ablation procedures have based their definitions of "anteroseptal" and "posteroseptal" APs on the fluoroscopic position of the ablation catheter, and with growing experience opted to introduce the "midseptal" AP.[6–11] Taking a semantic point of view, one would assume that any "septal" muscular accessory connection traverses the AV junction along or inside the cardiac septum. However, with regard to the electrophysiologists' terms "anteroseptal" and "posteroseptal," anatomists disagree.[12,13]

In view of the precision with which electrophysiologists need to position their electrode catheters under fluoroscopic guidance to ablate an accessory pathway and not destroy crucial adjacent structures such as the AV node or the bundle of His, it appears prudent to shortly review the anatomy of the AV junc-

From Huang SKS, Wilber DJ (eds.): *Radiofrequency Catheter Ablation of Cardiac Arrhythmias: Basic Concepts and Clinical Applications,* 2nd ed. Armonk, NY: Futura Publishing Company, Inc. ©2000.

tion in that region where the confluence of the AV annuli and the aortic valve apparatus makes for a highly complex situation.

Anatomic landmarks of particular importance for catheter ablation are the ostium of the coronary sinus and the compact AV node. Both are confined to the low right atrial area known as the triangle of Koch.[12] The ostium of the coronary sinus serves as its posterior border, while the compact AV node is located anteriorly at its apex where the tendon of Todaro (being the superior margin of Koch's triangle) merges with the central fibrous body. Slightly more anteriorly and superiorly is where the bundle of His penetrates the AV junction through the central fibrous body and the posterior aspect of the membranous AV septum. The attachment of the septal tricuspid valve leaflet forms the inferior margin of Koch's triangle.

There is no doubt that the triangle of Koch must be regarded as septal. In fact, it constitutes the right atrial surface of the muscular AV septum.[12] Because of the displacement of the attachment of the septal tricuspid valve leaflet relative to the attachment of the septal mitral valve leaflet, the muscular AV septum separates the right atrial cavity from the left ventricular outflow tract. The most anterior part of the AV septum consists of fibrous tissue and is part of the membranous septum. APs with an atrial insertion along the inferior margin of Koch's triangle, posteroinferior to the compact AV node and His bundle, have been labeled by electrophysiologists as midseptal, and they are indeed truly septal structures.

Anterosuperior to the AV septum, that is, anterosuperior to the compact AV node and the bundle of His, the tricuspid valve annulus diverges away from the septum to course along what is known as the supraventricular crest. This muscular anatomic structure interposes between the attachments of the leaflets of the tricuspid and pulmonary valves in the roof of the right ventricle.[12,13] Muscular strands connecting atrial and ventricular myocardium in this area have been labeled "anteroseptal" accessory pathways by electrophysiologists, but anatomically they do not belong to the septum. Rather, they must be considered (anterosuperior) paraseptal right-sided parietal accessory connections. The true anatomic background of a misleading electrophysiological nomenclature should be kept in mind when discussing catheter ablation of "anteroseptal" APs.

Patients

Between May 1987 and May 1997, 1320 patients with a total of 1427 accessory pathways underwent attempts at radiofrequency current catheter ablation of their accessory connection(s) at the University Hospital Eppendorf and the St. Georg Hospital in Hamburg, Germany. Among those patients, 76 (6%) and 58 (4%) were found to have accessory pathways defined electrophysiologically as anteroseptal and midseptal, respectively.

Patients with Anteroseptal Accessory Pathways

This patient group was comprised of 53 male and 23 female patients, with a mean (± 1 standard deviation) age of 33 ± 15 years (range, 7 to 70 years). All patients were free of an organic heart disease. Recurrent palpitations had been the predominant symptom in all patients, accompanied in some by dizziness, nausea, chest pain, and/or presyncope; 2 patients (3%) had survived an episode of cardiac arrest and 8 patients (11%) had experienced syncopal attacks. Orthodromic reentrant AV tachycardia was the prevailing arrhythmia responsible for the patients' symptoms. In addition to reentrant AV tachycardia, atrial fibrillation was documented in 20 patients (26%). Six patients (8%) had associated accessory pathways at other than anteroseptal locations. A median of 2 antiarrhythmic drugs (range, 1 to 6) were ineffective in 57 patients (75%).

Conduction through the accessory pathway was found to be bidirectional in 57 cases (75%), antegrade-only in 4 (5%) and concealed (retrograde-only) in the remaining 15 bypass tracts (20%).

Patients with Midseptal Accessory Pathways

This patient group was comprised of 37 male and 21 female patients, with a mean age of 30 ± 16 years (range, 2 to 75 years). One patient had Ebstein's anomaly of the tricuspid valve; the others were free of an organic heart disease. Next to palpitations and accompanying symptoms (see above), severe symptoms such as cardiac arrest and syncopal attacks were documented in 3 (5%) and 5 patients (9%), respectively. In the majority of patients, symptoms were caused by recurrent orthodromic reentrant AV tachycardia. Paroxysmal atrial fibrillation recurred in 14 patients (25%) and was the only documented arrhythmia in 8. The prevalence of multiple accessory pathways in this group of patients was, at 25%, significantly higher than among patients with anteroseptal accessory pathways. Up to 5 antiarrhythmic drugs (median, 1) had been ineffective in 41 patients (71%).

Conduction through midseptal AP was bidirectional in 45 cases (78%), antegrade-only in 3 (with 1 bypass tract exhibiting Mahaim-type preexcitation) and concealed in 10 (17%).

Catheter Ablation

The catheter ablation protocol used in our laboratories has been described in detail elsewhere.[14] In brief, multielectrode catheters were placed by way of a venous approach in the high right atrium, right ventricular apex, and inside the coronary sinus for electrical stimulation and recording purposes; another catheter was placed across the tricuspid valve to monitor electrical activation over the bundle of His. Mapping and ablation of APs was accomplished using a quadripolar catheter with a deflectable 4-mm tip electrode. This catheter was advanced towards the tricuspid valve annulus or into the coronary sinus using a femoral or jugular/subclavian venous approach, or towards the mitral valve annulus using a transaortic arterial approach.

Anteroseptal Accessory Pathways

APs are classified as anteroseptal if an AP activation potential and a His bundle potential are simultaneously recorded from the "diagnostic" catheter placed, by way of the femoral vein, at the His bundle region. With this catheter left in place, the precise location of the AP is verified by mapping this space in the 30° left anterior oblique projection using the ablation catheter which is almost always advanced by way of the right internal jugular vein (Figure 1). The optimal site chosen for RF current application is one from which atrial and ventricular potentials are recorded in conjunction with an AP activation potential, but with no or only a tiny His bundle potential (Figures 2 and 3). Rarely is ablation required in the presence of a marked His bundle potential recorded through the ablation catheter (see Figure 2).

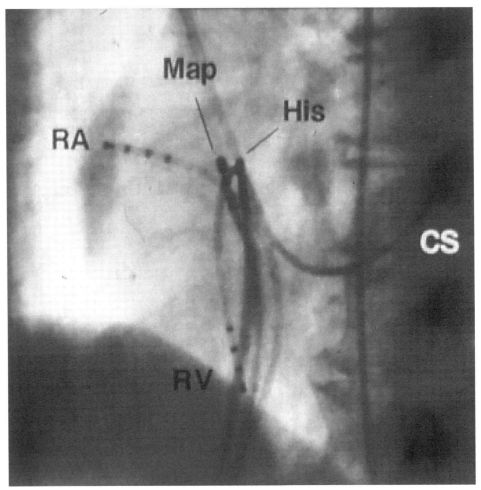

Figure 1. Radiographs in the left anterior oblique (top panel) and right anterior oblique projections (*continued*)

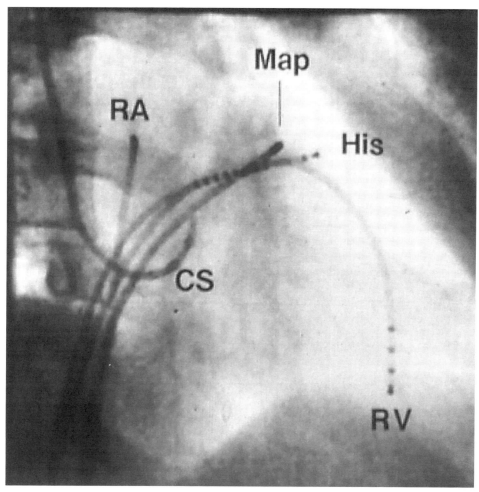

Figure 1. (*continued*) (bottom panel) showing catheter positions for ablation of an anteroseptal accessory pathway. Quadripolar "diagnostic" catheters are placed in the high right atrium (RA) and at the right ventricular apex (RV), a decapolar catheter is positioned at the bundle of His (His) and a "Jackman"-type catheter is advanced into the coronary sinus (CS). Note the proximity of the 4-mm tip electrode of the mapping/ablation catheter (Map) to the His bundle catheter.

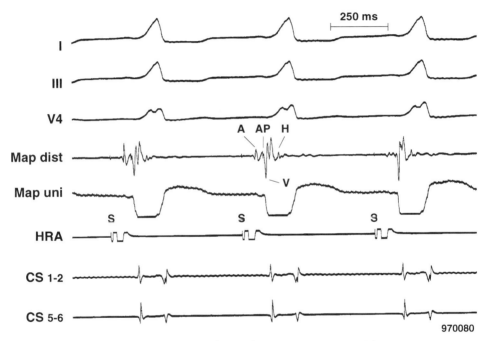

Figure 2. Preablation mapping during right atrial pacing in a patient with an overt anteroseptal accessory pathway. The distal electrode pair of the mapping/ablation catheter placed in the atrioventricular node/His bundle region as in Figure 1 records (Map dist) a distinct accessory pathway potential (AP) between the local atrial (A) and ventricular (V) potentials. Note marked His bundle potential (H) recorded after the local V potential because of slow antegrade conduction via the atrioventricular node/His bundle axis. CS = coronary sinus; dist = distal electrode pair; HRA = high right atrium; S = stimulus artifact; uni = unipolar recording.

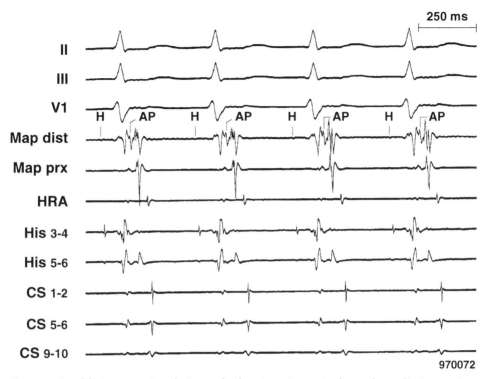

Figure 3. Preablation mapping during orthodromic atrioventricular tachycardia in a patient with a concealed anteroseptal accessory pathway. The distal electrode pair of the mapping/ablation catheter placed in the atrioventricular node/His bundle region as in Figure 1 continuously records (Map dist) a distinct accessory pathway potential (AP) between the local ventricular and atrial potentials, but only minute His bundle potentials (H) preceding the local V potentials. His = His bundle recording; prx = proximal electrode pair; other abbreviations as in Figure 2.

Midseptal Accessory Pathways

APs are classified as midseptal if ablation is achieved through the mapping/ablation catheter located in an area bounded anterosuperiorly by the tip electrode of the His bundle catheter and posteroinferiorly by the coronary sinus ostium as marked by the vortex of curvature in the coronary sinus catheter.[7] This area may be approached by way of a femoral transvenous route to the right atrium (if ablation is achieved here, the AP is labeled "right" midseptal) (Figure 4) or by way of a transaortic/transseptal route to the left ventricle/left atrium (if ablation is achieved here, the AP is labeled "left" midseptal) (Figure 5).

The optimal site for RF current applications to a "right" midseptal AP is one from which atrial and ventricular potentials are recorded simultaneously with an AP potential in between. Since the AV node may be in close proximity to the catheter tip, a catheter position more to the ventricular aspect of the tricuspid annulus should be attempted. Such a position is indicated by an

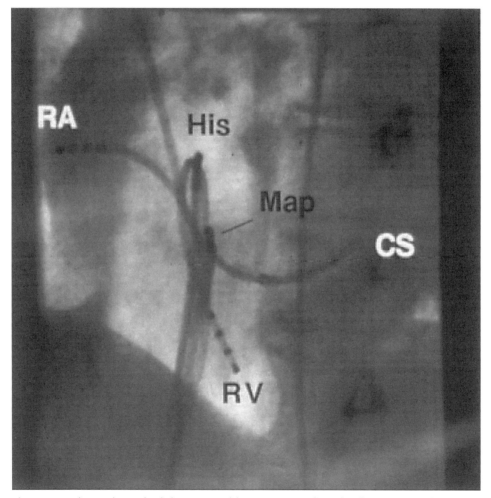

Figure 4. Radiographs in the left anterior oblique (top panel) and right anterior oblique projections (*continued*)

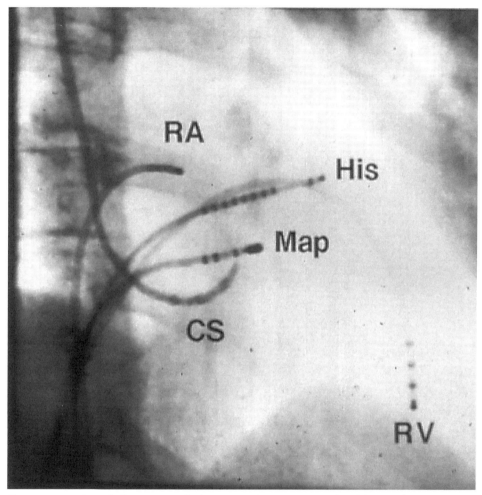

Figure 4. (*continued*) (bottom panel) showing catheter positions for ablation of a "right" midseptal accessory pathway. "Diagnostic" catheter positions as in Figure 1. The mapping/ablation catheter (Map) is advanced, by way of the femoral transvenous route, to a location at the atrial aspect of the tricuspid annulus midway between the tip of the His bundle catheter and the ostium of the coronary sinus (marked by the vortex of curvature in the catheter labeled CS).

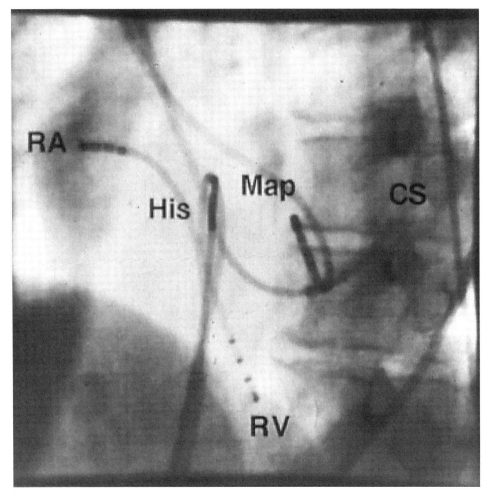

Figure 5. Radiographs in the left anterior oblique (top panel) and right anterior oblique projections (*continued*)

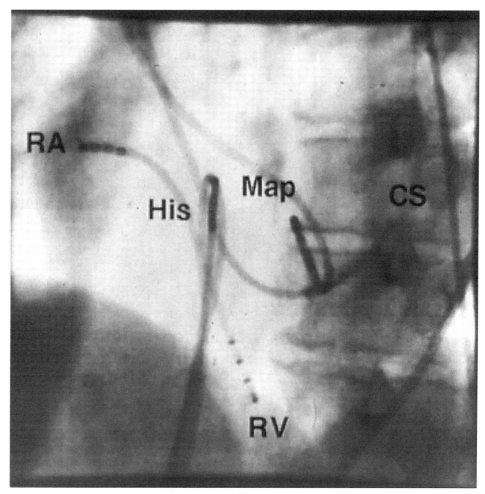

Figure 5. (*continued*) (bottom panel) showing catheter positions for ablation of a "left" midseptal accessory pathway. "Diagnostic" catheter positions as in Figure 1. The mapping/ablation catheter (Map) is advanced retrogradely into the left ventricle to a location beneath the mitral annulus midway between the tip of the His bundle catheter and the ostium of the coronary sinus (marked by the vortex of curvature in the catheter labeled CS).

amplitude of the local ventricular potential exceeding the amplitude of the local atrial potential (Figure 6). For a "left" midseptal AP, the ablation catheter is positioned at the mitral annulus within the area bounded by the His bundle and coronary sinus catheters (Figure 7).

For ablation, unmodulated 500-kHz (RF) alternating current was delivered in the unipolar mode through the tip electrode of the mapping/ablation catheter at sites of earliest antegrade ventricular activation or earliest retrograde atrial activation, preferably in the presence of a presumed AP activation potential. Provided that the ablation catheter was not displaced, presumed AP ablation was followed by the delivery of an additional "safety" application to

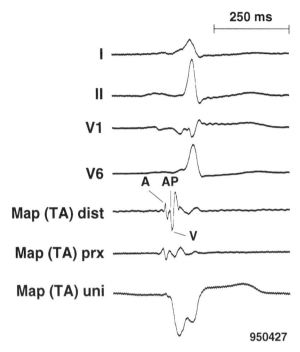

Figure 6. Preablation mapping during sinus rhythm in a patient with an overt "right" midseptal accessory pathway. The distal electrode pair of the mapping/ablation catheter placed at the tricuspid annulus as in Figure 4 records [Map (TA) dist] an accessory pathway potential (AP) between the local atrial (A) and ventricular (V) potentials. Note local V amplitude exceeding local A amplitude, indicative of a catheter position more to the ventricular aspect of the tricuspid annulus (TA).

the same site. The absence of residual antegrade AP conduction after a presumably successful RF current application was verified by right or left atrial (that is, coronary sinus) extrastimulus testing and pacing at increasing rates. During postablation right ventricular pacing close to the site of the AP and from a para-Hisian catheter position,[15] the following findings were regarded as indicative of the absence of residual retrograde AP conduction: 1) ventriculoatrial (VA) dissociation; 2) concentric retrograde atrial activation (could not be verified with the "single-catheter" technique in which only the ablation catheter was used to monitor retrograde atrial activation); 3) a marked prolongation of the local VA interval at the ablation site; and 4) decremental VA conduction.

Programmed electrical stimulation was performed with stimuli of 0.5-millisecond duration at twice diastolic threshold. Six surface electrocardiographic leads and at least 5 intracardiac leads were simultaneously recorded on a 16-channel paper recorder or by way of a dedicated computerized system (EPLab, Quinton Electrophysiology, Toronto, Ontario, Canada). Local intracardiac electrograms were filtered at 50–500 Hz.

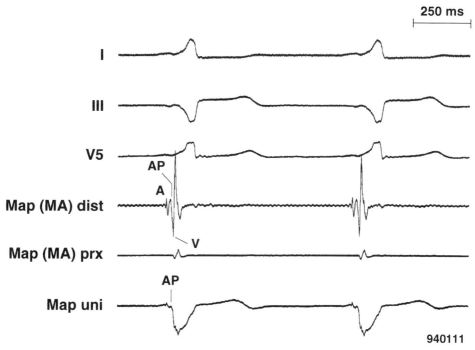

Figure 7. Preablation mapping during sinus rhythm in a patient with an overt "left" midseptal accessory pathway. The distal electrode pair of the mapping/ablation catheter placed beneath the mitral annulus as in Figure 5 records [Map (MA) dist] an accessory pathway potential (AP) between the local atrial (A) and ventricular (V) potentials.

Results

Surface Electrocardiogram

Anteroseptal Accessory Pathways

In patients with an accessory connection capable of antegrade conduction (Wolff-Parkinson-White syndrome), the 12-lead surface electrocardiogram (Table 1) showed a positive delta wave polarity in leads I, II, aVF, and V_4 to V_6, and a negative delta wave polarity in lead aVR; the delta wave polarity was predominantly negative (rarely positive) in lead V_1, predominantly positive in leads III, V_2 and V_3, and positive or isoelectric in lead aVL (Figure 8).

Midseptal Accessory Pathways

Antegradely conducting midseptal APs ablated from the right atrium gave rise to a delta wave polarity pattern in the 12-lead surface electrocardiogram

Table 1
Delta Wave Polarity Patterns for Antegradely conducting Accessory Pathways

	Anteroseptal	R Midseptal	L Midseptal
I	+	+	+
II	+	(+)	(+)
III	(+)	(−)	+, +/−
avR	−	(−)	(−)
aVL	+, +/−	+	+
aVF	+	(+/−), −	+, +/−
V1	(−)	(−)	+, +/−
V2	(+)	+	+
V3	(+)	+	+
V4	+	+	+
V5	+	+	+
V6	+	+	+

Abbreviations: L, left; R, right; +, positive; −, negative; +/−, isoelectric; (+), predominantly positive; (−), predominantly negative; (+/−), predominantly isoelectric.

which was positive in leads I, aVL, V_2 to V_6, predominantly positive (sometimes isoelectric) in lead II, and predominantly negative (sometimes isoelectric) in leads III, aVR and V_1; lead aVF was predominantly isoelectric (sometimes negative) (Figure 9). Overt midseptal accessory pathways ablated from the left ventricle had a positive or isoelectric, but never negative, delta wave polarity in leads III, aVF, and V_1 (Figure 10).

An isoelectric rather than negative delta wave polarity in leads III and aVF suggests an accessory pathway location closer to the AV node than to the ostium of the coronary sinus.[7]

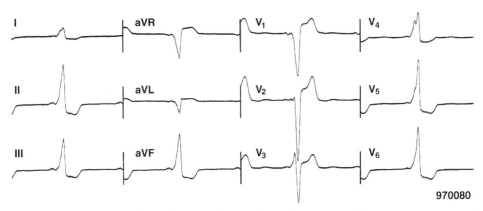

970080

Figure 8. Twelve-lead surface electrocardiogram from the patient with an overt anteroseptal accessory pathway whose intracardiac recordings are shown in Figure 2.

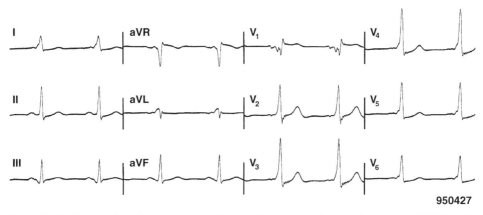

950427

Figure 9. Twelve-lead surface electrocardiogram from the patient with an overt "right" mid-septal accessory pathway whose intracardiac recordings are shown in Figure 6.

Ablation

Anteroseptal Accessory Pathways

Attempts at ablation of the 76 APs classified as anteroseptal were successful in 74 patients (97%); in 66 patients (87%), ablation was achieved in a single session. A median of 8 (range, 1–66) RF applications with a mean power of 26 ± 7 watts lasting for 28 ± 11 seconds were delivered. Session duration was 3.8 ± 1.5 hours, with a median fluoroscopy time of 37.2 minutes (range, 3.9–125.9 minutes). Impairment of AV node/His bundle conduction was not induced in any patient. In 3 patients, a right bundle branch block was noted postablation.

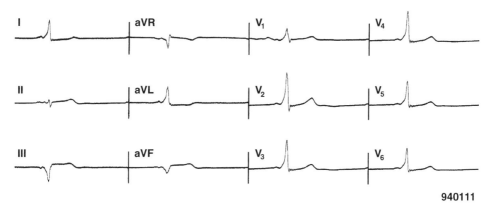

940111

Figure 10. Twelve-lead surface electrocardiogram from the patient with an overt "left" mid-septal accessory pathway whose intracardiac recordings are shown in Figure 7.

Midseptal Accessory Pathways

Attempts at ablation of the 58 APs classified as midseptal were successful in 57 patients (98%); in 50 patients (86%), ablation was achieved in a single session. A median of 6 (range, 1–49) RF applications with a mean power of 27 ± 7 watts lasting for 31 ± 12 seconds were delivered. Session duration was 3.8 ± 2.2 hours, with a median fluoroscopy time of 37.5 minutes (range, 5.0–121.3 minutes). In 8 patients, ablation was achieved from a left ventricular catheter position and in 2 patients from a left atrial catheter position (1 retrograde transaortic, 1 transseptal). In all other patients, a right atrial approach to the AP was chosen. Complications encountered were a first-degree AV conduction block in one patient and a persistent second-degree AV conduction block requiring pacemaker implantation in another.

Conclusion

Catheter ablation of anteroseptal and midseptal APs can be achieved effectively and safely despite the fact that these APs may be located perilously close to the specific conduction system. Great care must be taken to position the ablation catheter clearly away from the AV nodal area, either by verifying that no His bundle activation is recorded through the ablation catheter (specifically for anteroseptal APs) or that the ventricular activation potential exceeds that of the atrial activation potential in amplitude (for midseptal APs). It may also be advisable to titrate current delivery, starting at a low wattage.

References

1. Sealy WC, Gallagher JJ. The surgical approach to the septal area of the heart based on experience with 45 patients with Kent bundles. *J Thorac Cardiovasc Surg* 1980;79:542–551.
2. Sealy WC. Kent bundles in the anterior septal space. *Ann Thorac Surg* 1983;36:180–186.
3. Selle JG, Sealy WC, Gallagher JJ, et al. The complex posterior septal space in the Wolff-Parkinson-White syndrome: surgical experience with 47 patients. *J Thorac Cardiovasc Surg* 1989;37:299–304.
4. Gallagher JJ, Selle JG, Sealy WC, et al. Intermediate septal accessory pathways: a subset of preexcitation at risk for complete heart block/failure during WPW surgery [abstract]. *Circulation* 1986;74(suppl II):II387.
5. Epstein AE, Kirklin JK, Holman WL, et al. Intermediate septal accessory pathways: electrocardiographic characteristics, electrophysiologic observations and their surgical implications. *J Am Coll Cardiol* 1991;17:1570–1578.
6. Schlüter M, Kuck KH. Catheter ablation from right atrium of anteroseptal

accessory pathways using radiofrequency current. *J Am Coll Cardiol* 1992;19:663–670.

7. Kuck KH, Schlüter M, Gürsoy S. Preservation of atrioventricular nodal conduction during radiofrequency current catheter ablation of midseptal accessory pathways. *Circulation* 1992;86:1743–1752.

8. Xie B, Heald SC, Bashir Y, et al. Radiofrequency catheter ablation of septal accessory atrioventricular pathways. *Br Heart J* 1994;72:281–284.

9. Yeh SJ, Wang CC, Wen MS, et al. Characteristics and radiofrequency ablation therapy of intermediate septal accessory pathway. *Am J Cardiol* 1994;73:50–56.

10. Haïssaguerre M, Marcus F, Poquet F, et al. Electrocardiographic characteristics and catheter ablation of parahissian accessory pathways. *Circulation* 1994;90:1124–1128.

11. Tai CT, Chen SA, Chiang CE, et al. Electrocardiographic and electrophysiologic characteristics of anteroseptal, midseptal, and para-Hisian accessory pathways: implications for radiofrequency catheter ablation. *Chest* 1996; 109:730–740.

12. Dean JW, Ho SY, Rowland E, et al. Clinical anatomy of the atrioventricular junctions. *J Am Coll Cardiol* 1994;24:1725–1731.

13. Anderson RH, Ho SY. Anatomy of the atrioventricular junctions with regard to ventricular preexcitation. *PACE* 1997;20:2072–2076.

14. Schlüter M, Geiger M, Siebels J, et al. Catheter ablation using radiofrequency current to cure symptomatic patients with tachyarrhythmias related to an accessory atrioventricular pathway. *Circulation* 1991;84:1644–1661.

15. Hirao K, Otomo K, Wang X, et al. Para-Hisian pacing: a new method for differentiating retrograde conduction over an accessory AV pathway from conduction over the AV node. *Circulation* 1996;94:1027–1035.

Chapter 27

Ablation of Mahaim Fibers

John M. Miller, M.D., Steven A. Rothman, M.D.,
Henry H. Hsia, M.D., Alfred E. Buxton, M.D.

Introduction

Since the first description of anatomic connections in the septum bypassing the normal conduction system, considerable information has become available as to the electrophysiological behavior and clinical importance of these pathways. A subset of accessory pathways are those in which conduction time is prolonged and decremental (that is, the conduction time increases with more rapid paced rates) and in the anterograde direction only. The vast majority of these pathways have inserted into the right ventricle or right bundle branch, giving rise to a typical or slightly atypical left bundle branch block type QRS complex during preexcited beats or supraventricular tachycardia (SVT). Accessory pathways with these characteristics have been termed "Mahaim fibers" and the tachycardias in which they are used are referred to as "Mahaim tachycardia." The subject of this chapter is the diagnosis and catheter ablation of arrhythmias related to the several types of pathways that fit this overall description of Mahaim fibers.

History and Anatomy

In their original report, Mahaim and Benatt[1] described histological conduction tissue extending from the His bundle into basal septal ventricular myocardium (so-called fasciculoventricular fibers). With time, connections between the atrioventricular (AV) node and ventricular muscle were included under the rubric of Mahaim fibers. Anderson[2] proposed classifying these unusual pathways

From Huang SKS, Wilber DJ (eds.): *Radiofrequency Catheter Ablation of Cardiac Arrhythmias: Basic Concepts and Clinical Applications,* 2nd ed. Armonk, NY: Futura Publishing Company, Inc. ©2000.

anatomically into nodoventricular and fasciculoventricular types; this distinction also has electrophysiological implications, in that the typical Mahaim tachycardia would only be expected with the nodoventricular variety. Wellens[3] suggested a potential role for these fibers in clinical tachycardias. Subsequently, several investigators reported cases in which patients with Mahaim-type tachycardias underwent invasive electrophysiological studies.[4-9] The concept of electrophysiologically distinct "nodoventricular," "nodofascicular," and "fasciculoventricular" pathways became accepted into the differential diagnosis of wide QRS complex SVTs; the former 2 types of pathways were characterized by connections between a portion of the AV node and either ventricular muscle or specialized conduction tissue (right bundle branch, or RBB), respectively. With continued experience, however, it became clear that in some patients, these pathways did not always connect with the AV node. Gillette[10] and Klein[11] each reported on 2 patients with Mahaim-type tachycardias in whom a pathway that connected right atrial free wall with right ventricular free wall was found at surgery. Kou et al[12] reported a case in which they postulated a similar connection from the right atrial free wall to the right bundle in a patient with an atrial tachycardia. Tchou et al[13] demonstrated definitively in a patient with Mahaim tachycardia that the atrial insertion was in the right atrial free wall, rather than the AV node, by introducing programmed atrial extrastimuli during preexcited SVT from the lateral right atrium. They showed that ventricular activation over the accessory pathway could be advanced by premature atrial depolarizations that did not affect timing of atrial septal (peri-AV nodal) recordings, excluding a connection between the AV node and the pathway. They also showed that the pathway appeared to have a distal insertion into the RBB and thus was "insulated" along much of its ventricular course, since myocardial activation did not occur until after RBB activation. Subsequent studies have confirmed these findings and further elucidated the functional characteristics of these pathways.

It is now believed that atriofascicular fibers are composed of an intramural atrial portion that has features similar to the normal AV node (decremental conduction, adenosine sensitivity[14-16]) and a longer, thin fiber connecting this node-like structure to the right bundle branch, traversing the tricuspid annulus. This portion appears to be adenosine-insensitive and functionally similar to specialized conduction tissue (His or bundle branches), and similarly "insulated" from activating the immediately surrounding ventricular myocardium. Guiraudon et al[17] reported on histological findings from a patient who underwent successful surgical correction for a Mahaim fiber, showing morphological similarity of the surgical specimen to AV nodal tissue. Thus, it would appear that these pathways constitute a duplication of the normal septal conduction system.[18,19] The location of these pathways is typically along the lateral-most portion of the tricuspid annulus, but they have been reported along practically all of the annulus of the free wall. Although there is no reason these pathways should not also exist on the left side of the heart (along the mitral annulus), only rare cases compatible with this anatomy have been reported.[20,21]

In some of the earlier literature, the terms "nodoventricular" and "nodofascicular" were applied to clinical situations that would now be categorized as atriofascicular pathways. This can lead to some confusion in interpreting findings from these studies.

Electrocardiography

The ECG during SVT in patients with Mahaim-type tachycardia shows a wide QRS of the left bundle branch type; the precordial R wave transition is delayed until lead V_4 (Figure 1). Bardy et al [22] found that SVT cycle length is from 220 to 450 milliseconds and the QRS duration is ≤ 150 milliseconds with left axis deviation; wider QRS complexes, with more slurred upstrokes, are found in patients in whom the pathway inserts into ventricular myocardium as opposed to specialized conduction tissue (Figure 2). During sinus rhythm, the ECG shows a normal PR interval and minimal or no preexcitation in the majority of patients. Individuals with relatively slow AV nodal conduction may show a long PR interval with a variable degree of preexcitation.

Electrophysiology

In the electrophysiology lab, the accessory pathways in patients with Mahaim tachycardia are typically characterized by 1) unidirectional (anterograde-only) conduction; 2) long conduction times; and 3) decremental conduction (progressive increase in AV conduction time with incrementally faster atrial pacing or more closely-coupled atrial premature beats; see Figure 3). The conduction delay has been localized to the intra-atrial portion of the pathway; the interval from the inscription of the Mahaim fiber potential at the tricuspid annulus and the onset of ventricular activation remains constant. Adenosine administration results in loss of conduction over the pathway; with block occurring in the intra-atrial portion. The majority of these pathways are of the atriofascicular type; variations in the above features are found in some cases, as is detailed further below. The electrophysiological properties of atriofascicular pathways are thus consistent with their being a duplication of the normal AV node/His axis, including a distal insertion into the RBB.

A number of arrhythmias can be initiated in patients with Mahaim fibers. The most common type is a wide-QRS complex reentrant SVT in which ventricular activation occurs over an atriofascicular fiber inserting into the RBB, after which the impulse retrogradely activates the His and AV node, and exiting the AV node to the atria to complete the circuit. In this type of tachycardia, a Mahaim potential can usually be recorded at or beneath the tricuspid annulus; the distal RBB and His are sequentially activated thereafter. Proof of atrial involvement in the circuit comes from introducing late-coupled atrial premature depolarizations (APDs) during SVT from the lateral right atrium, which advance the timing of ventricular activation while not altering the timing of AV nodal activation (Figure 4). Proof of Mahaim fiber participation includes tachycardia termination when block occurs in the pathway (mechanical block from a catheter) and absence of tachycardia after pathway ablation. Proof of RBB participation in this tachycardia comes from transient mechanically-induced right bundle branch block resulting in prolongation of SVT cycle length and ventriculoatrial time due to a longer path length during tachycardia.[16]

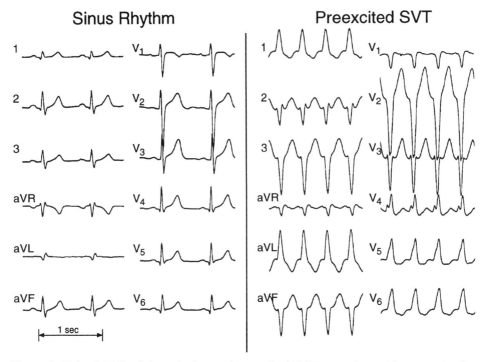

Figure 1. 12-lead ECGs of sinus rhythm and preexcited SVT in a patient with an atriofascicular fiber.

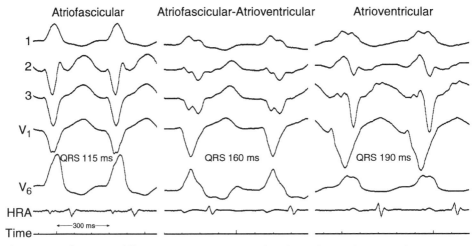

Figure 2. Surface ECG differences among preexcited tachycardias with ventricular activation over an atriofascicular fiber, both atriofascicular and atrioventricular, and atrioventricular only. QRS duration is shortest and initial forces most rapid when ventricular activation uses the His-Purkinje system (atriofascicular fiber). HRA = high right atrium.

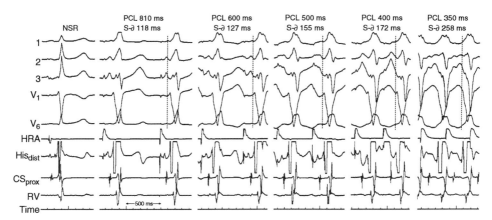

Figure 3. Progressive increase in AV conduction time over a decrementally-conducting atrio-ventricular pathway. Shown are 5 surface ECG leads and intracardiac recordings from high right atrium (HRA), distal His bundle (His$_{dist}$), proximal coronary sinus (CS$_{prox}$) and right ventricle (RV). Sinus rhythm is shown with panels of progressively more rapid right atrial pacing. The lengthening stimulus to delta (S-Δ) intervals are noted at each paced cycle length (PCL). Dashed vertical line denotes onset of QRS complex. Note that preexcitation is maximal at even 600 milliseconds PCL.

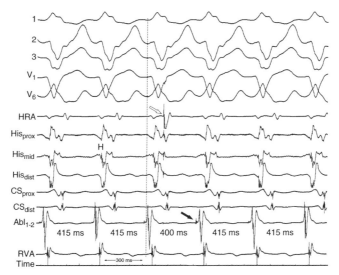

Figure 4. Atriofascicular tachycardia with proof of requirement of atrium during preexcited tachycardia. Abl$_{1-2}$ = recording from the distal electrode pair of the mapping/ablation catheter; H = His potential; RVA = RV apex. Surface and intracardiac recordings are as in previous figures. A wide QRS tachycardia is shown with an anterograde slowly conducting atriofascicular pathway for ventricular activation, retrograde conduction over the AV node; dotted vertical line denotes onset of surface QRS complex. The tachycardia is perfectly regular with a cycle length of 415 milliseconds; a sharp His potential is visible at the onset of the local ventricular activation in the His recording. An atrial extrastimulus (white arrow) is delivered after the inscription of the atrial electrogram in the His recordings, yet results in advancement of timing of occurrence of the next QRS complex (dark arrow, 400 milliseconds) without altering the timing of His or CS atrial recordings. This constitutes proof of a connection from lateral atrium to fascicles or ventricle rather than its originating in the AV node. The Abl recording contains a small Mahaim potential (dark arrow).

The other common type of tachycardia induced in these patients is one in which anterograde conduction occurs over the Mahaim fiber and retrograde conduction over a second accessory pathway (Figure 5).[20,23] Additional variations can also occur (anterograde fusion of Mahaim and AV node, retrograde second accessory pathway; anterograde Mahaim, retrograde fusion of AV node and second accessory pathway, and so on). A relatively large proportion of patients with Mahaim tachycardias have additional accessory pathways, either concealed or manifest; in some cases, the presence of a Mahaim-type connection is not evident until after a typical AV bypass tract is ablated.[10,23,24]

Mahaim fibers can also function as "bystanders," wholly or partly responsible for ventricular activation during other supraventricular arrhythmias. These include preexcited AV nodal reentry,[6,7,25–27] atrial tachycardia,[12] atrial flutter and fibrillation.[27–29]

Making the correct electrophysiological diagnosis in these complex cases is important in order to indicate what should be targeted for ablation. Obviously, ablating a Mahaim fiber that is only a bystander during a independent type of SVT accomplishes little.

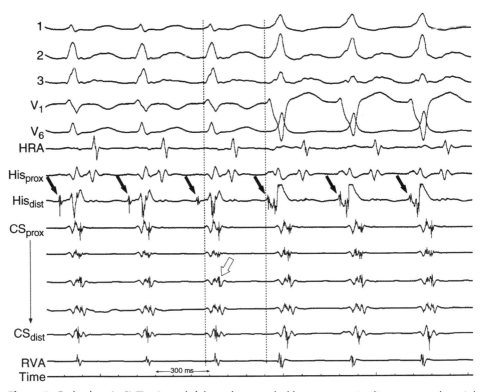

Figure 5. Orthodromic SVT using a left lateral concealed bypass tract (earliest retrograde atrial retrograde activation denoted by white arrow) and the AV node-His for anterograde conduction until the fourth beat, when fusion of anterograde conduction begins using a right lateral slowly conducting atrioventricular pathway (bystander). His potentials are indicated by dark arrows. Dashed vertical line denotes onset of QRS complex. Other recordings as in previous figures.

Anatomic and Electrophysiological Distinctions

The majority of cases of Mahaim tachycardias appear to incorporate a right lateral, anterograde-only, decrementally conducting atriofascicular fiber. Occasional cases are encountered in which an arrhythmia compatible with a Mahaim tachycardia is observed, but the electrophysiological properties of the anterograde limb differ from this typical description. Examples of these are as follows; Table 1 shows a comparison of electrophysiological features.

Atrioventricular Bypass Tracts with Slow/Decremental Properties

Several cases of bypass tracts that have slow or decremental conduction properties, but insert into ventricular muscle at the AV groove or further into the body of the ventricle, have appeared in the literature. These differ from more typical atriofascicular fibers in that the ventricular insertion is not in the distal normal conduction system. Relatively large accessory pathway potentials may be recorded at the tricuspid annulus (Figure 6). The physiology of these pathways is similar to that of the atriofascicular fiber (decremental conduction, adenosine sensitivity, ability to advance timing of QRS complexes by APDs that do not penetrate the AV node during preexcited tachycardia). Distinguishing the presence of these fibers as opposed to atriofascicular fibers may be difficult; in general, the preexcited QRS complex is relatively wider (since the insertion is into ventricular muscle instead of specialized conduction tissue), and the RB and His potentials occur later in the QRS complex (VH interval 37±9 milliseconds compared to 16±5 milliseconds for atriofascicular fibers).[29]

Nodoventricular and Nodofascicular Fibers

Although recent evidence indicates that atriofascicular fibers are most frequently responsible for what were earlier termed "nodoventricular" fibers, occasional patients have been reported in whom the Mahaim fiber is believed to arise from the region of the AV node and insert into ventricular myocardium as opposed to specialized conduction tissue. In these cases, the clinical and induced arrhythmia has been preexcited AV nodal reentry (bystander nodoventricular) or antidromic reentry with a second AV bypass tract forming the retrograde limb (integral nodoventricular).[20,23] When preexcited AV nodal reentry occurs, the nodoventricular fiber typically arises from the slow pathway, although cases have been reported in which the fiber exits from the fast pathway.[20] One feature suggesting participation of a nodoventricular fiber is the presence of a retrograde His deflection following, as opposed to preceding, the local ventricular potential in the His bundle recording during preexcited tachycardia (similar to antidromic SVT in typical AV bypass tracts). However, these findings may also be observed in atriofascicular tachycardia with retrograde

Table 1

Comparative features of different types of pathways associated with "Mahaim tachycardias."

Feature	Atriofascicular	Atrioventricular	Nodoventricular	Nodofascicular	Fasciculoventricular
PR in sinus rhythm	normal	short-normal	normal	normal	normal
QRS in sinus rhythm	normal or preexcited	preexcited	normal or preexcited	normal or preexcited	minimally preexcited
QRS with rapid atrial pacing	prolongs	prolongs	prolongs	prolongs	constant
QRS morphology when at maximum width	typical LBBB	preexcited	typical LBBB	typical LBBB	variable; minimal preexcitation
HV interval change with incremental rapid atrial pacing	decreases then fixed	decreases then fixed	decreases then fixed	decreases then fixed	short, constant
His position in SVT	onset of local HBE-V	variable	end of local HBE-V	onset of local HBE-V	—
Effect of APD during SVT delivered near atrial insertion of pathway (free wall RA)	advances V without septal A advancement	advances V without septal A advancement	may advance V (only after septal A advancement)	may advance V (only after septal A advancement)	none
AV dissociation in SVT	unlikely	unlikely	possible	possible	possible
Adenosine sensitivity	+++	+	+++	+++	—
Mahaim potential at tricuspid annulus	+++	++	—	—	—
Proximal insertion	atrial wall	atrial wall	AV node	AV node	His or RBB
Distal insertion	RBB	myocardium	myocardium	RBB	myocardium

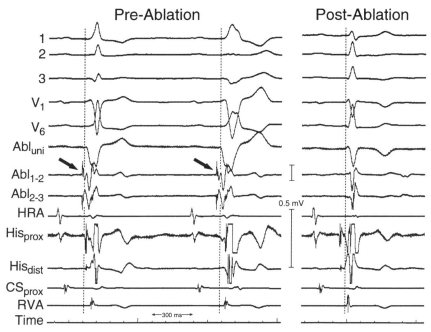

Figure 6. Large-amplitude Mahaim potentials recorded beneath the tricuspid annulus in a patient with a slowly conducting atrioventricular pathway, before and after ablation. Surface and intracardiac recordings as in previous figures. Arrows show Mahaim potentials with amplitude 0.5 mV, twice as large as the His potential. In preablation panel, 2 beats showing different degrees of preexcitation are shown. Note that although there is marked preexcitation on the second beat, the AV interval is still long due to slow AV nodal conduction. Abl_{uni} = unipolar recording from tip of ablation catheter; Abl_{2-3} = recording from second and third electrodes of ablation catheter. An amplitude scale is shown between panels for the Abl_{1-2} and His_{prox} recordings (both 0.5 mV).

right bundle branch block.[16] Due to the difficulty in obtaining definitive proof of the location of insertion sites of these pathways and the existence of plausible alternative explanations for observed phenomena, there is still controversy about whether distinct nodoventricular pathways actually exist.[30] On the other hand, there is better evidence for the existence of pathways that have electrophysiological features like those of atriofascicular pathways, but appear to have an atrial insertion in the septum near the AV node ("nodofascicular" fibers) instead of the right atrial free wall. Kottkamp et al[31] reported a case in which a catheter in the region of the AV node produced mechanical loss of preexcitation. During tachycardias in these cases, introduction of programmed atrial premature beats at the lateral right atrial wall does not advance subsequent ventricular activation during preexcited tachycardia, Mahaim potentials have not been recorded along the lateral tricuspid annulus and in some cases, ablation of the AV nodal slow pathway has effected cure of the tachycardia and elimination of Mahaim-type preexcitation.[26,32] The possibility remains that these cases actually represent atriofascicular pathways located in the septum as opposed to the free wall. The relative frequency of true nodofascicular fibers is unknown compared to more typical atriofascicular tracts, but they currently appear to form a small subset.

Fasciculoventricular Fibers

These rare pathways, consisting of an anomalous connection between the His or bundle branches and ventricular myocardium, differ from the fibers under consideration in this chapter. Although activation over these pathways results in a mildly abnormal (preexcited) QRS complex in sinus rhythm, the PR interval is normal, and the degree of preexcitation remains fixed and the HV interval constant over the range of atrial paced cycle lengths tested.[6,20,31] Perhaps most importantly, these fibers are not regarded as having an integral role in pathological tachyarrhythmias. These abnormal connections will not be discussed further in this chapter.

Fibers With Retrograde Conduction

Although the classical Mahaim physiology is characterized by unidirectional (anterograde) conduction, cases have been reported in which the pathway is not only capable of bidirectional conduction, but participates in orthodromic reentry.[23,33,34] Alternative explanations for these findings almost always exist and it is extremely difficult to prove conclusively that these fibers conduct retrogradely, since (in light of their slow anterograde conduction) one would anticipate a retrograde conduction time in excess of the retrograde AV nodal conduction time. There is reason to suspect that some of these pathways should be capable of retrograde conduction, like the normal conduction system to which they are analogous. A recent case report has clearly demonstrated this, although the pathway did not participate retrogradely in SVT.[35] Pacing at a site on or near the annulus from which a Mahaim potential can be recorded has not demonstrated retrograde conduction in several cases.[16]

Therapy: Pharmacological and Surgical

Pharmacological

It has already been noted that adenosine administration causes block in conduction over Mahaim fibers;[14] however, verapamil generally does not. Both oral flecainide[36] and encainide[37] have been shown to block conduction in Mahaim fibers and prevent tachycardia recurrences in small numbers of patients. Type Ia agents such as procainamide, quinidine, and disopyramide have had less consistent effects.[14,37,38]

Surgery

The first cases of curative therapy of patients with Mahaim tachycardias were from surgical reports.[10,11,17,39,40] These reports also added greatly to the understanding of the anatomy and intracardiac course of Mahaim fibers, as noted above. Because of the development of catheter ablation, surgical therapy is rarely used in current practice.

Therapy: Catheter Ablation

Mapping

Mapping principles for typical atrioventricular bypass tracts have been well characterized: searching for sites with earliest atrial activation during retrograde conduction, earliest anterograde conduction during sinus rhythm or atrial pacing, and pathway potentials along the AV groove. However, due to the unusual course and conduction properties of pathways involved in Mahaim tachycardias, these mapping techniques are largely inapplicable. Thus, successful ablation of these pathways requires different approaches than those which are used in the more common types of accessory AV connections.

Several catheter mapping strategies to guide RF ablation of these pathways have been reported; these are discussed below. Due to the relative rarity of patients with Mahaim physiology, there has not been a thorough comparison of techniques to determine which is superior. Certain situations make one or more methods preferable to others, however. The first 2 methods approximate the atrial insertion site; the next 2 localize the distal insertion site (fascicle or ventricle); and the last 2 localize the pathway directly as it crosses the tricuspid annulus. These mapping methods are:

1) Shortest stimulus-delta mapping:[15,28,41] the atrial site from which constant-rate pacing produces the shortest stimulus-delta is the site closest to the atrial insertion of the fiber. Using this technique, the mapping catheter is advanced from location to location along the atrial aspect of the tricuspid annulus while pacing from its distal electrode or electrode pair. The resulting interval stimulus-to-delta wave onset is measured; it should decrease progressively as the atrial insertion site is approached, and increase as it is passed. This method has several limitations, however. First, it is imperative that the mapping be performed at a constant paced cycle length; faster rates will result in a longer stimulus-to-delta interval even when pacing from the same site. Second, a constant distance of the mapping/pacing catheter from the tricuspid annulus must be maintained so as to diminish the influence of the time spent traversing intervening atrial tissue. Third, catheter manipulation during pacing can result in initiation of tachycardia that must then be terminated in order to continue mapping. Fourth, optimal sites may be overlooked if they cannot be consistently paced because of unstable catheter contact. In cases in which tachycardia is incessant or atrial fibrillation is present, this method cannot be applied.[27]

2) Extrastimulus mapping:[13,15] the atrial insertion site of the fiber is close to the site from which the longest-coupled (latest) extrastimulus during preexcited tachycardia advances the timing of the next ventricular

cycle. The same limitations apply to this method as to the shortest stimulus-delta method above; consistency of catheter-tissue contact and distance of the mapping/stimulation catheter from the tricuspid annulus are particularly important. This method is quite time-consuming and cannot be used during atrial fibrillation nor when SVT is difficult to initiate or nonsustained. It is also not particularly useful in cases of true nodofascicular pathways.

3) Determination of fascicular insertion (atriofascicular fiber):[27,29,42] the distal insertion of an atriofascicular fiber can be localized by carefully mapping along the lateral right ventricular wall toward the apex, seeking the earliest site of ventricular activation (Figure 7). A distal right bundle branch recording is usually present at this site. This method can be used to map in any rhythm during which consistent preexcitation is present (atrial pacing, preexcited SVT, atrial fibrillation). Seeking the distal insertion is less precise than in some other methods in that one may localize a distal right bundle recording, but not the portion into which the atriofascicular fiber inserts. It is most useful if the course of the atriofascicular fiber can be traced from the tricuspid annulus to its insertion into the right bundle,[16] but then ablation at the distal site con-

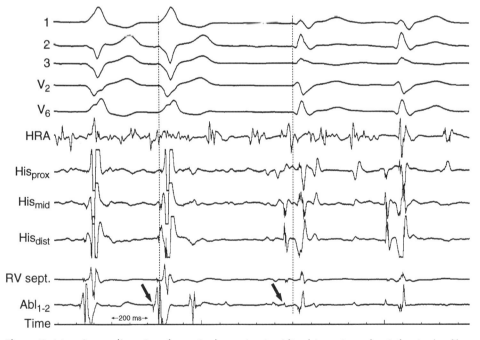

Figure 7. Mapping earliest site of ventricular activation/distal insertion of atriofascicular fiber during sustained atrial fibrillation. Surface and intracardiac recordings as in previous figures. Dark arrows denote Mahaim potential occurring before RBB potential and retrogradely activated His potential on 2 preexcited beats at left. Catheter movement halfway through the panel resulted in mechanical trauma to the pathway and conduction block lasting 8 seconds. Note change in activation sequence of His, RBB, and Mahaim potential during narrow QRS beats. Dashed vertical line denotes onset of QRS complex. Sept. = septum.

fers no advantage unless catheter stability is better at that location as opposed to the annulus. If the right bundle is ablated rather than the atriofascicular fiber, right bundle branch block will result; not only will this fail to eliminate the pathway and associated tachycardia, but it is possible that tachycardia will be facilitated because of increasing the path length.

4) Determination of earliest ventricular activation (atrioventricular fiber):[15] if a slowly-conducting pathway that inserts directly into ventricular muscle at the annulus or more distal ventricular myocardium has been diagnosed, the same principles apply to its precise localization as for more typical AV bypass tracts. Seeking a site with the earliest unipolar or bipolar ventricular recording or one with a sharp downstroke of a QS deflection is usually adequate for defining an appropriate target site for ablation. There is some evidence that a variable degree of arborization of the distal insertion site occurs in some patients.[29] This feature makes the ventricular insertion site a less attractive ablation target because of the potential for requiring ablation of relatively large amounts of ventricular myocardium in order to be effective.

5) Direct recording of Mahaim fiber at tricuspid annulus:[16,24,43,44] the most precise method of localizing Mahaim fibers is to record the activation of the fiber itself. The Mahaim potential is typically a low amplitude, high frequency recording made at the tricuspid annulus which resembles a His bundle potential (except that it is recorded several centimeters away from the usual His recording site; see Figures 6 and 8). This method has several advantages over other methods: it is generally less time-consuming than the inferential methods of locating the atrial insertion discussed above, and more precise than seeking the earliest ventricular activation of the atriofascicular fiber (which, as noted above, may undergo substantial branching). Only the annular and subannular (ventricular) portions of the fiber have been successfully recorded; attempts to record potentials from the atrial portion (corresponding to nodal-like tissue) have not borne fruit. Attempts to record a Mahaim potential can be used successfully during sinus rhythm, atrial pacing, or preexcited SVT; however, because of the relatively low amplitude of the Mahaim potential, attempting to localize it directly is difficult or impossible during atrial fibrillation.

6) Determination of site at which catheter trauma causes loss of preexcitation:[24,28,41] mechanically-induced loss of preexcitation has been used to guide catheter mapping and ablation of Mahaim fibers. This serendipitous finding is made during atrial pacing or preexcited SVT when standard catheter manipulation results in a sudden, transient loss of preexcitation (see Figure 7). This is observed during mapping on the ventricular aspect of the tricuspid annulus and generally lasts from a few beats to a few minutes, after which preexcitation resumes. Conduction block typically occurs while a Mahaim potential is still recorded; thus transmission is interrupted within its ventricular course. Transient mechanically-induced conduction block can also be observed during catheter manipulation and mapping of the atrial aspect of the tricuspid

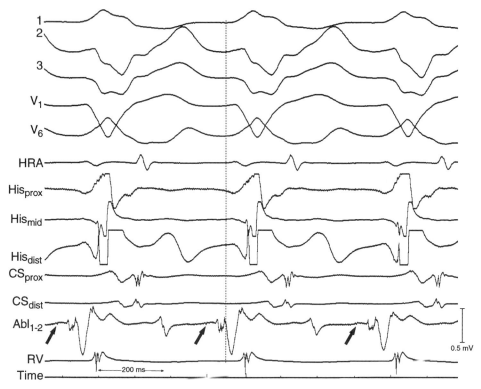

Figure 8. Multicomponent Mahaim potentials recorded from tricuspid annulus during preexcited tachycardia. Surface and intracardiac recordings as in previous figures. The Abl_{1-2} recording shows an atrial electrogram and Mahaim potential just prior to the QRS onset (dashed line); there is also a smaller potential 50 milliseconds prior to the larger Mahaim potential (arrows). Although the local ventricular electrogram onset is simultaneous with the QRS onset denoting some myocardial activation near the annulus, the Mahaim potential could be recorded all the way to the RV apex at its insertion to the RBB. An amplitude scale is at right for the Abl_{1-2} recording.

annulus. Catheter-induced block within the thinner discrete portion of the pathway below the tricuspid valve, and the more diffuse node-like structure within the atrial wall, are analogous to catheter-induced block in the normal His-Purkinje system[45] and AV node,[46] respectively. The mechanically-induced loss of preexcitation method can be used during any consistently preexcited rhythm (sinus, atrial pacing, atrial fibrillation, preexcited SVT). However, if mechanically-induced block occurs during preexcited SVT in which the Mahaim fiber is integrally involved, the tachycardia immediately terminates, which may lead to catheter displacement. Atriofascicular pathways appear to be more susceptible to mechanically-induced block than other types of bypass tracts. This may indicate that they are composed of a thinner strand, or are more superficially (endocardial surface) located than more typical bypass tracts. If one encounters a site at which catheter trauma produces conduction block, the location of the fiber has been specified precisely; however, if the catheter has moved from that spot, further mapping must be performed to relocalize the fiber. Conduction in the pathway may be successfully eliminated when RF energy is applied to a site at which catheter pressure caused loss of preexcitation,[28] but because of the possibility that the catheter position may have changed, it is best to wait to deliver energy until conduction has resumed.[24]

Using the above methods, the locations of successful ablation of Mahaim fibers have been shown to be along the lateral tricuspid annulus in the majority of cases, with a minority requiring ablation along the septal aspect of the tricuspid annulus or within the ventricle (Figure 9). Based on the reports in the literature of successful ablation sites, there is a statistically significant predilection for atriofascicular fibers to cross the tricuspid annulus in the lateral, anterolateral, or anterior regions, whereas atrioventricular fibers are roughly equally distributed between these and more posterior or septal regions (84% versus 53%, $P < 0.01$). Missing from the above list of mapping methods is attempting to localize the atrial insertion of the fiber by seeking the site of earliest retrograde atrial activation during ventricular pacing, since these pathways have only rarely been reported to have retrograde conduction.[23,33-35] The technical difficulties in determining whether or not retrograde conduction is proceeding over these pathways have been noted above.

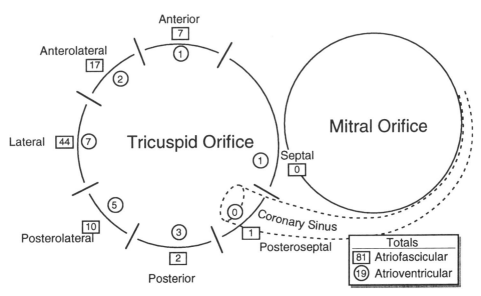

Figure 9. Locations of reported successful sites of RF ablation on the tricuspid annulus of 100 Mahaim fibers, viewed in a left anterior oblique projection.[13,15,16,23,24,26-29,31,32, 41,43,44,49] The number of atriofascicular pathways reported from each region is shown outside the annulus within a square, the number of atrioventricular Mahaim pathways inside the annulus (circled). Most pathways are successfully ablated at the lateral, posterolateral, or anterolateral regions. The prevalence of atriofascicular pathways is slightly higher toward the anterior wall, that of atrioventricular pathways more toward the posterior wall.

Results of Ablation

Once an appropriate target site for ablation has been identified, energy may be applied during sinus rhythm, atrial pacing, or preexcited SVT. Of these, atrial pacing may be preferable to ensure that enough preexcitation is evident to be able to assess efficacy (unlike sinus rhythm in many cases), and that the rhythm remains the same after elimination of preexcitation (unlike preexcited SVT). Direct current was used for ablation in some early reports;[47] since then, RF has been used almost exclusively. During energy delivery, an accelerated preexcited rhythm (presumably due to irritation of the pathway caused by heating) is often present (Figure 10).[16,24,48] Braun et al[48] observed this phenomenon in 36% of RF applications delivered in 15 patients with atriofascicular and slowly-conducting atrioventricular pathways. The accelerated preexcited rhythm lasted from 2 beats to more than 30 beats. The duration of RF delivery after cessation of this accelerated rhythm has been correlated with a successful outcome (that is, the longer RF was delivered after the arrhythmia appeared and ceased, the more likely was a permanent effect). Cappato et al reported a relatively high rate of recurrence of preexcitation during the first 24 hours postablation[28] but more recent reports have not had this problem. Acute success rates for catheter ablation approach 100% in the published literature, although the ease with which pathway conduc-

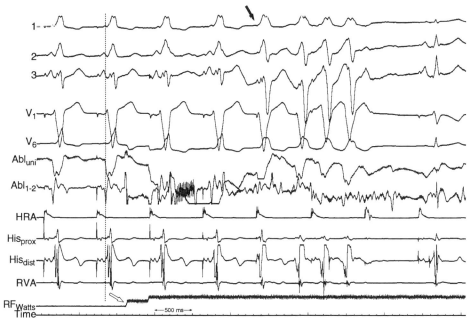

Figure 10. Ablation of a slowly conducting atrioventricular pathway (same patient as in Figure 3) with accelerated preexcited rhythm. Surface and intracardiac recordings as in previous figures; RF= radiofrequency. Dashed vertical line denotes onset of QRS complex. The white arrow marks the onset of RF energy delivery; 1.5 seconds later, premature QRS complexes with a morphology identical to the preexcited ones are seen (dark arrow) for 4 beats, after which preexcitation is permanently gone (last beat).

tion is eliminated varies greatly (requiring from 1 application to over 30 applications in up to 5 ablation sessions); recurrence rates are generally less than 5% during relatively short follow-up periods.[15,16,23,24,26–29,31,32,42–44,48,49] In cases of antidromic tachycardia (not bystander activation of the Mahaim), some investigators have resorted to AV nodal fast pathway ablation if the Mahaim fiber cannot be ablated directly. However, this must be performed with caution to make certain all AV nodal conduction is not interrupted. Thus, a variety of mapping and ablation strategies have been used successfully; most investigators agree that attempts to localize the actual Mahaim fiber potential as it crosses the tricuspid annulus is the preferred method.

Summary and Conclusions

Since their initial anatomic and electrophysiological descriptions, the characteristics of what have come to be called Mahaim fibers have been extensively explored. These unusual accessory pathways most often are shown to have slow and decremental conduction in the anterograde direction only and are associated with a variety of wide QRS complex tachycardias. Current evidence indicates that a so-called atriofascicular pathway, composed of an AV nodal-like intra-atrial portion and a longer, insulated fiber that inserts into the distal right bundle branch, is present in the majority of patients with Mahaim tachycardias. These features have led to the conclusion that such fibers represent a duplication of the AV node-His portion of the normal conduction system, the proximal portion of which is located in the lateral right atrial wall. Other less common variants include pathways with a septal rather than free wall atrial origin (possibly into a portion of the AV node) as well as those with long conduction times but a ventricular insertion just across the tricuspid annulus, as opposed to the right bundle branch. Isolated cases have been reported of similar fibers inserting into the left bundle branch as well as others capable of retrograde conduction. It is likely that in coming years, additional variants will continue to be described. Catheter ablation has been shown to be a highly effective means of permanently eliminating conduction over Mahaim fibers. A variety of mapping methods have been used to localize these unusual pathways; the preferred method is seeking sites on the tricuspid annulus from which Mahaim pathway potentials can be recorded. Since a significant proportion of patients with these pathways are found to have multiple mechanisms of tachycardia (including those in which the Mahaim fiber is merely a bystander), it is important to carefully determine what type or types one is working with before formulating an ablation strategy (in other words, which site to target).

References

1. Mahaim I, Benatt A. Nouvelles recherches sur les connexions supérieures de la branch gauche du faisceau de His-Tawara avec cloison interventriculaire. *Cardiologia* 1937;1:61–76.

2. Anderson RH, Becker AE, Brechenmacher C, et al. Ventricular preexcitation: a proposed nomenclature for its substrates. *Eur J Cardiol* 1975;3:27–36.

3. Wellens HJJ. The preexcitation syndrome. In: HJJ Wellens, ed. *Electrical Stimulation of the Heart in the Study and Treatment of Tachycardias.* Baltimore, MD: University Park Press, 1971. pp 97–109.

4. Touboul P, Vexler RM, Chatelain MT. Reentry via Mahaim fibres as a possible basis for tachycardia. *Br Heart J* 1978;40:806–811.

5. Ward DE, Camm AJ, Spurrell RA. Ventricular preexcitation due to anomalous nodo-ventricular pathways: report of 3 patients. *Eur J Cardiol* 1979;9:111–127.

6. Gallagher JJ, Smith WM, Kasell JH, et al. Role of Mahaim fibers in cardiac arrhythmias in man. *Circulation* 1981;64:176–189.

7. Morady F, Scheinman MM, Gonzalez R, et al. His-ventricular dissociation in a patient with reciprocating tachycardia and a nodoventricular bypass tract. *Circulation* 1981;64:839–844.

8. Weiss J, Cabeen WR, Roberts NK. Nodoventricular accessory atrioventricular connection associated with dual atrioventricular pathways: a case report and review of the literature. *J Electrocardiol* 1981;14:185–190.

9. Lerman BB, Waxman HL, Josephson ME. Supraventricular tachycardia associated with nodoventricular and concealed atrioventricular bypass tracts. *Am Heart J* 1982;104:1097–1102.

10. Gillette PC, Garson A Jr., Cooley DA, et al. Prolonged and decremental antegrade conduction properties in right anterior accessory connections: wide QRS antidromic tachycardia of left bundle branch block pattern without Wolff-Parkinson-White configuration in sinus rhythm. *Am Heart J* 1982; 103:66–74.

11. Klein GJ, Guiraudon GM, Kerr CR, et al. "Nodoventricular" accessory pathway: evidence for a distinct accessory atrioventricular pathway with atrioventricular node-like properties. *J Am Coll Cardiol* 1988;11:1035–1040.

12. Kou WH, Morady F, De Buitleir M, et al. Electrophysiology demonstration of an atriofascicular accessory pathway. *PACE* 1988;11:166–173.

13. Tchou P, Lehmann MH, Jazayeri M, et al. Atriofascicular connection or a nodoventricular Mahaim fiber? Electrophysiologic elucidation of the pathway and associated reentrant circuit. *Circulation* 1988;77:837–848.

14. Ellenbogen KA, Rogers R, Old W. Pharmacological characterization of conduction over a Mahaim fiber: evidence for adenosine sensitive conduction. *PACE* 1989;12:1396–1404.

15. Klein LS, Hackett FK, Zipes DP, et al. Radiofrequency catheter ablation of Mahaim fibers at the tricuspid annulus. *Circulation* 1993;87:738–747.

16. McClelland JH, Wang X, Beckman KJ, et al. Radiofrequency catheter ablation of right atriofascicular (Mahaim) accessory pathways guided by accessory pathway activation potentials. *Circulation* 1994;89:2655–2666.

17. Guiraudon CM, Guiraudon GM. "Nodal ventricular" Mahaim pathway: histological evidence for an accessory atrioventricular pathway with AV node-like morphology. *Circulation* 1988;78(suppl 2):40.

18. Tchou PJ, Keim SG, Kinn RM, et al. Electrophysiologic evidence for an ectopic node-His like atrioventricular conduction system in an atriofascicular pathway. *PACE* 1992;15:51.

19. Kuck KH, Siebels J, Braun E, et al. Mahaim fibers: a second atrioventricular conduction system. *PACE* 1997;20:1201.
20. Abbott JA, Scheinman MM, Morady F, et al. Coexistent Mahaim and Kent accessory connections: diagnostic and therapeutic implications. *J Am Coll Cardiol* 1987;10:364–372.
21. Yamabe H, Okumura K, Minoda K, et al. Nodoventricular Mahaim fiber connection to the left ventricle. *Am Heart J* 1991;122:232–234.
22. Bardy GH, Fedor JM, German LD, et al. Surface electrocardiographic clues suggesting presence of a nodofascicular Mahaim fiber. *J Am Coll Cardiol* 1984;3:1161–1168.
23. De Ponti R, Storti C, Stanke A, et al. Radiofrequency catheter ablation in patients with Mahaim-type slow-conduction accessory right atrioventricular pathway. *Cardiologia* 1994;39:169–180.
24. Heald SC, Davies DW, Ward DE, et al. Radiofrequency catheter ablation of Mahaim tachycardia by targeting Mahaim potentials at the tricuspid annulus. *Br Heart J* 1995;73:250–257.
25. Ward DE, Bennett DH, Camm J. Mechanisms of junctional tachycardia showing ventricular pre-excitation. *Br Heart J* 1984;52:369–376.
26. Grogin HR, Lee RJ, Kwasman M, et al. Radiofrequency catheter ablation of atriofascicular and nodoventricular Mahaim tracts. *Circulation* 1994;90:272–281.
27. Miller JM, Rothman SA, Harper GR, et al. Radiofrequency catheter ablation of an atriofascicular pathway during atrial fibrillation: a case report. *J Cardiovasc Electrophysiol* 1994;846–853.
28. Cappato R, Schlüter M, Weiss C, et al. Catheter-induced mechanical conduction block of right-sided accessory fibers with Mahaim-type preexcitation to guide radiofrequency ablation. *Circulation* 1994;90:282–290.
29. Haïssaguerre M, Cauchemez B, Marcus F, et al. Characteristics of the ventricular insertion sites of accessory pathways with anterograde decremental conduction properties. *Circulation* 1995;91:1077–1085.
30. Klein GJ, Guiraudon G, Guiraudon C, et al. The nodoventricular Mahaim pathway: an endangered concept? *Circulation* 1994;90:636–638.
31. Kottkamp H, Hindricks G, Shenasa H, et al. Variants of preexcitation—specialized atriofascicular pathways, nodofascicular pathways, and fasciculoventricular pathways: electrophysiologic findings and target sites for radiofrequency catheter ablation. *J Cardiovasc Electrophysiol* 1996;7:916–930.
32. Beurrier D, Brembilla-Perrot B, Bragard MF. Radiofrequency catheter ablation of a nodoventricular Mahaim tract. *Herz* 1996;21:314–319.
33. Shimizu A, Ohe T, Takaki H, et al. Narrow QRS complex tachycardia with atrioventricular dissociation. *PACE* 1988;11:384–393.
34. Wu D, Yeh SJ, Yamamoto T, et al. Participation of a concealed nodoventricular fiber in the genesis of paroxysmal tachycardias. *Am Heart J* 1990;119:583–591.
35. Kreiner G, Heinz G, Frey B, et al. Demonstration of retrograde conduction over and atriofascicular accessory pathway. *J Cardiovasc Electrophysiol* 1997;8:74–79.
36. Lau CP, Davies DW, Mehta D, et al. Flecainide acetate in the treatment of tachycardias associated with Mahaim fibres. *Eur Heart J* 1987;8:832–839.

37. Miles WM, Chang MS, Heger JJ, et al. Electrophysiologic and antiarrhythmic effects of oral encainide in patients with atrioventricular nodal reentry or nodoventricular reentry. *Am Heart J* 1987;114:26–33.

38. Strasberg B, Coelho A, Palileo E, et al. Pharmacological observations in patients with nodoventricular pathways. *Br Heart J* 1984;51:84–90.

39. Murdock CJ, Leitch JW, Klein GJ, et al. Epicardial mapping in patients with "nodoventricular" accessory pathways. *Am J Cardiol* 1991;68:208–214.

40. Sealy WC, Kopelman HE, Murphy DA. Accessory atrioventricular node and bundle: a cause of antidromic reentry tachycardia. *Ann Thorac Surg* 1992;54:306–310.

41. Okishige K, Strickberger SA, Walsh EP, et al. Catheter ablation of the atrial origin of a decrementally conducting atriofascicular accessory pathway by radiofrequency current. *J Cardiovasc Electrophysiol* 1991;2:465–475.

42. Haïssaguerre M, Warin JF, Le Metayer P, et al. Catheter ablation of Mahaim fibers with preservation of atrioventricular nodal conduction. *Circulation* 1990;82:418–427.

43. Mounsey JP, Griffith MJ, McComb JM. Radiofrequency ablation of a Mahaim fiber following localization of Mahaim pathway potentials. *J Cardiovasc Electrophysiol* 1994;5:432–437.

44. Brugada J, Martinez-Sanchez J, Kuzmicic B, et al. Radiofrequency catheter ablation of atriofascicular accessory pathways guided by discrete electrical potentials recorded at the tricuspid annulus. *PACE* 1995;18:1388–1394.

45. Suh IL, Cossú SF, Hsia IIII, et al. Catheter-induced bundle branch block: incidence and outcome. *Circulation* 1995;92(8):I–729.

46. Cossú SF, Rothman SA, Hsia HH, et al. Catheter-induced AV nodal block: a risk factor for developing heart block in patients undergoing slow pathway modification. *PACE* 1995;18:920.

47. Warin JF, Haïssaguerre M, D'Ivernois C, et al. Catheter ablation of accessory pathways: technique and results in 248 patients. *PACE* 1990;13:1609–1614.

48. Braun E, Siebels J, Volkmer M, et al. Radiofrequency-induced preexcited automatic rhythm during ablation of accessory pathways with Mahaim-type preexcitation: does it predict clinical outcome? *PACE* 1997;20:1124.

49. Tebbenjohanns J, Pfeiffer D, Jung W, et al. Radiofrequency catheter ablation of a right posterolateral atrioventricular accessory pathway with decremental conduction properties (Mahaim fiber). *Am Heart J* 1993;125:898–901.

Chapter 28

Radiofrequency Ablation of Multiple Accessory Pathways

Munther Homoud, M.D., N.A. Mark Estes III, M.D., Paul J. Wang, M.D.

Incidence of Multiple Accessory Bypass Tracts

Accessory atrioventricular (AV) bypass tracts are remnants of the AV connections due to failure of the fibrous separation between the atria and ventricles.[1] The overall incidence of atrioventricular bypass tracts is 0.1–0.3% of the general population.[2,3] The incidence of multiple bypass tracts is reported at 3–20% in the surgical series and at 5–18% in the radiofrequency ablation series (Table 1).[4–20] The incidence of multiple accessory pathways may vary based on selection bias and the definition used as discussed below.

The frequency of bypass tracts in first-degree relatives of patients with Wolff-Parkinson-White syndrome is greater than the incidence in the general population suggesting a familial form of this disorder.[21] Individuals with the familial form of Wolff-Parkinson-White syndrome have a greater incidence of multiple bypass tracts.[21]

Ebstein's anomaly, characterized by the downward displacement of the tricuspid valve, is the commonest congenital anomaly associated with the Wolff-Parkinson-White syndrome.[7,22] This syndrome is characterized by a higher incidence of multiple and right-sided bypass tracts compared to a control population of patients with Wolff-Parkinson-White syndrome and without congenital heart disease (50% versus 15.1% and 78.9% versus 21.6% respectively, $P < 0.001$).[14]

From Huang SKS, Wilber DJ (eds.): *Radiofrequency Catheter Ablation of Cardiac Arrhythmias: Basic Concepts and Clinical Applications,* 2nd ed. Armonk, NY: Futura Publishing Company, Inc. ©2000.

Table 1

	Number of Patients	Patients with Multiple Bypass Tracts	Comments
Gallagher et al (1976)	135	20 (15%)	
Iwa et al (1980)	35	5 (14%)	
Sealy et al (1981)	161	17 (10.6%)	
Cox et al (1985)	118	24 (20%)	
Selle et al (1987)	90	18 (20%)	
Colavita et al (1987)	388	52 (13%)	
de Buitleir et al (1991)	50	7 (14%)	
Leather et al (1991)	75	8 (11%)	
Schlüter et al (1991)	92	4 (4.3%)	
Jackman et al (1991)	166	10 (6%)	
Langberg et al (1992)	130	12 (9%)	25% of recurrence had MBPT vs. 10% SBPT
Lesh et al (1992)	100	8 (8%)	1 pt. with 3 BPT had Ebstein's anomaly
Pressley et al (1992)	422	77 (18%)	38 pts. with Ebstein's anomaly; 50% MBPT
Calkins et al (1992)	250	15 (6%)	
Yeh et al (1993)	210	24 (11%)	RFW and LFW commoner combination
Swartz et al (1993)	114	8 (7%)	
Chen et al (1993)	145	20 (13.8%)	
Haïssaguerre et al (1994)	512	25 (4.9%)	
Huang et al (1996)	858	73 (8.5%)	2 LFW BPT commonest combination

MBPT = multiple bypass tracts; RFW = right free wall; LFW = left free wall.

Definition and Identification of Multiple Accessory Pathways

The definition of multiple accessory pathways is based on an approximation of the distance between accessory pathways during intraoperative or catheter-based mapping. Accessory pathways separated by 1–3 centimeters have been defined as being multiple. This variability of definition has contributed to the range in the incidence reported for multiple accessory pathways. In a series of 24 patients with multiple bypass tracts reported by Yeh et al, 93% (50 of 54) of the bypass tracts were uncovered before radiofrequency ablation by using 1 or more of the aforementioned strategies.[16] The distance from 1 ipsilateral bypass tract to the other is an important criterion for identifying multiple bypass tracts. While Yeh et al defined the distance as greater than 1 centimeter, Chen et al defined the separation as greater than 3 centimeters.[16,18] Reports of multistranded or broad-banded bypass tracts as wide as 3 centimeters led Chen et al to use the 3-centimeter cutoff.[18] The 3-centimeter cutoff also has its origins in the surgical literature where surgical incisions are made approximately 1.5 centimeters to each side of the bypass tract to incorporate wide multistranded accessory pathways.[4]

There are a number of limitations to the mapping-based identification of multiple accessory pathways based on these definitions of distance. Many accessory pathways may have broad atrial or ventricular insertions. A broad insertion may lead to the diagnosis of 2 or more accessory pathways. This is particularly true in catheter-based mapping, more so than in intraoperative mapping. An accessory pathway with a broad insertion may require 2 anatomically separate lesions in order to abolish retrograde or antegrade conduction, and therefore might be incorrectly classified as 2 accessory pathways. In the surgical treatment of accessory pathways, an anatomic region, for example the posterior septal space, is dissected. Therefore, a broad insertion would not be interpreted as 2 separate accessory pathways. At the same, 2 distinct accessory pathways in the same anatomic region might be interpreted as 1 accessory pathway if conduction preferentially traveled via 1 accessory pathway.

The identification of multiple accessory pathways is based on these measurements of distance rather than on differences in the surface morphological appearance, since the latter may vary with the degree of fusion and may not indicate distinct accessory pathway structures. Nevertheless, clues to multiple accessory pathways include: 1) several ECG morphologies (for manifest pathways) during sinus rhythm, atrial premature beats, atrial pacing, or pre-excited tachycardias; 2) varying retrograde atrial activation sequences during ventricular pacing or antidromic or orthodromic tachycardia; 3) appearance of new pre-excitation patterns or retrograde atrial activation sequences after surgical dissection, catheter ablation, or adenosine administration (Table 2).

Multiple pre-excited ECG morphologies may be clues to multiple accessory pathways. Changing morphologies in atrial fibrillation provide evidence of multiple morphologies because of the potential for varying R-R intervals. However, the sensitivity of this technique may be limited since 1 of the accessory pathways may have a particularly short antegrade refractory period and therefore be responsible for nearly all of the conduction in atrial fibrillation (Figure 1). Multiple accessory pathways may also be misdiagnosed during atrial fibrillation because of the frequent occurrence of bundle branch aberrancy during atrial fibrillation. Also varying degrees of fusion with normal antegrade conduction may be mistaken for multiple accessory pathways.

Atrial premature beats or atrial premature stimulation may also provide a clue of multiple accessory pathways. Figure 2 demonstrates the presence of 2

Table 2

Electrocardiographic Clues to Multiple Accessory Pathways

- Variations in pre-excited QRS morphology especially during atrial fibrillation
- Atypical patterns of pre-excitation
- Antidromic AVRT using a posterior septal accessory bypass tract
- Orthodromic AVRT with changing retrograde P wave morphologies
- Antidromic AVRT with varying degrees of antegrade fusion

Electrophysiologic Evidence of Multiple Accessory Pathways

- Change in pre-excited morphology at different pacing cycle lengths and sites
- Differing patterns of antegrade and retrograde conduction
- Appearance of an accessory bypass tract after drug induced block of conduction or ablation of an accessory bypass tract
- Varying patterns of retrograde atrial activation sequence during AVRT or ventricular pacing or from orthodromic to antidromic AVRT

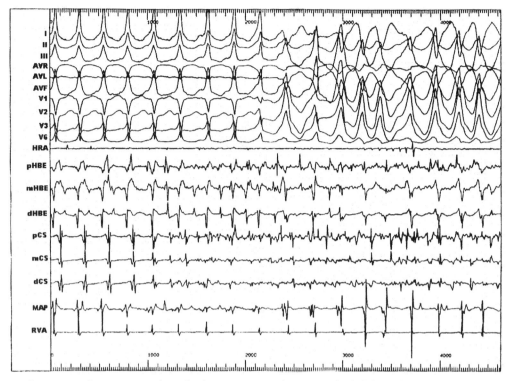

Figure 1. In this patient with multiple accessory pathways, in the left lateral, posterior septal, and anterior septal spaces, only conduction via the left free wall accessory pathway is observed during atrial fibrillation. The shortest pre-excited R-R interval is 180 milliseconds.

distinct ECG patterns during sinus rhythm and following an atrial premature complex. Atrial pacing at varying cycle lengths and sites may be particularly useful in identifying multiple accessory pathways. While some differences in the pre-excited pattern are common, it is important that careful mapping be performed to determine that the accessory pathways are anatomically distinct rather than part of a broad ventricular insertion. Figures 3A and 3B demonstrate a subtle change in the pre-excited pattern. In contrast, atrial pacing in the same patient in Figure 4 demonstrates a very different pattern consistent predominantly with an anterior septal accessory pathway. If the pattern of pre-excitation is not consistent with an established pattern, one must suspect the presence of multiple accessory pathways. Caution should be used since fusion among several accessory pathways may lead one to conclude incorrectly that additional accessory pathways are present.

Pre-excited tachycardias having more than 1 morphology suggest that multiple accessory pathways may be present. Patients with clinically documented pre-excited atrioventricular reentrant tachycardia have a higher incidence of multiple accessory pathways since many pre-excited tachycardias use an accessory pathway rather than the A-V junction in the retrograde limb.[23] Since a critical distance between the 2 limbs of the reentrant tachycardia must be no less than 4 centimeters, a pre-excited tachycardia with a morphology

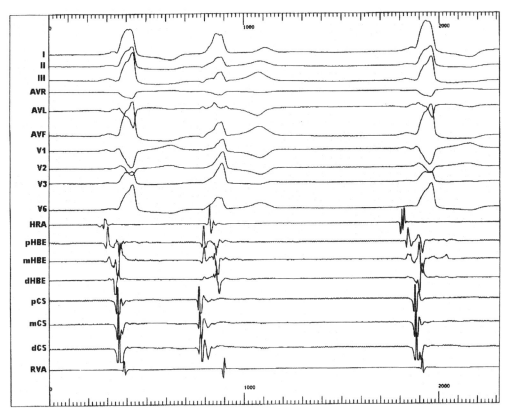

Figure 2. The first beat in sinus rhythm demonstrated a pre-excited pattern consistent with an anterior septal accessory pathway. However, the second beat indicates from a left-sided atrial premature complex exhibits a pre-excited pattern consistent with a left posterior septal accessory pathway. This is from the same patient as in Figure 1, demonstrating evidence of a left free wall accessory pathway conduction during atrial fibrillation.

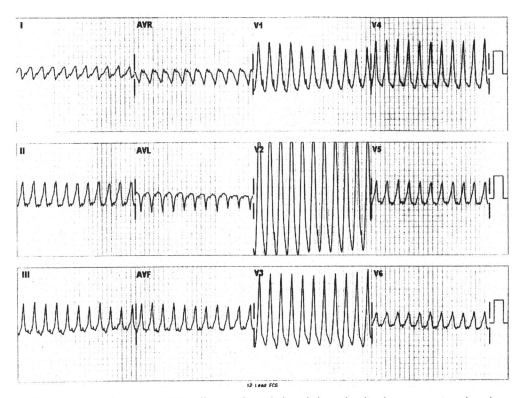

Figure 3A. Atrial pacing at 230 milliseconds cycle length from the distal coronary sinus length demonstrates a pattern consistent with a left-sided accessory pathway. The delta waves are positive from V_1 to V_6 and in the inferior leads. However, the delta wave is negative in avL and predominantly positive in lead I. It likely represents a fusion of a left lateral and a left posterior accessory pathway.

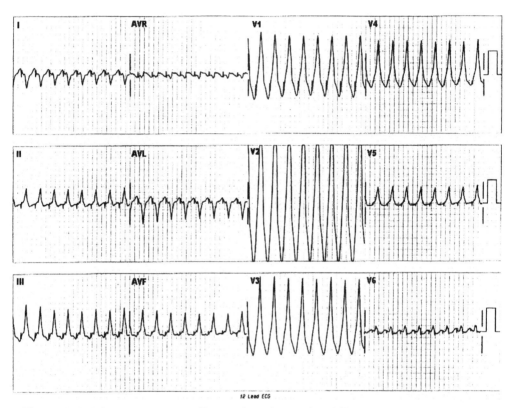

Figure 3B. Atrial pacing at a 300 milliseconds cycle reveals a different pattern. The precordial leads are also consistent with a left-sided accessory pathway. The direction of the delta waves is most consistent with a left lateral accessory pathway. The relatively narrow QRS complex in the front plane suggests fusion.

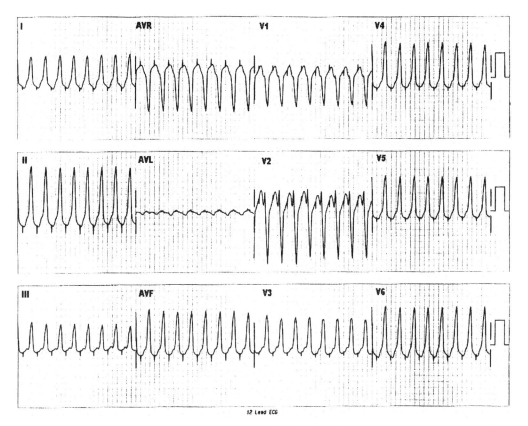

Figure 4. Atrial pacing at 300 milliseconds cycle length reveals a pattern most consistent with an anterior septal accessory pathway. However, anterior septal accessory pathways do not typically have a negative delta wave in lead avL, suggestion fusion with a left lateral accessory pathway.

suggestive of a posterior septal bypass tract should raise suspicion of a second bypass tract acting as the retrograde limb of the circuit.[23] Figure 5 demonstrates initiation of a pre-excited tachycardia that uses an anterior septal accessory pathway as the antegrade limb. Retrograde conduction is concentric, consistent with either posterior septal or A-V junction conduction. In Figure 6 there is an example of a pre-excited tachycardia using 2 accessory pathways. Once again, the anterior septal accessory pathway is the antegrade limb but a left lateral accessory pathway is now the retrograde limb.

Multiple accessory pathways may also be identified by changes in the retrograde atrial activation sequence during ventricular stimulation or circus movement tachycardia. Ventricular pacing may reveal a retrograde activation sequence different from that expected based on the antegrade pre-excitation pattern. In Figure 7A, there is evidence of an anterior septal accessory pathway. However, in Figure 7B, during ventricular pacing the earliest retrograde atrial activation is seen in the coronary sinus, consistent with presence of a left-sided accessory pathway.

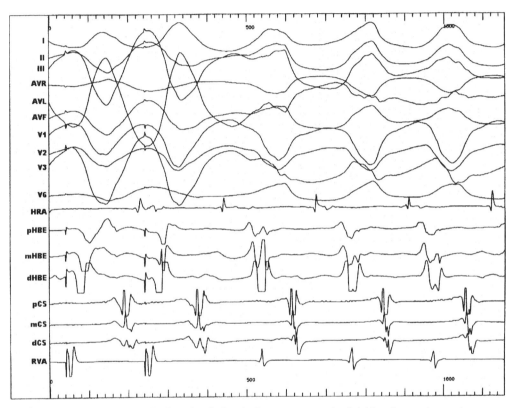

Figure 5. Premature ventricular stimulation induces a pre-excited A-V reciprocating tachycardia that uses an anterior septal accessory pathway as the antegrade limb. The retrograde sequence is concentric and may represent conduction via the A-V junction or a posterior septal accessory pathway.

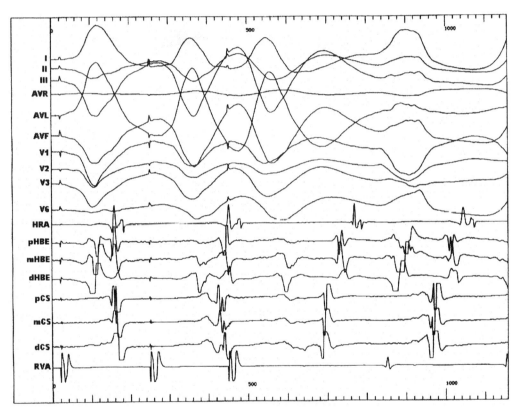

Figure 6. Premature ventricular stimulation induces a pre-excited AVRT that uses 2 accessory pathways. An anterior septal accessory pathway is the antegrade limb and a left lateral accessory pathway is the retrograde limb with the earliest atrial activity in the distal coronary sinus.

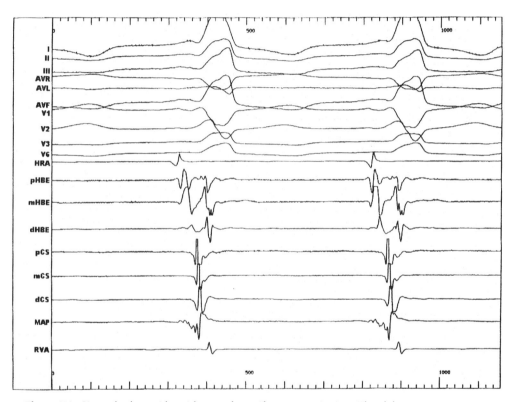

Figure 7A. Sinus rhythm with evidence of manifest pre-excitation. The delta waves are negative in leads V_1, V_2, and avL. The delta waves are positive in leads I, II, III, avF, and V_3-V_6. This suggests an anterior septal accessory pathway. There may be fusion with conduction from a left-sided accessory pathway because the delta wave is negative in avL.

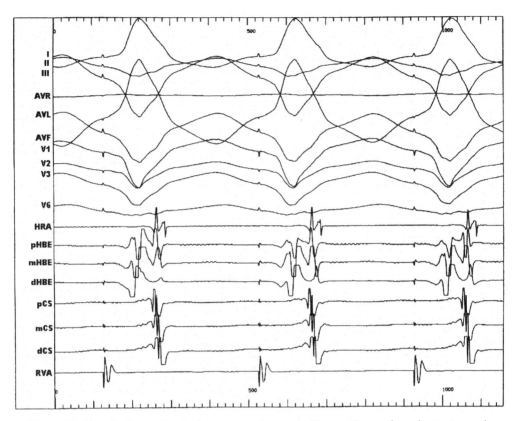

Figure 7B. Ventricular pacing in the same patient as in Figure 7A reveals earliest retrograde atrial activation sequence in the distal coronary sinus, consistent with a left lateral accessory pathway.

The retrograde activation sequence during AV reciprocating tachycardia (AVRT) also may be important in identifying multiple accessory pathways. During initiation of the tachycardia, during the same tachycardia, or during tachycardias, there may be evidence of a change in the retrograde atrial activation sequence. Figure 8 demonstrates the ventricular premature stimulation with retrograde atrial activation initially earliest in the distal coronary sinus. The sequence changes to the proximal coronary sinus being earliest, suggesting presence of a left posterior as well as a left lateral accessory pathway. There may also be shifts from antidromic tachycardia to orthodromic tachycardia.[18] The greater incidence of concealed bypass tracts in patients with multiple bypass tracts should lead to a thorough invasive evaluation for evidence of eccentric ventriculo-atrial conduction pre- or postablation.[20,24] Variation of the morphology of the retrograde P wave during reentrant tachycardia should also suggest multiple bypass tracts.[16]

Despite these various methods of identifying possible multiple accessory pathways, many accessory pathways are not identified until after catheter ablation or surgical dissection of 1 or more pathways.[16] Failure to detect the pres-

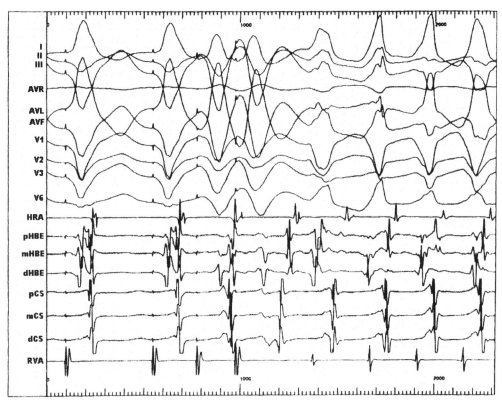

Figure 8. At the left side of the panel ventricular premature stimulation with 2 extrastimuli is shown. The retrograde atrial activation sequence following the second premature extrastimulus is earliest in the distal coronary sinus, indicating presence of a left lateral accessory pathway. The coronary sinus catheter is held constant. On the right side of the panel, the earliest atrial activation has shifted to the proximal coronary sinus, indicating presence also of a left posterior accessory pathway.

ence of multiple accessory pathways during preoperative electrophysiological study has been reported in as many as 25–35% of the surgical series and up to 40% of patients of patients in the catheter ablation series.[4,18,25] There may be a number of reasons for failure to identify these accessory pathways. The changes in pre-excitation pattern may be subtle in shifting from 1 accessory pathway to another. One accessory pathway may preferentially conduct during atrial pacing or participate in pre-excited tachycardias. Similarly, 1 accessory pathway may be responsible for the retrograde limb during reciprocating tachycardia or for conduction during ventricular pacing. There also may be fusion of accessory pathway conduction antegrade or retrograde. Repetitive concealed conduction into the bypass tract during AVRT may preclude identification of that pathway before ablation of the first accessory bypass tract.[7,26] The relative frequency of concealed bypass tracts in patients with multiple bypass tracts lends credence to this theory, since antegrade mapping is precluded. Bypass tracts that are close to each other are difficult to separate from each other and the trauma incurred by mapping for one may temporarily interrupt the conduction properties of the other.[18,20] The relative frequency of concealed bypass tracts in patients with multiple bypass tracts limits mapping to ventricular pacing with a reduced chance of using accessory bypass potentials to localize the pathway.[20] Using pace mapping in patients with bilateral concealed pathways leads to different sequences of retrograde conduction depending upon the site of pacing.[18] Septal pathways may not lend themselves to electrophysiological detection because of confusion with midline retrograde conduction.[7] The use of intravenous verapamil or adenosine may assist in differentiating one from the other. A shift in pre-excitation pattern or retrograde atrial activation sequence during adenosine administration may reflect the contribution of conduction via the A-V junction as well as that of adenosine-sensitive accessory pathways.

Distribution of Multiple Accessory Bypass Tracts

In patients with multiple accessory atrioventricular pathways, the commonest combination is right free wall and posteroseptal bypass tracts.[5,7,8] Other common combinations have been reported such as left and right free wall and ipsilateral, multiple left free wall.[16,20] A critical distance needs to separate the 2 limbs of AVRT to allow it to sustain itself. Hence a posterior septal bypass tract, due to its proximity to the AV node, can be a limb of an antidromic reciprocating tachycardia only if another bypass tract is present.[23]

Arrhythmias Associated with Multiple Accessory Bypass Tracts

Multiple accessory pathways may participate in each of the 4 types of arrhythmias: 1) orthodromic AVRT; 2) antidromic AVRT; 3) atrial fibrillation; and 4) other arrhythmias such as A-V nodal reentry with accessory pathway as a bystander. The presence of 2 or more accessory pathways, along with the AV node-His bundle, allows for a large number of possible reentrant tachycardias. The accessory pathways involved in the reentrant circuit must have disparate electrophysiological characteristics that would satisfy the conditions of reentry such as unidirectional block. In addition multiple accessory pathways may act as bystanders, creating varying degrees of fusion antegrade or retrograde. The observed rapid conduction properties of pathways in patients with multiple bypass tracts probably lends these pathways to a myriad of arrhythmias.[18,20,27]

In orthodromic AVRT, the antegrade conduction occurs down the AV node with the bypass tract acting as the retrograde limb and is the most common associated arrhythmia. There may be a shift from 1 accessory pathway as the retrograde limb to another accessory pathway or there may fusion between 2 accessory pathways in the retrograde limb.

In antidromic reciprocating tachycardia, characterized by a pre-excited wide complex QRS, antegrade conduction occurs down the accessory bypass tract, while the AV node or a second accessory pathway may act as the retrograde limb of the tachycardia circuit. There is a higher incidence of multiple bypass tracts in those patients with antidromic reciprocating tachycardia where 22 of 374 (6%) of patients with single bypass tracts had antidromic reciprocating tachycardia induced compared to 20 of 61 (33%) patients with multiple bypass tracts.[23] Multiple bypass tracts have also been reported in patients with the permanent form of junctional reciprocating tachycardia.[28] During antidromic tachycardia, there may be a shift from 1 accessory pathway to another in the antegrade limb or the retrograde limb.

Rapid antegrade conduction via accessory pathways in atrial fibrillation may lead to ventricular fibrillation (VF) and sudden cardiac death. Data from Olmsted County, Minnesota, suggest that this incidence is 0.15% per patient-year.[29] Although the incidence is low, patients with multiple bypass tracts are at greater risk of sudden cardiac death.[27,30,31] Patients with multiple bypass tracts have shorter R-R interval during atrial fibrillation.[7,20,27] The shortest R-R intervals during atrial fibrillation and antegrade and retrograde refractory periods were significantly shorter in patients with multiple bypass tracts (228 ± 16 milliseconds versus 250 ± 21 milliseconds, 233 ± 18 milliseconds versus 270 ± 32 milliseconds, and 238 ± 10 milliseconds versus 262 ± 21 milliseconds respectively, $P<0.05$).[18] Antegrade and retrograde accessory bypass tract refractory periods are also significantly shorter in patients with multiple bypass tracts (278 ± 67 milliseconds versus 299 ± 81 milliseconds, $P<0.05$ and 259 ± 39 milliseconds versus 273 ± 61 milliseconds, $P<0.05$ respectively).[20] In a series of 251 patients with the Wolff-Parkinson-White syndrome reported by Teo et al, the 31 (12.4%) patients with multiple accessory pathways had a 3-fold increase in risk for VF.[27] Although an RR interval of less than 250 milliseconds in atrial fibrillation was found to be the only independent risk factor associated with VF, the presence of multiple bypass tracts increased the positive predictive value of RR less than 250 milliseconds in atrial fibrillation from 9% to 22%.[27]

On the other hand, in a series of 690 patients with Wolff-Parkinson-White syndrome, sudden cardiac death was reported in 15 patients (2.2%).[32] Of the 16 bypass tracts identified, 11 were septal; only 1 patient had multiple bypass tracts, a left lateral and a left posteroseptal bypass tract. The presence of septal bypass tract, factors that increase adrenergic tone and male sex but not multiple bypass tracts, were associated with a history of aborted sudden cardiac death.[32] The small number of patients with multiple accessory pathways may have limited this analysis. In the series reported by Huang et al, the presence of multiple bypass tracts was not significantly associated with VF.[20]

Atrial fibrillation is also more common in patients with multiple bypass tracts.[18] This may be in part due to the potential for rapid retrograde conduction during AVRT which may act to induce atrial fibrillation.

Patients with multiple accessory pathways may also have arrhythmias such as AV nodal reentrant tachycardia (AVNRT) with the accessory pathways serving as bystanders. The ECG pattern may reflect fusion among several accessory pathways.

Radiofrequency of Multiple Bypass Tracts

Radiofrequency ablation of accessory atrioventricular bypass tracts has become a safe and successful method of treating patients with the Wolff-Parkinson-White syndrome.[11,13] Radiofrequency ablation may be performed more frequently in patients with multiple accessory pathways than single accessory pathways. In the series reported by Chen et al, 20 patients among 145 consecutive patients with Wolff-Parkinson-White syndrome had multiple accessory pathways.[18] These patients had a greater incidence of atrial fibrillation and antidromic reentrant tachycardia (40% versus 12.8% and 15% versus 0.8% respectively, $P<0.05$). In a series of 858 patients with the Wolff-Parkinson-White syndrome, Huang et al[20] found 73 patients (8.5%) with multiple bypass tracts. Concealed bypass tracts were commoner than manifest and the commonest combination was 2 left free wall bypass tracts. Separation distance had been defined as greater than 3 centimeters between pathways. The success of radiofrequency ablation and the incidence of complications in some series is comparable between single and multiple accessory pathways (99% versus 98% and 1.1% versus 2.7% respectively).[20] In other series the success rate for ablation was lower for multiple accessory pathways than the rate for single bypass tracts (89% versus 98%, $P<0.01$).[16]

The procedure time (2.0 ± 1.1 hours versus 3.1 ± 1.2 hours, $P<0.05$) and radiation time (29 ± 19 minutes versus 48 ± 26 minutes $P<0.05$) are greater for the ablation of the multiple accessory pathways.[20] Although the recurrence rate per patient with multiple bypass tracts was higher (2.5% versus 9.5%, $P<0.05$), the recurrence rate per pathway was not (2.5% versus 4.5%, $P>0.05$).[20] In another series the overall recurrence rate was 12% or 5% recurrence per tract, similar to the recurrence rate for single bypass tract radiofrequency ablation.[16] In the series by Huang et al of the 7 pathways that recurred, 2 were new.[20] Their location close to formerly ablated pathways pointed to catheter trauma as a possible cause for failure of earlier detection after the original ablation. These pathways may also have represented part of a broad insertion of a single accessory pathway.

Although dual AV nodal pathways are seen in 10–20% of patients undergoing electrophysiological evaluation,[33,34] AVNRT in patients with multiple accessory pathways is unusual. Among 402 patients with accessory bypass tracts who had undergone pathway ablation, 32 (8%) patients had either AVNRT, AV nodal reentrant echoes, or dual AV nodal pathways.[35] Following the successful ablation of the atrioventricular bypass tracts, only 1 patient developed AVNRT. Patients found to have the substrate for AVNRT should have ablation directed at eliminating the tachycardia only if it had been documented clinically.

Summary

The presence of multiple bypass tracts is not an infrequent occurrence in patients with the Wolff-Parkinson-White syndrome. With radiofrequency catheter ablation becoming a popular therapeutic tool, recognition of the existence of multiple bypass tracts in anticipation of ablation would reduce the recurrence of supraventricular tachycardia. Clues can be derived from observing the 12-lead electrocardiogram at baseline and during atrial pacing, atrial stimulation, atrial fibrillation, atrial premature complexes, and AVRT. The relatively greater incidence of concealed bypass tracts in patients with multiple bypass tracts emphasizes the need for a thorough electrophysiological evaluation at the end of each radiofrequency ablation to exclude this possibility.

Multiple bypass tracts have rapid conduction properties and a higher incidence of antidromic AVRT as well as atrial fibrillation. Controversy exists as to whether multiple bypass tracts are associated with a higher incidence of sudden cardiac death. Certain congenital heart disorders such as Ebstein's anomaly and the clinical occurrence of pre-excited reentrant tachycardia are associated with an increased incidence of multiple bypass tracts. Right free wall, anterior septal, and septal bypass tracts occur more frequently in patients with multiple bypass tracts.

Although the ablation of multiple bypass tracts carries a high success rate, the rate of recurrence per patient is relatively high. The number of lesions required, the length of the procedure and exposure to radiation are also increased. Although careful electrophysiological evaluation, especially after ablating the first bypass tract, is necessary to exclude the presence of multiple bypass tracts, late reappearance may be unavoidable.

References

1. Lunel AA. Significance of annulus fibrosus of heart in relation to AV conduction and ventricular activation in cases of Wolff-Parkinson-White syndrome. *Br Heart J* 1972;34:1263–1271.
2. Chung KY, Walsh TJ, Massie E. Wolff-Parkinson-White syndrome. *Am Heart J* 1965;69:116–133.
3. Krahn AD, Manfreda J, Tate RB, et al. The natural history of preexcitation in men: the Manitoba follow-up study. *Ann Intern Med* 1992;116:456–460.
4. Sealy WC, Gallagher JJ. Surgical problems with multiple accessory pathways of atrioventricular conduction. *J Cardiovasc Surg* 1981;81:707–717.
5. Selle JG, Sealy WC, Gallagher JJ, et al. Technical considerations in the surgical approach to multiple accessory pathways in the Wolff-Parkinson-White syndrome. *Ann Thorac Surg* 1987;43:579–584.
6. Iwa T, Magara T, Watanabe Y, et al. Interruption of multiple accessory conduction pathways in the Wolff-Parkinson-White syndrome. *Ann Thorac Surg* 1980;30:313–325.
7. Colavita PG, Packer DL, Pressley JC, et al. Frequency, diagnosis, and clinical characteristics of patients with multiple accessory atrioventricular pathways. *Am J Cardiol* 1987;59:601–606.
8. Gallagher JJ, Sealy WC, Kasell J, et al. Multiple accessory pathways in patients with the pre-excitation syndrome. *Circulation* 1976;54:571–591.
9. de Buitleir M, Sousa J, Bolling SF, et al. Reduction in medical care cost associated with radiofrequency catheter ablation of accessory pathways. *Am J Cardiol* 1991;68:1656–1661.

10. Leather RA, Leitch JW, Klein GJ, et al. Radiofrequency catheter ablation of accessory pathways: a learning experience. *Am J Cardiol* 1991;68: 1651–1655.

11. Jackman WM, Wang X, Friday KJ, et al. Catheter ablation of accessory atrioventricular pathways (Wolff-Parkinson-White syndrome) by radiofrequency current. *N Engl J Med* 1991;324:1605–1611.

12. Langberg JJ, Calkins H, Kim YN, et al. Recurrence of conduction in accessory atrioventricular connections after initially successful radiofrequency catheter ablation. *J Am Coll Cardiol* 1992;19:1588–1592.

13. Lesh MD, Van Hare GF, Schamp DJ, et al. Curative percutaneous catheter ablation using radiofrequency energy for accessory pathways in all locations: results in 100 consecutive patients. *J Am Coll Cardiol* 1992;19: 1303–1309.

14. Pressley JC, Wharton JM, Tang ASL, et al. Effect of Ebstein's anomaly on short- and long-term outcome of surgically treated patients with Wolff-Parkinson-White syndrome. *Circulation* 1992;86:1147–1155.

15. Calkins H, Prystowsky E, Berger RD, et al. Recurrence of conduction following radiofrequency catheter ablation procedures: relationship to ablation target and electrode temperature. *J Cardiovasc Electrophysiol* 1996;7: 704–712.

16. Yeh SJ, Wang CC, Wen MS, et al. Radiofrequency ablation in multiple accessory pathways and the physiologic implications. *Am J Cardiol* 1993;71: 1174–1180.

17. Swartz JF, Tracy CM, Fletcher RD. Radiofrequency endocardial catheter ablation of accessory atrioventricular pathway atrial insertion sites. *Circulation* 1993;87:487–499.

18. Chen SA, Hsia CP, Chiang CE, et al. Reappraisal of radiofrequency ablation of multiple accessory pathways. *Am Heart J* 1993;125:760–771.

19. Haïssaguerre M, Gaïta F, Marcus FI, et al. Radiofrequency catheter ablation of accessory pathways: a contemporary review. *J Cardiovasc Electrophysiol* 1994;5:532–552.

20. Huang JL, Chen SA, Tai CT, et al. Long-term results of radiofrequency catheter ablation in patients with multiple accessory pathways. *Am J Cardiol* 1996;78:1375–1379.

21. Vidaillet HJ Jr, Pressley JC, Henke E, et al. Familial occurrence of accessory atrioventricular pathways (preexcitation syndrome). *N Engl J Med* 1987;317:65–69.

22. Porter CJ, Holmes DR. Preexcitation syndromes associated with congenital heart disease. In: Benditt DG, Benson DW, eds. *Cardiac Preexcitation Syndrome: Origins, Evaluation and Treatment*. Boston, MA: Martinus Nijhoff, 1986. p. 291

23. Bardy GH, Parker DC, German LD, et al. Preexcited reciprocating tachycardia in patients with Wolff-Parkinson-White syndrome: incidence and mechanisms. *Circulation* 1984;70:377–391.

24. Yeh SJ, Wang CC, Lin FC, et al. Usefulness of predischarge electrophysiologic study in predicting late outcome after surgical ablation of the accessory pathway in the Wolff-Parkinson-White syndrome. *Am J Cardiol* 1992;69:909–912.

25. Guiraudon GM, Klein GJ, Sharma AD, et al. Surgery for the Wolff-Parkinson-White syndrome, the epicardial approach. In: Zipes DP, Jalife J, eds. Cardiac Electrophysiology: From Cell to Bedside. Philadelphia, PA: WB Saunders,1990. pp 907–915.
26. Klein GJ, Yee R, Sharma AD. Concealed conduction in accessory atrioventricular pathways: an important determinant of the expression of arrhythmias in patients with Wolff-Parkinson-White syndrome. *Circulation* 1984; 70:402–411.
27. Teo WS, Klein GJ, Guiraudon GM, et al. Multiple accessory pathways in the Wolff-Parkinson-White syndrome as a risk factor for ventricular fibrillation. *Am J Cardiol* 1991;67:889–891.
28. Shih HT, Miles WM, Klein LS, ct al. Multiple accessory pathways in the permanent form of junctional reciprocating tachycardia. *Am J Cardiol* 1994;73:361–367.
29. Munger TM, Packer DL, Hammill SC, et al. A population study of the natural history of Wolff-Parkinson-White syndrome in Olmsted County, Minnesota, 1953–1989. *Circulation* 1993;87:866–873.
30. Klein GJ, Bashore TM, Sellers TD, et al. Ventricualr fibrillation in the Wolff-Parkinson-White syndrome. *N Engl J Med* 1979;301:1080–1085.
31. Montoya PT, Brugada P, Smeets J, et al. Ventricular fibrillation in the Wolff-Parkinson-White syndrome. *Eur Heart J* 1991;12:144–150.
32. Timmermans C, Smeets JLRM, Rodriguez LM, et al. Aborted sudden death in the Wolff-Parkinson-White syndrome. *Am J Cardiol* 1995;76:492–494.
33. Denes P, Wu D, Dhingra R, et al. Dual atrioventricular nodal pathways: a common electrophysiological response. *Br Heart J* 1975;37:1069–1086.
34. Reyes WJ, Milstein S, Dunnigan A, et al. Surgical implications of dual atrioventricular nodal physiology in patients with accessory atrioventricular connections [abstract]. *Circulation* 1989;80:II-41.
35. Zardini M, Leitch JW, Guiraudon GM, et al. Atrioventricular nodal reentry and dual atrioventricular node physiology in patients undergoing accessory pathway ablation. *Am J Cardiol* 1990;66:1388–1389.
36. Calkins H, Sousa J, El-Atassi R, et al. Diagnosis and cure of the Wolff-Parkinson-White syndrome or paroxysmal supraventricular tachycardias during a single electrophysiologic test. *N Engl J Med* 1991;324:1612–1618.
37. Josephson ME. Preexcitation syndromes. In: Josephson ME. *Clinical Cardiac Electrophysiology, Techniques and Interpretations* . Philadelphia, PA: Lea & Febiger, 1993. pp 311–416.
38. Wellens HJJ, Durrer D. Effect of procainamide, quinidine, and ajmaline in the Wolff-Parkinson-White syndrome. *Circulation* 1974;50:114–120.

Part VI

Radiofrequency Catheter Ablation of Ventricular Tachycardia

Chapter 29

Ablation of Idiopathic Left Ventricular Tachycardia

Delon Wu, M.D., Ming-Shien Wen, M.D., San-Jou Yeh, M.D.

Ventricular tachycardia occurs in patients without structural heart disease. In 1979, Zipes et al[1] reported 3 patients with no significant cardiac abnormalities, in whom ventricular tachycardia was inducible with rapid atrial pacing. The tachycardia had a QRS configuration of complete right bundle branch block and left axis deviation. They suggested that the origin of this tachycardia was from a small area near the posteroinferior portion of the left ventricle and the mechanism was either reentrant excitation or triggered activity. In 1981, Belhassen et al[2] reported the effectiveness of verapamil on ventricular tachycardia displaying a QRS of right bundle branch block and left axis deviation in a young man with no organic heart disease. However, it was Lin et al[3] who first designated the tachycardia with a QRS of right bundle branch block and superior axis as a unique clinical entity with specific properties in 1983. This tachycardia occurs predominantly in young male patients and is responsive to verapamil but usually not to adenosine. It can be induced and terminated by programmed stimulation.[1-6] A sharp high-frequency Purkinje potential is registered before the local electrogram from the middle or lower portion of the left interventricular septum during tachycardia.[5,6] Reentry is likely to be the operative mechanism.[3,4] Idiopathic ventricular tachycardia with a QRS pattern of right bundle branch block may occasionally display an inferior axis.[4] This tachycardia is identical to the tachycardia with a superior axis. Rarely, idiopathic ventricular tachycardia originating from the left ventricle may present with a QRS of atypical left or right bundle branch block and inferior axis.[7,8] The latter tachycardia is provocable by exercise, is responsive to

From Huang SKS, Wilber DJ (eds.): *Radiofrequency Catheter Ablation of Cardiac Arrhythmias: Basic Concepts and Clinical Applications,* 2nd ed. Armonk, NY: Futura Publishing Company, Inc. ©2000.

Supported in part by grants from the National Science Council (NSC 86–2314-B-182–033 and NSC 86–2314-B-182–061) of the Republic of China, Taipei, Taiwan

both verapamil and adenosine,[9,10] and is different from the tachycardia with a QRS of right bundle branch block and a superior or an inferior axis.

Clinical Characteristics

Idiopathic left ventricular tachycardia occurs predominantly in young male patients with the age of onset usually between 15 and 40 years and a male to female ratio of about 3 to 1.[3,4,10–13] The heart rate during tachycardia is usually between 150 and 200 beats per minute, but it may be as slow as 120 beats per min or as fast as 250 beats per min. Alternans of the cycle length is noted frequently during tachycardia;[3,13,14] otherwise, the rate of tachycardia is rather stable. The QRS morphology is that of complete right bundle branch block with an R/S ratio of less than one in leads V_5 and V_6 (Figure 1). The QRS duration is narrower than that of the ventricular tachycardia due to previous myocardial infarction or dilated cardiomyopathy. Most patients display a superior or an indeterminate QRS axis during tachycardia, but an inferior QRS axis is seen occasionally. The resting electrocardiogram during sinus rhythm is normal; however, a symmetrical T-wave inversion may be seen in inferior and lateral precordial leads following attacks of tachycardia (Figure 2).[3,15] The attack of tachycardia is paroxysmal without a precipitating factor and may last for minutes to hours; rarely it may persist for days. Sometimes, the tachycardia may be incessant. Most patients experience only palpitation or mild dizziness during tachycardia; syncope occurs infrequently. Exercise or isoproterenol infusion

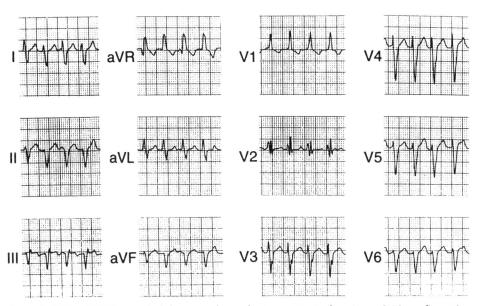

Figure 1. 12-lead ECG recorded during tachycardia in a patient, showing a QRS configuration of complete right bundle branch block (QRS duration, 0.12 seconds), superior axis (-120°), and atrioventricular dissociation. Note an R/S ratio of less than one in lateral precordial leads.

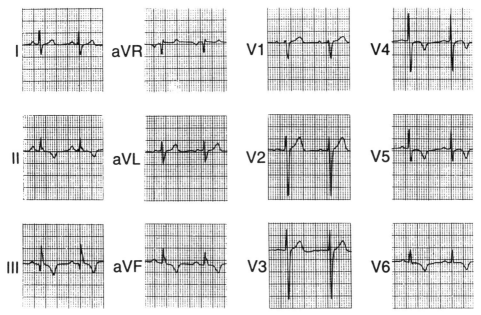

Figure 2. 12-lead ECG recorded during sinus rhythm following termination of tachycardia in the same patient as in Figure 1, showing symmetrical T wave inversion in inferior (leads II, III & aVF) and lateral precordial (leads V_4-V_6) leads.

may occasionally provoke attack of tachycardia.[1,13,16,17] Carotid sinus massage or Valsalva maneuver has no effect on this tachycardia.[15,17,18] This tachycardia has a benign course. It may decrease in frequency and disappear as the time goes by.[19] It is unusual to see this tachycardia in patients aged more than 55. However, cardiomegaly with congestive heart failure may result in patients with incessant tachycardia. Our experience includes 49 patients, who underwent radiofrequency ablation therapy for tachycardia between July 1991 and May 1997. There are 43 men and 6 women with a mean age of 28 ± 11 (standard deviation, SD) years (range, 12–57). All patients had no obvious structural heart disease by cardiovascular examination, chest radiograph, and two-dimensional Doppler echocardiographic examination, although 2 had mild hypertension, 1 had uremia, 15 had echocardiographic evidence of mitral valve prolapse, 4 had mitral valve prolapse with mild mitral regurgitation, and 3 had a decreased left ventricular ejection fraction as a result of incessant tachycardia. The left ventricular size and the ejection fraction returned to normal during follow-up period after successful ablation of the tachycardia in the latter 3 patients. Three patients presented with syncope, 10 patients with dizziness, and the others with palpitations. The duration of symptoms ranged from 1 month to 20 years. All 49 patients had clinically documented ventricular tachycardia that was responsive to verapamil, and all received from 1 to 4 antiarrhythmic drugs with variable effects prior to referral. The QRS configuration during tachycardia was of complete right bundle branch block and a superior QRS axis in 35 patients, indeterminate QRS axis in 12 patients, and an inferior QRS axis in 3 patients. The rate of tachycardia was 164 ± 24 beats per min (range, 125–214).

Electrophysiological Properties

Idiopathic left ventricular tachycardia is inducible by programmed stimulation with incremental atrial or ventricular pacing or delivery of atrial or ventricular extrastimulus.[3–6,20–22] However, electrical induction of this tachycardia is slightly less reproducible as compared to that of ischemic ventricular tachycardia. Manipulation of the catheter in the left ventricle may render this tachycardia noninducible. Infusion of isoproterenol is frequently necessary for induction of the tachycardia. An inverse relationship between the first coupling interval of the induced tachycardia and the coupling interval of the initiating extrastimulus or the paced cycle length is usually noted.[3,4] The cycle length of the induced tachycardia is rather stable without a concordant shortening in relating to the paced cycle length or the coupling interval of the extrastimulus that induces the tachycardia. Alternans of the cycle length occurs occasionally.[3,13,14] The most unique finding of this tachycardia is the registration of a sharp high frequency Purkinje potential preceding the local electrogram over the middle and lower portion of the left interventricular septum during tachycardia.[5,6,11,23] Of the 49 patients studied in our laboratory, the earliest registered high frequency Purkinje spike was located at the inferoapical septum in 29, at the midseptum in 17, at the anterolateral free wall in 2, and at the high anterior free wall in 1. The interval between the Purkinje spike and the onset of QRS was 32.3 ± 4.8 milliseconds (range, 25–43). Unlike ischemic ventricular tachycardia, fragmented or continuous potentials were not seen during diastole.[11,12] Entrainment of the tachycardia can be demonstrated readily by overdrive pacing from sites in both right and left ventricles, especially from the right ventricular outflow tract.[4,23–25] The tachycardia is terminable by programmed stimulation.

Pharmacological Responses

Intravenous verapamil slows the rate of tachycardia progressively and then terminates the tachycardia.[3–5,21,22] However, nonsustained tachycardia may continue to occur for a while after termination. The tachycardia is usually rendered noninducible after verapamil. Chronic oral verapamil is effective in preventing the recurrence of tachycardia.[3,19,20] We have also observed that intravenous diltiazem or oral diltiazem is equally effective in terminating the tachycardia or preventing the recurrence of tachycardia. Responses to other antiarrhythmic agents such as lidocaine, procainamide, propranolol, ajimaline, sotalol, esmolol, or amiodarone are less consistent and usually ineffective.[3,19,20] The effect of adenosine on tachycardia is controversial. Ng et al[9] administered adenosine triphosphate intravenously to 15 patients in incremental doses, from 2.5 mg to a maximum of 30 mg, and none showed a response. Griffith et al[10] gave intravenous adenosine to 7 patients in incremental doses to a maximum of 0.25 mg/kg and none responded. In contrast, DeLacey et al[26] reported response to adenosine in a patient with idiopathic ventricular tachycardia of right bundle branch block and superior axis and Lee et al[13] noted a response to adenosine in 6 of 22 patients with verapamil-sensitive idiopathic left ventricular tachycardia.

Catheter Ablation

Radiofrequency ablation is an effective therapeutic modality for idiopathic left ventricular tachycardia.[11,23] With this therapy, radiofrequency current is delivered to a site over middle or inferoapical portion of the left interventricular septum, where the high frequency Purkinje spike is registered the earliest and where the pace map 12-lead ECG displays a QRS morphology resembling that during tachycardia. Klein et al,[27] using this technique, delivered radiofrequency currents to the mid-posterior portion of the left ventricular septum and successfully ablated a patient with idiopathic ventricular tachycardia that exhibited a QRS pattern of right bundle branch block and superior axis. Page et al[28] successfully ablated 2 patients by delivery of radiofrequency currents to a site approximately two thirds of the way toward the apex at the left interventricular septum, where a sharp spike was registered at 35 and 45 milliseconds respectively before the onset of QRS complex during tachycardia. Pacing at this site produced a QRS pattern that closely resembled the pattern seen during tachycardia. However, pacing at several sites without successful ablation also produced an ECG pattern indistinguishable from that at the successful ablation site. Nakagawa et al[11] studied 8 patients with idiopathic left ventricular tachycardia. In these patients, the earliest Purkinje potential was registered at the posteroapical left ventricular septum and preceded the QRS during tachycardia by 15 to 42 milliseconds (mean±SD, 27±9). In 7 of the 8 patients, successful ablation was obtained at a site which showed a registration of the earliest Purkinje potential at the posterior left ventricular septum, while in one patient, ablation was successful at a site recording a late Purkinje potential fusing with the earliest ventricular activation. Pace mapping during tachycardia at the successful ablation site displayed a similar QRS configuration and a stimulus-QRS interval equal to the spike-QRS interval during tachycardia. However, a similar QRS pattern by pacing at nearby sites that registered a late spike potential was also observed. Coggins et al[12] conducted radiofrequency ablation in 8 patients with idiopathic left ventricular tachycardia. Successful ablation was obtained at posterior left ventricular septum midway between apex and base in 7 patients and at the anteroseptal site in 1 patient. High frequency Purkinje potentials were not observed at the local electrogram from the successful ablation site in 7 of 8 patients, while in 1 patient a Purkinje spike was registered 10 to 29 milliseconds before the QRS during tachycardia at the successful ablation site. They noted that at the successful ablation site, at least 11 of 12 leads displayed a pace map R/S ratio matched to the 12-lead ECG of clinical ventricular tachycardia. Kottkamp et al[17] studied 5 patients with idiopathic left ventricular tachycardia with a QRS pattern of right bundle branch block and left axis deviation. One of these 5 patients also had a tachycardia with a QRS pattern of right bundle branch block and right axis deviation. Activation mapping during tachycardia revealed that the earliest activation site was recorded in the left ventricular septum, and was distributed over a wide area from the base to the mid-apical region. Delivery of radiofrequency currents to the earliest endocardial activation site was successful in eliminating the tachycardia in only 2 of the 5 patients. In 2 patients, mid-diastolic fragmented potentials were recorded in a small area at the mid-apical inferior region and at the basal septum respectively; delivery of radiofrequency currents to the area showing fragmented mid-diastolic potentials resulted in elimination of the tachycardia in both patients.

Between July 1991 and May 1997, a total of 49 consecutive patients with verapamil-sensitive idiopathic left ventricular tachycardia underwent radiofrequency ablation therapy in our laboratory. All 49 patients received programmed ventricular stimulation to a maximum of 3 ventricular extrastimuli at 2 different driven cycle lengths from the right ventricular apex and outflow tract. If tachycardia was not induced, the stimulation was repeated after isoproterenol infusion (1 to 4 µg/min to achieve a 20% increase in sinus rate). If ventricular tachycardia was induced, the potential ablation sites were searched by both the activation and pace mapping techniques in 42 patients (Figures 3–8). The ablation catheter was introduced to a femoral artery and advanced retrogradely into the left ventricle. The mapping efforts were initially concentrated at the inferoapical septum. If an ideal ablation site was not found in this area, the tip of the ablation catheter was then moved upward to the midseptal area. The endocardial activation time was mapped by comparing the high frequency Purkinje potential to the onset of QRS during tachycardia. The radiofrequency currents were delivered to a site considered to be the tachycardia exit, where the endocardial activation was the earliest and preceded the onset of QRS by ≥25 milliseconds, and where pace map 12-lead ECG resembled that during ventricular tachycardia. A current strength of 20 to 35 watts for 10 to 20 seconds was delivered initially. If the tachycardia was terminated in 10 seconds, additional currents were applied to the same site for another 60 to 120 seconds. Programmed stimulation was repeated after ablation. If tachycardia was not inducible, the stimulation was repeated after isoproterenol infusion. Successful ablation was defined as inability to induce tachycardia by programmed stimulation with or without isoproterenol infusion. In the other 7 patients, radiofrequency ablation was attempted intentionally at a site away from the tachycardia exit in order to better define the circuit.[29] In these 7 patients, after the putative tachycardia exit site was defined, potential target site was searched at the midseptal area proximal to the exit site. The potential target site was the site where application of mechanical pressure to the catheter tip resulted in termination of ventricular tachycardia without inducing ventricular ectopies.[30] Test currents were then delivered to this site during induced tachycardia. If the tachycardia was terminated in 10 seconds, additional currents were applied to the same site for 60 to 120 seconds. The postablation stimulation protocol was conducted similarly as described above.

Successful ablation was achieved in 46 of 49 patients (94%). The successful ablation site was the inferoapical septum in 21 patients, the midseptum in

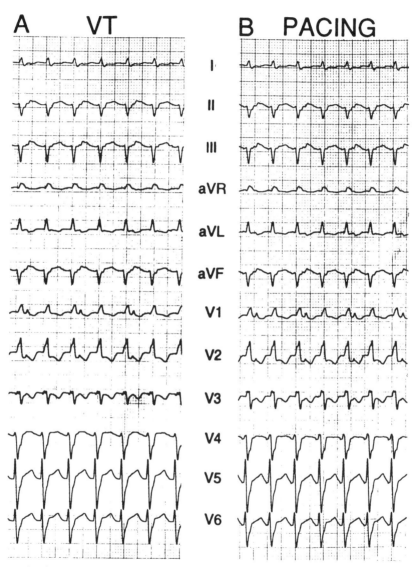

Figure 3. 12-lead ECG from a patient with a ventricular tachycardia originating from the inferoapical left ventricular septum, showing QRS configuration during spontaneous tachycardia (panel A) and during pace mapping at the successful ablation site (panel B). Note that the pace map QRS matches to that of the spontaneous tachycardia, and is of right bundle branch block and superior axis. VT = ventricular tachycardia.

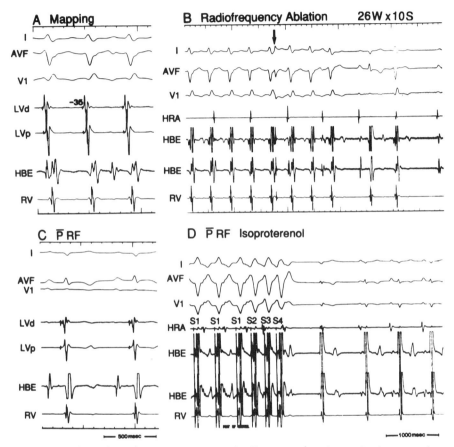

Figure 4. Recordings from the same patient as in Figure 3, showing activation mapping, radiofrequency ablation, and postablation electrogram and programmed stimulation. *A* shows recording of the earliest Purkinje spike that preceded the local electrogram and occurred 35 milliseconds before the onset of QRS during tachycardia at the successful ablation site in the inferoapical septum of the left ventricle. *B* shows delivery of radiofrequency currents 26 watts to this site for 10 seconds, resulting in termination of the tachycardia in 1.2 seconds. *C* shows persistence of the Purkinje spike at the successful ablation site during sinus rhythm after ablation. *D* shows no induction of ventricular tachycardia during isoproterenol infusion with programmed ventricular stimulation after ablation. I, AVF & V_1 = ECG leads I, AVF & V_1; HRA, HBE, LVd, LVp and RV = bipolar electrogram recorded from high right atrium, His bundle recording site, distal 2 electrodes of the ablation catheter in the left ventricle, proximal 2 electrodes of the ablation catheter in the left ventricle, and right ventricular apex; S_1 = basic driven stimulus; S_2 = the first extrastimulus; S_3 = the second extrastimulus; S_4 = the third extrastimulus.

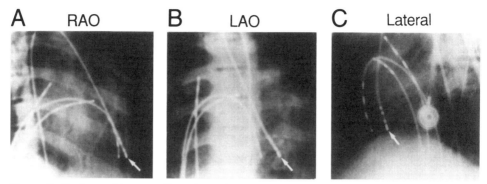

Figure 5. Radiographic recordings from the same patient as in Figures 3 and 4, showing catheter positions. Three electrode catheters were positioned in the high right atrium, across the tricuspid valve and in the right ventricular apex respectively. The tip of the ablation electrode was positioned at the inferoapical left ventricular septum (indicated by an arrow), where successful ablation was obtained. *A* was recorded at the right anterior oblique projection (RAO), *B* at the left anterior oblique projection (LAO), and *C* at the left lateral projection.

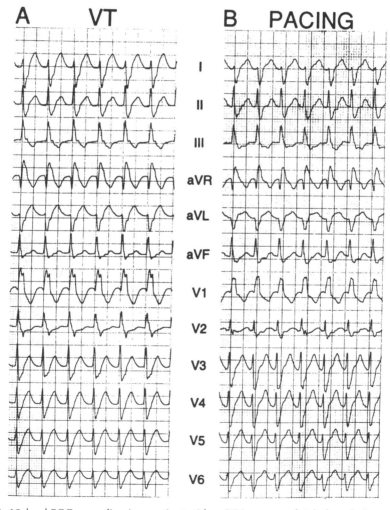

Figure 6. 12-lead ECG recording in a patient with a QRS pattern of right bundle branch block and inferior axis during spontaneous tachycardia (A), pacing at the successful ablation site in the high anterior left ventricular free wall (B). Note the paced QRS matches to that of the spontaneous tachycardia.

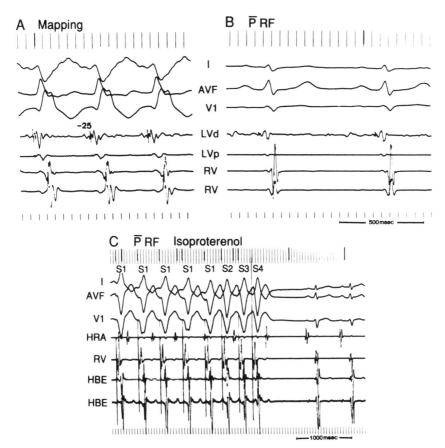

Figure 7. Recordings from the same patient as in Figure 6, showing activation mapping, postablation recording and postablation programmed stimulation. *A* shows the earliest registration of the Purkinje spike that preceded the onset of QRS by 25 milliseconds at the superior anterior left ventricular wall, where delivery of radiofrequency currents resulted in elimination of the tachycardia. *B* shows persistence of the Purkinje spike during sinus rhythm at the ablation site after successful ablation. *C* shows no induction of tachycardia during isoproterenol infusion after ablation.

15 patients, the anterior lateral wall in 2 patients, the high anterior wall in 1 patient, and a distant site at the midseptal area 3.1±0.7 cm away from the tachycardia exit in 7 patients. Patients with a superior or indeterminate QRS axis during tachycardia were ablated from inferoapical septum or midseptum (see Figures 3–5), while patients with an inferior QRS axis were ablated from anterolateral or high anterior left ventricular free wall (see Figures 6–8). The total procedure time, fluoroscopic time, and median number of current applications were 168±46 minutes, 44±32 minutes, and 3±5 respectively. There were no complications except for one patient who developed ventricular fibrillation during postablation programmed stimulation, which was converted to sinus rhythm by DC shock without sequela. During a follow-up duration of 38±14 months (range, 4–69), recurrence of tachycardia occurred in 5 of 46 pa-

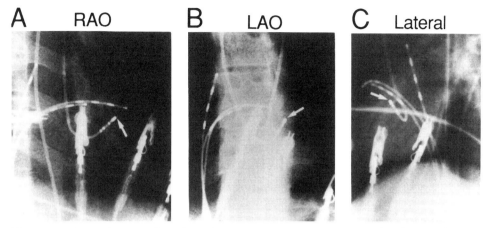

Figure 8. Radiographic recordings from the same patient as in Figures 6 and 7, showing the successful ablation site. The ablation catheter was introduced to a femoral artery and advanced retrogradely through the aorta into the left ventricle. The tip of the catheter was positioned at the successful ablation site in the superior anterior left ventricular free wall (indicated by an arrow).

tients (11%) who had successful ablation. All 5 patients with tachycardia recurrence were successfully ablated by a second trial.

Operative Mechanism

Triggered activity related to delayed afterdepolarizations has been suggested to be the operative mechanism in some patients with verapamil-sensitive idiopathic left ventricular tachycardia that displays a QRS configuration of right bundle branch block and superior axis by Zipes et al,[1] Sung et al,[16,31] and Bhandari et al.[32] These patients showed a concordant shortening of the initiating coupling interval of the tachycardia to the paced cycle length that induced tachycardia, but the cycle length of tachycardia was similar. In contrast, studies from several laboratories including our laboratory have unanimously demonstrated an inverse relation between the initiating coupling interval of the tachycardia and the paced cycle length that induced the tachycardia, and that entrainment can readily be demonstrated by overdrive ventricular pacing in almost every patient.[3,4,24,25] These observations strongly suggest that reentry is likely to be the operative mechanism of this tachycardia. Since the tachycardia could have been induced and entrained during rapid atrial or ventricular pacing, a concordant shortening of the first coupling interval of the tachycardia without affecting subsequent cycle length may be noted following cessation of rapid pacing. As to the nature of the reentry circuit, Ward et al[6] and Kottkamp et al[17] have suggested that it is a microreentry circuit confined to the territory of the posterior fascicle. Aizawa et al[33] conducted an entrainment study and compared the postpacing interval, measured from the last stimulus artifact to the high frequency Purkinje spike at the tachycardia exit site, and found that the postpacing interval was shorter at the right ventricular outflow tract than the right ventricular apex. They suggested that the right ventricular outflow tract is closer to the entrance of the reentry circuit, whereas the right ventricular apex is closer to the exit site. Findings from our laboratory that the tachycardia can be ablated from a distant site, 2 to 4 cm away from the tachycardia exit, suggest that the reentry circuit of this tachycardia is of considerable size not confined to a small area in the territory of the posterior fascicle.[29] Whether the Purkinje system is an essential portion of the tachycardia circuit has remained unanswered. The Purkinje spikes that preceded the local electrogram at the successful ablation site persist after ablation and are not specific to this tachycardia.[23] They are also recorded along the fascicular networks of the left bundle branch system in patients with no structural heart disease and no idiopathic left ventricular tachycardia. Thus, the Purkinje spike that is recorded over a wide area in the inferior and mid-left ventricular septum reflects the endocardial activation after emergence of the impulse from the exit site.[23,34] Regarding the anatomic substrate of this tachycardia, Suwa et al[35] and Thakur et al[36] implicated that the left ventricular fibromuscular band may be the essential part of the circuit as it is found in patients with idiopathic left ventricular tachycardia. However, our laboratory has shown that the left ventricular fibromuscular band is also present in patients with no structural heart disease and no idiopathic left ventricular tachycardia and therefore is not a specific arrhythmogenic substrate for this tachycardia.[37]

Idiopathic Ventricular Tachycardia Due to Triggered Activity from the Anterobasal Left Ventricle

A specific type of tachycardia originating from the right ventricular outflow tract is characterized by provocation of the tachycardia by exercise, emotional stress, or isoproterenol infusion.[38–41] This tachycardia is responsive to vagal maneuver, edrophonium, adenosine, dipyridamole, verapamil, and β-blocker.[9,10,13,18,39,42] It may be induced by programmed stimulation, especially during isoproterenol infusion, but cannot be entrained by overdrive pacing. Triggered activity due to delayed afterdepolarization has been suggested to be the operative mechanism by Wu et al in 1981.[39] This tachycardia shares some similarities with the idiopathic left ventricular tachycardia with a QRS pattern of right bundle branch and superior axis; however, differences between these two tachycardias can be identified. The rate of this tachycardia oscillates widely depending on the level of sympathetic tone and the circulating catecholamine, while the rate of the idiopathic left ventricular tachycardia is stable. Provocation of idiopathic left ventricular tachycardia by exercise or isoproterenol infusion occurs only rarely and appears to be related to achievement of a critical sinus rate. Cycle length alternans is common in idiopathic left ventricular tachycardia, but is rarely seen in exercise-provocable tachycardia from the right ventricular outflow tract. The first coupling interval of tachycardia has an inverse relationship to the paced cycle length or the coupling interval that induced the tachycardia in idiopathic left ventricular tachycardia, whereas a concordant relationship may be noted in the exercise-provocable right ventricular outflow tract tachycardia. Entrainment is demonstrable in idiopathic left ventricular tachycardia but not in the exercise-provocable right ventricular outflow tract tachycardia.

A new type of tachycardia originating from the anterobasal left ventricle and with characteristics similar to the exercise-provocable right ventricular outflow tract tachycardia has been noted recently.[7,8,43] Kobayashi et al[9] reported 2 male patients with idiopathic left ventricular tachycardia, in whom the QRS configuration was of atypical right bundle branch block and inferior axis, and the rate of tachycardia oscillated widely. The tachycardia was responsive to verapamil, adenosine, dipyridamole, acetylcholine and vagal maneuvers. The earliest endocardial activation was noted at the anterobasal or upper midseptal region of the left ventricle, and there was no recordable Purkinje spike before the local electrogram during tachycardia; entrainment could not be demonstrated. Callans et al[10] reported 4 patients (3 males and 1 female) in whom the tachycardia was exacerbated by exercise and inducible on isoproterenol infusion. In 2 of these 4 patients, the tachycardia displayed a pattern

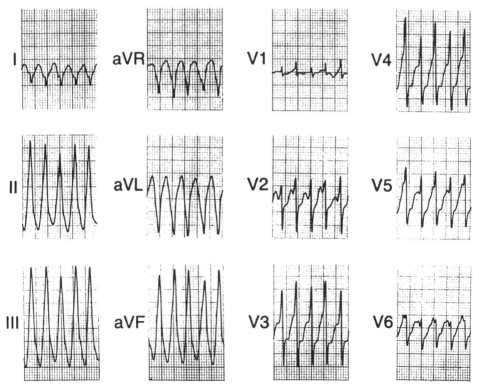

Figure 9. 12-lead ECG from a patient, showing idiopathic tachycardia due to triggered activity from the anterobasal left ventricle. Note the QRS pattern is of atypical left bundle branch block and inferior axis.

of atypical right bundle branch block, inferior axis, and a dominant R wave in V_1. Pace mapping from the mediosuperior aspect of the mitral annulus reproduced an ECG pattern identical to the clinical tachycardia. Application of radiofrequency current to this site successfully eliminated the tachycardia in both patients. In the 2 other patients, the tachycardia had a pattern of atypical left bundle branch block, inferior axis, and a precordial transition of the R wave at lead V_2. Pacing at the basal aspect of the superior left ventricular septum near the His bundle recording site reproduced an ECG pattern resembling that of the clinical tachycardia. Catheter ablation was not conducted in these 2 patients. We have also observed 4 female patients with idiopathic left ventricular tachycardia, in whom the attack of tachycardia was related to exercise and emotional stress and the tachycardia was sensitive to adenosine and verapamil.[43] The tachycardia exhibited a QRS pattern of atypical left (1 patient) (Figure 9) or right (3 patients) (Figure 10) bundle branch block, inferior axis, and wide oscillation of rate. Atrial or ventricular stimulation induced tachycardia in all 4 patients (3 with and 1 without isoproterenol infusion). Entrainment was not demonstrated in any of the 4 patients. The earliest endocardial activation was noted at the anterobasal aspect of the left ventricle just below the mitral annulus adjacent to the left ventricular outflow tract (Figures 11 and 12). Radiofrequency currents applied to this site resulted in elimination of the tachycardia in 3 of the 4 patients (see Figure 11).

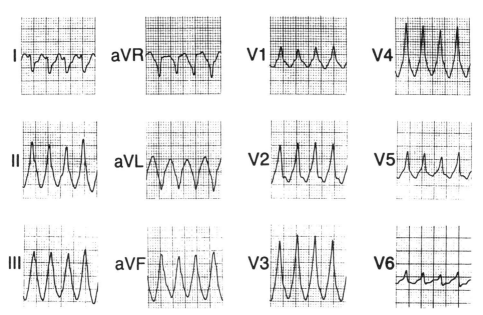

Figure 10. 12-lead ECG from a patient, showing idiopathic tachycardia due to triggered activity from the anterobasal left ventricle. Note the QRS pattern is of atypical right bundle branch block and inferior axis

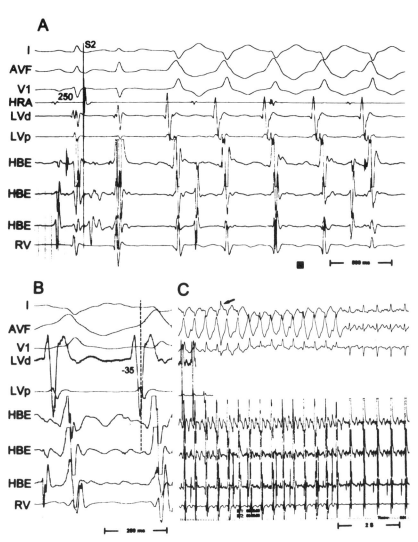

Figure 11. Recordings from the same patient as in Figure 10 showing induction, mapping and radiofrequency ablation of the ventricular tachycardia. *A* shows induction of ventricular tachycardia with delivery of an atrial extrastimulus during sinus rhythm at a coupling interval of 250 ms. *B* shows endocardial activation mapping during tachycardia with the earliest activation registered 35 ms before the onset of QRS at the anterobasal left ventricle. *C* shows termination and successful ablation of the ventricular tachycardia following delivery of radiofrequency current (indicated by an arrow).

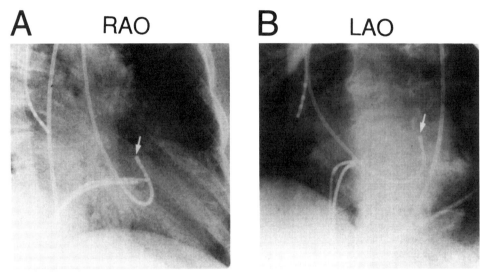

Figure 12. Radiographic recordings from the same patient as in Figures 10 and 11, showing the successful ablation site, which was located at the anterobasal left ventricle just below the mitral annulus and adjacent to the left ventricular outflow tract.

References

1. Zipes DP, Foster PR, Troup PJ, et al. Atrial induction of ventricular tachycardia: reentry versus triggered automaticity. *Am J Cardiol* 1979;44:1–8.
2. Belhassen B, Rotmensch HH, Laniado S. Response of recurrent sustained ventricular tachycardia to verapamil. *Br Heart J* 1981;46:679–682.
3. Lin FC, Finley CD, Rahimtoola SH, et al. Idiopathic paroxysmal ventricular tachycardia with a QRS pattern of right bundle branch block and left axis deviation: a unique clinical entity with specific properties. *Am J Cardiol* 1983;52:95–100.
4. Ohe T, Shimomura K, Aihara N, et al. Idiopathic sustained left ventricular tachycardia: clinical and electrophysiologic characteristics. *Circulation* 1988;77:560–568.
5. German LD, Packer DL, Bardy GH, et al. Ventricular tachycardia induced by atrial stimulation in patients without symptomatic cardiac disease. *Am J Cardiol* 1983;52:1202–1207.
6. Ward DE, Nathan AW, Camm AJ. Fascicular tachycardia sensitive to calcium antagonists. *Eur Heart J* 1984;65:896–905.
7. Kobayashi Y, Kikushima S, Tanno K, et al. Sustained left ventricular tachycardia terminated by dipyridamole: cyclic AMP-mediated triggered activity as a possible mechanism. *PACE* 1994;17:377–385.
8. Callans DJ, Menz V, Schwartzman D, et al. Repetitive monomorphic tachycardia from the left ventricular outflow tract: electrocardiographic patterns consistent with a left ventricular site of origin. *J Am Coll Cardiol* 1997;29:1023–1027.

9. Ng KS, Wen MS, Yeh SJ, et al. The effects of adenosine on idiopathic left ventricular tachycardia. *Am J Cardiol* 1994;74:195–197.
10. Griffith MJ, Garratt CJ, Rowland E, et al. Effects of intravenous adenosine on verapamil-sensitive "idiopathic" ventricular tachycardia. *Am J Cardiol* 1994;73:759–764.
11. Nakagawa H, Beckman KJ, McClelland JH, et al. Radiofrequency catheter ablation of idiopathic left ventricular tachycardia guided by a Purkinje potential. *Circulation* 1993;88:2607–2617.
12. Coggins DL, Lee RJ, Sweeney J, et al. Radiofrequency catheter ablation as a cure for idiopathic tachycardia of both left and right ventricular origin. *J Am Coll Cardiol* 1994;23:1333–1341.
13. Lee KL, Lauer MR, Young C, et al. Spectrum of electrophysiologic and electropharmacologic characteristics of verapamil-sensitive ventricular tachycardia in patients without structural heart disease. *Am J Cardiol* 1996;77: 967–973.
14. Tai YT, Fong PC, Lau CP, et al. Reentrant fascicular tachycardia with cycle length alternans: insights into the tachycardia mechanism and origin. *PACE* 1990;13:900–907.
15. Belhassen B, Shapira I, Pelley A, et al. Idiopathic recurrent sustained ventricular tachycardia responsive to verapamil; an ECG-electrophysiologic entity. *Am Heart J* 1984;108:1034–1037.
16. Sung RJ, Shapiro WA, Shen EN, et al. Effects of verapamil on ventricular tachycardia possibly caused by reentry, automaticity and triggered activity. *J Clin Invest* 1983;72:350–360.
17. Kottkamp H, Chen X, Hindricks G, et al. Radiofrequency catheter ablation of idiopathic left ventricular tachycardia: further evidence for microreentry as the underlying mechanism. *J Cardiovasc Electrophyiol* 1994;5:268–273.
18. Lerman BB, Belardinelli L, West A, et al. Adenosine-sensitive ventricular tachycardia: evidence suggesting cyclic AMP-mediated triggered activity. *Circulation* 1986;74:270–280.
19. Ohe T, Aihara N, Kamakura S, et al. Long-term outcome of verapamil-sensitive sustained left ventricular tachycardia in patterns without structural heart disease. *J Am Coll Cardiol* 1995;25:54–58.
20. Mont L, Seixas T, Brugada P, et al. The electrocardiographic, clinical, and electrophysiologic spectrum of idiopathic monomorphic ventricular tachycardia. *Am Heart J* 1992;124:746–753.
21. Klein GJ, Milman PJ, Yee R. Recurrent ventricular tachycardia responsive to verapamil. *PACE* 1984;7:938–948.
22. Sethi KK, Monoharan S, Mohan JC, et al. Verapamil in idiopathic ventricular tachycardia of right bundle branch block morphology: observations during electrophysiologic and exercise testing. *PACE* 1986;9:8–16.
23. Wen MS, Yeh SJ, Wang CC, et al. Radiofrequency ablation therapy in idiopathic left ventricular tachycardia with no obvious structural heart disease. *Circulation* 1994;89:1690–1696.
24. Okumura K, Matsuyama K, Miyagi H, et al. Entrainment of idiopathic ventricular tachycardia of left ventricular origin with evidence of reentry with an area of slow conduction and effect of verapamil. *Am J Cardiol* 1988;62: 727–732.

25. Okumura K, Yamabe H, Tsuchiya T, et al. Characteristics of slow conduction zone demonstrated during entrainment of idiopathic ventricular tachycardia of left ventricular origin. *Am J Cardiol* 1996;77:379–383.

26. DeLacey WA, Nath S, Haines DE, et al. Adenosine and verapamil-sensitive ventricular tachycardia originating from the left ventricle: radiofrequency catheter ablation. *PACE* 1992;15:2240–2243.

27. Klein LS, Shih HT, Hackelt FK, et al. Radiofrequency catheter ablation of ventricular tachycardia in patients without structural heart disease. *Circulation* 1992;85:1066–1074.

28. Page RL, Shenasa H, Evans JJ, et al. Radiofrequency catheter ablation of idiopathic recurrent ventricular tachycardia with right bundle branch block, left axis morphology. *PACE* 1993;16:327–336.

29. Wen MS, Yeh SJ, Wang CC, et al. Successful radiofrequency ablation of idiopathic left ventricular tachycardia at a site away from the tachycardia exit. *J Am Coll Cardiol* 1997;30:1024–1031.

30. Blomstrom-Lundgvist C, Blomstrom P, Beckman-Suurkula M. Incessant ventricular tachycardia with a right bundle-branch block pattern and left axis deviation abolished by catheter manipulation. *PACE* 1990;13:11–16.

31. Sung RJ, Kenng EC, Nguyen NX, et al. Effects of β-adrenergic blockade on verapamil-responsive and verapamil-irresponsive sustained ventricular tachycardia. *J Clin Invest* 1988;81:688–699.

32. Bhandari A, Hong RA, Rahimtoola S. Triggered activity as a mechanism of recurrent ventricular tachycardia. *Br Heart J* 1988;59:501–505.

33. Aizawa Y, Chinushi M, Kitazawa H, et al. Spatial orientation of the reentrant circuit of idiopathic left ventricular tachycardia. *Am J Cardiol* 1995;76:316–319.

34. Peters NS, Jackman WM, Schilling RJ, et al. Human ventricular endocardial activation mapping using a novel noncontact catheter. *Circulation* 1997;95:1658–1660.

35. Suwa M, Yoneda Y, Nagao H, et al. Surgical correction of idiopathic paroxysmal ventricular tachycardia possibly related to left ventricular false tendon. *Am J Cardiol* 1989;15:1217–1220.

36. Thakur RK, Klein GJ, Sivaram C, et al. Anatomic substrate for idiopathic left ventricular tachycardia. *Circulation* 1996;93:497–501.

37. Lin FC, Wen MS, Wang CC, et al. Left ventricular fibromuscular band is not a specific substrate for idiopathic left ventricular tachycardia. *Circulation* 1996;93:525–528.

38. Wilson FN, Wishart SW, Macleod AG, et al. A clinical type of paroxysmal tachycardia of ventricular origin in which paroxysms are induced by exertion. *Am Heart J* 1932;8:155–169.

39. Wu D, Kou HC, Hung JS. Exercise-triggered paroxysmal ventricular tachycardia: a repetitive rhythmic activity possibly related to afterdepolarization. *Ann Intern Med* 1981;95;410–414.

40. Buxton AE, Waxman HL, Marchlinski FE, et al. Right ventricular tachycardia: clinical and electrophysiologic characteristics. *Circulation* 1983;68:917–927.

41. Palileo EV, Ashley WW, Swiryn S, et al. Exercise-provocable right ventricular outflow tract tachycardia. *Am Heart J* 1982;104:185–193.
42. Lerman BB. Response of nonreentrant catecholamine-mediated ventricular tachycardia to endogenous adenosine and acetylcholine: evidence for myocardial receptor-mediated effects. *Circulation* 1993;87:382–390.
43. Yeh SJ, Wen MS, Wang CC, et al. Adenosine-sensitive ventricular tachycardia from the anteroseptal left ventricle. *J Am Coll Cardiol* (in press).

Chapter 30

Ablation of Idiopathic Right Ventricular Tachycardia

David J. Wilber, M.D.

Ventricular tachycardia arising from the right ventricle (RV) in the absence of overt structural heart disease is a common entity, representing up to 10% of all ventricular tachycardias evaluated by specialized arrhythmia services.[1,2] Clinical presentation is heterogenous, ranging from asymptomatic findings during routine examination, to episodic palpitations, dizziness, and syncope. Symptom onset is variable, typically between the ages of 20 and 40 years, although the arrhythmia is occasionally seen in preadolescents and older patients. Nonsustained tachycardias are more frequent, comprising 60–92% of reported series.[3–9] In these patients, episodes may be sporadic, but more often occur as repetitive salvos (the electrocardiographic pattern of repetitive monomorphic ventricular tachycardia).[10–12] Occasionally, runs of ventricular tachycardia are incessant, and premature ventricular complexes comprise a substantial proportion of all beats in a 24-hour period.[2,9] Of repetitive monomorphic ventricular tachycardia arising from the RV, more than 80% have a left bundle inferior QRS axis configuration.[3,11]

Less commonly, patients present with paroxysmal sustained tachycardias, separated by relatively long intervals of infrequent premature ventricular complexes.[2,13–17] Episodes tend to increase in frequency and duration during exercise and emotional stress. In addition, some patients with repetitive monomorphic tachycardia may develop more prolonged runs during exercise or catecholamine provocation.[3,17–19] Similar to nonsustained tachycardias, the vast majority of sustained episodes manifest a left bundle inferior axis QRS configuration.

From Huang SKS, Wilber DJ (eds.): *Radiofrequency Catheter Ablation of Cardiac Arrhythmias: Basic Concepts and Clinical Applications,* 2nd ed. Armonk, NY: Futura Publishing Company, Inc. ©2000.

Diagnostic Evaluation and Prognosis

The diagnosis of idiopathic RV tachycardia is one of exclusion. It has become apparent that subtle forms of RV disease (right ventricular dysplasia or cardiomyopathy [RVC]) may not always be detected on the basis of clinical examination and routine echocardiography.[20–26] Ventricular tachycardia associated with RVC often manifests multiple QRS configurations during different episodes, including tachycardias with a superior QRS axis (both uncommon in idiopathic RV tachycardia). However, many patients with RVC present with a left bundle inferior QRS axis tachycardia alone.[27,28] Exclusion of RVC in patients considered for catheter ablation is more than an academic exercise, since both long-term prognosis[28–31] and response to catheter ablation[31–33] may be less favorable.

Initial reports of idiopathic ventricular tachycardia with a left bundle inferior axis QRS configuration indicated that 10–40% of patients had right ventricular abnormalities by contrast cineangiography or quantitative echocardiography (generalized right ventricular enlargement or hypokinesis, focal dilation, or wall motion abnormalities). Many of these abnormalities were subtle, and their clinical significance was questioned.[5,6] However, in the early report of Peitras et al, sudden death occurred in 2 of 15 patients with right ventricular abnormalities not considered diagnostic of RVC, while no deaths occurred in 23 patients with completely normal RVs.[4] Similar findings were reported by Deal et al.[23]

An abnormal SAECG is uncommon in patients with idiopathic right ventricular outflow tachycardia. In 4 reported series, only 3 of 72 patients (14%) had an abnormal SAECG by standard time domain analysis, and usually only 1 of 3 criteria were abnormal.[3,8,17,34] In contrast, an abnormal time domain SAECG is present in 50–80% of patients with RVC.[34,35] Similar differences are evident by frequency domain analysis.[36] The 12-lead electrocardiogram (ECG) is usually normal. Widespread T wave abnormalities should raise suspicion of associated structural heart disease. Similarly, myocardial biopsy is rarely revealing in this group of patients, although mild nonspecific findings are not uncommon. Occasionally, more prominent biopsy abnormalities are found (fibrosis >10% by morphometric analysis with or without adipose tissue).[7,8] However, in these cases, right ventricular imaging techniques usually identify significant abnormalities. Cardiac magnetic resonance imaging (MRI) provides more detailed information with respect to cardiac structure and tissue characteristics, and in conjunction with cine imaging can detect subtle wall thinning and contraction abnormalities not readily appreciated by other techniques. Recently, several groups have reported a substantial incidence of MRI abnormalities (65–76%) in patients with idiopathic RV outflow tachycardia who are considered not to have RVC.[37–39] These abnormalities included focal thinning and segmental contraction abnormalities, and were equally distributed between the outflow tract and the anterior free wall. In addition, focal fatty infiltration was observed in approximately 25% of patients. Correlation of MRI abnormalities to the site of tachycardia origin as determined by successful ablation was variable.[38,39] At the present time, the clinical significance of these abnormalities, both in the pathogenesis of tachycardia and as prognostic markers, is uncertain.

"Idiopathic" left bundle superior axis tachycardias are much less frequently observed. In contrast to tachycardias with an inferior QRS axis, a superior axis is associated with a very high incidence of occult structural abnormalities. Mehta found right ventricular structural abnormalities on echocardiography in 6 of 6 patients with left bundle superior axis sustained ventricular tachycardia. In addition, 5 of 6 patients had more than 10% fibrous replacement of myocardium by morphometric analysis of biopsy specimens.[7] In subsequent study, these investigators found an abnormal SAECG in 7 of 9 patients with left bundle superior axis tachycardias.[8] The probability of an abnormal SAECG was strongly correlated with the degree of fibrosis found in biopsy specimens.[40] Wellens reported progression from normal right ventricular structure to typical RVC on serial echocardiograms during long-term follow-up in 2 of 5 patients with left bundle superior axis tachycardias.[25] Collectively, these observations underscore the importance of close follow-up in this group of patients.

Long-term prognosis in patients with truly idiopathic RV tachycardia is excellent, despite frequent recurrences of tachycardia.[3–9,13–19,23,41–43] Sudden death is rare in patients with initially normal left and right ventricular function;[18,23–25,43,44] in such patients, occult cardiomyopathy is usually identified on postmortem examination. Similarly, progression to diffuse cardiomyopathy is rare. However, in patients presenting with at least some evidence of structural heart disease (right ventricular contraction abnormalities by echocardiography or angiography, abnormal biopsy, abnormal SAECG), progression to a more generalized cardiomyopathy within the initial 6 months of clinical presentation may occur, as may sudden death.[4,23,26]

At present, there is no universally accepted standard for the diagnostic evaluation of RV tachycardia. It is our practice to obtain echocardiograms with special attention to the right ventricle in all patients. Coronary artery disease is excluded by noninvasive testing or angiography depending on the degree of clinical suspicion. Cine MRI and/or first-pass radionuclide right ventriculograms are also obtained routinely. Myocardial biopsy is reserved for patients in whom diagnostic uncertainty remains after initial evaluation. The diagnosis of RVC is made following recently established guidelines.[45a] Patients with completely normal results of diagnostic evaluation, particularly those with a relatively long history of tachycardia, can be reassured of their benign prognosis. Patients with recent onset of tachycardia associated with multiple minor abnormalities not meeting criteria for RVC, and those with a non-outflow tract site of origin, are followed closely with periodic clinical examination and assessment of right and left ventricular function.

Electrophysiological Evaluation

Convincing evidence has accumulated that the large majority of outflow tract tachycardias are due to cAMP-mediated triggered activity.[45b] The diagnostic use of adenosine, as initially proposed by Lerman and colleagues, has been particularly helpful in this regard.[15] Of 81 patients with RV outflow tract tachycardia in 5 reported series, intravenous adenosine resulted in termination in 95%.[46-50] Ventricular tachycardia due to cAMP-dependent triggered activity occasionally originates from right ventricular sites outside the outflow tract[19,47] or from the left ventricle.[51] Adenosine rarely influences tachycardias due to reentry,[15,47] and in particular has no effect on tachycardias associated with RVC.

In patients who present with sustained ventricular tachycardias due to triggered activity, the tachycardia usually can be reproduced by programmed stimulation.[15,17,47-50] Burst pacing is usually more effective than ventricular extrastimuli, and a critical range of paced cycle lengths for induction is often observed, which may shift with changing levels of adrenergic activation. The tachycardia can occasionally be induced in the baseline state.[17,48,49] However, catecholamine infusion is generally required to facilitate induction, and may result in spontaneous onset of tachycardia. Epinephrine is occasionally more effective than isoproterenol. Tachycardia induction may be inconsistent,[17] reflecting the complex interplay between heart rate, degree of adrenergic activation, and coupling intervals during ventricular pacing. Deep sedation may suppress this tachycardia, particularly that which results from the use of benzodiazepines. Aminophylline and atropine may occasionally facilitate tachycardia induction. Tachycardia rates are frequently rapid (cycle lengths of less than 300 milliseconds), but may be highly variable.

The QRS morphology during RV outflow tachycardia typically has a left bundle configuration with QS or rS patterns in leads V_1 and V_2, and a right or left inferior axis (Figures 1–11). Minor variations in QRS morphology between complexes during tachycardia are not infrequently observed (see figure 8) and may be associated with minor variations in local electrograms recorded near the site of tachycardia origin.[52] However, multiple morphologically distinct tachycardias due to triggered activity are rare and should raise suspicion of alternate mechanisms and occult underlying heart disease. We have observed 2 distinct tachycardia morphologies in only 2 of 42 patients with adenosine-sensitive RV outflow tachycardia. One patient had 2 widely separated foci in the outflow tract. The second had both right and left bundle QRS configurations with inferior QRS axes. In the latter case, the 2 tachycardias appeared to arise from a single focus in the deep septum, with exit to either the right or left side of the septum during different episodes.

In a small number of patients, idiopathic RV tachycardias may be due to catecholamine-enhanced automaticity or reentry. These mechanisms appear to be an uncommon cause of sustained RV outflow tachycardia, but may be observed more frequently in tachycardias originating from other RV sites.[46] Typically, enhanced automaticity is initiated by catecholamine infusion, but not programmed stimulation.[14,16] Pacing during tachycardia may result in transient suppression, but not termination. Convincing evidence of a reentrant mechanism is available in only a few cases. Aziwa et al reported 3 patients with idiopathic RV tachycardia localized to the septal portion of the inflow tract within 1 cm of the His bundle, one of which also had an additional right bundle tachycardia.[53] All tachycardias were initiated and terminated by programmed stimulation in the absence of isoproterenol, and in each, entrainment was demonstrated. Similar tachycardias have been reported by others.[54,55] Sustained idiopathic RV tachycardias presumed to be reentrant have also been reported to arise from the anterior and posterobasal RV free wall.[55,56]

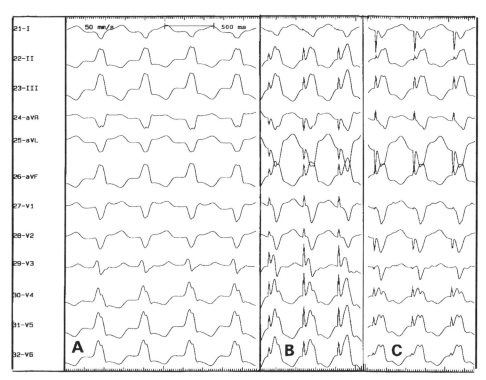

Figure 1. Twelve-lead electrocardiograms from a patient with idiopathic right ventricular out-flow tachycardia arising from the anterior septal outflow tract. Panel A: Induced tachycardia with a CL of 450 milliseconds. Note the QS complex in lead I and R=S in lead V_3. Panel B: Pacing from the site of successful ablation. Pacing at a rate 100 milliseconds faster than the tachycardia CL produces an exact match on the first 2 complexes, but widespread minor dif-ferences on the third complex, most likely related to the relatively large mismatch of pacing rate and tachycardia rate. During pacing at a cycle length of 400 at the same site, all complexes appeared similar to the first 2 of this example. This underscores the potential for large differ-ences between pacing and tachycardia rates to produce significant alterations in morphology at even a successful ablation site. Panel C: Pacing from a different site approximately 1.5 cm caudal on the septum produces a similar QRS configuration in all leads except for lead V_3, un-derscoring the importance of requiring an exact match to select target sites for ablation.

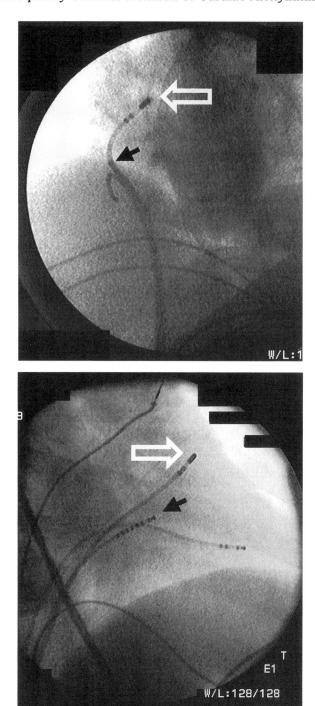

Figure 2. Catheter positions at the successful ablation site for the septal tachycardia illustrated in Figure 1. Top panel: 60° left anterior oblique. Bottom panel: 30° right anterior oblique. The open arrow indicates the ablation catheter and the closed arrow the His catheter. The third catheter is positioned on the midanterior septum. Note the position of the ablation electrode to the right of the His position in the LAO projection.

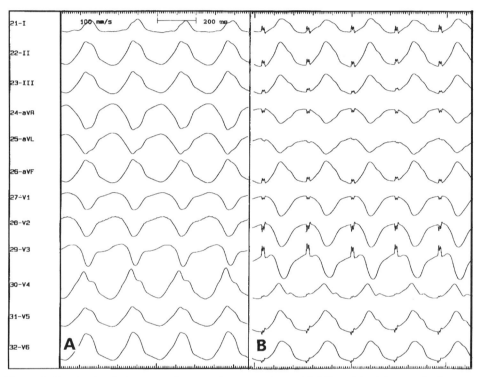

Figure 3. Twelve-lead electrocardiograms from a patient with idiopathic right ventricular outflow tachycardia arising from the midanterior free wall. Panel A: Induced tachycardia with a CL of 250 milliseconds. Note the monophasic R wave in lead I and precordial transition zone at lead V_4. Panel B: Pacing from the site of successful ablation on exactly reproduces the tachycardia morphology.

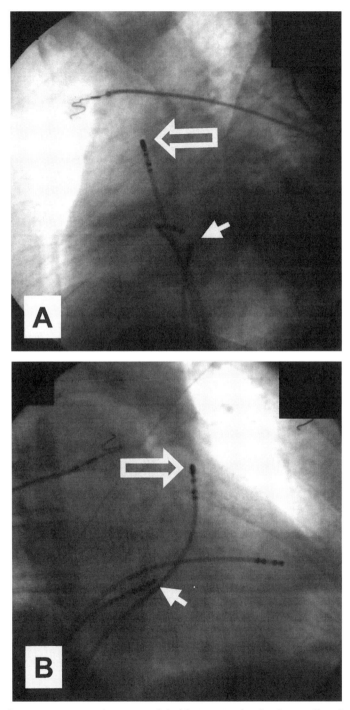

Figure 4. Catheter positions at the successful ablation site for the free wall tachycardia illustrated in Figure 3. Panel A: 60° left anterior oblique. Panel B: 30° right anterior oblique. The open arrow indicates the ablation catheter and the closed arrow the His catheter. The third catheter is positioned on the midanterior septum. Note the position of the ablation electrode to the left of the His position in the LAO projection.

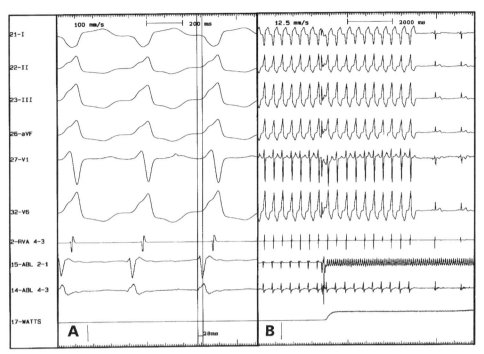

Figure 5. Surface electrocardiograms and intracardiac electrograms during idiopathic right ventricular outflow tachycardia. Panel A: Electrograms from the ablation site (ABL) have rapid slew rates with onset 28 milliseconds prior to the surface QRS. Panel B: Onset of RF energy application at this site resulted in termination of the tachycardia within 4 seconds.

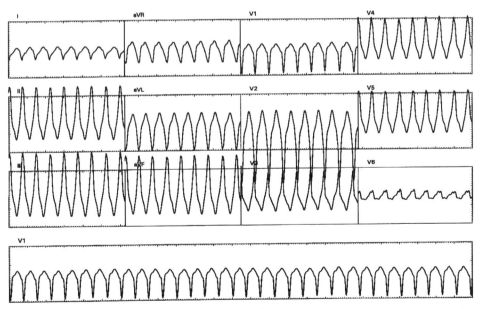

Figure 6. Electrocardiogram of tachycardia arising from the anterior septum. Note QS complex in lead I, and precordial transition zone between V_2 and V_3.

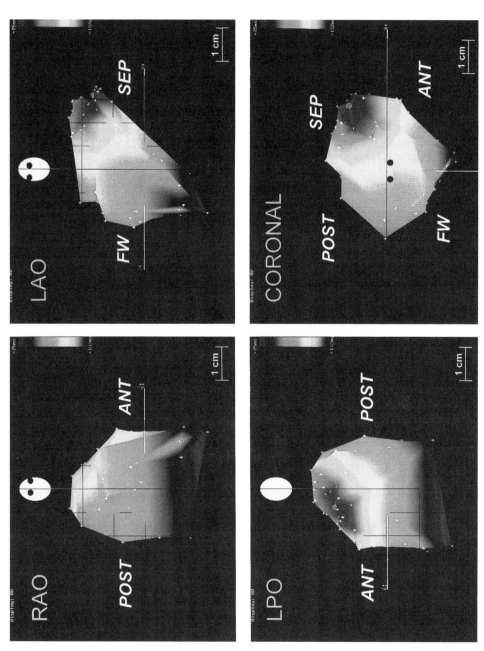

Figure 7. Electroanatomic map in multiple projections of the tachycardia illustrated in Figure 6. The color-coded isochrones represent activation times during tachycardia with peak QRS voltage in lead II as the fiducial point. The green dot represents the site of ablation. ANT = anterior; FW = free wall; POST = posterior; LAO = left anterior oblique (45°); LPO = left posterior oblique (45°); RAO = right anterior oblique (45°); SEP = septal. See color plate.

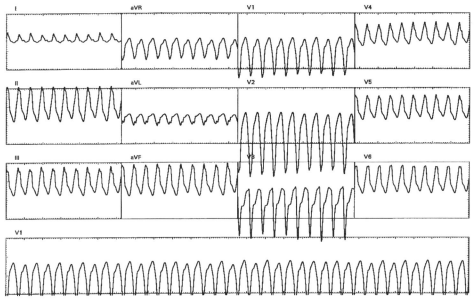

Figure 8. Electrocardiogram of tachycardia arising from the mid/posterior free wall. Note monophasic R waves in lead I, and precordial transition zone at V_4.

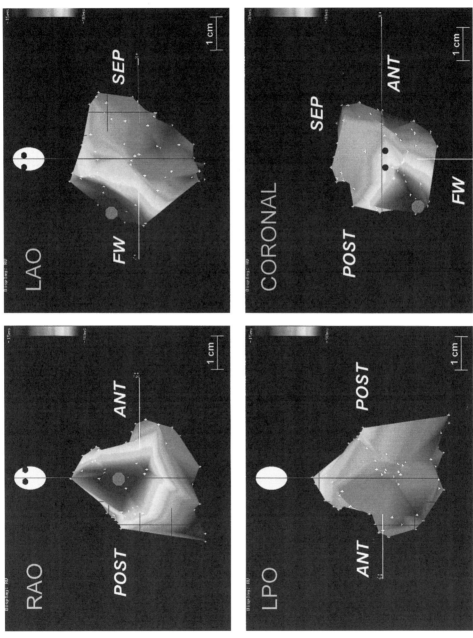

Figure 9. Electroanatomic map in multiple projections of the tachycardia illustrated in Figure 8. The format is the same as in Figure 7. See color plate.

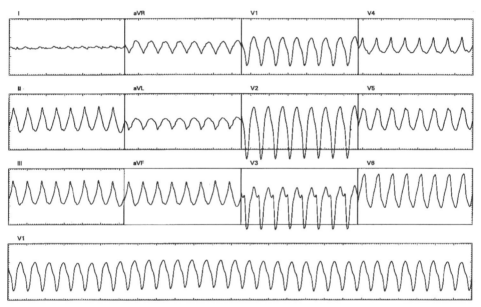

Figure 10. Electrocardiogram of tachycardia arising from the anterior free wall. Note nearly iso-electric QRS in lead I typical of this location, and precordial transition zone at V_4.

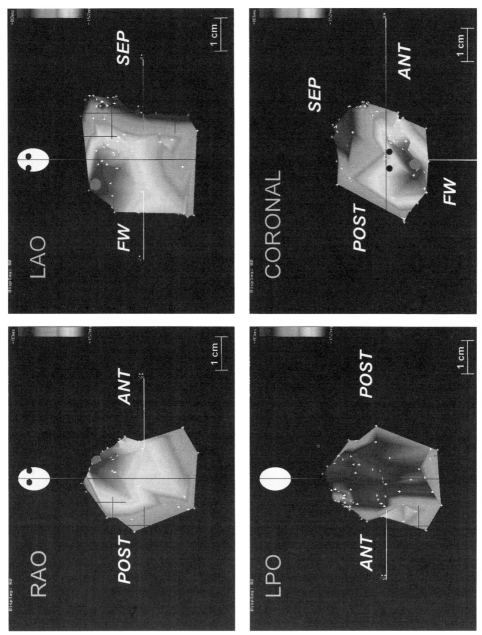

Figure 11. Electroanatomic map in multiple projections of the tachycardia illustrated in Figure 10. The format is the same as Figure 7. See color plate.

In contrast to patients with spontaneous sustained RV tachycardia, induction of sustained tachycardia is considerably less common during programmed stimulation in patients presenting clinically with at most nonsustained runs.[3,5,6,8,9,11,12,57] Evidence of catecholamine responsiveness is usually present, although a complex relationship exists between mean heart rate, the length of the RR interval preceding the first ectopic beat, and the coupling interval of the first ectopic beat.[10,11] However, in selected patients with the electrocardiographic pattern of repetitive monomorphic ventricular tachycardia, sustained tachycardias with characteristics typical of cAMP-mediated triggered activity can be induced by programmed ventricular stimulation following autonomic and pharmacological manipulation.[19]

Endocardial Mapping

Optimal techniques for localizing the site of origin of idiopathic RV tachycardia have received considerable attention. As expected for focal rhythms, endocardial activation at successful ablation sites tends to be only modestly early, ranging from 10–60 milliseconds prior to onset of the surface QRS.[17,52-55,58–63] Bipolar endocardial electrograms have high amplitudes and rapid slew rates (see Figure 5). Fractionated complex electrograms and diastolic potentials are rarely, if ever, seen, and should raise suspicion of underlying structural disease.

The morphology of the unipolar electrogram has potential utility for localization of focal sources of activation. Amerandal and colleagues[59] noted that the presence of a QS complex was highly sensitive in identifying successful ablation sites. However, nearly 70% of unsuccessful sites also manifested a QS unipolar complex. Man et al examined the unipolar electrogram morphology at various distances from the site of origin of mechanically induced RV premature complexes.[64] A QS complex was recorded at the origin of the premature complex in all patients, but was also recorded from electrodes located more than 1 cm away in 65% of patients. Thus, unipolar electrogram morphology with standard ablation electrodes is a highly sensitive but nonspecific marker for target sites in patients with idiopathic RV tachycardia.

Pace mapping has generally been more useful as a means of localizing target sites, with most investigators reporting successful ablation at sites with identical or near identical matches in all 12 surface leads.[17,54,55,58-61] Differences in QRS configuration between pacing and spontaneous tachycardia in a single lead may be critical (see Figure 1). The use of additional ECG leads or body surface mapping may improve the precision of pace mapping.[65]

Several factors influencing the precision and spatial resolution of RV pace mapping in structurally normal hearts have been examined. Kadish et al examined the spatial resolution of unipolar pacing with respect to the degree of pace map matching.[66] Pacing at a site 5 millimeters from the index pacing site resulted in minor differences in configuration (notching, new small component, change in amplitude of individual component, or overall change in QRS shape) in at least one lead in 24 of 29 patients. In contrast, if only major changes in QRS configuration were considered, pacing sites separated by as much as 15 millimeters could appear similar. Current strength up to 10 mA had little effect on unipolar paced ECG configuration. These results suggest that under optimal conditions, the spatial resolution of an exact pace map match may be less than 5 millimeters. Bipolar pacing may introduce additional variability in the RV paced electrocardiogram, but these changes can be minimized by low pacing outputs and small interelectrode distances (≤ 5 mm).[67] Goyal and colleagues demonstrated that significant changes in paced QRS configuration occur during bipolar pacing at the same RV site when differences in paced cycle length exceed 80 milliseconds.[68] Rate-dependent aberration due to increasing degrees of incomplete repolarization and fusion with the preceding T wave during shorter cycle lengths may both play a role. These data suggest that pace mapping should be performed as close as possible to the cycle length of the spontaneous tachycardia or the coupling interval of single premature ventricular complexes to maximize the ability to obtain an exact pace map at the site of tachycardia origin (see Figure 1). Finally, isoproterenol infusion, which is frequently required to initiate ventricular tachycardia in the laboratory, is reported to have no significant effect on QRS configuration.[69]

Additional insight into activation during idiopathic RV tachycardia can be gained by inspection of electroanatomic maps generated by magnetic catheter tracking techniques.[70] A more detailed discussion of this technique is presented in Chapter 36. Maps of the right ventricular outflow tract obtained in 3 different patients during sustained RV outflow tachycardia are illustrated in Figures 7, 9, and 11. These maps were limited to the 3–4 cm of the right ventricle immediately inferior to the pulmonary valve. Activation away from the site of origin tends to be rapid. An early activation zone, consisting of all electrograms within 10 milliseconds of the earliest recorded electrogram (red and orange isochrones on each map) can be observed over areas of 2–4 cm². Given interobserver variability of up to 5 milliseconds or more in the manual assignment of activation time, it is not surprising that electrogram timing alone is reported to have relatively limited utility as a predictor of successful ablation sites. However, high density simultaneous display of activation time and anatomic location facilitates discrimination between minor differences in timing and "smooths over" potential measurement errors. Ablation directed at the center of the early activation zone terminated the tachycardia in each patient. Exact pace map matches were most likely to be recorded from the center of the early activation zone identified by the electroanatomic map, but nearly similar matches could be obtained at sites 1–2 cm away (but still within 10 milliseconds of the earliest activation). These findings suggest that a combination of exact pace map match and earliest recorded activation time may best identify the optimal target site for ablation.

Location of Tachycardia Focus and Role of the 12-Lead Electrocardiogram

The reported location of tachycardias within the outflow tract varies widely. Both Movsowitz[61] and Gumbrielle[60] reported that all successfully ablated outflow tachycardias arose from a relatively well-circumscribed area on the superior midseptal and anterior septal surfaces, just under the pulmonary valve. However, in an early report of surgical treatment of adenosine-sensitive RV outflow tachycardia, epicardial mapping identified a mid-free wall focus that was successfully cryoablated.[71] Subsequently, a free wall focus was reported in 55 of 183 patients (22%) with RV outflow tachycardia where specific information is available, but varied between 5–63% of individual series (Table 1).[9,52,54,58,59,62,63,72,73] Figures 3, 8, and 10 are examples of free wall tachycardias. While a majority of septal tachycardias are located in the anterior septum within 1 cm of the pulmonary valve, more inferior and posterior foci can occur.[63,72] The reported variability in tachycardia localization may reflect differences in patient characteristics and selection, disagreement over the interpretation of fluoroscopic catheter positions, or the inherent imprecision of fluoroscopic localization of anatomic sites.

The predictive value of the QRS configuration to identify the site of tachycardia origin has also been controversial. Jadonath et al evaluated QRS configuration at 9 standard pacing sites on the septal surface of the outflow tract in 11 normal patients.[74] Pacing at anteroseptal sites produced a QS or Qr in lead I and a QS in lead aVL. Pacing at posteroseptal sites produced an Rs or R in lead I and a QS in aVL. Precordial R wave transition (R≥S) moved leftward from V_3 to V_4 as pacing sites moved from superior to inferior. No data were obtained during free wall pacing. Shima et al evaluated paced electrocardiogram morphology at 8 standard sites identified by biplane fluoroscopy on both the septum and free wall in 13 patients.[75] The schematic in Figure 12 illustrates the orientation and terminology used in the following discussion. Pacing at anterior sites near the septal free wall junction generally displayed QS complexes in lead I similar to the findings of Jandonath et al. However, pacing from septal, posterior, and free wall sites each produced R>S complexes in lead I, with the largest R/S ratio at posterior sites. The precordial transition zone was significantly later in free wall sites compared to septal sites (≥ V4 versus ≤ V3),

Table 1
Location of Right Ventricular Outflow Tachycardia in Patients Undergoing Radiofrequency Catheter Ablation

	Year	N	Septal	Free Wall	Unsuccessful/ Unknown
Almendral et al[59]	1998	15	11 (74%)	2 (13%)	2 (13%)
Chinushi et al[52]	1997	13	9 (69%)	4 (31%)	0
Coggins et al[58]	1994	20	16 (80%)	1 (5%)	1 (15%)
Gumbrielle et al[60]	1997	10	10 (100%)	0	0
Kamakura et al[73]	1998	35	27 (77%)	8 (23%)	NA
Klein et al[54]	1992	12	10 (83%)	2 (17%)	0
Lerman et al[19]	1995	8	2 (25%)	5 (63%)	1 (12%)
Movsowitz et al[61]	1996	18	16 (89%)	0	2 (11%)
O'Conner et al[62]	1996	6	3 (50%)	2 (33%)	1 (17%)
Rodriguez et al[63]	1997	35	22 (63%)	7 (20%)	6 (17%)
Wen et al[72]	1998	44	30 (68%)	9 (20%)	5 (11%)
Authors	1998	45	27 (60%)	17 (38%)	1 (2%)
			183 (71%)	55 (22%)	19 (7%)

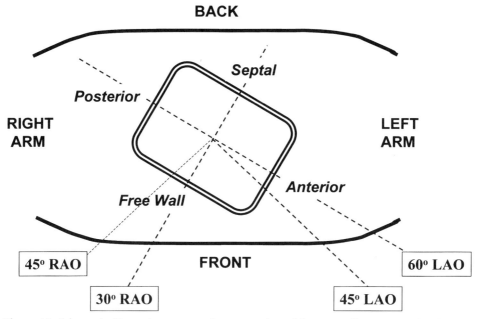

Figure 12. Schematic illustrating a coronal cross-section of the RV outflow tract with reference to standard imaging planes.

and this difference became more prominent as the pacing site moved away from the pulmonary valve.

Finally, Kamakura and colleagues,[73] using a mapping scheme similar to that of Shima (though with slightly different terminology), reported that leftward sites in the RAO view produced negative complexes (QS), while rightward sites produced positive complexes (R), irrespective of location on the septum or free wall. R waves were larger in lead V_1 and V_2 at septal and superior sites compared to free wall and inferior sites. These investigators did not specifically examine the polarity of lead I or the location of the precordial transition zone in septal versus free wall tachycardia, but noted that free wall tachycardias were significantly more likely to have notching of the the the R wave (RR', Rr') in leads II and III, while septal tachycardias generally displayed monophasic R waves in these leads. As in our own experience, these investigators also noted that lead aVL is invariably negative in patients with RV outflow tachycardias irrespective of location. However, the amplitude in lead aVL is generally greater in tachycardias of septal origin (see Figure 6) than in tachycardias of free wall origin (see Figures 8 and 10).

These data indicate that the surface electrocardiogram contains useful clues for localizing RV outflow tachycardias, but they must be interpreted carefully. Specific characteristics in individual leads may not be associated with a single unique site. Individual differences in the orientation of the heart within the chest, and the imprecision of radiographic localization, introduce additional variability. In general, a QS complex in lead I is generated from sites at or near the anterior septum (the most leftward portion of the RV outflow tract in the

Table 2
Guidelines for the Localization of Right Ventricular Outflow
Tachycardia Based on the Surface Electrocardiogram

Lead I	
negative deflection (QS):	rightward sites (septal >> free wall)
positive deflection (R):	leftward sites (free wall >> septum)
Precordial Leads	
V_1, V_2 voltage	higher at septal and superior sites
precordial transition (R≥S):	later (usually ≥ V_4) at inferior and free wall sites
Other Leads	
notching in leads II, III	favors free wall site
amplitude of a VL	greater amplitude favors septal site

See text for details and references.

supine, anteroposterior orientation). As the site of origin moves rightward (either on the septum or on the free wall) R waves appear and become progressively predominant. In the precordial leads, R wave amplitudes tend to be larger in V_1 and V_2 at superior and leftward (septal) sites, with a trend toward lower right precordial R amplitude and a shift in the precordial transition zone to the left as sites shift to the right (free wall) or inferiorly. These guidelines are summarized in Table 2. In our own experience, and that of others[73,76] they provide a reliable first approximation for localizing tachycardias within the outflow tract. Finally, idiopathic RV tachycardias with a superior QRS axis are generally located in the body of the right ventricle on the anterior free wall, or mid- and distal septum (Figure 13).

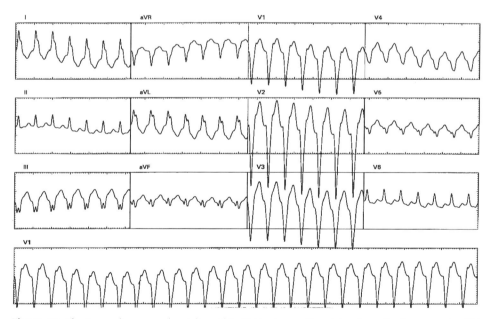

Figure 13. Electrocardiogram of an idiopathic RV tachycardia arising from the low anterior RV free wall. Note the left superior QRS axis.

Until recently, tachycardias with an inferior QRS axis and a very early precordial transition zone (RS ratios ≥ 1 in leads V_1 or V_2), the so-called atypical left bundle pattern, were a source of confusion. These tachycardias almost universally arise from the left ventricular outflow tract (basal septum, aortic commissures or adjacent free wall), may be epicardial in location, and are most appropriately classified as left ventricular tachycardias.[51,77]

Approach to Ablation

We generally begin mapping by placing the ablation catheter in the proximal pulmonary artery and slowly withdrawing it into the outflow tract until the first local endocardial electrogram is recorded. This site is just below the pulmonary valve, and it is at this level that the majority of RV outflow tachycardias originate. Torque is applied to the catheter for circumferential mapping of the outflow tract within 1 cm of the pulmonary valve, with a minimum of 4 sites—anterior and posterior septal, and anterior and posterior free wall, as determined by biplane fluoroscopy (see Figure 12). The plane of the septum in the LAO projection is nearly perpendicular to the imaging plane (Figure 14), with slight variability introduced by the exact degree of angulation and the anatomic orientation of the heart. Based on the results of mapping and pacing at these initial sites, and guided by surface QRS configuration, attention is then directed to specific regions of early activation and best pace map matches. A catheter positioned at the proximal His bundle and/or midanterior septum aids in accurate anatomic localization, as septal sites are nearly always within the same vertical plane or further rightward relative to these catheter positions in the LAO projection, even accounting for slight leftward bulging of the septum (see Figures 2 and 14).[78] We avoid placing a catheter in the most distal portion of the RV apex. This area may be more vulnerable to perforation, particularly given the frequent need for isoproterenol infusion to initiate or maintain tachycardia. Many clinicians prefer to use a 2 catheter "leapfrog" method. In this approach, the catheter associated with the best pace map and activation time is left in place and a second catheter is used to explore the surrounding area. Once a site with better characteristics is located, the roving catheter is left in place, and the initial catheter is used for the next step in mapping. The "leapfrog" process continues until an optimal site is selected.

It is our preference to perform mapping during sustained tachycardia where possible, at cycle lengths 20–40 milliseconds shorter than the tachycardia cycle length. This method facilitates rapid comparison of tachycardia and paced QRS configurations at the end of the pacing train in simultaneously displayed 12-lead electrocardiograms which are available with most contemporary recording systems. Either unipolar or closely spaced bipolar pacing may be used. Mapping of spontaneous nonsustained tachycardias or isolated premature beats may be performed when no other arrhythmia can be initiated, provided that documentation of an exact 12-lead match of QRS configuration during spontaneous tachycardia and premature complexes is obtained. In this latter instance appropriate attention must be given to the matching of pacing

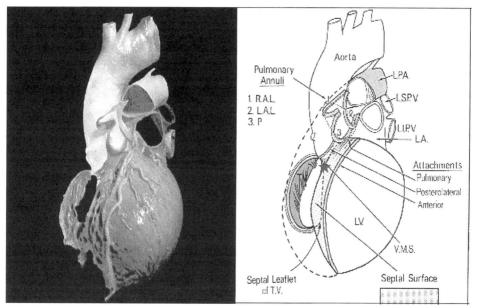

Figure 14. Perfusion fixed heart demonstrating the disposition of the right ventricular outflow tract in the 45° LAO imaging plane. The right ventricular free wall has been dissected free, leaving only the attachments to the septum and tricuspid and pulmonary annuli. Note that the entire septal surface of the outflow tract in this projection is to the right of the His bundle region (red star). As the imaging plane moves toward the 60° LAO, the septal surface becomes nearly perpendicular to the imaging plane, but because of the septal curvature as one moves closer to the pulmonary valve, septal points remain to the right or at most vertical to the His bundle region. LA = left atrium; LAL = left anterolateral; LIPV = left inferior pulmonary vein; LPA = left pulmonary artery; LSPV = left superior pulmonary vein; LV = left ventricle; P = posterior; R = right anterolateral; TV = tricuspid valve; VMS = ventricular membranous septum. (Adapted with permission from McAlpine WA. *The Heart and Coronary Arteries*. Berlin, Germany: Springer-Verlag, 1975. p 119.) See color plate.

rate to the coupling intervals of premature complexes. As previously discussed, a combination of earliest activation time and exact pace map match optimizes target site selection.

We prefer to use temperature-guided radiofrequency (RF) application where possible for ablation of idiopathic RV tachycardias, using a cutoff point of 60°C to 70°C. Cooling of the catheter tip by circulating blood flow is relatively poor in some regions of the RV, particularly in the presence of prominent trabeculations, and at the anterior septal free wall junction; electrode tip temperature may increase rapidly with relatively low power applications. In the absence of temperature monitoring, gradual power titration with close attention to the impedance curve is essential. In our experience, and that of Wen and colleagues,[72] termination of tachycardia at ultimately successful sites is generally within 10 seconds (see Figure 5). Acceleration of the tachycardia during RF application followed by gradual slowing or abrupt termination may also be observed.[17] Application of RF energy in sinus rhythm at sites near the tachycardia origin also may result in induction of repetitive responses or tachycardia with QRS characteristics similar to that seen during spontaneous tachycardia.[79] These observations may be due to thermal facilitation of triggered activity[80,81] but may also simply reflect thermally-induced abnormal automaticity.[82] Neither phenomenon is a specific marker for a successful ablation site, although they are more commonly observed within 1–2 cm of the ultimately successful site.

Potential Pitfalls in Localization and Ablation

Persistent difficulty in identifying optimal target sites, or in eliminating tachycardia during ablation is uncommon, but may arise for several reasons. The induced tachycardia may not be of RV origin. Occasionally, preexcited tachycardia with antegrade conduction through a right sided accessory AV connection (either passively or as the antegrade limb of AV reciprocating tachycardia) may cause diagnostic confusion, particularly when preexcitation is intermittent or latent.[83] As previously discussed, atypical left bundle patterns ($R \geq S$ in V_1 or V_2) indicate an origin in the left ventricle, either endocardial or epicardial. Inadequate exploration of all potential sites within the outflow tract, particularly those located more inferiorly on the septum or on the free wall, may also result in inability to identify optimal sites.

Finally, a small number of RV outflow tachycardias with typical left bundle (QS or rS in leads V_1 and V_2) inferior QRS pattern may arise from intramural sites in the deep or subepicardial septum with preferential exit to the RV endocardium.[84] We recently performed high-density septal mapping, including recordings from the anterior interventricular vein and left ventricle in 3 patients with medically refractory ventricular tachycardia and previous failed ablation. In each patient, early activation times were identified on the endocardium of the RV outflow tract within 1 cm of the pulmonary valve (-18 to -35 milliseconds). Epicardial activation times were also presystolic (-25 to -40 milliseconds); left ventricular sites were uniformly late. In 2 patients, sites were identified in the mid- or posterior RV septal endocardium where activation times equaled or preceded those from the epicardium and where pacing produced an exact pace map. While application of RF energy with a 4 millimeter electrode failed to terminate tachycardia in either patient, subsequent RF application with an 8 millimeter electrode at the same site resulted in permanent elimination of the tachycardia without adverse sequella. While both large tip and irrigated tip electrodes produce wider and deeper lesions than standard 4 millimeter electrodes, experience with these newer electrodes in the RV outflow tract is limited. Considerable care should be exercised in catheter placement and lesion monitoring to minimize the risk of perforation. In the third patient, the earliest RV endocardial activation was on the anterior septum, but an exact pace map match could not be obtained. Earlier activation was recorded in the anterior interventricular vein, and this patient subsequently underwent successful surgical epicardial cryoablation. It remains to be determined whether experimental nonsurgical approaches to epicardial foci adjacent to the septum, either through the coronary venous system, or transpericardially, will prove clinically safe and effective.

Outcome of Ablation

Initial success with direct current shocks for ablation of idiopathic RV tachycardia[85,86] was followed by widespread use of RF energy sources for catheter ablation. Table 3 summarizes available data with respect to the outcome of RF catheter ablation of RV outflow tract tachycardia. Series of greater than 5 patients were included if adequate outcome data were provided. The most recent series representing the largest number of patients was selected for each institution. Acute procedural success was obtained in 246 of 268 patients (92%).[52,54–56,58–63,72,87] In patients with successful ablation, 7% recurred during a variable period of follow-up. Of note is the fact that approximately 40% of the recurrences occurred prior to hospital discharge. The large majority of patients with recurrences underwent repeat ablation procedure with long-term freedom from additional recurrences. The remaining recurrences were within the first year of follow-up; recurrence more than 1 year postablation was rare despite follow-up of greater than 3 years in a substantial number of patients. Procedural variables influencing the probability of recurrence following initially successful ablation were examined by Wen et al. Poor pace map matches (less than 12 of 12), and later activation at the target site, as well as reliance on pace mapping alone, were each significant predictors of recurrence.[72]

Serious complications occurred in 3 patients (1%) in these series, each related to cardiac perforation and tamponade. All events occurred prior to the availability of electrode tip temperature monitoring, and in 2 of 3 patients, they were directly associated with an impedance rise during RF energy application.

Table 3
Outcome of a Radiofrequency Catheter Ablation in Patients With
Idiopathic Right Ventricular Outflow Tachycardia

	Year	N	Acute Success	Mean Follow-up (mo)	Recurrence
Almendral et al[59]	1998	15	13/15*	21	1/13
Calkins et al[55]	1993	10	10/10	8	0/10
Chinushi et al[52]	1997	13	13/13	28	1/13
Coggins et al[58]	1994	20	17/20	10	1/17
Gumbrielle et al[60]	1997	10	10/10	16	0/10
Lerman et al	1995	8	7/8	13	0/7
Mandrola et al[56]	1995	35	35/35*	24	0/35
Movsowitz et al[61]	1996	18	16/18	12	5/16
O'Conner et al[62]	1996	6	5/6*	13	0/5
Rodriguez et al[63]	1997	35	29/35	30	4/28
Vohra et al[87]	1997	9	8/9	9	0/8
Wen et al[72]	1998	44	39/44	41	4/39
Authors	1998	45	44/45	37	2/44
		215	246/268 (92%)		18/246 (7%)

* Acute success determined at hospital discharge, with one or more patients undergoing repeat procedures due to early recurrence or initial failure. In all other series, success was determined at the end of the initial procedure.

Table 4
Outcome of Radiofrequency Catheter Ablation in Patients With Idiopathic Right Ventricular Tachycardia From Non-Outflow Sites

	Year	Acute Success	Location	Recurrence
Aizawa et al[53]	1993	3/3	IT-3	0/3
Calkins et al[55]	1993	2/4	IT-2, PB-1, AFW-1	0/2
Mandrola et al[56]	1995	5/8	IT-6, AFW-2	0/5
Vohra et al et al[87]	1996	1/3	RVA-2, AFW-1	0/1
Authors	1998	3/5	RVA-1, PB-2, AFW-2	0/3
		14/23 (61%)		0/14

AFW=anterior free wall; IT=inflow tract; PB=posterobasal

Two of the 3 patients were aged older than 50, and the age of the remaining patient was not reported. Routine use of thermometry and careful attention to the positioning of diagnostic catheters should minimize the risk of this complication. Persistent right bundle branch block occurred in 5 patients (2%), although the relationship to RF energy delivery was not always clearly defined.

Published data regarding outcome in non-outflow tract idiopathic RV tachycardia is limited, as these patients comprise less than 10% of all reported patients with RV tachycardias undergoing ablation. Available data are compiled in Table 4.[53,55,56,87] In general, ablation of these tachycardias has been less successful, potentially reflecting a greater diversity of mechanisms as well as a greater likelihood of occult structural heart disease.

The number of patients undergoing ablation of RV tachycardias may be considerably larger than has been suggested by published series. In a voluntary survey of 157 electrophysiology laboratories, 463 patients underwent ablation of idiopathic ventricular tachycardia in 1993 alone; the large majority of these was for RV tachycardias.[88] The overall success rate was reported as 85%, with an incidence of tamponade of approximately 1%. More contemporary surveys are not yet available.

Selection of Patients for Catheter Ablation

Given the generally benign prognosis of idiopathic RV tachycardia, reasonable concerns have been raised with respect to the selection of appropriate candidates for RF ablation.[89] In a substantial number of patients, symptoms are absent or minor, often despite frequent repetitive ectopic activity on ambulatory monitoring.

For patients with symptomatic and bothersome palpitations, the tachycardia may respond to several different drugs. Data on pharmacological therapy is available primarily for outflow tract tachycardias, and the results have been variable. Verapamil is reported to be effective during acute drug testing in up to 60% of patients, particularly those with only nonsustained runs;[90] others have reported less favorable results during long-term therapy.[3,5,6,18] As monotherapy, β-blockers have modest efficacy (25–50%).[3,5,14] Between 20–50% of patients may respond to Class Ia or Ic drugs.[3,18,91] The class III agent sotalol is reported to be effective in approximately 50% of patients.[6,18,91] However in a direct comparison with verapamil and flecainide, sotalol was not demonstrated to be clearly superior.[91] Overall recurrent tachycardia or symptoms are reported in 30–40% of patients during long-term follow-up on pharmacological therapy.[9,18,43]

In patients with hemodynamic compromise associated with tachycardia (syncope and presyncope), catheter ablation should be considered early in the course of the patient's care, even as primary therapy. These patients comprise a substantial proportion of previously reported ablation series. When symptoms are less severe, multiple factors, including side effects and inconvenience associated with long-term drug therapy, response to prior drug trials, and patient preference must be balanced against the potential risks and benefits of the ablation procedure.

Several specific circumstances merit additional comment. Ablation of frequent, highly symptomatic, single premature ventricular complexes arising from the RV has been reported by several centers.[92–94] The techniques and outcome were similar to those reported for RV tachycardias. Such an approach merits consideration in the rare patient who is disabled by symptomatic ectopic beats and is unresponsive or intolerant to drug therapy. However, reassurance and judicious use of antiarrhythmic drugs remains the mainstay for the vast majority of such patients. Initial data suggest that ablation of RV tachycardias may be safely performed in children and adolescents. No complications were reported in 6 patients (aged 6–16) by O'Conner and colleagues,[62] in 2 patients (ages 7–16) by Smeets and colleagues,[95] or in our own experience with 7 patients (aged 8–17). Safety in the very young has not been established, and experimental data raise concern with respect to lesion enlargement over time following RF application in the immature heart.[96] Finally, patients in whom runs of ventricular tachycardia persist for a substantial portion of the day may be at risk of developing tachycardia-mediated myopathy.[97] Well-documented tachycardiomyopathy secondary to idiopathic RV tachycardia is rare and when reported is usually due to incessant tachycardia.[9,98–100] Little objective data exist with respect to serial changes in ventricular function in patients with repetitive monomorphic VT of high density (> 20–50% of each 24-hour period), but long-term follow-up generally indicates little change in clinical status.[9] Whether high density alone, irrespective of symptoms, should prompt earlier consideration of catheter ablation remains unsettled.

With current technology, and in experienced centers, catheter ablation of most forms of idiopathic RV tachycardia can be accomplished with low morbidity and excellent immediate and long-term outcome. These results approach those reported for ablation of atrioventricular nodal reentry and accessory pathways.

References

1. Brooks F, Burgess H. Idiopathic ventricular tachycardia: a review. *Medicine* 1988;67:271–294.
2. Slama R, Leclercq JF, Coumel PH. Paroxysmal ventricular tachycardia in patients with apparently normal hearts. In: Zipes DP, Jalife J, eds. *Cardiac*

Electrophysiology and Arrhythmias. Orlando, FL: Grune & Stratton, 1985. pp 545–552.

3. Buxton A, Waxman H, Marchlinski F, et al. Right ventricular tachycardia: clinical and electrophysiologic characteristics. *Circulation* 1983;68:917–827.

4. Pietras R, Lam W, Bauernfeind R, et al. Chronic recurrent right ventricular tachycardia in patients without ischemic heart disease: clinical, hemodynamic, and angiographic findings. *Am Heart J* 1983;105:357–371.

5. Ritchie A, Kerr C, Qi A, et al. Nonsustained ventricular tachycardia arising from the right ventricular outflow tract. *Am J Cardiol* 1989;64:594–598.

6. Proclemer A, Ciani R, Geruglio G. Right ventricular tachycardia with left bundle branch block and inferior axis morphology: clinical and arrhythmological characteristics in 15 patients. *PACE* 1989;12:977–989.

7. Mehta D, Odawara H, Ward DE, et al. Echocardiographic and histologic evaluation of the right ventricle in ventricular tachycardias of left bundle branch block morphology without overt cardiac abnormality. *Am J Cardiol* 1989;63:939–944.

8. Mehta D, McKenna WJ, Ward DE, et al. Significance of signal-averaged electrocardiography in relation to endomyocardial biopsy and ventricular stimulation studies in patients with ventricular tachycardia without clinically apparent heart disease. J Am Coll Cardiol 1989;14:372–379.

9. Lemery R, Brugada P, Bella PD, et al. Nonischemic ventricular tachycardia: clinical course and long-term follow-up in patients without clinically overt heart disease. *Circulation* 1989; 79: 990–999.

10. Zimmerman M, Maisonblanche P, Cauchemex B, et al. Determinants of the spontaneous ectopic activity in repetitive monomorphic idiopathic ventricular tachycardia. *J Am Coll Cardiol* 1986;7:1219–1227

11. Coumel P, Leclercq JF, Slama R. Repetitive monomorphic idiopathic ventricular tachycardia. In Zipes DP, Jalife J, eds. *Cardiac Electrophysiology and Arrhythmias.* Orlando, FL: Grune & Stratton, 1985. pp 457–468.

12. Rahilly GT, Prystowsky EN, Zipes DP, et al. Clinical and electrophysiologic findings in patients with repetitive monomorphic ventricular tachycardia and otherwise normal electrocardiogram. *Am J Cardiol* 1982;50;459–468.

13. Wu D, Kou H, Hung J. Exercise-triggered paroxysmal ventricular tachycardia: a repetitive rhythmic activity possibly related to afterdepolarization. *Ann Intern Med* 1981;95:410–414.

14. Palileo EV, Ashley WW, Swiryn S, et al. Exercise provocable right ventricular outflow tract tachycardia. *Am Heart J* 1982;104:185–193.

15. Lerman BB, Belardinelli L, West A, et al. Adenosine-sensitive ventricular tachycardia evidence suggesting cyclic AMP-medicated triggered activity. *Circulation* 1986;74:270–280.

16. Sung RJ, Keung EC, Nguyen NX, et al. Effects of β-adrenergic blockade on verapamil-responsive and verapamil-irresponsive sustained ventricular tachycardias. *J Clin Invest* 1988;81:688–699.

17. Wilber DJ, Baerman J, Olshansky B, et al. Adenosine-sensitive ventricular tachycardia: clinical characteristics and response to catheter ablation. *Circulation* 1993;87:126–134.

18. Mont L, Seixas T, Brugada P, et al. The electrocardiographic, clinical, and electrophysiologic spectrum of idiopathic monomorphic ventricular tachycardia. *Am Heart J* 1992;124:746–753.

19. Lerman BB, Stein K, Engelstein ED, et al. Mechanism of repetitive monomorphic ventricular tachycardia. *Circulation* 1995;92:421–429.

20. Nava A, Thiene G, Canciani B, et al. Clinical profile of concealed form of arrhythmogenic right ventricular cardiomyopathy presenting with apparently idiopathic ventricular arrhythmias. *Int J Cardiol* 1992;35:195–206.

21. Orlov MV, Brodsky MS, Allen BJ, et al. Spectrum of right heart involvement in patients with ventricular tachycardia unrelated to coronary artery disease or left ventricular dysfunction. *Am Heart J* 1993;126:1348–1356.

22. Breithardt G, Borggrefe M, Wichter T. Catheter ablation of idiopathic right ventricular tachycardia. *Circulation* 1990;82:2273–2276.

23. Deal BJ, Miller SM, Scagliotti D, et al. Ventricular tachycardia in a young population without overt heart disease. *Circulation* 1986:6;1111–1118.

24. Rowland T, Schweiger M. Repetitive paroxysmal ventricular tachycardia and sudden death in a child. *Am J Cardiol* 1984;53:1729.

25. Wellens HJJ, Rodrigues LM, Smeets JL. Ventricular tachycardia in structurally normal hearts. In Zipes DP, Jalife J, eds. *Cardiac Electrophysiology.* Philadelphia, PA: Harcourt Brace & Co., 1995. pp 780–788.

26. Gill JS, Poloniecki J, Ward DE, et al. Survival and cardiac status in patients presenting with idiopathic ventricular tachycardia on long term follow-up [abstract]. *PACE* 1994;17:766.

27. Marcus FI, Fontaine GH, Guiraudon G, et al. Right ventricular dysplasia: a report of 24 adult cases. *Circulation* 1982;65:384–398.

28. Leclercq JF, Coumel P. Characteristics, prognosis, and treatment of the ventricular arrhythmias in right ventricular dysplasia. *Eur Heart J* 1989; 10:61–67.

29. Kullo IJ, Edwards WD, Seward JB. Right ventricular dysplasia: the Mayo Clinic experience. *Mayo Clin Proc* 1995;70:541–548.

30. Berder V, Vauthier M, Mabo P, et al. Characteristics and outcome in arrhythmogenic right ventricular dysplasia. *Am J Cardiol* 1995;75:411–414.

31. Marcus FI, Fontaine G. Arrhythmogenic right ventricular cardiomyopathy: a review. *PACE* 1995;18:1298–1314.

32. Ellison KE, Friedman PL, Ganz LI, et al. Entrainment mapping and radiofrequency catheter ablation of ventricular tachycardia in right ventricular dysplasia. *J Am Coll Cardiol* 1998;32:724–728.

33. Wichter T, Haverkamp W, Block M. Management of arrhythmogenic right ventricular cardiomyopathy [abstract]. *Circulation* 1994;90:I–340.

34. Blomstrom-Lundqvist C, Hirsch I, Olsson B, et al. Quantitative analysis of the signal-averaged QRS in patients with arrhythmogenic right ventricular dysplasia. *Eur Heart J* 1988;9:303–312.

35. Kinoshita O, Fontaine G, Rosas F, et al. Time and frequency domain analysis of the signal- averaged ECG in patients with arrhythmogenic right ventricular dysplasia. *Circulation* 1995;91:715–721.

36. Kinoshita O, Kmamkura S, Ohe T, et al. Frequency analysis of signal-averaged electrocard-iogram in patients with right ventricular tachycardia. *J Am Coll Cardiol* 1992;20:1230–1237.

37. White RD, Trohman RG, Flamm SD, et al. Right ventricular arrhythmia in the absence of arrhythmogenic dysplasia: MR imaging of myocardial abnormalities. *Radiology* 1998;207:743–751.

38. Globits S, Kreiner G, Frank H, et al. Significance of morphological abnormalities detected by MRI in patients undergoing successful ablation of right ventricular outflow tract tachycardia. *Circulation* 1997;96:2633–2640.

39. Markowitz SM, Litvak BL, Ramirez de Arellano EA, et al. Adenosine sensitive ventricular tachycardia: right ventricular abnormalities delineated by magnetic resonance imaging. *Circulation* 1997:96:1192–2000.

40. Gill JS, Davies MJ, Rowland E, et al. Histologic features related to the presence of late potentials in patients with "idiopathic" right ventricular tachycardia [abstract]. *PACE* 1995;18:796.

41. Tanabe T, Goto Y. Long-term prognostic assessment of ventricular-tachycardia with respect to sudden death in patients with and without overt heart disease. *Jpn Circulation J* 1989;53:1557–1564.

42. Noh C, Gillette PC, Case CL, et al. Clinical and electrophysiological characteristics of ventricular tachycardia in children with normal hearts. *Am Heart J* 1990;120:1326–1332.

43. Goy JJ, Tauxe F, Fromer M, et al. Ten years follow-up of 20 patients with idiopathic ventricular tachycardia. *PACE* 1990;13:1142–1147.

44. Tada H, Ohe T, Yutani C, et al. Sudden death in a patient with apparent idiopathic ventricular tachycardia. *Jpn Circ J* 1996;60:133–136.

45a. McKenna WJ, Thiene G, Nava A, et al. Diagnosis of arrhythmogenic right ventricular dysplasia/cardiomyopathy. *Br Heart J* 1994;71:215–218.

45b. Lerman BB, Stein KM, Markowitz SM. Adenosine sensitive ventricular tachycardia: a conceptual approach. *J Cardiovasc Electrophysiol* 1996;7:559–569.

46. Wilber D, Kall J, Kinder C, et al. Sustained right ventricular tachycardia: relationship of mechanism to underlying heart disease [abstract]. *PACE* 1996;19:600.

47. Lerman BB. Response of nonreentrant catecholamine-mediated ventricular tachycardia to endogenous adenosine and acetylcholine. *Circulation* 1993;87:382–390.

48. Griffith MJ, Garratt CJ, Rowland E, et al. Effects of intravenous adenosine on verapamil-sensitive "idiopathic" ventricular tachycardia. *Am J Cardiol* 1994;74:759–764.

49. Ng KS, Wen MS, Yeh SJ, et al. The effects of adenosine on idiopathic ventricular tachycardia. *Am J Cardiol* 1994;74:195–197.

50. Lee KLF, Lai WT, Tai YT, et al. Adenosine sensitivity of verapamil-responsive ventricular tachycardia: role of catecholamines [abstract]. *J Am Coll Cardiol* 1994;24:397A.

51. Yeh SJ, Wen MS, Wang CC, et al. Adenosine sensitive ventricular tachycardia from the anterobasal left ventricle. *J Am Coll Cardiol* 1997;30:1339–1345.

52. Chinushi M, Aizawa Y, Takahashi K, et al. Radiofrequency catheter ablation for idiopathic right ventricular tachycardia with special reference to morphological variation and long-term outcome. *Heart* 1997;78:255–261.

53. Aizawa Y, Chinushi M, Naitoh N, et al. Catheter ablation with radiofre-

quency current of ventricular tachycardia originating from the right ventricle. *Am Heart J* 1993;125:1269–1275.

54. Klein LS, Shih HT, Hackett FK, et al. Radiofrequency catheter ablation of ventricular tachycardia in patients without structural heart disease. *Circulation* 1992;85:1666–1674.

55. Calkins H, Kalbfleisch SJ, El-Atassi R, et al. Relation between efficacy of radiofrequency catheter ablation and site of origin of idiopathic ventricular tachycardia. *Am J Cardiol* 1993;71:827–833.

56. Mandrola JM, Klein LS, Miles WM, et al. Radiofrequency catheter ablation of idiopathic ventricular tachycardia in 57 patients: acute success and long term follow-up [abstract]. *J Am Coll Cardiol* 1995;19A.

57. Brodsky MA, Orlov MV, Winters RJ, et al. Determinants of inducible ventricular tachycardia in patients with clinical ventricular tachyarrhythmia and no apparent structural heart disease. *Am Heart J* 1993;126:1113–1120.

58. Coggins DL, Lee RJ, Sweeney J, et al. Radiofrequency catheter ablation as a cure for idiopathic ventricular tachycardia of both right and left ventricular origin. *J Am Coll Cardiol* 1994;23:1333–1341.

59. Amerendral J, Peinado R. Radiofrequency catheter ablation of idiopathic right ventricular outflow tract tachycardia. In: Farre J, Concepcion M, eds. *Ten Years of Radiofrequency Catheter Ablation*. Armonk, NY: Futura Publishing Co., 1998. pp 249–262.

60. Gumbrielle TP, Bourke JP, Doig JC, et al. Electrocardiographic features of septal location of right ventricular outflow tract tachycardia. *Am J Cardiol* 1997;79:213–216.

61. Movsowitz C, Schwartzman D, Callans DJ, et al. Idiopathic right ventricular outflow tract tachycardia: narrowing the anatomic location for successful ablation. *Am Heart J* 1996;131:930–936.

62. O'Conner BK, Case CL, Sokoloski MC, et al. Radiofrequency catheter ablation of right ventricular outflow tachycardia in children and adolescents. *J Am Coll Cardiol* 1996;27:869–874.

63. Rodriguez LM, Smeets JL, Timmermans C, et al. Predictors for successful ablation of right-and left-sided idiopathic ventricular tachycardia. *Am J Cardiol* 1997;79:309–314.

64. Man KC, Daoud EG, Knight BP, et al. Accuracy of the unipolar electrogram for identification of the site of origin of ventricular activation. *J Cardiovasc Electrophysiol* 1997:8:774–779.

65. Klug D, Ferracci A, Molin F, et al. Body surface potential distributions during idiopathic ventricular tachycardia. *Circulation* 1995;91:2002–2009.

66. Kadish AH, Childs K, Schmaltz S, et al. Differences in QRS configuration during unipolar pacing from adjacent sites: implications for the spatial resolution of pace-mapping. *J Am Coll Cardiol* 1991;17:143–151.

67. Kadish AH, Schmaltz S, Morady F. A comparison of QRS complexes resulting from unipolar and bipolar pacing: implications for pace-mapping. *PACE* 1991;15:823–832.

68. Goyal R, Harvey M, Daoud EG, et al. Effect of coupling interval and pacing cycle length on morphology of paced ventricular complexes: implications for pace mapping. *Circulation* 1996;94:2843–2849.

69. Goyal R, Mukhopadhyay PS, Syed ZA, et al. Effect of isoproterenol on QRS

morphology during ventricular pacing: implications for pace mapping. *J Electrocardiol* 1998;31:133–136.

70. Gepstein L, Hayam G, Ben-Haim SA. A novel method for nonfluoroscopic electroanatomic mapping of the heart: in vivo and in vitro accuracy results. *Circulation* 1997;95:1611–1620.

71. Wilber DJ, Blakeman BM, Pifarre R, et al. Catecholamine sensitive right ventricular outflow tract tachycardia: intraoperative mapping and ablation of a free-wall focus. *PACE* 1989;12:1851–1856.

72. Wen MS, Taniguchi Y, Yeh SJ, et al. Determinants of tachycardia recurrences after radiofrequency ablation of idiopathic ventricular tachycardia. *Am J Cardiol* 1998;81(4):500–503.

73. Kamakura S, Shimizu W, Matsuo K, et al. Localization of optimal ablation site of idiopathic ventricular tachycardia from and left ventricular outflow tract by body surface ECG. *Circulation* 1998;98:1525–1533.

74. Jadonath RL, Schwartzman DS, Preminger MW, et al. Utility of the 12-lead electrocardiogram in localizing the origin of right ventricular outflow tract tachycardia. *Am Heart J* 1995;130(5):1107–1113.

75. Shima T, Ohnishi H, Inoue T, et al. The relation between pacing sites in the right ventricular outflow tract and QRS morphology in the 12-lead ECG. *Jpn Circ J* 1998;62:399–404.

76. Rodriguez LM, Smeets JL, Weide A, et al. The 12-Lead ECG for localizing origin of idiopathic ventricular tachycardia [abstract]. *Circulation* 1993;88:643.

77. Callans DJ, Menz V, Schwartzman D, et al. Repetitive monomorphic tachycardia from the left ventricular outflow tract: electrocardiographic patterns consistent with a left ventricular site of origin. *J Am Coll Cardiol* 1997;29:1023–1027.

78. McAlpine WA. *The Heart and Coronary Arteries*. Berlin, Germany: Springer-Verlag, 1975.

79. Chinushi M, Aizawa Y, Ohhira K, et al. Repetitive ventricular response induced by radiofrequency ablation for idiopathic ventricular tachycardia originating from the outflow tract of the right ventricle. *PACE* 1998;21:669–678.

80. Mugelli A, Cerbai E, Amerini S, et al. The role of temperature on the development of oscillatory afterpotentials and triggered activity. *J Mol Cell Cardiol* 1986;18:1313–1316.

81. Gambassi G, Cerbai E, Pahor M, et al. Temperature modulates calcium homeostasis and ventricular arrhythmias in myocardial preparations. *Cardiovasc Res* 1994;28:391–399.

82. Nath S, Lynch C, Whayne JG, et al. Cellular electrophysiological effects of hyperthermia on isolated guinea pig papillary muscle. *Circulation* 1993;88:1826–1831.

83. Goldberger JJ, Pederson DN, Damle RS, et al. Antidromic tachycardia utilizing decremental, latent accessory atrioventricular fibers: differentiation from adenosine-sensitive ventricular tachycardia. *J Am Coll Cardiol* 1994;24:732–738.

84. Wilber DJ, Lin AC, Burke MC, et al. High density septal mapping in pa

tients with idiopathic right ventricular outflow tract tachycardia and prior failed ablation. [abstract] *PACE* 1999;22:733.

85. Stevenson WG, Nademanee K, Weiss JN, et al. Treatment of catecholamine-sensitive right ventricular tachycardia by endocardial catheter ablation. *J Am Coll Cardiol* 1990;16:752–755.

86. Morady F, Kadish AH, DiCarlo L, et al. Long-term results of catheter ablation of idiopathic right ventricular tachycardia. *Circulation* 1990;82:2093–2099.

87. Vohra J, Shah A, Hua W, et al. Radiofrequency ablation of idiopathic ventricular tachyardia. *Aust N Z J Med* 1996;26:186–194.

88. Scheinman M. NASPE survey on catheter ablation. *PACE* 1995;18:1474–1478.

89. Silka MJ, Kron J. Radiofrequency catheter ablation for idiopathic right ventricular tachycardia: first, last, or only therapy—who decides? *J Am Coll Cardiol* 1996;27:875–876.

90. Gill JS, Blaszyk K, Ward DE, et al. Verapamil for the suppression of idiopathic ventricular tachycardia of left bundle branch block-like morphology. *Am Heart J* 1993;126:1126–1133.

91. Gill JS, Mehta D, Ward D, et al. Efficacy of flecainide, sotalol, and verapamil in the treatment of right ventricular tachycardia in patients without overt cardiac abnormality. *Br Heart J* 1992;68:392–397.

92. Zhu DW, Maloney JD, Simmons TW, et al. Radiofrequency catheter ablation for management of symptomatic ventricular ectopic activity. *J Am Coll Cardiol* 1995;26:843–849.

93. Gursoy S, Brugada J, Souza O, et al. Radiofrequency ablation of symptomatic but benign ventricular arrhythmias. *PACE* 1992;15:738–741.

94. Gumbrielle T, Bourke JP, Furniss SS. Is ventricular ectopy a legitimate target for ablation? *Br Heart J* 1994;72:492–494.

95. Smeets JL, Rodriguez LM, Timmermans C, et al. Radiofrequency catheter ablation of idiopathic ventricular tachycardias in children. *PACE* 1997;20:2068–2071.

96. Saul JP, Hulse JE, Papagiannis J, et al. Late enlargement of radiofrequency lesions in infant lambs: implications for ablation procedures in small children. *Circulation* 1994;90:942–949.

97. Fenelon G, Wijns W, Andries E, et al. Tachycardiomyopathy: mechanisms and clinical implications. *PACE* 1996;19:95–106.

98. Maia IG, Cruz Filho F, Costa AM, et al. Repetitive monomorphic ventricular tachycardia. *Arq Bras Cardiol* 1994;62:11–15.

99. Kim YH, Goldberger J, Kadish A. Treatment of ventricular tachycardia induced cardiomyopathy by transcatheter radiofrequency ablation. *Heart* 1996;76:550–552.

100. Vijgen J, Mill P, Biblo LA, et al. Tachycardia-induced cardiomyopathy secondary to right ventricular outflow tract ventricular tachycardia: improvement of left ventricular systolic function after radiofrequency catheter ablation of the arrhythmia. *J Cardiovasc Electrophysiol* 1997;8:445–450.

Chapter 31

Catheter Ablation of Bundle Branch Reentrant Ventricular Tachycardia

Ali A. Mehdirad, M.D., Patrick J. Tchou, M.D.

Introduction

Single bundle branch reentry beats in the human heart were first described in the 1970s.[1-2] These authors reported that a stimulated ventricular premature beat (V$_2$) frequently elicited a spontaneous ventricular response, the "V$_3$ phenomenon."

Bundle branch reentry can also be a potential mechanism for sustained ventricular tachycardia in patients with conduction delay within the His-Purkinje system (HPS) which is usually associated with structural heart disease. Several reports have described sustained ventricular tachycardia attributed to reentry within the HPS.[3-10]

Electrophysiological characteristics of sustained bundle branch reentry were first described by Welch et al[8] and subsequently by other authors.[11-13] The diagnostic criteria for bundle branch reentry are summarized in Table 1. An example of such tachycardia initiated with right ventricular programmed stimulation is shown in Figure 1.

Substrate for Bundle Branch Reentry

While the anatomic structures consisting of the His bundle, the right and left bundle, and the myocardium form a potential reentrant circuit, the electrophysiological characteristics of the HPS (namely, rapid conduction with long

From Huang SKS, Wilber DJ (eds.): *Radiofrequency Catheter Ablation of Cardiac Arrhythmias: Basic Concepts and Clinical Applications,* 2nd ed. Armonk, NY: Futura Publishing Company, Inc. ©2000.

Table 1
Diagnostic Criteria for Bundle Branch Reentry Ventricular Tachycardia

1. Prolonged HV interval during sinus rhythm (>60 milliseconds) and usually somewhat longer during tachycardia. This further HV interval prolongation during tachycardia may be dependent in part on the recording site of the His bundle catheter. A proximal His bundle recording site may in fact slightly shorten the HV interval during tachycardia (when the recording site is more proximal than the site where the impulse turns around to descend the contralateral bundle branch).
2. Spontaneous variation in ventricle-to-ventricle (VV) intervals usually seen at initiation of tachycardia is preceded, rather than followed, by similar changes in H-H or RB-RB intervals.
3. Similar His-to-ventricle (HV) relations during tachycardia even if different programmed stimulation method was used for induction.
4. Single or multiple premature ventricular beats especially using a short-to-long sequence in the basic drive cycle length can usually induce the tachycardia. The first beat of tachycardia and all subsequent beats are preceded by H or RB potentials.
5. Resetting of tachycardia with a single premature ventricular beat by advancing the His or RB electrogram, indicative of association of HPS with the reentrant circuit of tachycardia.
6. Surface QRS morphology, as well as activation sequence of intracardiac electrograms, must be consistent with depolarization of the ventricle through 1 of the bundle branches.
7. Termination of tachycardia with retrograde conduction block within the HPS (V with no His or RB electrogram).
8. Absence of consistent H or RB deflection between QRS complexes during ventricular pacing at the cycle length of tachycardia.

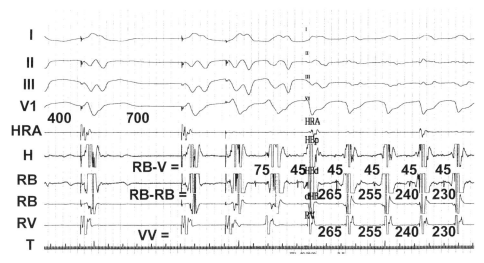

Figure 1. Initiation of bundle branch reentrant VT with right ventricular programmed stimulation. This figure illustrates initiation of a sustained VT with a single premature beat from the right ventricular apex. A short-to-long basic drive (400–700) was used prior to delivery of the premature stimulus. Such short-to-long basic drives can facilitate the initiation of bundle branch reentry as it promotes longer HPS refractory periods in the last beat of the drive, thus facilitating block and conduction delay within the HPS. Following the premature beat, delayed retrograde activation of the HPS via the left bundle occurs followed by anterograde activation of the right bundle and then the right ventricle giving the first reentrant beat of the tachycardia. The first RBV interval of the tachycardia is prolonged due to concealed retrograde penetration of the right bundle from the premature stimulated ventricular beat. Subsequent RBV intervals remain constant. Once the RBV interval became constant, changes in the VV interval was preceded by similar changes in the RBRB interval confirming that this tachycardia has a bundle branch reentrant mechanism.

refractory periods) prevent sustained reentry in the normal heart. The typical electrophysiological substrate in patients with inducible sustained bundle branch reentry tachycardia is conduction delay within the HPS as manifested by intraventricular conduction delay or bundle branch block pattern seen in the 12-lead electrocardiogram.[11–13] Such bundle branch block pattern is not necessarily indicative of actual conduction block in the particular bundle. Sufficient conduction delay within that bundle would produce ventricular activation via the contralateral bundle branch. However, complete anterograde bundle branch block in one bundle does not exclude the possibility of sustained bundle branch reentry using that bundle for conduction in the retrograde direction during tachycardia.

Patients with sustained bundle branch reentry tachycardia typically have dilated hearts due to underlying disease. While the incidence of bundle branch reentrant ventricular tachycardia appears to be highest in patients with non-ischemic dilated cardiomyopathy, approximately half of the patients reported in the largest published series had ischemic cardiomyopathy due to the prevalence of coronary artery disease.[14] Furthermore, cases of bundle branch reentry ventricular tachycardia have been reported in patients with isolated conduction disease of the HPS and no other structural heart disease.[15]

Clinical Characteristics

The cycle length of bundle branch reentry ventricular tachycardia in general is below 300 milliseconds. The most common QRS morphology in clinical and laboratory-induced tachycardia has a typical left bundle branch block pattern. This is consistent with retrograde conduction via the left bundle branch and anterograde conduction within the right bundle branch. However, there have been a few reports of tachycardia with a right bundle branch block pattern QRS morphology.[10,11,14,16]

A recent study in the human heart without HPS disease reported preferential retrograde conduction of ventricular premature beats via the left bundle branch regardless of the source of such premature beats. This observation may in part explain the preponderance of clinical and laboratory induced tachycardia with left bundle branch block QRS morphology.[17] Based on these authors' observations, the circuit of HPS reentry can be categorized into 3 types (Figure 2). Type A is the typical reentry with retrograde conduction via the left bundle branch and anterograde conduction via the right bundle branch resulting in a QRS morphology of left bundle branch block pattern. Obviously, ablation of either the right or the left bundle branch can interrupt this reentrant circuit and prevent the tachycardia. Type B is fascicular reentry where retrograde conduction is via a left-sided fascicle and anterograde conduction via the other fascicle resulting in a QRS morphology having a right bundle branch block pattern. An example is shown in Figure 3. It is clear that the right bundle branch is not a part of the reentry circuit and its ablation does not affect the tachycardia. Ablation of either the left anterior or the left posterior fascicle is needed to interrupt the tachycardia circuit. Type C has a reversed reen-

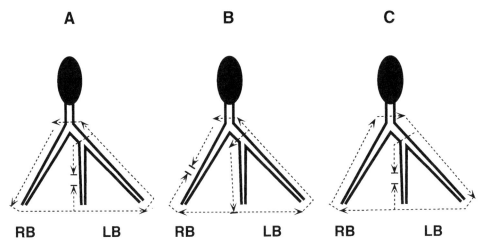

Figure 2. Three types of HPS reentrant circuits. Type A is the most commonly seen clinical form of bundle branch reentrant VT. This circuit has a counterclockwise rotation with retrograde activation via the left bundle branches and anterograde activation via the right bundle. Type B is fascicular reentry wherein retrograde activation is via 1 fascicle and anterograde is via the other. The His bundle and the right bundle are activated in a bystander fashion. Type C is the opposite of Type A having a clockwise rotation of the reentrant circuit. The QRS morphology of Type B and Type C can be the same because ventricular activation during tachycardia is from the left bundle branch system. Reproduced with permission from Tchou P, Mehdirad AA. Bundle branch reentry ventricular tachycardia. *PACE* 1995;18:1427–1437.

trant circuit of type A. That is, retrograde conduction is via the right bundle branch and anterograde conduction is via the left bundle branch, resulting in a right bundle branch block QRS pattern. Similar to type A, interruption of the reentrant circuit can be achieved by ablating either the right or the left bundle branch.

Ventricular tachycardia originating from the myocardium with incidental "bystander" activation of the HPS can mimic HPS reentrant ventricular tachycardia. However, spontaneous VV interval changes in such instances would be expected to be followed by similar HH interval changes rather than preceded by them.

HPS reentry tachycardia with a right bundle branch QRS morphology should be distinguished from idiopathic left ventricular tachycardia seen in the normal heart. This tachycardia occurs in the presence of normal QRS duration in sinus rhythm and is inducible using programmed atrial or ventricular stimulation or during atrial and ventricular pacing. This tachycardia will frequently have a His potential preceding the QRS or within the early portion of the QRS suggesting a fascicular origin of the tachycardia. Intravenous administration of verapamil usually terminates this arrhythmia and oral administration can prevent recurrence in some patients. Another tachycardia that should be distinguished from HPS reentry tachycardia is fascicular tachycardia caused by digoxin toxicity. The latter has a right bundle branch block pattern QRS morphology with an axis in the frontal plane that is deviated

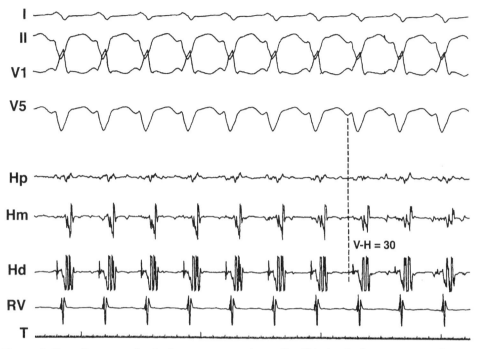

Figure 3. Type B reentry: fascicular reentrant tachycardia. This fascicular reentrant tachycardia was initiated with programmed stimulation in a patient with a dilated cardiomyopathy who also had a typical bundle branch reentrant VT induced during the electrophysiology study. While the tachycardia has a right bundle branch block QRS morphology, it is not a Type C bundle branch reentry. The fascicular origin of this tachycardia could be deduced from the fact that RB activation occurs following the QRS rather than preceding the QRS. This pattern is consistent with retrograde His Bundle activation with bystander RB activation during a fascicular reentrant rhythm. Reproduced with permission from Tchou P, Mehdirad AA. Bundle branch reentry ventricular tachycardia. *PACE* 1995;18:1427–1437.

rightward or leftward, and not uncommonly there is a beat to beat shift in the frontal plane axis. Data from studies in isolated Purkinje fibers and in the intact dog heart strongly suggest triggered activity as the mechanism of this arrhythmia.[18,19] Intravenous verapamil will slow and terminate this tachycardia but tachycardia will resume as the verapamil effect wears off. Digoxin-specific FAB fragment administration causes gradual slowing of the tachycardia before termination.

Catheter Ablation

Right Bundle Branch Ablation

Direct current catheter ablation was the initial reported approach to right bundle ablation.[11,13,20] However, because of concerns with potential complications

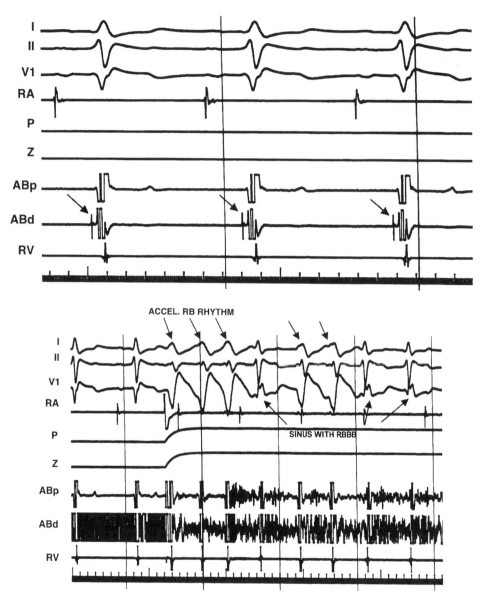

Figure 4A,B. Mapping and ablation of the right bundle. Upper panel shows a right bundle recording from the tip of the ablation catheter. To obtain this electrogram, the catheter is positioned at the typical His bundle location and its tip gradually advanced. The tip deflection can be adjusted with each advancement so as to obtain the optimal His-RB recordings. From a His bundle recording position, the catheter would need to be advanced about 1 cm so that the tip of the catheter is over the discrete right bundle branch and beyond the bifurcation of the left bundle fibers. With close bipolar recording (2–5 mm interelectrode spacing), there should be no atrial electrogram at all on the right bundle electrogram. With 1-cm interelectrode distances, a small atrial electrogram may be seen. Lower panel shows the delivery of radiofrequency energy to the right bundle branch. Occasionally, an accelerated right bundle rhythm can be seen at the initiation of energy delivery as shown on this panel. Right bundle branch block develops quickly when the catheter tip is properly positioned. Reproduced with permission from Tchou P, Mehdirad AA. Bundle branch reentry ventricular tachycardia. *PACE* 1995;18:1427–1437.

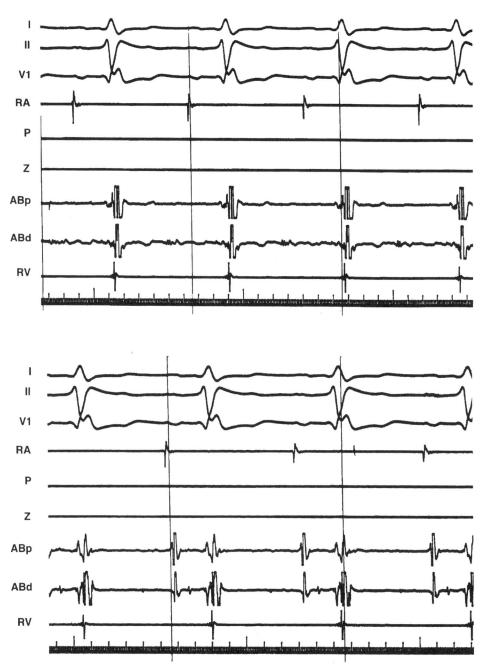

Figure 4C,D. At the end of the ablation, the local right bundle recording is no longer visible (upper panel) and a right bundle branch block QRS morphology is present on the surface ECG. Withdrawal of the catheter to the His bundle position (lower panel) demonstrates that the His bundle recording is still intact. When patients have a left bundle branch block type of intra-ventricular conduction delay on their 12-lead ECG prior to ablation, the HV interval is likely to prolong somewhat after the ablation. The extent of prolongation depends on the amount of conduction delay present in the left bundle branches.[28] Reproduced with permission from Tchou P, Mehdirad AA. Bundle branch reentry ventricular tachycardia. *PACE* 1995;18:1427–1437.

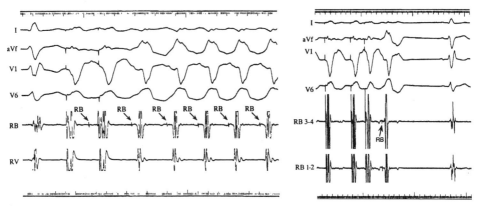

Figure 5. Concealed RB potentials during sinus rhythm. Recording of the right bundle potential could be difficult during sinus rhythm in patients with right bundle branch conduction delay at baseline. This example shows that the right bundle potential could not be recorded during sinus rhythm as the patient has an underlying incomplete right bundle branch block QRS pattern. While the right bundle clearly can conduct in the anterograde direction since the patient has the typical form of bundle branch reentrant tachycardia, the distal right bundle electrogram activated late during sinus rhythm due to the right bundle conduction delay and is obscured by the septal ventricular electrogram activated via the left side. However, the RB potential can readily be observed during tachycardia or during a single bundle branch reentrant beat elicited with right ventricular premature stimulation because ventricular activation is exclusively via the right bundle during those beats. Reproduced with permission from Wang, et al.[22]

(depression of ventricular function, barotrauma, myocardial rupture, large lesions, and the need for general anesthesia) radiofrequency ablation has become the method of choice. Radiofrequency catheter ablation of the right bundle branch was first reported by Langberg et al in 1989 and has become the method of choice since then.[21] This technique can be used with minimal sedation and the development of right bundle branch block can be used to monitor energy delivery and thereby avoid excessive amount of tissue damage. A femoral vein approach and the use of a steerable catheter are essential. The standard technique for ablating the right bundle includes identification of the area of the septum where the largest His potential is recorded. Using anterior-posterior or, preferably, a right anterior oblique view, the catheter should gradually be advanced superiorly and to the patient's left with continuous adjustment of catheter curvature, until a right bundle potential is recorded. The right bundle potential can be distinguished from the His potential by the following: 1) absence of or minimal atrial electrogram on the recording; and 2) an HRB interval of at least 15 milliseconds.[2] Attempts should be made to obtain a distal right bundle recording in order to ensure that the catheter tip is well away from the His bundle and left bundle system. Slight amounts of clockwise torque will ensure adequate catheter tip contact with the septum and the right bundle branch.

The delivery of radiofrequency energy should be started at low levels (5 watts or 20 volts) and gradually increased at 10-second intervals. In general, right bundle branch block develops at around 15–20 watts or 40 volts. The output can then be increased by 5 watts to ensure successful ablation. Alternatively, the catheter tip may be set to 60°C in ablation systems where temperature feedback control of power delivery is available. Figure 4 demonstrates typical electrogram recording before and after ablation of the right bundle branch. In some circumstances, ablation of the right bundle may be difficult due to inability to map the right bundle potential. When HPS disease produces right bundle branch conduction delay, the right bundle potential could be hidden within the ventricular electrogram during sinus rhythm.[22] Thus, when the 12-lead ECG shows a complete or incomplete right bundle branch block pattern, mapping of the right bundle potential may be impossible during sinus rhythm. However, the potential should be readily observed during single macro-reentrant ventricular beats elicited by right ventricular premature stimulation, or during sustained bundle branch reentrant tachycardia (Figure 5). In this scenario, mapping of the right bundle branch potential should be done during the ventricular tachycardia or during single macro reentrant ventricular beats. After successful right bundle ablation, aggressive ventricular pacing and extrastimulation protocols should be used to investigate the inducibility of the tachycardia. In addition, decremental atrial stimulation should be used to evaluate the conduction properties of the HPS and to assess the propensity to develop infra-Hisian block. Anterograde HPS conduction can also be assessed following atropine infusion and procainamide infusion of up to 10 milligrams per kilogram. Should atrioventricular block below the His bundle occur after the ablation or if the HV interval is greater than 100 milliseconds, permanent pacing should be considered.

Left Bundle Branch Ablation

In the majority of patients with bundle branch reentrant tachycardia, the conduction abnormality in the left bundle is more severe than that in the right bundle branch.[11] However, in most patients, the conduction properties of the left bundle branch after right bundle ablation are still sufficient enough for maintaining 1-to-1 atrioventricular conduction during sinus rhythm. For those occasional patients in whom anterograde conduction down the left bundle is known to be inadequate for maintaining atrioventricular conduction, ablation of the conducting right bundle will commit the patient to a permanent pacemaker. Under such condition, ablation of the left bundle can prevent bundle branch reentry and still preserve anterograde conduction through the atrioventricular conduction system, obviating the need for possible pacemaker implantation. Because catheter placement in the left ventricle and left bundle ablation are technically more difficult and associated with potentially more serious complications, left bundle ablation should be pursued only in those patients who are likely to develop marked HV interval prolongation or atrioventricular block after right bundle ablation. The presence of complete left bundle branch block in sinus rhythm would suggest the possibility of anterograde conduction block within the left bundle. However, such a QRS pattern may only indicate left bundle conduction delay rather than block. During the electrophysiological study or during mapping of the right bundle potential, transient right bundle branch block may develop due to mechanical trauma of the right bundle from the catheter tip. If such transient right bundle branch block is accompanied by high-grade or complete atrioventricular block below the His bundle, one can surmise that anterograde conduction down the left bundle will not be adequate to maintain 1-to-1 atrioventricular conduction after right bundle ablation.[23] The presence of a left bundle potential following the V electrogram either intermittently or during every sinus beat would indicate anterograde conduction block in the left bundle with delayed retrograde activation of the left bundle recording site via the transeptal conduction from the right side. When these electrophysiological signs are present, ablation of the left bundle may be preferable in order to preserve conduction within the better conducting right bundle and to avoid the need for a permanent pacemaker.

Technique for Left Bundle Ablation

When ablating the left bundle or its fascicles, it is important to appreciate the difference in the anatomy of the right versus the left bundle branch. While the right bundle is, anatomically, a continuation of the His bundle, the left bundle arises as a broad band of fibers from the His bundle virtually in a perpendicular direction towards the inferior septum.[24] The posterior fascicle arises more proximally while the anterior fascicle arises more distally (Figure 6). Because the left bundle is a broad band of fibers, it is more difficult to ablate with a single radiofrequency application. Furthermore, the fascicle may diverge quite proximally so that the common left bundle extends only a short distance from the His bundle. Thus, ablation of the common left bundle may be difficult without harming the His bundle. In these circumstances, it may be necessary to deliver several lesions along the left side of the septum in an arc distal to the His bundle extending from the anterior superior septum, a point that is radiographically near the right bundle in the RAO view, to the inferior basilar septum so as to transect both fascicles. Transsection of both fascicles is the preferred approach when both a bundle branch reentrant VT and a fascicular reentrant VT coexist. An approach to selectively ablating the left bundle branch has been previously demonstrated in the canine heart.[25] A similar approach can be used in the human heart. The mapping catheter should be placed towards the inferior apical septum and the catheter gradually withdrawn towards the His bundle until a discrete left bundle potential is observed. The LBV interval should be less than or equal to 20 milliseconds and the A:V electrogram ratio should be 1:10 or less. At this position, the tip of the ablation catheter should be 1 to 1.5 centimeters inferior to the optimal His bundle recording site near the distal portion of the common left bundle. In contrast to right bundle ablation, a single radiofrequency lesion is not as likely to ablate the entire left bundle. Several applications of radiofrequency energy in this region may be needed to accomplish complete left bundle branch block due to the broader anatomy of the left bundle branch in comparison to the right bundle.

It is more difficult to monitor the progress of left bundle ablation during delivery of radiofrequency energy when compared to right bundle ablation.

Most patients will already have some intraventricular conduction delay localized to the left bundle system. As opposed to the usually clear development of right bundle branch block in lead V_1 during right bundle ablation, the development of a complete left bundle branch block may produce relatively subtle ECG changes primarily manifesting as widening of the QRS and changes in the QRS axis. One can also monitor the presence of retrograde conduction during a ventricular premature beat after each application of a radiofrequency lesion. Elimination of the retrograde V_2H_2 conduction that was present prior to ablation is a good indication that sufficient ablation of the left bundle has been performed to eliminate bundle branch reentry.

Ablation of anterior or posterior fasciles for prevention of fascicular reentrant tachycardia is more difficult as the catheter would have to be inserted into the left ventricle. Because the fasciles are not as discrete anatomically as the right bundle, mapping their locations is more complex and more applications of radiofrequency energy are generally needed to achieve successful ablation.

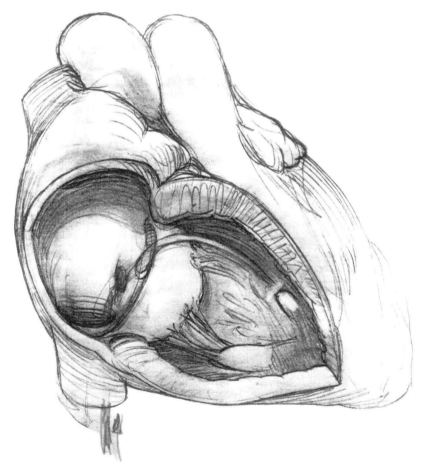

Figure 6. Anatomy of the right and left bundle branches. These drawings show the anatomy of the right (this page) and (*continued*)

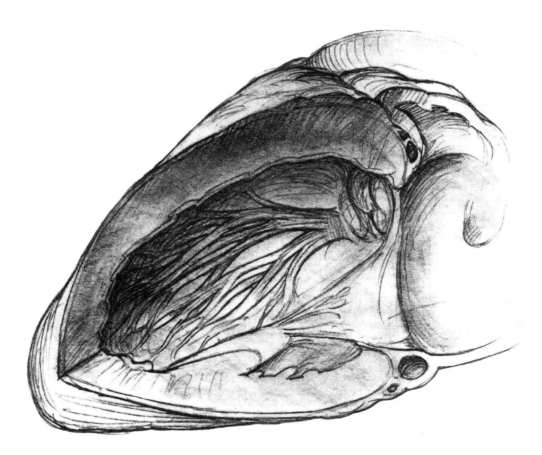

Figure 6. (*continued*) left (this page) bundle branches. While the right bundle has a very discrete course over the right side of the septum and can be easily ablated, the left bundle branches are more difficult to ablate for several reasons. The common left bundle does not exist as a discrete structure. Since the left bundle fibers separate from the common His bundle over a relatively long segment, the common left bundle is comparatively wide and quite short. Thus, ablation of the common left bundle is associated with a higher risk of His bundle damage. When left bundle ablation is contemplated, it is best to ablate in a wider arc along the proximal fascicular branches.

Viewing the heart from an RAO angle, the posterior fascicle extends inferiorly from the His bundle towards the inferior diaphragmatic wall. The anterior fascicle extends towards the apex of the heart. However, there is considerable variation of this anatomy and the exact distance from the His bundle where the left bundle branches can vary significantly from person to person.

Long Term Success and Additional Antitachycardia Therapy

Right bundle branch ablation using radiofrequency energy is safe and effective and recurrence of conduction via the ablated bundle is extremely unlikely. Therefore, recurrence of bundle branch reentry tachycardia is not seen clinically. The only complication is development of complete atrioventricular block (10–15%), which can readily be dealt with by implantation of a pacemaker.[17] These patients may be at risk for other types of ventricular tachycardia and careful screening should be conducted during follow-up electrophysiology studies to assess for the presence of any other sustained ventricular tachycardia. Experience with left bundle ablation of bundle branch reentry and fascicular reentry tachycardia associated with HPS disease is still limited. Therefore, it is difficult to state with confidence the complication and recurrence rate.[14,26,27] In the recent experience at the Cleveland Clinic, ablation of the left bundle was associated with hemodynamic deterioration in 1 case which may have been related to the worsening systolic septal movement associated with the newly created left bundle branch block. Thus, caution should be exercised in patients with severe left vnetricular dysfunction and the absence of a marked intraventricular conduction delay of the left bundle branch block type in whom the creation of a new left bundle branch block may worsen an already marginally compensated ventricular function.

Long-term survival in these patients depends ultimately on the underlying cardiac disease and identification, and appropriate treatment of other ventricular tachycardia.[12,14,23] Where these tachycardia are present, the implantable defibrillator can be an important additional therapy. Similarly, catheter ablation may be a useful additional therapy in patients who already have an implantable defibrillator. When such a patient experiences excessively frequent device discharges, the ablation of a demonstrable bundle branch or fascicular reentrant tachycardia can readily allow control of frequent shocks without the need for antiarrhythmic drug administration. A recent analysis of survival among 16 patients undergoing radiofrequency ablation of the right bundle and followed for a mean duration of 22 ± 10 months showed 1 sudden death and 1 death due to heart failure.[23] Three of these patients had implantable defibrillators, 2 of which were implanted prior to the ablation. Two patients underwent heart transplant during their follow-up. Certainly, a majority of these patients have significantly depressed ventricular function in association with the HPS disease. Thus, it can be argued that these patients are at risk for other ventricular tachycardia. Whether it is beneficial to implant defibrillators or treat with amiodarone on a routine basis in the absence of identifying another tachycardia remains to be demonstrated. However, in patients presenting with cardiac arrests where the initially identified rhythm was ventricular fibrillation, it would appear prudent to procede with a device implant as the laboratory induced rhythm may not be the one responsible for the clinical event.

References

1. Akhtar M, Damato AN, Batsford WP, et al. Demonstration of reentry within the His-Purkinje system in man. *Circulation* 1974;50:1150.
2. Akhtar M, Gilbert CJ, Wolf FG, et al. Reentry within the His-Purkinje system: elucidation of reentrant circuit using the right bundle and His bundle recordings. *Circulation* 1978;58:295.
3. Spurrell RAJ, Sowton E, Deuchar DC. Ventricular tachycardia in 4 patients evaluated by programmed electrical stimulation of heart and treated in 2 patients by surgical division of anterior radiation of left bundle branch. *Br Heart J* 1973;35:1014.
4. Guerot CL, Valere PE, Castillo-Fenoy A, et al. Tachycardia par reentree de branche a branche. *Arch Mal Coeur* 1974;67:1.
5. Gavrilescu S, Luca C. Recurrent ventricular tachycardia due to reentry within the bundle branches. *Chest* 1976;70:387.
6. Brechenmacher C, Mossard JM, Voegtlin R. Reentree ventricular permanente cachee et tachycardie ventriculaire paroxystique par mouvement circulaire. *Arch Mal Coeur* 1977;70:61.
7. Reddy CP, Slack JD. Recurrent sustained ventricular tachycardia: report of a case with His bundle branches reentry as the mechanism. *Eur J Cardiol* 1980;11:23.
8. Welch WJ, Strasberg B, Coelho A, et al. Sustained macroreentrant ventricular tachycardia. *Am Heart J* 1982;104(1):166.
9. Lloyd EA, Zipes DP, Heger JJ, et al. Sustained ventricular tachycardia due to bundle branch reentry. *Am Heart J* 1982;104:1095.
10. Touboul P, Kirkorian G, Atallah G, et al. Bundle branch reentry: a possible mechanism of ventricular tachycardia. *Circulation* 1983;67:674.
11. Caceres J, Jazayeri M, McKinnie J, et al. Sustained bundle branch reentry as a mechanism of clinical tachycardia. *Circulation* 1989;79:256.
12. Cohen TJ, Chien WW, Lurie KG, et al. Radiofrequency catheter ablation for treatment of bundle branch reentrant ventricular tachycardia: results and long-term follow-up. *J Am Coll Cardiol* 1991;7:1767–1773.
13. Tchou P, Jazayeri M, Denker S, et al. Transcatheter electrical ablation of right bundle branch: a method of treating macroreentrant ventricular tachycardia attributed to bundle branch reentry. *Circulation* 1988;78:246.
14. Blanck Z, Dhala A, Deshpande S, et al. Bundle branch reentrant ventricular tachycardia: cumulative experience in 48 patients. *J Cardiovasc Electrophysiol* 1993;4:253.
15. Blanck Z, Jazayeri M, Dhala A, et al. Bundle branch reentry: a mechanism of ventricular tachycardia in the absence of myocardial or valvular dysfunction. *J Am Coll Cardiol* 1993;22:1718.

16. Chien WW, Scheinman MM, Cohen TJ, et al. Importance of recording the right bundle branch deflection in the diagnosis of His-Purkinje reentrant tachycardia. *PACE* 1992;15:1015.

17. Mehdirad AA, Keim S, Rist K, et al. Asymmetry of retrograde conduction and reentry within the His-Purkinje system: a comparative analysis of left and right ventricular stimulation. *J Am Coll Cardiol* 1994;24:177.

18. Gorgels AP, Beekman HD, Brugada P, el al. Extrastimulus-related shortening of the first post-pacing interval in digitalis-induced ventricular tachycardia: observations during programmed electrical stimulation in the conscious dog. *J Am Coll Cardiol* 1983;1:840–857.

19. Wellen HJJ. The electrocardiogram in digitalis intoxication. In: Yu PN, Goodwin JF, eds. *Progress in Cardiology*. Philadelphia, PA: Lea & Febiger, 1976. pp 271–290.

20. Touboul P, Kirkorian G, Atallah G, et al. Bundle branch reentrant tachycardia treated by electrical ablation of the right bundle branch. *J Am Coll Cardiol* 1986;7:1404.

21. Langberg JJ, Desai J, Dullet N, et al. Treatment of macroreentrant ventricular tachycardia with radiofrequency ablation of the right bundle branch. *J Am Coll Cardiol* 1989;63:1010–1013.

22. Wang C, Sterba R, Tchou P. Bundle branch reentry ventricular tachycardia with two distinct left bundle branch block morphologies. *J Cardiovasc Electrophysiol* 1997;8:688–693.

23. Mehdirad AA, Keim S, Rist K, et al. Long-term clinical outcome of right bundle branch radiofrequency catheter ablation for treatment of bundle branch reentrant ventricular tachycardia. *PACE* 1995;18:2135–2143.

24. Massing GK, James TN. Anatomical configuration of the His bundle and bundle branches in the human heart. *Circulation* 1976;4:609–621.

25. Helguera ME, Trohman RG, Tchou P. Radiofrequency catheter ablation of the left bundle branch in a canine model. *J Cardiovasc Electrophysiol* 1996;7:406–414.

26. Berger RD, Orias D, Kasper EK, et al. Catheter ablation of coexistent bundle branch and interfascicular reentrant ventricular tachycardias. *J Cardiovasc Electrophysiol* 1996;7:341–347.

27. Crijns HJGM, Smeets JLRM, Rodriguez LM, et al. Cure of interfascicular reentrant ventricular tachycardia by ablation of the anterior fascicle of the left bundle branch. *J Cardiovasc Electrophysiol* 1995;6:486–492.

28. Mehdirad AA, Curtiss E, Tchou P. Interrelations between QRS morphology, duration, and HV interval changes following right bundle branch radiofrequency catheter ablation. *PACE* 1998;21(6):1180–1188.

Chapter 32

Ablation of Ventricular Tachycardia Late After Myocardial Infarction: Techniques for Localizing Target Sites

William G. Stevenson, M.D., Dusan Kocovic, M.D., and Peter L. Friedman, M.D., Ph.D.

Reentry Circuits in Infarct Scars

Sustained monomorphic ventricular tachycardia (VT) in humans is commonly caused by reentry.[1-5] A common feature of many of these reentry circuits is the presence of a region of slow conduction that is a critical component of the reentry circuit and a desirable target for catheter ablation. Slow conduction regions located in the infarct region or border zone contain surviving myocyte bundles surrounded by fibrosis. Conduction slowing is caused by decreased cell-to-cell coupling and/or by circuitous paths for wavefront propagation through isolated fiber bundles.[6] Among patients, and even in an individual patient, a variety of reentry circuit configurations may occur (Figure 1); a single region of slow conduction can give rise to more than 1 reentry circuit. [7-9] Reentry circuits vary in size and shape. The reentry paths are defined by either regions of functional conduction block or fibrosis. [1-5] The circuit may contain narrow isthmuses that can be transected by a focal lesion, or broad sheets that require a series of lesions for interruption.[3,10,11]

The location of the reentry circuit, or critical components of the reentry circuit, has important implications for catheter ablation. In the majority of

From Huang SKS, Wilber DJ (eds.): *Radiofrequency Catheter Ablation of Cardiac Arrhythmias: Basic Concepts and Clinical Applications,* 2nd ed. Armonk, NY: Futura Publishing Company, Inc. ©2000.

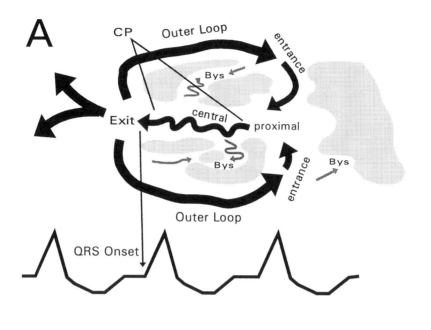

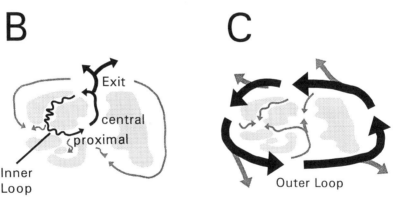

Figure 1. Three different theoretical reentry circuits are shown originating from the same chronic infarct. In each panel gray stippled areas are inexcitable regions in the infarct. The reentry circuit is indicated by the black arrows. Gray arrows indicate excitation wavefronts from the circuit that depolarize bystander regions that are not in the circuit. The circuit in panel A contains 2 loops and a common pathway (CP) creating a figure 8 configuration. The common pathway is a relatively small mass of tissue depolarization which generates low amplitude signals that are not detectable in the standard body surface electrocardiogram. The common pathway has an exit, central, and proximal regions. The QRS complex is inscribed after the excitation wavefront leaves the common pathway at the exit (arrow to the QRS onset at the bottom of the panel) and begins propagating around the border of the scar through 2 outer loops. The excitation wavefronts then enter the infarct region to reach the proximal portion of the common pathway. Several regions in the chronic infarct are bystanders that are electrically excitable but not in the circuit. The circuit in panel B is contained entirely within the chronic infarct. This circuit consists of exit, central, proximal, and inner loop regions. The circuit in panel C is a single outer loop in which the reentry wavefront circulates around the margins of the chronic infarct. Excitation wavefronts collide in the paths within the chronic infarct, which are bystanders. Bys = bystander; CP = common pathway. From Stevenson et al.[14]

cases a portion of the reentry circuit is contained in the subendocardium, accessible to intracavitary catheter ablation techniques. In up to a third of patients, reentry circuits involve the subepicardium.[12,13] Portions of the reentry circuit are often intramural, and in some cases the entire circuit may be intramural.[4]

Types of Reentry Circuit Sites

For catheter mapping, a working classification of reentry circuit sites that defines each mapping site according to its likely relation to regions of slow conduction in the circuit has been developed.[14] Examples of these sites are illustrated for theoretical reentry circuits in Figure 1. In the circuit in panel A, the circulating reentrant wavefront propagates through a region of slow conduction in a narrow isthmus in the scar. Depolarization of tissue in this isthmus generates low amplitude electrical signals that are not detected in the electrocardiogram recorded from the body surface. The wavefront leaves the isthmus region at the reentry circuit exit and propagates out, away from the exit, to depolarize the remainder of the ventricles, producing the QRS complex. The excitation wavefront may return to the slow conduction region or narrow isthmus through 1 of 2 different types of loops. An *outer* loop is a broad sheet of myocardium along the border of the infarct (see Figure 1, panel A). Depolarization of tissue in an outer loop may be detectable in the electrocardiogram recorded from the body surface. A second type of reentry loop is contained within the scar and is designated an *inner* loop (see Figure 1, panel B). In the example in Figure 1, panel A, 2 outer loops share a common pathway. The proximal portion of the common pathway is the *entrance,* and the distal portion is the *exit.* When there are 2 loops sharing a common pathway, as in Figure 1, panel A, the circuit has a figure 8 configuration, as has been described in animal models and humans.[12,15] In the figure 8 type of circuit, slow conduction may occur at the proximal and distal ends of the common pathway, rather than occurring centrally in the common pathway.[16] A variety of other reentry circuit types are theoretically possible. Circuits may contain only a single loop (see Figure 1, panel B) or more than 2 loops. A region of scar may serve as an anatomic obstacle for a single outer loop with no common pathway (see Figure 1, panel C).[17]

Sites that are not in the reentry circuit are designated bystanders. Identification of target sites for catheter ablation is complicated by the existence of electrically abnormal bystander regions that are not participating in the reentry circuit, but which give rise to fractionated electrograms with a timing that falsely suggests they are located in the reentry circuit (Figure 2).[5,18,19] Various types of bystander sites are theoretically possible. Blind alleys or dead-end pathways may be connected to any point in the circuit (see Figure 1, panel A). If multiple possible loops exist for the circuit, the loop with the shortest conduction time determines the tachycardia cycle length and is therefore the dominant loop.[5] Any loop with a longer conduction time behaves as a bystander.

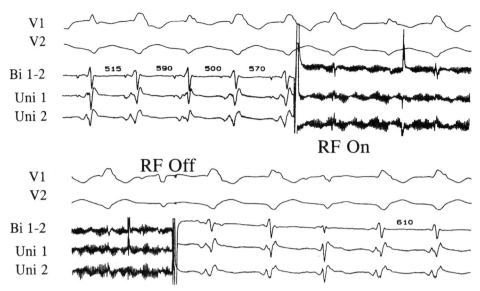

Figure 2. RF application at a site with an isolated potential abolishes the isolated potential without terminating tachycardia, suggesting that the isolated potential arose from a bystander. From the top are surface ECG leads V_1 and V_2 and intracardiac recordings from the ablation catheter distal electrodes 1 and 2 (Bi 1–2), and high-pass unipolar filtered recordings from electrodes 1 (Uni 1) and 2 (Uni 2). Tachycardia has a somewhat variable cycle length and QRS morphology. An isolated potential precedes each QRS. Following RF (lower panel) the isolated potential is abolished with little change in the larger component of the electrogram. From Stevenson et al. Radiofrequency catheter ablation of ventricular tachycardia late after myocardial infarction. *J Cardiovasc Electrophyiol* 1997;8:1309–1319.

Identifying Target Sites for Catheter Ablation

QRS Morphology During Ventricular Tachycardia and Pace Mapping

For VT that contains regions of slow conduction or isthmuses, the onset of the QRS occurs when the circulating excitation wavefront emerges from the reentry circuit exit (see Figure 1, panel A) and depolarizes a sufficient mass of myocardium to be detected from the body surface electrocardiogram recording. The morphology of the QRS complex often reflects the location of the reentry circuit exit.[20,21] A left bundle branch block-like configuration in lead V_1, with a large dominant S wave, usually indicates an exit in the left ventricular septum, or in the right ventricle. Left ventricular sites that are not septal generally cause a right bundle branch block QRS configuration in V_1. The frontal plane axis is also useful. Anterior wall exits, high in the ventricle, give rise to an inferiorly directed QRS axis, with dominant R waves in II, III, and aVF. Exits along the inferior wall give rise to a superiorly directed frontal plane axis. Exits along the lateral left ventricular wall, remote from the septum, give rise to a rightward QRS axis.

Analysis of the QRS morphology produced by pacing from the mapping catheter during sinus rhythm (pace mapping) can also be used to suggest the approximate region containing the reentry circuit exit. Pace mapping, which is performed during sinus rhythm, should not be confused with analysis of the QRS morphology during entrainment, for which pacing is performed during VT (see below). Sites where pace mapping produces a QRS morphology that matches that of VT are often near the reentry circuit exit.[22,23]

There are a number of nuances that can affect the QRS morphology during pace mapping. The pacing rate, or prematurity of stimuli can alter the QRS morphology.[24] At fast pacing rates, conduction slowing or regions of functional block may alter the sequence of ventricular activation. Depending on the pacing rate, portions of the QRS complex become superimposed on the T wave of the preceding beat, altering the QRS morphology. For analysis of the QRS morphology pacing should ideally be performed at a rate that approximates that of the VT. During bipolar pacing capture of underlying myocardium may occur at the cathode, anode, or both electrodes simultaneously depending on tissue contact, stimulus strength, and stimulus prematurity.[25] When pacing is performed in normal tissue using narrow interelectrode distances of ≤ 5 millimeters, changes in the site of capture are unlikely to cause major alterations in QRS morphology.[26] Unipolar pacing avoids capture at the proximal ring electrodes, but it produces a large stimulus artifact that can interfere with assessment of the QRS morphology. The clinical significance of these theoretical concerns has not been determined. The QRS morphology is only a crude guide to the location of the reentry circuit exit, and in some cases is frankly misleading: the circuit exit is remote from the region expected. The QRS morphology correlates best with the epicardial, rather than the endocardial, ventricular activation sequence, which is determined not only by the location of the reentry circuit exit, but also by the location of areas of conduction block.[20,21,27] Pace mapping can also be misleading. At many sites in the reentry circuit, the QRS complex during pace mapping does not resemble that of the VT (Figure 3). Thus a pace map that does not resemble VT does not indicate that the site is outside of the reentry circuit.[22] The specificity of pace mapping may be improved by body surface mapping.[28]

Pace Mapping to Identify Slow Conduction

Areas of slow conduction can sometimes be detected by pace mapping; abnormal conduction causes a delay between the stimulus and QRS onset (Figure 4).[22] It is important to assess the stimulus-to-QRS delay in all 12 electrocardiogram leads, as the initial portion of the QRS can be isoelectric in 1 or more individual leads. A stimulus-to-QRS delay of greater than 40 milliseconds is associated with sites is in the reentry circuit, but is not a reliable guide. The stimulus-to-QRS interval is short at many sites that are in the reentry circuit and long SQRS intervals can occur at bystander sites.

In summary, analysis of the tachycardia QRS morphology and pace mapping can be used to focus initial mapping to regions likely to contain the reentry circuit exit or abnormal conduction but may not be sufficiently specific or sensitive to be the sole guide for ablation.

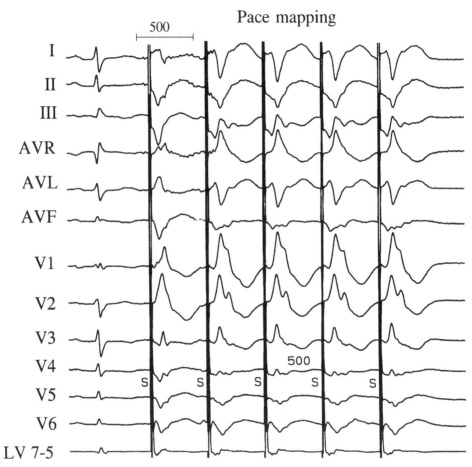

Figure 3. Pace mapping during sinus rhythm (right panel) and entrainment from the same site during ventricular tachycardia (*continued*)

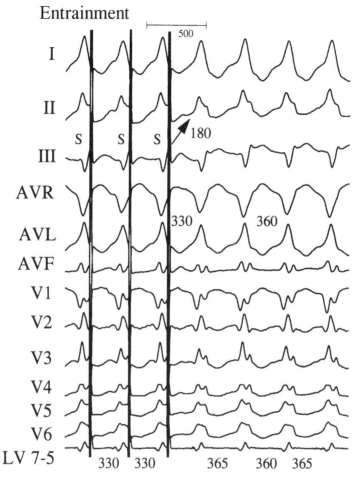

Figure 3. (*continued*) (left panel) often produce markedly different QRS morphologies. From the top of each panel are surface electrocardiogram leads I to V_6 and a filtered unipolar recording from the mapping catheter electrode (LV 7–5), which is 2 millimeters proximal to the pacing electrode. In the left panel, unipolar pacing is performed at a midinferior wall site (site 7–5) in a patient with prior inferior wall myocardial infraction. The paced QRS complex has a right bundle branch block configuration with a frontal plane axis directed superiorly and to the right. There is no conduction delay (SQRS < 40 ms). In the right panel, pacing is performed at this site during VT. The tachycardia cycle length is 360 to 365 ms. The tachycardia QRS morphology has a left bundle branch block configuration with a frontal plane axis directed inferiorly and to the left. Dominant R waves in V_2—V_6 suggest a basal exit. The last 3 stimuli of a stimulus train having a cycle length of 330 ms is shown. Pacing entrains the tachycardia with concealed fusion, with no change in the QRS morphology. (Additional intracardiac tracings are shown in Figures 8 and 10, below). The SQRS interval is 180 ms, consistent with a proximal site in this reentry circuit. RF application at this site terminated VT.

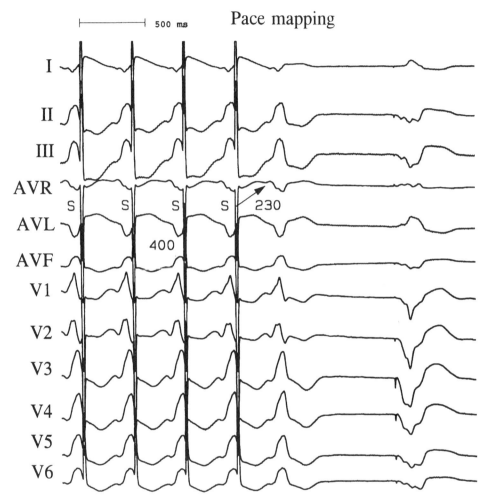

Figure 4. Evidence of conduction delay during pace mapping is shown. The underlying rhythm is atrial fibrillation with VVI pacing from a right ventricular permanent pacemaker (last beat on the right side of the panel). Unipolar pacing at a cycle length of 400 ms from an inferoseptal left ventricular site is shown (left side of panel). A markedly long SQRS interval of 230 ms is present, consistent with abnormal conduction from the pacing site in the region of infarction, to the margin of the infarct region.

Recording and Interpreting Electrograms

Recordings from electrode catheters can be obtained in either a unipolar or bipolar mode.[29] For unipolar recordings the catheter electrode is connected to the positive amplifier input. The negative input is traditionally the Wilson central terminal, or an electrode that is remote from the heart. A catheter placed in the inferior vena cava provides an indifferent electrode that is usually associated with lower noise recordings than the Wilson central terminals.[30] The amplifier is placed in a bipolar mode, but recordings are obtained between the electrode of interest on the mapping catheter and the electrode in the inferior vena cava. Traditionally, unipolar recordings are "near DC" recordings that are not filtered, or are high-pass filtered at .5 Hz or less to reduce baseline drift. These "unfiltered" unipolar recordings have a relatively wide field of view, including potentials generated by adjacent as well as remote myocardium.[31] Low amplitude signals, in regions of abnormal conduction, can be obscured by large amplitude "far field" potentials in unipolar recordings (Figure 5).[2,3,6,31,32] High-pass filtering can be used to reduce the "far field" component in unipolar recordings.[33] After high-pass filtering, however, the unipolar electrogram morphology no longer indicates the direction of wavefront propagation.

Bipolar recordings are the differential recordings between 2 electrodes in the heart. Much of the far field signal is subtracted out, improving detection of low amplitude potentials (see Figure 5). In normal tissue, local depolarization

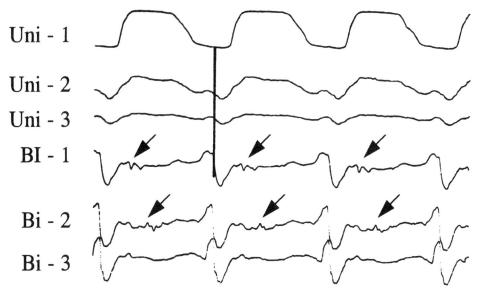

Figure 5. Simultaneous unfiltered unipolar and bipolar recordings obtained during intraoperative mapping of ventricular tachycardia are shown. From the top are 3 unfiltered unipolar recordings, followed by bipolar recordings from the same region. The vertical line indicates the maximal negative slope of the bipolar electrogram. Unipolar electrograms are substantially broader due to the contribution of far field signals. Low amplitude isolated potentials (arrows) present in the bipolar tracings are absent in the unipolar tracings. From Kimber et al[31] with permission.

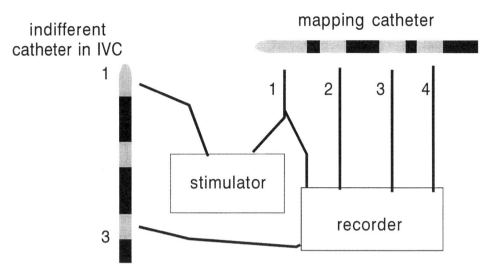

Figure 6. A setup for unipolar pacing with simultaneous unipolar and bipolar recordings is shown. An indifferent catheter is positioned in the inferior vena cava. The output from the mapping catheter electrode 1 is split into the cathodal (negative) output of the stimulator, and into the amplifier. Pacing is performed between the mapping catheter electrode 1 (cathode) and 1 of the electrodes on the IVC catheter (anode). Bipolar recordings are obtained between electrodes 1 and 2 and any other desired electrode pairs. Unipolar recordings are obtained by selecting electrode 1 as the positive input and 1 of the IVC catheter electrodes as the negative input for the desired channel.

coincides with a peak negative or positive deflection.[34] Bipolar recordings also have limitations. The amplitude of the signal is influenced by the direction of wavefront propagation. A wavefront that is perpendicular to the axis of the recording bipole may not generate a potential difference between the 2 recording electrodes, and go undetected. A signal of interest in the bipolar recording may originate from tissue beneath the distal recording electrode, beneath the proximal electrode, or beneath both electrodes. This is of importance because the ablation energy is usually applied to the distal electrode alone. Ablation may be unsuccessful because the target was beneath the proximal electrode. The source of the signal can often be ascertained from examination of simultaneously recorded, high-pass filtered, unipolar signals. For mapping of VT in infarct scars, our practice is to record both bipolar and unipolar electrograms high-pass filtered at 30 Hz or 100 Hz (Figure 6).

Sinus Rhythm Electrograms

Slow conduction through infarcts produces electrograms which are abnormal during sinus rhythm as well as during VT (Figure 7, panel C).[35,36] Fractionated and/or low-amplitude electrograms are often recorded from a relatively large region in and around the infarct scar and can be used to mark the infarct region. Surgical resection of subendocardial regions giving rise to frac-

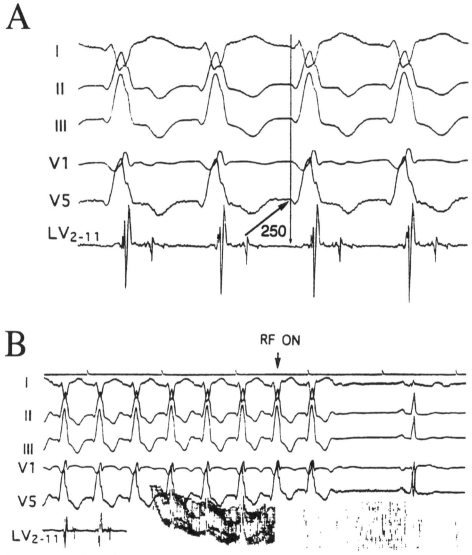

Figure 7. Recordings obtained during VT (panels A and B) and sinus rhythm before and after ablation (*continued*)

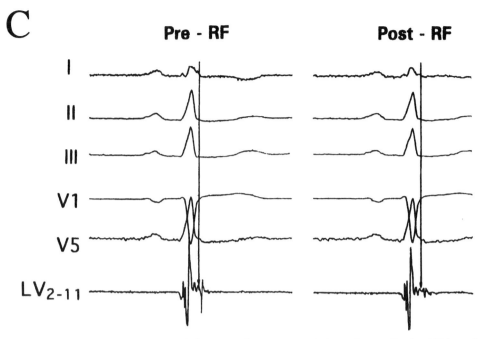

Figure 7. (*continued*) (panel C) at a left ventricular site (LV 2–11) are shown. During VT (panel A) isolated potentials are present; the largest precedes the QRS onset by 250 ms. RF ablation at this site terminates VT (panel B). During sinus rhythm, a late potential is recorded from this site; the signal extends beyond the end of the QRS complex (arrow). Following ablation, the amplitude of the late potential signal is markedly reduced. These findings suggest that the tissue giving rise to the late potential was also the source of the isolated potential observed during VT, which was damaged by ablation which terminated tachycardia. From Harada et al[41] with permission.

tionated signals often abolishes VT, but results in resection of large areas.[37,38] Fractionated electrograms can also be due to motion artifact, particularly when recording at high gain.[39]

Late potentials, defined as signals inscribed after the end of the sinus rhythm QRS complex (see Figure 7, panel C), indicate delayed depolarization and are potential markers of slow conduction.[40,41] Late potentials are present at 23% of reentry circuit exit sites, and increase in prevalence to 71% at sites that are in the central or proximal region of the reentry circuit as determined by entrainment (see below) (Table 1). In some cases a late potential marks an isthmus, which during VT is the source of an isolated diastolic potential (see Figure 7). However, late potentials are also frequently present at adjacent bystander sites.

In summary, low amplitude fractionated electrograms and late potentials during sinus rhythm are markers of the infarct region that are useful for identifying regions for further interrogation during VT. Care must be taken to ensure that catheter position is stable and that a fractionated electrogram is not due to artifact.

Table 1
Predictors of Radiofrequency Termination of Ventricular Tachycardia

	N	Radiofrequency Termination	%	Odds Ratio	95% CI
ECF					
Yes	86	15	17	3.4	1.4–8.3
No	155	9	6		
PPI-VTCL <30 msec					
Yes	64	13	20	4.6	1.6–12.9
No	114	4	4		
DP or CEA					
Yes	19	6	32	5.2	1.8–15.5
No	222	18	8		
S-QRS <70% VTCL >60 msec					
Yes	132	19	14	4.9	1.4–17.1
No	83	3	4		
ECF + PPI-VTCL <30 ms*					
Yes	40	10	25	5.3	2.0–13.8
No	168	11	7		
ECF + PPI + S-QRS <70% >60 ms					
Yes	22	8	36	8.8	3.1–25.2
No	186	12	6		
ECF + DP + CEA					
Yes	11	5	45	9.3	2.6–33.4
No	230	19	8		
DP or CEA + PPI					
Yes	11	6	55	13.9	3.8–50.2
No	226	18	8		

Electrograms During Tachycardia

If multiple sites in a reentry circuit can be recorded, the circuit can be identified by reconstructing the sequence of depolarization. Because portions of reentry circuits are often intramural or epicardial, entire reentry circuits are rarely delineated. Activation time at endocardial sites is commonly referenced to the onset of the QRS complex in the surface electrocardiogram. In the pioneering studies of Josephson and coworkers, electrical activity that preceded the QRS onset was termed presystolic, and the earliest presystolic electrical activity was designated the tachycardia site of origin.[42] Presystolic electrical activity (see Figure 2) occurs at and proximal to the reentry circuit exit, but does not reliably identify successful ablation sites.[5,9]

Several factors reduce the reliability of electrogram timing as a guide for catheter ablation.[31,43,44] The timing of local activation cannot be reliably de-

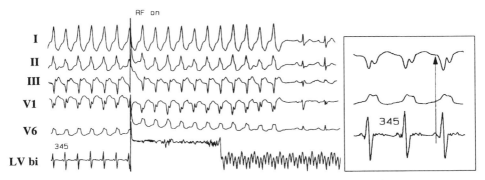

Figure 8. Application of RF current at the same site shown in Figures 3 and 15 terminates VT. At the right side of the figure the tracings from ECG leads V_1 and V_6 and the bipolar recording from electrodes 1 and 2 of the mapping catheter are shown at greater magnification. A high amplitude deflection follows the QRS onset (arrow). Low amplitude fractionated electrical activity extends from the QRS into early diastole. Despite absence of "presystolic electrical activity" this was a central site in the reentry circuit (entrainment from this site is shown in Figure 11) and ablation terminated tachycardia as shown.

termined from electrograms with multiple peaks (see Figure 11 below). Far field electrical activity can confuse assessment of local activation.[31,33] If the catheter is in a relatively narrow path in the reentry circuit, the signal generated by that source may produce a low amplitude potential that is obscured by the signal generated by activation of larger masses of adjacent myocardium (see Figures 5 and 8). Abnormal bystander regions can have presystolic or diastolic electrical activity, falsely suggesting that they are in the reentry circuit (see Figure 2).[5,18,19,45] Finally, at any given moment an excitation wavefront is passing through some portion of the reentry circuit, and thus there is no truly "early" or "late" segment in the circuit; searching for presystolic electrical activity ignores portions of the reentry circuit (see Figure 8).[45]

Isolated Diastolic Potentials

Isolated diastolic potentials are short duration low-amplitude deflections inscribed between the QRS offset and subsequent QRS onset (see Figure 2 and Figure 7, panel A).[46-48] They can be due to depolarization of narrow isthmuses of tissue in the reentry circuit and are useful markers of target sites for ablation.[2,3,5,7,41-49] They are frequently present at exit, central, and proximal reentry circuit sites, but also occur at adjacent bystander regions (see Figure 2). It is important to assess stability of the potential. Isolated potentials that are not consistently related to the tachycardia QRS complex are probably caused by artifact or depolarization of bystander pathways.[47]

At selected sites where pacing entrains tachycardia with concealed fusion, Bogen and coworkers found that the presence of an isolated potential that was not dissociated from the tachycardia by pacing from the right ventricular apex increased successful ablation from 54% to 89%.[46] Kocovic and coworkers found that the presence of an isolated potential at reentry circuit site identified by entrainment increases the likelihood that radiofrequency (RF) application will interrupt VT.[48]

RF Current for Thermal Mapping

The effect of RFcurrent application during VT can be used to provide further confirmation that the site is critical to the maintenance of tachycardia. Application of RF current heats the tissue and usually does not produce propagated depolarizations.[5,50] In patients with the Wolff-Parkinson-White syndrome, conduction block is observed at catheter tip temperatures exceeding 48°C. Interruption of tachycardia (see Figures 7 and 8) suggests that the ablation site is in the reentry circuit.[12,13] Ventricular tachycardia may terminate abruptly, or by gradual slowing. At exit, central, and proximal reentry circuit sites, the mean time to tachycardia termination is 10 ± 11 seconds; when RF application at other sites terminates VT, the average time to termination is 19 ± 16 seconds, which suggests that a larger region must be heated for interruption of reentry.[14] When RF application fails to terminate VT at a site that appears to be in the reentry circuit by entrainment or electrogram criteria, the site may be a bystander, with false positive mapping criteria. Alternatively, the size of the RF lesion may not be sufficient to interrupt conduction because the reentry path is relatively broad.

Programmed Electrical Stimulation for Mapping

Electrical stimulation at the mapping site can be used to assess the relation of the site to a reentry circuit. Stimulation may reset, entrain, terminate, or have no effect on tachycardia. To use entrainment for mapping, the patient must have sustained monomorphic VT that is hemodynamically tolerated for some period of time. Furthermore, tachycardia must be due to reentry, and sufficiently stable such that pacing does not terminate or alter the tachycardia. Use of unipolar stimulation avoids the potential for cardiac stimulation at electrodes other than the tip electrode that is used for ablation, but the large stimulus artifact sometimes interferes with analysis of the QRS morphology (see Figure 3, panel B and Figure 4).[25] It is not clear that unipolar pacing is superior to bipolar pacing; the 2 methods have not been directly compared. The pacing current strength determines, in part, the size of the virtual electrode (cathode or anode) that is directly depolarized by the stimulus.[51] In regions of infarction, relatively high current strengths may be required for capture (e.g., 10 mA at 2 to 9 ms pulse width). The optimal stimulus strength for mapping purposes has not been defined.

Entrainment Mapping

The majority of VTs that allow mapping can be reset or entrained by pacing stimuli, enabling these features to be used for mapping. Before applying these methods it is important to determine that the tachycardia can be entrained, indicating that reentry is the likely tachycardia mechanism.[5,52–55]

The ability to entrain or reset a tachycardia is due to the presence of an excitable gap at each point in the tachycardia circuit. The excitable gap is the time between recovery of the site from depolarization and arrival of the next depolarizing wavefront (Figure 9). During the excitable gap an appropriately timed stimulus can capture and produce a stimulated excitation wavefront that travels in 2 directions in the circuit (see Figure 9, panel B). The stimulated antidromic wavefront propagates in the reverse direction in the circuit, collides with a returning orthodromic wavefront, and is extinguished. The stimulated orthodromic wavefront travels in the same direction as the circulating antidromic wavefronts and resets the circuit. If a train of several stimuli is applied at a cycle length shorter than the tachycardia cycle length, but longer than the refractory period of the site, each stimulus will reset the reentry circuit (Figure 10). Continuous resetting of the reentry circuit is entrainment.

During entrainment a portion of the tissue is captured by the antidromic wavefront and a portion is captured by the orthodromic wavefront (see Figure 10, panels C and D). If depolarization from both the orthodromic and antidromic wavefronts is evident in the surface electrocardiogram recordings, the result is QRS fusion during entrainment (Figure 10). The QRS produced by the last stimulated orthodromic wavefront finds no stimulated antidromic wavefront to collide with. Thus the last entrained beat which occurs at the pacing

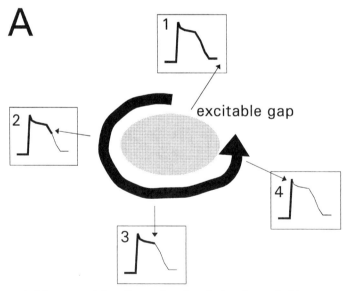

Figure 9. An excitable gap and the effects of pacing during the excitable gap are shown for a simple theoretical reentry circuit consisting of a wavefront (black arrow) circulating around an obstacle (gray oval). In panel A, the leading edge of the circulating wavefront is indicated by the head of the arrows. Representative action potentials recorded at 1 point in time from different sites around the circuit are shown in boxes 1 to 4. Near the leading edge of the circulating wavefront the action potential upstroke has been inscribed (dark line in box 4). Sites 3 and 4 are in later stages of repolarization. Site 1 has fully repolarized. At this point in time there is an excitable gap between the head and tail of the arrow. (*continued*)

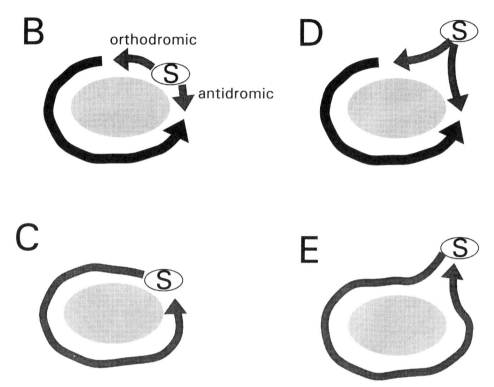

Figure 9. (*continued*) Panels B and C show the effects of a premature stimulus at the region of the excitable gap. The suprathreshold stimulus captures, depolarizing tissue and producing an antidromic wavefront and an orthodromic wavefront. The antidromic wavefront collides with the circulating orthodromic wavefront and is extinguished. The stimulated orthodromic wavefront propagates through the circuit resetting the circuit. Panel C shows that the stimulated orthodromic wavefront returns to the initial site of stimulation after making 1 complete revolution through the circuit. Thus the time from the stimulus to the following depolarization (postpacing interval) equals the revolution time through the reentry circuit (tachycardia cycle length). Panels D and E show the effects of a capturing stimulus at a site remote from the circuit. An appropriately timed stimulus captures and produces excitation wavefronts (gray arrow) that reach the reentry circuit during the excitable gap; these split into orthodromic and antidromic wavefronts in the circuit. The antidromic wavefront collides with the returning orthodromic wavefront (black arrow) and is extinguished. The stimulated orthodromic wavefront continues through the circuit resetting the tachycardia. Panel E shows that the stimulated orthodromic wavefront returns to the initial site of stimulation after propagating to the circuit, then making 1 revolution through the circuit and returning back to the stimulation site. Thus the time from the stimulus to the following depolarization (postpacing interval) exceeds the revolution time through the reentry circuit. From Stevenson et al[14] with permission.

rate does not have QRS fusion. At a given pacing rate the degree of fusion is constant; that is, the QRS morphology is the same from beat to beat. When the pacing rate is increased, each stimulus falls earlier during the excitable gap. The stimulated antidromic wavefront then propagates a greater distance before colliding with a returning orthodromic wavefront. Because the stimulated antidromic wavefront depolarizes a greater mass of tissue at the faster rate, the fusion QRS complexes begin to resemble QRS complexes produced by pacing in the absence of tachycardia (Figure 10, panel B). Figure 10, panels A and B show progressive fusion. The QRS morphology changes as the pacing rate is increased. Constant fusion and progressive fusion are hallmarks of entrainment. Their demonstration is sufficient to presume that reentry is the tachycardia mechanism.[52–54] Termination of tachycardia by pacing associated with conduction block is the third classical sign of entrainment.[53]

Postpacing Interval During Entrainment

At sites where pacing entrains or resets the tachycardia, the postpacing interval can be used to determine if the site is in the reentry circuit.[5,14] Figure 9 panels B and C illustrate capture of a single stimulus at a site in the reentry

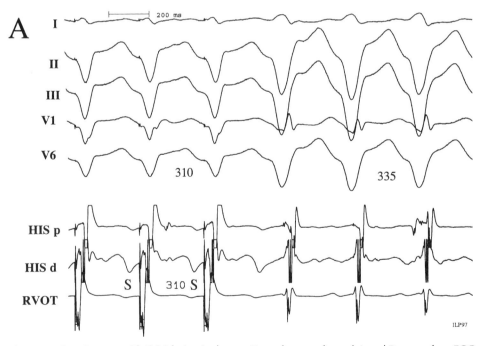

Figure 10. Entrainment with QRS fusion is shown. From the top of panel A and B are surface ECG leads and intracardiac recordings from the His bundle HIS p and HIS d and right ventricular outflow tract (RVOT). Tachycardia has a cycle length of 335 ms. The last 3 stimuli of the pacing train are shown. In the top panel pacing is performed at a cycle length of 310 ms. (*continued*)

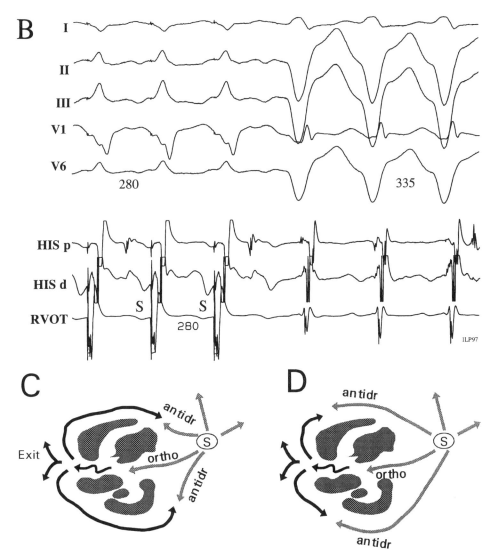

Figure 10. (*continued*) In the bottom panel pacing is performed at a cycle length of 280 ms. At each paced cycle length the QRS morphology is constant (constant fusion). At the faster paced cycle length the QRS morphology more closely resembles that of pacing from the right ventricular outflow tract, with an inferiorly directed frontal plane axis (R waves in leads II and III). Thus fusion is progressive. The mechanism of these findings is shown schematically in panels C and D. The reentry circuit has the same configuration and in Figure 1, panel A. Pacing is performed at a site remote from the circuit. Pacing produces wavefronts that reach the circuit and propagate in antidromic (antidr) and orthodromic (ortho) directions in the circuit. The change in QRS morphology during pacing is due to myocardium depolarized by antidromic wavefronts directly from the pacing site. When pacing at a shorter cycle length (panel D) the antidromic wavefronts propagate a greater distance, depolarizing more myocardium, and producing a greater change in the QRS configuration as compared to that of VT.

circuit. The stimulus produces an antidromic wavefront that is contained in or near the circuit. The stimulated orthodromic wavefront propagates through the circuit, resetting the tachycardia, and returning to the pacing site. The time from the stimulus to the subsequent depolarization at the pacing site is therefore equal to the revolution time through the reentry circuit, which is the tachycardia cycle length. Thus, the postpacing interval, which is measured from the stimulus that resets the tachycardia to the following electrogram that indicates depolarization at the pacing site, is equal to the tachycardia cycle length. In contrast, when pacing at a site remote from the reentry circuit entrains tachycardia, the postpacing interval is longer than the tachycardia cycle length (see Figure 9, panels D and E). The pacing stimulus produces a wavefront that propagates to the circuit and then splits into orthodromic and antidromic wavefronts. The stimulated orthodromic wavefront propagates through the circuit and back to the stimulation site. Thus the postpacing interval is the conduction time from the stimulus site to the reentry circuit, then through the circuit and back to the pacing site. The greater the conduction time between the circuit and the pacing site, the longer the postpacing interval. For infarct-related tachycardias, the likelihood of tachycardia termination by ablation decreases substantially when the postpacing interval exceeds the tachycardia cycle length by ≥30 ms.[5] The postpacing interval reflects the conduction time between the pacing site and the reentry circuit regardless of whether entrainment occurs with or without QRS fusion. However, the postpacing interval does not distinguish between broad regions where interruption of reentry is difficult, such as outer loops, and narrow isthmuses in the reentry circuit.

There are many potential pitfalls in the analysis of the postpacing interval.[5,56,57] If pacing prolongs the conduction time or alters the path through the reentry circuit, the postpacing interval lengthens, exceeding the tachycardia cycle length. Conduction slowing during pacing can be evident as a progressive increase in the postpacing interval during entrainment at progressively faster pacing rates, or oscillation of the tachycardia cycle length after termination of pacing. To avoid altering conduction times and the reentry path, the slowest stimulus trains or latest single stimuli that reliably entrain or reset the tachycardia should be analyzed. Termination of stimulation must be followed by resumption of the same tachycardia; a change in QRS morphology or tachycardia cycle length may indicate that the reentry circuit has been altered.

The postpacing interval analysis is unreliable if electrogram timing does not reflect local activation at the site.[5,56,57] Fractionated electrograms and the potential for far field electrograms (discussed above) can complicate interpretation of the postpacing interval. Often it is not possible to be certain which deflection in a fragmented electrogram indicates local depolarization (Figures 8 and 11). Our approach has been to measure the interval equal to 1 tachycardia cycle length after the stimulus, and then to determine the time from that point to the nearest electrogram. The minimum difference between the postpacing interval and the tachycardia cycle length is determined. This approach likely increases the number of false positive sites at the expense of minimizing false negative sites.

The postpacing interval should ideally be assessed in electrograms

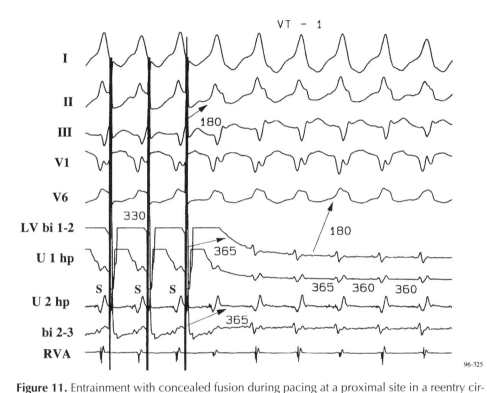

Figure 11. Entrainment with concealed fusion during pacing at a proximal site in a reentry circuit is shown. These recordings are from the same site as in figures 4 and 10. From the top are surface ECG leads (I, II, III, V1, and V6) and intracardiac recordings from the mapping catheter distal electrodes (LV bi 1–2), unipolar electrode 1 high-pass filtered (U 1 hp), unipolar electrode 2 high-pass filtered (U 2 hp), bipolar recordings from electrodes 2–3 (bi 2–3), and the bipolar recording from the right ventricular apex (RVA). Ventricular tachycardia with a cycle length of 360 to 365 ms is present. Unipolar pacing is performed from electrode 1 of the mapping catheter. The last 3 stimuli (S) of a stimulus train at a cycle length of 330 ms are shown. Pacing entrains tachycardia with concealed fusion; the 12 lead ECG during entrainment is shown in Figure 4, panel B. Arrows indicate the interval 365 ms from the last stimulus; which occurs at the time of a very low amplitude signal in LV bi 1–2 and U 2 hp. The postpacing interval measured to this low amplitude signal matches the tachycardia cycle length, consistent with pacing at a reentry circuit site. That pacing stimuli capture the tissue generating this low amplitude signal rather than the larger amplitude component of the electrogram is indicated by the fact that the large electrogram, which remains evident in the unipolar electrode 2 recording precedes the stimulus and has the same morphology during pacing and tachycardia. The SQRS is 180 ms and the low amplitude signal precedes the QRS by 180 ms, consistent with a reentry circuit site. The SQRS is 50% of the tachycardia cycle length consistent with a central site in the reentry circuit. RF ablation at this site terminated tachycardia, as shown in Figure 8). (A high gain recording of the LV bipolar electrogram is shown in Figure 10.) At the bottom of the figure, panels A, B, and C show the mechanism of entrainment with concealed fusion illustrated for the reentry circuit shown in Figure 1, panel A. Pacing is performed at a central/proximal site in the common pathway. In panel A, stimuli capture producing an antidromic wavefront (gray arrows) that collides with a returning orthodromic wavefront in the circuit. The stimulated orthodromic wavefront propagates to the exit. The conduction time between the stimulation site and the exit is 180 ms, as indicated by the SQRS interval. (*continued*)

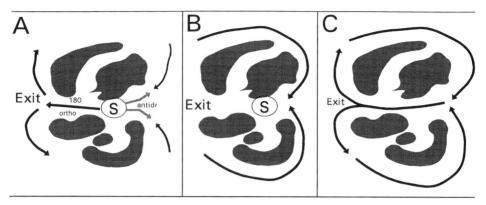

Figure 11. (*continued*) Following the last stimulus, the orthodromic wavefronts continue through the circuit, resetting the tachycardia (panel B). The complete reentry circuit is shown in panel C.

recorded from the mapping catheter electrode(s) used for stimulation. During stimulation electrical noise is introduced that may saturate the recording amplifiers or otherwise obscure these electrograms (see Figure 11, top). Recording from the proximal electrodes introduces an error, the magnitude of which is determined by the distance between the pacing and recording sites, the angle of the catheter relative to the excitation wavefront, and the conduction velocity in the tissue.[57] The error is small in tissue with normal conduction velocity, but increases markedly if conduction is slow. Even greater error occurs when a low amplitude isolated potential is present in the recordings at the stimulation site but not in those obtained from the proximal electrodes. If the signal present in recordings from the distal electrode has the same timing as that in the proximal electrodes, the error introduced by measuring the post-pacing interval from the proximal electrodes 2 to 6 millimeters from the stimulation site is probably small.

QRS Morphology During Entrainment:
Concealed Fusion and the Stimulus-to-QRS Interval

During entrainment the QRS morphology depends on the location of the pacing site relative to the reentry circuit, and the pacing rate. During pacing at some sites, the stimulated antidromic wavefront captures the vast majority of the ventricle, such that the QRS complexes are the same as those produced by pacing in the absence of tachycardia. The reentry circuit may still be entrained, but there is no electrocardiographic evidence to confirm that the circuit is being captured. This is concealed entrainment.[53,55] Pacing at some sites that are in or near the reentry circuit entrains tachycardia without altering the QRS morphology as compared to that of the tachycardia (Figures 3,11–14). The stimulated antidromic wavefronts are contained in or near the circuit and ventricular activation occurs entirely by the stimulated orthodromic wavefronts which propagate away from the reentry circuit exit.[5,8,58] The QRS morphology remains the same during pacing and tachycardia; QRS fusion must be "concealed" in or near the reentry circuit. This type of entrainment has been referred to as entrainment with concealed QRS fusion,[5,8] a form of concealed entrainment,[58] or exact entrainment.[12]

Entrainment with concealed fusion is associated with a 17% to 50% incidence of tachycardia termination by ablation.[5,58] Although entrainment with concealed fusion occurs more frequently during pacing at sites in or near the reentry circuit, it can also occur at bystander sites that are not in the circuit. Furthermore, entrainment with QRS fusion occurs during pacing at some outer

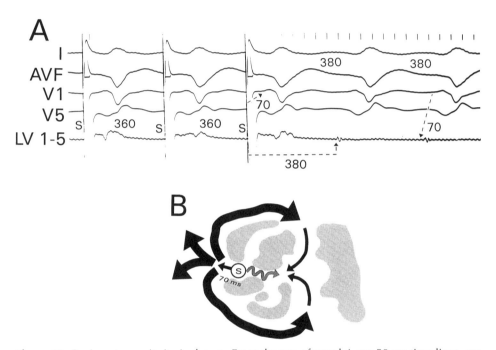

Figure 12. Pacing at an exit site is shown. From the top of panel A are 50 ms time lines, surface electrocardiogram leads I, AVF, V_1, V_5, and an intracardiac bipolar recording from the mapping catheter (LV 1–5). VT with a cycle length of 380 ms is present. The last 3 stimuli (S) of a stimulus train at a cycle length of 360 ms are shown. Pacing entrains tachycardia with concealed fusion. Following the last stimulus, the postpacing interval therefore matches the VT cycle length of 380 ms consistent with a reentry circuit site. Also, the SQRS interval of 70 ms approximates the electrogram to QRS interval during tachycardia as indicated by the dashed arrow from the last QRS complex. The SQRS interval is 70 ms, which is 19% of the tachycardia cycle length, consistent with an exit site. Panel B illustrates these findings for a theoretical reentry circuit. The stimulated antidromic wavefront (gray arrow) collides in the infarct with a returning orthodromic wavefront and is extinguished. The stimulated orthodromic wavefront (black arrow) exits the infarct from the same site as the tachycardia wavefronts, advancing the QRS complex without altering the QRS morphology (entrainment with concealed fusion). The next depolarization at the pacing site after the last stimulus occurs after the stimulated orthodromic wave-front has made 1 complete revolution through the reentry circuit. Thus the postpacing interval approximates the tachycardia cycle length. The electrogram to QRS interval during tachycardia reflects the conduction time from the mapping site to the point where the wave-front exits the circuit and begins to inscribe the QRS complex. This approximates the SQRS interval during pacing. From Stevenson et al[14] with permission.

loop sites that are in the reentry circuit, but not usually critical isthmuses. The postpacing interval and analysis of the SQRS interval are useful for determining whether the site is in the reentry circuit.

During entrainment with concealed fusion the SQRS interval indicates the conduction time from the stimulation site to the reentry circuit exit (see Figure 11).[5,59] When the site is in the reentry circuit the electrogram recorded from the site during tachycardia precedes the QRS onset by this same interval; the SQRS during entrainment with concealed fusion matches the electrogram to QRS recorded during tachycardia (see Figures 11, 12, and 14). In contrast, at adjacent bystander sites where pacing entrains tachycardia with concealed fu-

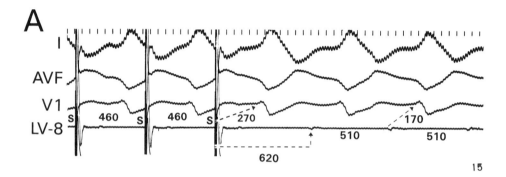

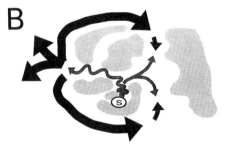

Figure 13. Pacing at an adjacent bystander is shown. From the top of panel A are 50 ms time lines, surface electrocardiogram leads I, AVF, V_1 and a bipolar recording from the distal electrode pair of the left ventricular mapping catheter LV-8. Ventricular tachycardia has a cycle length of 510 ms (last 2 beats of the panel). The last 3 stimuli (S) of a stimulus train at the mapping site are shown. Pacing at a cycle length of 460 ms entrains tachycardia with concealed fusion. In the LV-8 recording the postpacing interval of 620 ms indicated by the dashed arrow, exceeds the tachycardia cycle length by 110 ms, consistent with a bystander site. The SQRS interval of 270 ms exceeds the electrogram to QRS interval of 170 ms. The effects of pacing at an adjacent bystander site in a theoretical circuit is illustrated in panel B. The stimulated wavefronts (gray arrows) reach the reentry circuit common pathway and then propagate in both directions in the circuit. The antidromic wavefronts collide with returning orthodromic wavefronts and are contained in the chronic infarct. The stimulated orthodromic wavefront entrains the tachycardia with concealed fusion. The postpacing interval is the conduction time from the pacing site to the circuit, through the circuit and back to the pacing site and exceeds the tachycardia cycle length. From Stevenson et al[14] with permission.

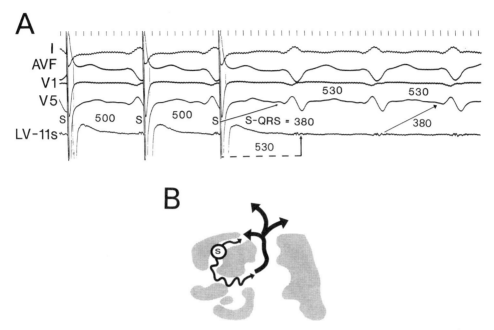

Figure 14. Pacing at an inner loop site is shown. From the top of panel A are 50 ms time lines, surface electrocardiogram leads I, AVF, V_1, V_5, and a bipolar recording from the distal electrode pair of the left ventricular mapping catheter at site 11s. Ventricular tachycardia with a cycle length of 530 ms is present. Pacing at a cycle length of 500 ms entrains tachycardia with concealed fusion. The postpacing interval (dashed arrow approximates the tachycardia cycle length consistent with a reentry circuit site. Also, the SQRS interval approximates the electrogram to QRS interval. The SQRS interval is 380 ms, which is 71% of the tachycardia cycle length, consistent with an inner loop site. Panel B illustrates stimulation at an inner loop site in a theoretical reentry circuit. The stimulated antidromic wave-front (gray arrow) collides with an orthodromic wavefront and is contained in the chronic infarct. The stimulated orthodromic wavefront resets the tachycardia. The long SQRS interval is due to the long conduction time between the pacing site and the exit of the excitation wavefronts from the scar. From Stevenson et al[14] with permission.

sion, the SQRS interval usually exceeds the electrogram to QRS interval (see Figure 13). Theoretically, the SQRS interval will match the electrogram—QRS at 2 types of bystander sites: those for which the conduction time from the site to the reentry circuit is equal to half of the tachycardia cycle length, and those that are in a path between the reentry circuit and the margin of the infarct scar.[5] These exceptions are rare. Analysis of the SQRS is particularly useful when the postpacing interval can not be assessed due to electrical noise at the recording site during pacing. Analysis of the SQRS and electrogram-QRS intervals is subject to limitations similar to those discussed earlier for the postpacing interval.

At reentry circuit sites where pacing entrains tachycardia with concealed fusion the SQRS interval also provides a means of identifying the likely relation of the site to the reentry circuit exit. A short stimulus to QRS interval indicates that the conduction time between the pacing site and exit is short (see Figure 12). As the pacing site is moved further from the exit, but remains in the circuit the SQRS becomes longer (see Figures 11 and 14). Accordingly, these sites have been subdivided into exit, central, proximal, and inner loop sites (Figure 15).

Effects of "Nonpropagating" Stimuli

Occasionally a stimulus terminates tachycardia without producing an excitation wavefront that propagates beyond the scar (Figure 16–18).[60-64] This finding can be mimicked by spontaneous tachycardia termination; it is important to demonstrate reproducibility. Often, stimuli applied at a longer coupling interval reset the tachycardia with concealed fusion, suggesting that stimuli can capture the site. The mechanism of tachycardia termination could be capture with block of all propagating wavefronts within the scar, or prolongation of refractoriness. In either case, the stimulus site is likely to be in or near the tachycardia circuit.

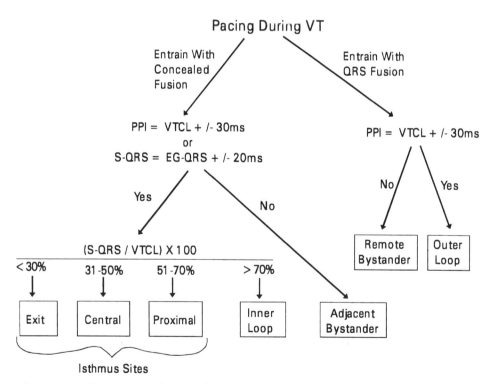

Figure 15. A flow diagram for classifying sites in a VT reentry circuit using entrainment is shown. PPI = postpacing interval; VTCL = VT cycle length; EQ-QRS = the interval from the electrogram recorded at the pacing site during VT to the QRS onset. See text for discussion. From Stevenson et al[14] with permission.

Integration of Catheter Mapping Strategies

It is desirable to minimize the time spent with the patient in tachycardia. One strategy is to identify the infarct region based on wall motion abnormalities and abnormal low amplitude sinus rhythm electrograms, then to focus on the likely exit region based on QRS morphology of tachycardia and pace mapping. Once the catheter is positioned at a likely exit region, VT is initiated by right ventricular stimulation. Recordings are examined for diastolic potentials. Pacing is then performed from the mapping catheter to classify the site and attempt to dissociate any diastolic potentials from the tachycardia. Based on these findings, either RF is applied during tachycardia to assess termination or the catheter is moved to a new site. This approach does not require sampling from other sites when a desirable target site is identified. The entire reentry circuit does not need to be delineated. The relation of the different types of sites to acute termination by a single RF lesion applied during VT has been analyzed for 398 sites during 75 different monomorphic VTs in 37 patients (Table 2).[14] The characteristics of different types of sites are summarized in Table 2.[5,14,22,41,48]

Future Improvements

For many patients with VT after myocardial infarction, mapping is a long, difficult procedure complicated by hemodynamically poorly tolerated tachycardias, multiple morphologies of tachycardias, and tachycardias originating deep to the endocardium that are difficult to localize and ablate. A number of technological advances aimed at solving some of these problems are entering clinical trials in humans.[65–67] Basket electrodes and noncontact electrodes may al-

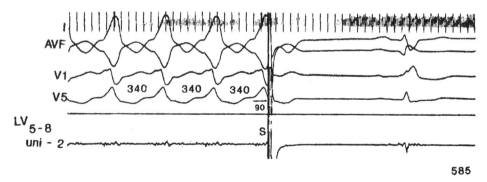

Figure 16. Termination of VT by a stimulus that does not produce a QRS complex is shown. From the top are 50-milliseconds time lines (longest vertical lines); electrocardiogram leads 1, AVF, V_1, and V_5; stimulus marker channel; and a unipolar recording from the electrode 2.5 millimeters from the tip of the mapping catheter (LV 5–8 uni-2). Sustained monomorphic VT has a cycle length of 340 milliseconds. A stimulus (S) 90 milliseconds after the QRS onset is applied to the distal electrode of the mapping catheter. The stimulus terminates tachycardia without producing a wavefront that propagates out of the scar. Application of RF current at this site terminates VT (not shown). From Stevenson W et al.[64]

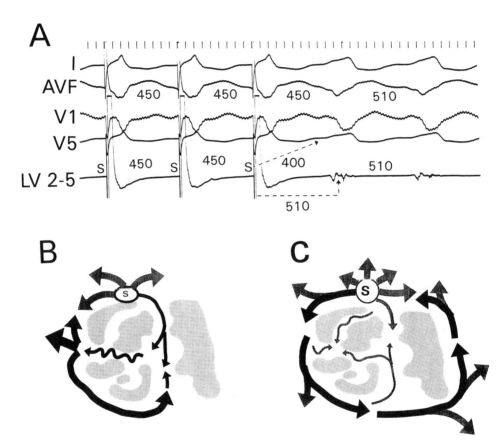

Figure 17. Pacing at an outer loop site is shown. From the top of panel A are 50 ms time lines, surface electrocardiogram leads I, AVF, V_1, and V_5, and a bipolar recording from the distal electrode pair of the left ventricular mapping catheter at site 2–5. VT with a cycle length of 510 ms is present. The last 3 stimuli (S) of a stimulus train at the mapping site are shown. Pacing entrains tachycardia with QRS fusion. The postpacing interval in the recording from the pacing site (LV 2–5) matches the tachycardia cycle length of 510 ms, consistent with a reentry circuit site. Panel B shows stimulation is performed at an outer loop site (S) in a theoretical reentry circuit. Stimulated antidromic wavefronts (gray arrows) propagate away from the infarct border, altering the activation sequence distant from the infarct, causing fusion QRS complexes. The stimulated orthodromic wavefront resets the reentry circuit. After the last stimulus, the pacing site is next depolarized by the orthodromic wavefront that has made 1 revolution through the circuit. The postpacing interval therefore approximates the tachycardia cycle length. From Stevenson et al[14] with permission.

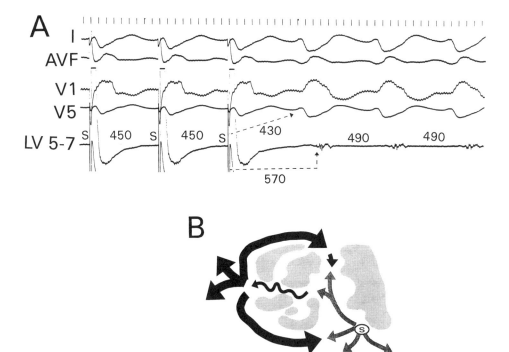

Figure 18. Pacing at a remote bystander is shown. From the top of panel A are 50 ms time lines, surface electrocardiogram leads I, AVF, V_1, and V_5 and a bipolar recording from the distal electrode pair of the left ventricular mapping catheter at site 5–7. VT with a cycle length of 490 ms is present. Pacing at a cycle length of 450 ms entrains tachycardia with QRS fusion. The postpacing interval in the left ventricular recording (LV 5–7) is 570 ms, exceeding the tachycardia cycle length by 80 ms consistent with a bystander site. Panel B illustrates that pacing is at a bystander site in a schematic reentry circuit. The stimulated wavefronts (gray arrows) propagate away from the border of the scar, altering the QRS morphology. Stimulated wavefronts also reach the reentry circuit and propagate through the circuit, resetting it. The postpacing interval is the conduction time from the pacing site to the circuit, through the circuit and back to the pacing site and exceeds the tachycardia cycle length.

Table 2
Mapping Findings at Reentry Circuit Sites

	Entrainment				Sinus Rhythm		VT	
	ECF	PPI = VTCL	S-QRS = EG-QRS	S-QRS/VTCL	Late Potential	Pace-map Match VT	IP	RF Term
Exit	+	+	+	≤.3	23%	often	52%	37%
Central	+	+	+	.31 − .5	70%	uncommon	58%	23%
Proximal	+	+	+	.51 − .7	70%	uncommon	55%	25%
Inner loop	+	+	+	>.7	15%	uncommon	2%	9%
Outer Loop	−	+	N/A	Variable	6%	variable	8%	10%
Adjacent bystander	+	−	−	Variable	75%	−	48%	11%
Remote bystander	−	−	N/A	Variable	15%	uncommon	2%	3%

From references 5, 14, 22, 41, and 48.

low sampling from multiple sites simultaneously. A nonfluoroscopic catheter navigation system may allow better integration of anatomy with electrophysiologic information. Small-diameter catheters for mapping the epicardium through branches of the coronary venous system could aid in identifying epicardial reentry circuit regions.

References

1. de Bakker JMT, van Capelle FJL, Janse MJ, et al. Macroreentry in the infarcted human heart: mechanism of ventricular tachycardias with a focal activation pattern. *J Am Coll Cardiol* 1991;18:1005–1014.
2. de Bakker JMT, van Capelle FJL, Janse MJ, et al. Reentry as a cause of ventricular tachycardia in patients with chronic ischemic heart disease: electrophysiologic and anatomic correlation. *Circulation* 1988;77:589–606.
3. Downar E, Kimber S, Harris L, et al. Endocardial mapping of ventricular tachycardia in the intact human heart. II. evidence for multiuse reentry in a function sheet of surviving myocardium. *J Am Coll Cardiol* 1992;20:869–878.
4. Pogwizd SM, Hoyt RH, Saffitz JE, et al. Reentrant and focal mechanisms underlying ventricular tachycardia in the human heart. *Circulation* 1992;86:1872–1887.
5. Stevenson WG, Khan H, Sager P, et al. Identification of reentry circuit sites during catheter mapping and radiofrequency ablation of ventricular tachycardia late after myocardial infarction. *Circulation* 1993;88:1647–1670.
6. de Bakker JMT, van Capelle FJL, Janse MJ, et al. Slow conduction in the infarcted human heart, "zigzag" course of activation. *Circulation* 1993;88:915–926.
7. Fitzgerald D, Friday KJ, Yeung-Lai-Wah J, et al. Myocardial regions of slow conduction participating in the reentrant circuit of multiple ventricular tachycardias: report on ten patients. *J Cardiovasc Electrophysiol* 1991;2;193–206.
8. Stevenson WG, Weiss J, Wiener I, et al. Localization of slow conduction in a ventricular tachycardia circuit: implications for catheter ablation. *Am Heart J* 1987;114:1253–1258.
9. Morady F, Harvey M, Kalbfleisch SJ, et al. Radiofrequency catheter ablation of ventricular tachycardia in patients with coronary artery disease. *Circulation* 1993;87:363–372.
10. Bartlett TG, Mitchell R, Friedman PL, et al. Histological evolution of radiofrequency lesions in an old human myocardial infarct causing ventricular tachycardia. *J Cardiovasc Electrophysiol* 1995;6:625–629.
11. Ellison KE, Stevenson WG, Couper GS, et al. Ablation of ventricular tachycardia due to a post-infarct ventricular septal defect: identification and transection of a broad reentry loop. *J Cardiovasc Electrophysiol* 1997;8(10):1163–1166.
12. Littman L, Svenson RH, Gallagher JJ, et al. Functional role of the epicardium in post-infarction ventricular tachycardia: observations derived from computerized epicardial activation mapping, entrainment, and epicardial laser photoablation. *Circulation* 1991;83:1577–1591.

13. Svenson RH, Littmann L, Gallagher JJ, et al. Termination of ventricular tachycardia with epicardial laser photocoagulation: a clinical comparison with patients undergoing successful endocardial photocoagulation alone. *J Am Coll Cardiol* 1990;15:163–170.

14. Stevenson WG, Friedman PL, Sager PT, et al. Exploring post-infarct reentrant ventricular tachycardia with entrainment mapping. *J Am Coll Cardiol* 1997;29:1180–1189.

15. El-Sherif N, Mehra R, Gough WB, et al. Reentrant ventricular arrhythmias in the late myocardial infarction period. Interruption of reentrant circuits by cryothermal techniques. *Circulation* 1983;68:644–656.

16. Dillon SM, Allessie MA, Ursell PC, et al. Influence of anisotropic tissue structure on reentrant circuits in the epicardial border zone of subacute canine infarcts. *Circ Res* 1988;63:182–206.

17. Miller JM, Harken SH, Hargrove WC, et al. Patterns of endocardial activation during sustained ventricular tachycardia. *J Am Coll Cardiol* 1985; 6:1280–1287.

18. Miller JM, Vassallo JA, Hargrove WC, et al. Intermittent failure of local conduction during VT. *Circulation* 1985;72:1286–1292.

19. Brugada P, Abdollah H, Wellens HJJ. Continuous electrical activity during sustained monomorphic ventricular tachycardia: observations on its dynamic behavior during the arrhythmia. *Am J Cardiol* 1985;55:402–411.

20. Miller JM, Marchlinski FE, Buxton AE, et al. Relationship between the 12-lead electrocardiogram during ventricular tachycardia and endocardial site of origin in patients with coronary artery disease. *Circulation* 1988;77: 759–766.

21. Kuchar DL, Ruskin JN, Garan H. Electrocardiographic localization of the site of origin of ventricular tachycardia in patients with prior myocardial infarction. *J Am Coll Cardiol* 1989;13:893–900.

22. Stevenson WG, Sager P, Natterson PD, et al. Relation of pace-mapping QRS morphology and conduction delay to ventricular tachycardia reentry circuits in human infarct scars. *J Am Coll Cardiol* 1995;26:481–488.

23. Josephson ME, Waxman HL, Cain ME, et al. Ventricular activation during ventricular endocardial pacing. II. Role of pacemapping to localize origin of ventricular tachycardia. *Am J Cardiol* 1982;50:11–22.

24. Goyal R, Harvey M, Doud EG, et al. Effect of coupling interval and pacing cycle length on morphology of paced ventricular complexes: implications for pace mapping. *Circulation* 1996;94:2843–2849.

25. Stevenson WG, Wiener I, Weiss JN. Contribution of the anode to ventricular excitation during programmed electrical stimulation in humans. *Am J Cardiol* 1986;57:582–586.

26. Kadish AH, Childs K, Schmaltz S, et al. Differences in QRS configuration during unipolar pacing from adjacent sites: implications for the spatial resolution of pace-mapping. *J Am Coll Cardiol* 1991;17:143–151.

27. Kimber SK, Downer E, Harris L, et al. Mechanisms of spontaneous shift of surface electrocardiographic configuration during ventricular tachycardia. *J Am Coll Cardiol* 1992;20:1397–1404.

28. SippenGroenewegen A, Spekhorst H, van Hemel NM, et al. Value of body surface mapping in localizing the site of origin of ventricular tachycardia

in patients with previous myocardial infarction. *J Am Coll Cardiol* 1994;24: 1708–1724.

29. de Bakker JMT, Hauer RNW, Simmers TA. Activation mapping: unipolar versus bipolar recording. In: Zipes DP, Jalife J, eds. *Cardiac Electrophysiology: From Cell to Bedside.* Philadelphia, PA: WB Saunders, 1995. p 1068.

30. Kadish AH, Morady F, Rosenheck S, et al. The effect of electrode configuration on the unipolar his-bundle electrogram. *PACE* 1989;12:1445–1450.

31. Kimber S, Downar E, Masse S, et al. A comparison of unipolar and bipolar electrodes during cardiac mapping studies. *PACE* 1996;19:1196–1204.

32. Ino T, Fishbein MC, Mandel WJ, et al. Cellular mechanisms of ventricular bipolar electrograms showing double and fractionated potentials. *J Am Coll Cardiol* 1995;26:1080–1089.

33. Gottipaty VK, Abrol R, Friedman PL, et al. Use of filtering to distinguish local from distant electrical signals in unipolar electrograms. *Circulation* 1994;90(4, part 2):I-596a.

34. Anderson KP, Walker R, Ershler PR, et al. Determination of local myocardial electrical activation for activation sequence mapping: a statistical approach. *Circ Res* 1991;69:898–917.

35. Stevenson WG, Weiss JN, Wiener I, et al. Fractionated endocardial electrograms are associated with slow conduction in humans: evidence from pace-mapping. *J Am Coll Cardiol* 1989;13:369–374.

36. Miller JM, Tyson GS, Hargrove WC, et al. Effect of subendocardial resection on sinus rhythm endocardial electrogram abnormalities. *Circulation* 1995;91:2385–2391.

37. Wiener I, Mindich B, Pintchon R. Determinants of ventricular tachycardia in patients with ventricular aneurysms: results of intraoperative epicardial and endocardial mapping. *Circulation* 1982;65:856–861.

38. Bourke JP, Campbell RWF, Renzulli A, et al. Surgery for ventricular tachycardia based on fragmentation mapping in sinus rhythm alone. *Eur J Cardiothorac Surg* 1989;3:401–407.

39. Ideker RE, Lofland GK, Bardy GH, et al. Late fractionated potentials and continuous electrical activity caused by electrode motion. *PACE* 1983;6: 908–914.

40. Hood MA, Pogwizd SM, Peirick J, et al. Contribution of myocardium responsible for ventricular tachycardia to abnormalities detected by analysis of signal-averaged ECGs. *Circulation* 1992;86:1888–1901.

41. Harada T, Stevenson WG, Kocovic DZ, et al. Catheter ablation of ventricular tachycardia after myocardial infarction: relationship of endocardial sinus rhythm late potentials to the reentry circuit. *J Am Coll Cardiol* 1997;30:1015–1023.

42. Josephson ME, Horowitz LN, Scott R, et al. Role of catheter mapping in the preoperative evaluation of ventricular tachycardia. *Am J Cardiol* 1982;49: 207–220.

43. Berbari EJ, Lander P, Scherlag BJ, et al. Ambiguities of epicardial mapping. *J Electrocardiol* 1992;24:16–20.

44. Ideker RE, Smith WM, Blanchard SM, et al. The assumptions of isochronal cardiac mapping. *PACE* 1989;12:456.

45. Brackman J, Kabell G, Scherlag B, et al. Analysis of interectopic activation

patterns during sustained ventricular tachycardia. *Circulation* 1983;67: 449–456.

46. Bogun F, Bahu M, Knight BP, et al. Comparison of effective and ineffective target sites that demonstrate concealed entrainment in patients with coronary artery disease undergoing radiofrequency ablation of ventricular tachycardia. *Circulation* 1997;95:183–190.

47. Fitzgerald DM, Friday KJ, Wah JAYL, et al. Electrogram patterns predicting successful catheter ablation of ventricular tachycardia. *Circulation* 1988;77:806–814.

48. Kocovic DZ, Harada T, Friedman PL, et al. Characteristics of electrograms recorded at reentry circuit sites and bystanders during ventricular tachycardia after myocardial infarction. *J Am Coll Cardiol* 1999;34(2):381–388.

49. Kuck KH, Schlüter M, Geiger M, et al. Successful catheter ablation of human ventricular tachycardia with radiofrequency current guided by endocardial mapping of the area of slow conduction. *PACE* 1991;14(6):1060–1071.

50. Langberg JJ, Calkins H, El-Atassi R, et al. Temperature monitoring during radiofrequency catheter ablation of accessory pathways. *Circulation* 1992; 86:1469–1474.

51. Wikswo JP. Tissue anisotropy, the cardiac bidomain, and the virtual cathode effect. In: Zipes DP and Jalife J, eds. *Cardiac Electrophysiology: From Cell to Bedside.* Philadelphia, PA: WB Saunders, 1995. pp 348–361.

52. Okumura K, Olshansky B, Henthorn RW, et al. Demonstration of the presence of slow conduction during sustained ventricular tachycardia in man: use of transient entrainment of the tachycardia. *Circulation* 1987;75:369–378.

53. Okumura K, Henthora RW, Epstein AE, et al. Further observation on transient entrainment: importance of pacing site and properties of the components of the reentry circuit. *Circulation* 1985;72:1293–1307.

54. Henthorn RW, Okumura K, Olshansky B, et al. A fourth criteria for transient entrainment: the electrogram equivalent of progressive fusion. *Circulation* 1988;77:1003–1012.

55. Stevenson WG, Nademanee K, Weiss JN, et al. Programmed electrical stimulation at sites in ventricular reentry circuits: comparison of predictions from computer simulations with observations in humans. *Circulation* 1989;80:793–806.

56. Khan HH, Stevenson WG. Activation times in and adjacent to reentry circuits during entrainment: implications for mapping ventricular tachycardia. *Am Heart J* 1994;127:833–842.

57. Hadjis TA, Harada T, Stevenson WG, et al. Effect of recording site on postpacing interval measurement during catheter mapping and entrainment of postinfarction ventricular tachycardia. *J Cardiovasc Electrophysiol* 1997; 8:398–404.

58. Morady F, Kadish A, Rosenheck S, et al. Concealed entrainment as a guide for catheter ablation of ventricular tachycardia in patients with prior myocardial infarction. *J Am Coll Cardiol* 1991;17:678–689.

59. Fontaine G, Frank R, Tonet J, et al. Identification of a zone of slow conduction appropriate for ventricular tachycardia ablation: theoretical considerations. *PACE* 1989;12:262–267.

60. Garan H, Ruskin JN. Reproducible termination of ventricular tachycardia

by a single extrastimulus within the reentry circuit during the ventricular effective refractory period. *Am Heart J* 1988;116:546–550.

61. Shenasa M, Cardinal R, Kus T, et al. Termination of sustained ventricular tachycardia by ultrarapid subthreshold stimulation in humans. *Circulation* 1988;78:1135–1143.

62. Shoda M, Kasanuki H, Ohnishi S, et al. Determination of the site for catheter ablation based on termination of ventricular tachycardia by a non-propagated stimulus: results of the long-term follow-up period [abstract]. *J Am Coll Cardiol* 1993;21:264A.

63. Stevenson WG, Sager P, Nademanee K, et al. Identifying sites for catheter ablation of ventricular tachycardia. *Herz* 1992:17:158–170.

64. Garan H, Fallon JT, Rosenthal S, et al. Endocardial, intramural, and epicardial activation patterns during sustained monomorphic ventricular tachycardia in late canine myocardial infarction. *Circ Res* 1987;60: 887–897.

65. Greenspan AJ, Hsu SS, Datorre S. Successful radiofrequency catheter ablation of sustained ventricular tachycardia postmyocardial infarction in man guided by a multielectrode "basket" catheter. *J Cardiovasc Electrophysiol* 1997;8:565–570.

66. Gepstein L, Hayam G, Ben-Haim SA. A novel method for nonfluoroscopic catheter-based electroanatomical mapping of the heart: in vitro and in vivo accuracy results. *Circulation* 1997;95:1611–1622.

67. Peters NS, Jackman WM, Schilling RJ, et al. Human left ventricular endocardial activation mapping using a novel noncontact catheter. *Circulation* 1997;95:1658–1660.

Chapter 33

Ablation of Ventricular Tachycardia Associated with Nonischemic Structural Heart Disease

Robert F. Coyne, M.D., Francis E. Marchlinski, M.D.

Introduction

Most experience with catheter ablation for ventricular tachycardia (VT) with structural heart disease has been in the setting of coronary artery disease. This chapter will discuss radiofrequency ablation in the adult patient with noncoronary structural heart disease, specifically 1) arrhythmogenic right ventricular dysplasia, 2) repaired tetralogy of Fallot, 3) "idiopathic" dilated cardiomyopathy, and 4) other infiltrative myopathies such as sarcoidosis and Chagas' disease. For each specific disease process, we will describe the epidemiological considerations related to the development of sustained VT. We will also describe the anatomic substrate and the electrophysiological nature of this substrate both in sinus rhythm and with the development of VT. Our own as well as previously published experience with radiofrequency ablation for VT in these disease processes will be provided, with emphasis on special considerations that apply to each unique disease substrate and VT syndrome. Finally, we will conclude with a summary and a description of recommendations for future investigation that may permit more generalized applicability of ablative therapy for VT associated with noncoronary structural heart disease.

From Huang SKS, Wilber DJ (eds.): *Radiofrequency Catheter Ablation of Cardiac Arrhythmias: Basic Concepts and Clinical Applications,* 2nd ed. Armonk, NY: Futura Publishing Company, Inc. ©2000.

Arrhythmogenic Right Ventricular Dysplasia

Pathological, Epidemiological, and Diagnostic Considerations

Right ventricular dysplasia, a pathological condition primarily affecting the right ventricle, involves replacement of myocardium to a variable extent by fatty and fibrous tissue.[1] The arrhythmogenic subset, characterized by relatively frequent and recurrent VT, was first described by Fontaine et al in 1977.[2] This arrhythmogenic right ventricular dysplasia (ARVD) should be distinguished from Uhl's anomaly. Patients with the latter have "paper-thin" right ventricles, direct apposition of epicardial and endocardial surfaces, congestive heart failure during infancy and childhood, and a low propensity for sustained ventricular arrhythmias.[3–5] Pathologically, ARVD predominantly affects 3 areas of the right ventricle (the so-called triangle of dysplasia): the anterior infundibulum, the apex, and the basal inferior wall.[6] Histological appearance may vary from myocyte degeneration and necrosis with foci of inflammation to myocardial replacement with fibrous or lipomatous tissue.[6,7] Although the right ventricle is primarily affected, there have been reports of left ventricular involvement in ARVD as well.[8–12]

Epidemiologically, ARVD usually affects males and is sporadic,[6,7,13] although familial clusterings have been reported.[3,14–19] Among affected family members, pathological involvement may vary greatly.[3] Owing perhaps to the heterogenous nature of the disease, the clinical course is variable with up to 10% of patients experiencing sudden death in 1 series.[20] ARVD may be present in as many as 20% of people under 35 years of age who experience sudden death.[7] Some investigators have suggested a more benign prognosis in those ARVD patients presenting with VT and subsequently treated with antiarrhythmic agents.[21,22] However, 5-year recurrence of arrhythmic events may be as high as 40% and appears to correlate with extent of disease, presence of late potentials, and inducible VT.[23]

The diagnosis of ARVD may be suggested by 3 features of the 12-lead ECG: 1) incomplete or complete RBBB (50% of affected individuals); 2) inverted T-waves in V_1-V_3 (90% of affected individuals); 3) "epsilon" waves (see Figure 1) in the anterior precordial leads in 15–60% of affected individuals.[6,22,24–26] The signal-averaged ECG is typically abnormal, although a normal SAECG does not preclude the diagnosis.[27,28] Echocardiography may show diffuse right ventricular dilatation or localized aneurysmal segments; however, these findings may also be observed in other myopathies.[29,30] ^{123}I-MIBG scintigraphy, which quantifies myocardial sympathetic activity by measuring presynaptic norepinephrine uptake, shows regional sympathetic denervation in 83% of patients with ARVD.[31] Magnetic resonance imaging (MRI) may be particularly helpful in diagnosing subtle cases in which relatively small areas of fatty infiltration exist,[32–34] and can often obviate the need for either biopsy or right ventricular angiography.[35] However, the right ventricular free wall is a relatively thin structure and normal epicardial fat overlying the free wall may be easily misinterpreted as fatty infiltration with MRI, particularly if imaging experience is lacking. Thus, right ventricular angiography remains the gold standard for confirming the presence of ARVD.

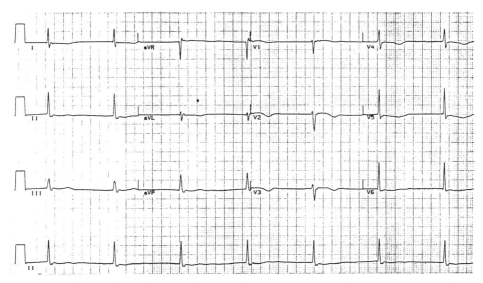

Figure 1. Surface 12-lead electrocardiogram from a patient with features suggestive of arrhythmogenic right ventricular dysplasia, including incomplete RBBB, inverted T waves in V_1–V_3, and epsilon waves (arrow).

Electrophysiological Considerations

During sinus rhythm, local ventricular electrograms of areas involved with ARVD typically show broadened deflections and late, sharp, high-frequency terminal deflections representing delayed myocardial activation and slow conduction.[6] These late electrograms, which correlate with epsilon waves on the surface ECG or late potentials on the SAECG, should be differentiated from the normal "late" electrograms observed in the right ventricular infundibulum of normal hearts. In patients with ARVD, the delayed myocardial activation and slow conduction in affected areas provide the anatomic substrate for reentry, the mechanism for ventricular tachycardia due to ARVD.

The relationship of exercise to arrhythmogenesis is well documented in patients with ARVD.[3,6,7,21,36,37] Haïssaguerre and colleagues have shown that continuous infusion of high dose isoproterenol can induce VT in the majority of patients with ARVD (85%), versus 2% of control subjects.[38] VT due to ARVD facilitated by catecholamines should be distinguished from catecholamine-induced right ventricular outflow tract (RVOT) VT; the former is reentrant while the latter is triggered or automatic (see Figure 2). In one series, Wichter et al have suggested that focal sympathetic denervation in the outflow tract corresponded to catecholamine-provoked VT in patients with ARVD; however, it apepars in retrospect that most of their patients had RVOT VT rather than ARVD VT per se.[31] Whether regional abnormalities in sympathetic innervation are important in ARVD VT remains unknown.

At electrophysiological study, over 90% of patients with ARVD have VT inducible with programmed stimulation.[6,13,22,29] Inducibility of VT in patients

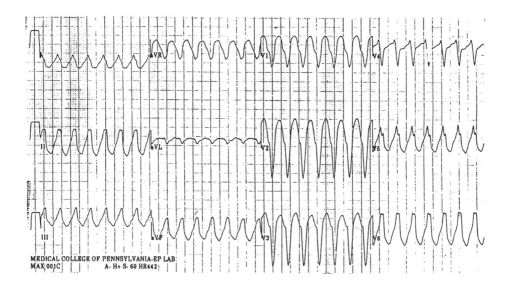

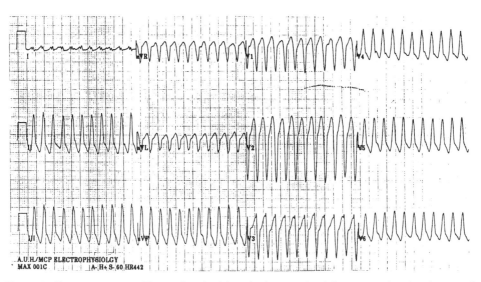

Figure 2. Figure contrasts VT associated with arrhythmogenic right ventricular dysplasia and catecholamine-sensitive right ventricular outflow tract ventricular tachycardia. Top panel: ARVD VT. Note precordial transition and frontal plane axis. This tachycardia was mapped to the superior right ventricular free wall. Bottom panel: RVOT VT. Note precordial transition and frontal plane axis. This tachycardia was mapped to the most supero-leftward portion of the RVOT under the pulmonic valve.

with ARVD appears to be highly reproducible over time.[40] VT associated with ARVD can be entrained, but may or may not demonstrate either mid-diastolic potentials or continuous electrical activity.[41,42] Frequently, multiple morphologies of tachycardia can be induced in the same individual. Almost all VTs have LBBB morphology, poor R wave progression across the precordial leads, and a variable frontal plane axis consistent with a site of origin from the described right ventricular free wall sites (see Figure 3).[6] Occasionally, VT with RBBB morphology may be seen, presumably reflecting left ventricular involvement or left sided epicardial breakthrough; however, the majority of ARVD VTs map to the right ventricular anterior infundibulum, apex, and basal inferior wall.

Experience with Catheter Ablation

Early surgical ablation attempts at treating refractory tachyarrhythmias associated with ARVD included surgical incisions with or without cryoablation, and, in the extreme, right ventricular disarticulation.[43–47] Surgical incisions were generally associated with a high rate of recurrence despite additional antiarrhythmic therapy,[21,48] while disarticulation conferred a substantial perioperative mortality.[22,46] Attempts at direct-current ablation, despite high acute

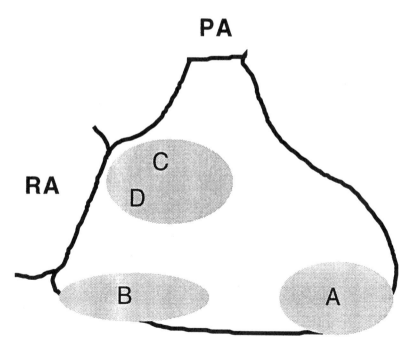

Figure 3. Four different morphologies of VT from a patient with arrhythmogenic right ventricular dysplasia. The site of origin for each tachycardia is represented in the schematic of the right ventricular free all (RAO projection), which also depicts the anatomic areas commonly involved with the dysplastic process (shaded areas). Panel A: VT arising from the apical free wall. Note strongly negative QRS morphology in the precordial leads. The leftward forces as manifested by R waves in leads I and aVL reflect depolarization of the apical left ventricle. (*continued*)

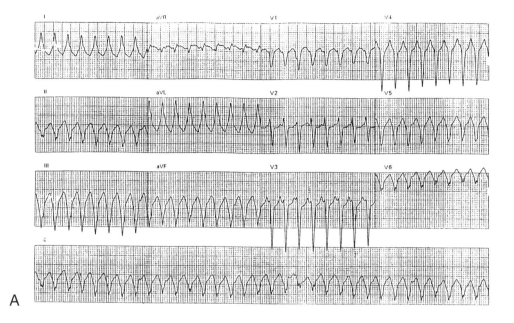

A

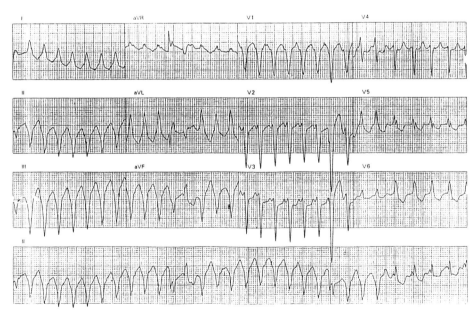

B

Figure 3. (*continued*) Panel B: VT arising from the diaphragmatic free wall. Note leftward and superior forces in the inferior leads. A different slower tachycardia with a morphology similar to the tachycardia depicted in Panel D is present during the last 5 complexes of the tracing. (*continued*)

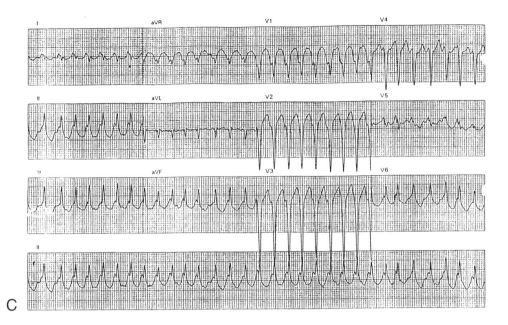

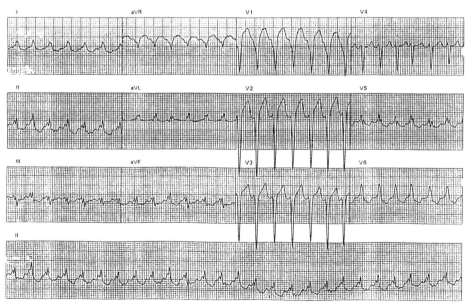

Figure 3. (*continued*) Panel C: VT arising from the superior aspect of the infundibulum. Note strongly positive forces in the inferior leads. Panel D: VT arising from a less superior area of the infundibulum.

success rates (greater than 90%),[45,49,50] were complicated by substantial arrhythmia recurrence.[49,50] Shoda et al reported a 50% incidence of new VT in 8–20 months of follow-up, despite noninducibility at follow-up electrophysiological study 2 weeks post direct current ablation.[50]

The limited data describing radiofrequency ablation in treating ARVD ventricular tachycardia are summarized in Table 1. In early 1995, Asso and colleagues reported using earliest detectable endocardial activation during VT (mean 112 ± 74 milliseconds pre-QRS, range 36–260) to successfully ablate 7 tachycardias in 4 of 6 patients with syncopal VT in whom the procedure was attempted.[51] Most remained on antiarrhythmic therapy. No midterm recurrences were noted in 22 ± 6 months of follow-up, and repeat electrophysiological study more than 6 months postprocedure showed no inducible VT. In another small series of patients with ARVD and VT reported by Stabile et al,[52] radiofrequency energy was delivered based upon both pace mapping and earliest activation (mean 37.9 ± 7.4 milliseconds pre-QRS). The site of tachycardia origin was the right ventricular apex in 3 patients, the right ventricular infundibulum in 2 patients, the right ventricular anterior free wall in 1 patient, and the right ventricular basal inferior wall in 2 patients. In 7 of 8 patients, the procedure was acutely successful, and only 1 recurrence was noted in 19 ± 9 months of follow-up.[52] In contrast to these promising results, however, Haverkamp and colleagues have reported a 60% recurrence in 14 patients with drug-refractory VT in whom radiofrequency ablation was acutely successful using both earliest detectable endocardial activation and pace mapping.[53] Of note, only 5 of their patients had VT inducible by programmed stimulation, and 9 required catecholamine infusion. The difference in outcome of the series reported to date may be related to the small number of patients, site of origin of the targeted tachycardia (e.g., infundibulum versus inferior wall), differences in mapping endpoints for energy delivery, and, possibly, disease progression causing new tachycardias. In our experience, loss of the late, fractionated electrogram at the tachycardia site of origin is sometimes observed following acutely successful radiofrequency ablation; the specificity and predictive value of this finding with respect to tachycardia recurrence is unknown.

In summary, the limited data suggests that radiofrequency ablation for VT associated with ARVD can be accomplished safely with a relatively high acute success rate. Particular care to catheter selection and technique should be used when typical right ventricular free wall sites of origin are targeted. VT occur-

Table 1
Acute success and long-term outcome in patients undergoing
radiofrequency ablation for VT associated with ARVD.

Author	Year	Patients, n	Ablation Criteria	Acute Success, %	Follow-Up, months	Recurrence, %
Asso[51]	1995	6	EA	66%	22 ± 6	0
Stabile[52]	1995	8	EA, PM	88%	19 ± 9	12.5%
Haverkamp[53]	1993	14	EA, PM	71%	22 ± 13	60%

EA = earliest (presystolic) activation; PM = pacemapping; EN = entrainment.

rence may occur following acutely successful ablation; whether such occurrences reflect disease extent or progression, site of origin of ablated VT, or differences in mapping end points is unknown.

VT Associated with Repaired Tetralogy of Fallot

Epidemiological Considerations

Tetralogy of Fallot is the most common intrinsic cyanotic congenital heart lesion, comprising 6% of congenital cardiac births.[54] The tetrad consists of infundibular stenosis, an overriding aorta, a ventricular septal defect, and right ventricular hypertrophy. In 1955, the first patient with tetralogy of Fallot had the defect corrected by open intracardiac surgery.[55] Currently, complete repair is associated with an excellent long-term prognosis,[56] with actuarial survival rates approaching those of the normal population. The major late complication or risk after surgical repair appears to be recurrent VT and/or sudden death.[57–59] In older reported series, sudden death accounted for 30–75% of late deaths.[59–62] Even in patients without bifascicular block or transient complete heart block immediately following surgery, retrospective data suggests a 1–6% incidence of sudden death, probably due to malignant ventricular arrhythmias.[57,59,61]

Electrophysiological Considerations

In patients with tetralogy of Fallot, complete repair involves patching of the ventricular septal defect and a right ventriculotomy or infundibulotomy. Subsequent scarring and fibrosis from the incisions and patching provides the anatomic substrate for macro-reentrant VT observed in adult patients.[63–67] During sinus rhythm in these patients, fractionated and late local electrograms may be recorded from the region of the ventriculotomy or near the ventricular septal defect patch.[65,66,68] With initiation of tachycardia, further electrogram fragmentation, mid-diastolic potentials, and continuous electrical activity may be observed in these areas.[63,65,66,69–71] Typically, the VT circuit is associated with the right ventriculotomy or infundibulotomy scar;[63–65,67,69,70,72] less commonly, reentry is associated with the septal patch.[66,67] In either case, VTs associated with repaired tetralogy of Fallot have varying cycle lengths (190–400+ milliseconds have been reported in the literature), can be invariably initiated and terminated by programmed stimulation, and can be entrained.[63,65,73] For initiation of ventriculotomy-associated tachycardia, high-density open-chest intracardiac "balloon" catheter mapping has shown that creation of a line of block located in the vicinity of the ventriculotomy scar is necessary.[63] During ongoing ventriculotomy-associated tachycardia, intraoperative mapping studies by Josephson and colleagues have shown a zone of slow conduction extending superiorly from the ventriculotomy scar to the pulmonic valve.[71] Clockwise rotation about the ventriculotomy scar generally results in an inferior axis tachycardia (both LBBB and RBBB morphologies have been described), while counterclockwise rotation usually causes a LBBB superior axis tachycardia.[71] Patch-associated tachycardia is usually RBBB in morphology and superiorly directed (Figure 4).[66]

Radiofrequency Ablation Consideration

Early surgical ablation approaches advocated for VT associated with repaired tetralogy of Fallot included transmural ventriculotomy from the region of the previous ventriculotomy scar to the pulmonic valve and resection of myocardium with cryoablation at sites of earliest activation.[63,64,71] Catheter ablation using direct current shock has also been reported to be successful using earliest-activation mapping.[74]

Published data describing radiofrequency ablation is limited to case reports and small series, which are summarized in Table 2. The first successful ablations were described in 2 patients by Burton and Leon in 1993.[58] The investigators used pace mapping during tachycardia (entrainment) and during sinus rhythm to identify likely sites for delivery of radiofrequency energy; successful ablation sites demonstrated concealed (surface 12-lead) entrainment during tachycardia and a 12/12 perfect pace map during sinus rhythm. Multiple radiofrequency lesions were necessary (mean 7). The authors did not report on presence or absence of diastolic potentials or continuous electrical activity during tachycardia at these sites. Other investigators have also reported success using pace mapping in sinus rhythm; again, multiple radiofrequency lesions were necessary.[72]

In our experience as well as that of others, mid-diastolic potentials during tachycardia may be more useful to identify likely slow conduction zone targets for radiofrequency energy delivery.[69] However, at least for ventriculotomy-associated tachycardia, the slow conduction zone may be too broad to be spanned by discrete anatomic lesions.[70] Instead, an "anatomic approach" may be required to create a fixed line of block connecting the ventriculotomy scar to an anatomic boundary (i.e., the pulmonic valve).[70] This anatomic approach, similar in principle to older surgical approaches, is analogous to radiofrequency ablation of Type 1 atrial flutter, where an anatomic line of block is created across the "isthmus" that the flutter wavefront obligatorily traverses. To date, however, there is no data regarding which patient subsets with ventriculotomy-associated tachycardia might benfit from such an anatomic approach, how block in these patients should be determined, and whether anatomic block, as opposed to very slow conduction, is necessary to prevent tachycardia recurrence. Furthermore, there has been no systematic appraisal of other methods' relative utility in determining targets for delivery of radiofrequency energy (pace mapping, entrainment, mid-diastolic potentials, or, potentially, exit site criteria analogous to those developed for VT associated with coronary artery disease (see Chapter 32). However, regardless of the method used for targeting ablation sites, preliminary data suggests acute procedural success is associated with a good medium-term outcome, with no recurrent ventricular tachycardia in up to 15-month mean follow-up.[67,75]

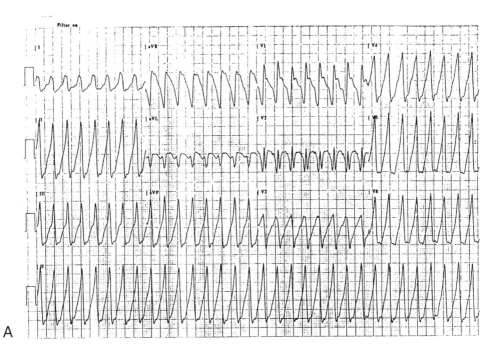

A

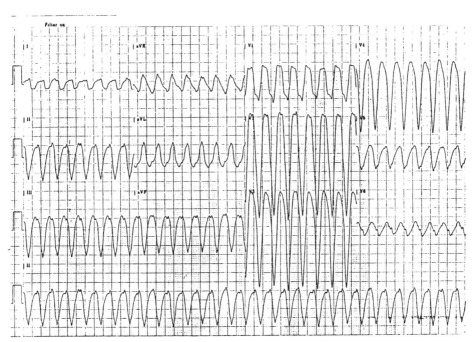

B

Figure 4. Typical 12-lead electrocardiogram morphologies of VT associated with the infundibulotomy scar in a patient with repaired tetralogy of Fallot. Paper speed is 25 mm/sec. Panel A: VT associated with clockwise rotation about infundibulotomy scar. Note inferiorly directed axis. Panel B: VT associated with counterclockwise rotation about the infundibulotomy scar.

Table 2
Acute success and long-term outcome in patients undergoing
radiofrequency ablation for VT associated with tetralogy of Fallot.

Author	Year	Patients, n; VTs, n	Ablation Criteria	Acute Success, %	Follow-Up, Months	Recurrence, %
Burton[58]	1993	2;2	PM, EN	100%	4 ± 2	0
Goldner[72]	1994	1;1	PM	100%	7	0
Biblo[69]	1994	1;2	EA, MDP	100%[†]	28	0
Hebe[67]	1995	3;3	EA, ?MDP	100%	15	0
Chinushi[70]	1995	1;2	EA, AN*	100%[‡]	—	—
Horton[§]	1995	1;1	AN**	100%	—	—

PM = pace mapping; EN = entrainment; EA = earliest (presystolic) activation; MDP = mid-diastolic potential; AN = anatomically guided

§Personal communication.

*Ablation guided by earliest activation unsuccesful; subsequent anatomically-guided ablation successful (scar to pulmonic valve)

**Anatomically-guided ablation from the ventriculotomy scar to the tricuspid annulus.

†Recurrence of 1 of 2 ablated morphologies of VT after 4 months. Following repeat ablation, no VT for 28 months.

‡Acute success achieved only after anatomic ablation was performed (scar to pulmonic valve).

In summary, ventricular arrhythmias are a known late complication following successful repair of tetralogy of Fallot. These arrhythmias have been shown to be reentrant in mechanism by a number of criteria. In most cases, tachycardia originates from the vicinity of the ventriculotomy scar; however, septal origins corresponding to the ventricular septal defect patch have also been described. Although limited data exist, radiofrequency ablation using pace mapping/entrainment, mid-diastolic potentials, or anatomic considerations may be successful in acutely eliminating VT. In limited series, acute procedural success seems to suggest a good medium-term outcome.

Nonischemic Dilated Cardiomyopathy

Nonischemic dilated cardiomyopathy may be caused by myriad conditions, including but not limited to toxic, endocrinologic, mechanical, autoimmune, pregnancy-related, infectious, and idiopathic causes. As such, any discussion regarding tachyarrhythmia disturbances and their treatment with radiofrequency ablation in this cohort is limited by the heterogeneity of the disease processes involved. After brief discussions of VT-induced cardiomyopathy and bundle branch reentry, this section will focus on VTs of myocardial origin associated with idiopathic dilated cardiomyopathy.

Cardiomyopathy Secondary to VT

It is well known that chronic surpaventricular tachyarrhythmias may result in progressive ventricular dilatation and failure.[76–79] Additionally, chronic

VT can lead to a dilated cardiomyopathy in both animal models[80,81] as well as in humans.[82–84] Because myocardial mechanics normalize within 3 months in the majority of patients following elimination of the tachyarrhythmia,[81] it is important to discern the individual patient presenting with VT as the cause of his or her "idiopathic" dilated cardiomyopathy. Successful resolution of cardiomyopathy following radiofrequency ablation for frequent (approximately 30% of waking hours by Holter monitoring) or incessant VT has been described for typical right ventricular outflow tract tachycardia[86,87] as well as for idiopathic left VT.[88] The pathophysiology of and approach to radiofrequency ablation of these ventricular tachycardias are more fully discussed in Chapters 29 and 30.

Bundle Branch Reentry VT

The incidence of inducible bundle branch reentry is approximately 40% in patients with dilated cardiomyopathy who present with sustained ventricular arrhythmias or sudden death.[89] Although the vast majority of patients with inducible bundle branch reentry have dilated cardiomyopathy,[89,90] bundle branch reentry may also occur in the absence of any structural heart disease.[91] "Typical" bundle branch reentry utilizes the right bundle branch and the left bunde branch as the antegrade and retrograde limbs of a macro-reentrant circuit, respectively. Other forms of macro-reentry involving the His-Purkinje system have been described, including "reverse" bundle branch reentry, interfascicular reentry, and "typical" bundle branch reentry with more than one exit site from the right bundle branch.[92] Recognizing typical bundle branch reentry in the patient with dilated cardiomyopathy is critically important becuase radiofrequency ablation of the right bundle branch offers a potentially curative approach. Some investigators have suggested successful RF ablation of the right bundle branch may help to avoid ICD implantation in patients with cardiomyopathy and bundle branch reentry;[90] however, our institution favors ICD implantation regardless of acute procedural success. The pathophysiology of and radiofrequency ablation approach to bundle branch reentry are fully discussed in Chapter 31.

VT of Myocardial Origin in Dilated Cardiomyopathy

Epidemiological and Pathological Considerations

Ventricular tachyarrhythmias are quite frequent in dilated cardiomyopathy, with between 42–60% of patients showing at least nonsustained VT on 24-hour Holter monitoring.[93–95] However, the utility of electrophysiology study in risk-stratifying these patients is limited, with lower sensitivity and specificity than for the cohort with coronary artery disease.[96–98] Signal-average ECG may be helpful in predicting adverse outcome,[99] but this is controversial.

In idiopathic cardiomyopathy, evidence suggests that the degree of interstitial fibrosis as detected by biopsy is associated with spontaneous VT as documented by 48-hour Holter monitoring.[100] Additionally, the degree of myocyte hypertrophy and myofibrillar degeneration has been shown to strongly correlate with spontaneous ventricular ectopy and nonsustained VT.[101] In contrast, ejection fraction, wall stress, and left ventricle mass and dimension are less well correlated with arrhythmogenesis.[100] Patchy myocardial fibrosis is extremely common in patients with idiopathic dilated cardiomyopathy. In a large autopsy series of over 150 patients, grossly visible scars were identified in 14% of patients, and histologically evident fibrosis was noted in 57%. Generally, the left ventricle is more affected by fibrosis.[102] The myocardial fibrosis and myofibrillar destruction, which may be variably located, provide the anatomic substrate for sustained VTs.

Electrophysiological Considerations

Endocardial mapping studies during sinus rhythm have shown that abnormal, fractionated, and/or late electrograms are less frequently seen in patients with dilated cardiomyopathy and monomorphic VT than in patients with VT related to coronary artery disease.[103] However, the incidence of abnormal *epicardial* electrograms roughly equals the incidence of abnormal *endocardial* electrograms in patients with dilated cardiomyopathy and monomorphic VT.[104] Presumably, these electrogram abnormalities correspond to areas of focal fibrosis and myofibrillar destruction, which provide the substrate for tachycardia. As a result, VTs associated with dilated myopathy may have deep myocardial or epicardial exit sites, as well as the endocardial sites more typically assoicated with infarct-related VT. This may help explain the relatively low success of endocardial catheter ablation in patients with dilated myopathies compared to those with ischemic myopathies.

In certain animal models of dilated cardiomyopathy, high density mapping has shown that VT is not due to reentry.[105] However, data in humans shows that reentry is an important mechanism for at least some monomorphic VTs in patients with dilated cardiomyopathy.[106,107] First, high degrees of fibrosis can decrease electrical coupling between adjacent myocytes and cause conduction slowing and reentry. Second, in cardiomyopathy patients presenting with sustained VT, clinical VTs may be inducible by programmed stimulation in most patients.[96–98,108–110] Finally, induced tachycardias may manifest mid-diastolic potentials and demonstrate entrainment.[106]

Because of the heterogenous and patchy nature of the interstitial fibrosis observed in patients with idiopathic cardiomyopathy, monomorphic VT may arise from virtually any location. Therefore, there is a wide spectrum of QRS morphologies among patients with tachycardia. Although most VTs appear to arise from the left ventricle, perhaps due to the relative predominance of interstitial fibrotic changes in the left ventricle compared to the right ventricle, right VTs originating from the septum and free wall have been noted in patients with cardiomyopathy involving both the left and right ventricles.[102]

Ablation Considerations

Early experience with direct current ablation of VT showed that rates of acute procedural success and subsequent freedom from tachycardia recurrence were lower in patients with idiopathic cardiomyopathy than in patients with coronary artery disease.[111] Overall, radiofrequency ablation has been similarly less successful in the cohort of patients with idiopathic cardiomyopathy; results from published series as well as our own data are summarized in Table 3. In selected patient subgroups, acute ablation success rates may be higher. Kottkamp et al have reported a 67% acute success rate in 8 patients with 9 targeted monomorphic VTs.[106] In this highly selected group (the 8 patients were selected from a group of 115 patients with idiopathic cardiomyopathy referred for electrophysiological evaluation), prerequisites for inclusion included incessant or frequently recurrent VT that was reproducibly induced with programmed stimulation. Eight of the 9 tachycardias were mapped to the left ventricle; 1 tachycardia mapped to the midbasal septum of the right ventricle. The primary criterion for identifying the site for ablation was the presence of mid-diastolic potentials and/or concealed entrainment; the secondary criterion was earliest detectable pre-systolic activity (range −60 to −110-milliseconds); and the tertiary criterion was pace mapping. Follow-up testing was performed at 6–12 weeks. Overall, 6 of 9 VTs were successfully ablated, including all 4 tachycardias that manifested primary mapping criteria of mid-diastolic potentials and/or entrainment (mean 5 radiofrequency energy deliveries per site). When only early activation or pace mapping was used to target radiofrequency energy

Table 3
Acute success and long-term outcome in patients undergoing
radiofrequency ablation for VT assoicated with dilated cardiomyopathy

Author	Year	Patients, n; VTs, n	Ablation Criteria	Acute Success, %	Follow-Up, Months	Recurrence, %
Kottkamp[106]	1995	8;9	MDP, EN, EA, PM**	66%†	8 ± 5	66%#
Wilber[107]	1995	7;7	MDP, EN, EA, PM***	86%‡	3–10	0

Abbreviations: MDP = mid-diastolic potential; EN = entrainment; EA = earliest activity; PM = pace mapping

*Unpublished data

**Entrainment and mid-diastolic potentials primary criteria for energy delivery, earliest activity secondary, and pace mapping tertiary.

***Entrainment and mid-diastolic potentials criteria for energy delivery in the 3 patients in whom tachycardia was inducible by programmed stimulation; earliest activity and pace mapping criteria in 4 other patients in whom tachycardia was inducible only with burst pacing and/or isoproterenol.

†All four tachycardias manifesting primary criteria successfully ablated; two of five tachycardias manifesting only secondary or tertiary criteria successfully ablated.

‡All four tachycardias inducible only by burst pacing/isoproterenol successfully ablated. Two tachycardias induced with programmed stimulation and manifesting entrainment/mid-diastolic potentials also successfully ablated. Ablation unsuccessful in one patient whose tachycardia was induced by programmed stimulation but did not demonstrate entrainment or mid-diastolic potentials.

#Two of 6 patients had no VT at all in follow-up; unknown whether tachycardia occurrence in remaining patients represented recurrence of targeted VTs.

delivery, just 3 of 5 tachycardias were successfully ablated. None of the acutely ablated tachycardias was inducible at follow-up electrophysiology study; however, the majority of patients experienced different VT in short-term follow-up. Of the 4 patients who presented with incessant VT, no patient had recurrence of incessant tachycardia.

In another small series of 7 patients with VT and dilated cardiomyopathy, Wilber and colleagues reported similar findings in a 3-patient subgroup in whom VT was inducible with programmed stimulation.[107] In 2 of these 3 patients, target sites for ablation manifested mid-diastolic potentials (80–128 milliseconds pre-QRS) and concealed entrainment. Ablation of these sites was

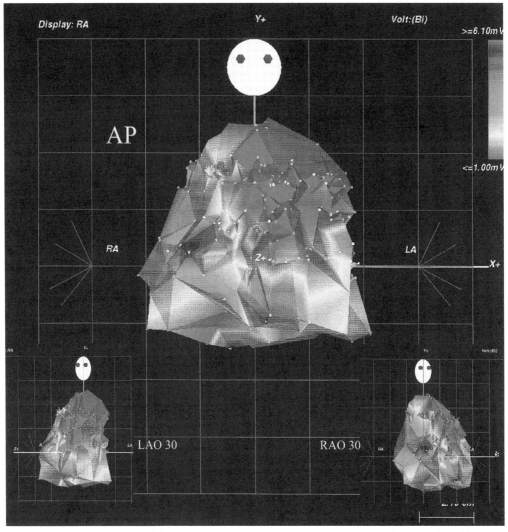

Figure 5. Voltage maps of the right ventricular free wall in 2 patients with idiopathic dilated cardiomyopathy. Each map displays a voltage color scale (upper right) and AP, LAO, and RAO views. The interventricular septum is not displayed. Both patients had multiple morphologies of ventricular tachycardia. See color plate. (*continued*)

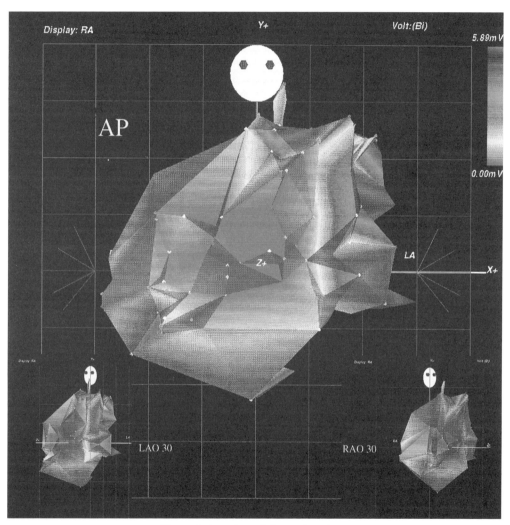

Figure 5. (*continued*) See color plate.

acutely successful. In the third patient, no sites demonstrated either mid-diastolic potentials or concealed entrainment; ablation was unsuccessful. In 4 other patients, VT was inducible by burst pacing and/or catecholamine infusion but not by programmed stimulation, suggesting a mechanism other than reentry. In all 4 of these patients, ablation at sites with presystolic activity in the −10 to −35 millisecond range and perfect pace maps was acutely successful. No site manifested either mid-diastolic potentials or entrainment. In the overall series of 7 patients, 6 procedures were acutely successful, with no clinical tachycardia recurrence in 3–10 month follow-up.

In summary, radiofrequency ablation for VT in patients with dilated cardiomyopathy may be successful in highly selected subgroups. The ability to generalize the results in these subgroups to the overall population with dilated cardiomyopathy is likely limited by the patchy nature of myocardial fibrosis in idiopathic cardiomyopathy, allowing for epicardial and deep myocardial "breakthrough" sites. Emerging technology for mapping and targeting epicardial surfaces may help improve success rates. Because of the limited data available, optimal criteria for ablation site selection are not known. We typically attempt to define the earliest presystolic site site recorded during VT. In selected patients, after identifying the extent of endocardial scar defined by isopotential mapping during sinus rhythm (see Figure 5), we have attempted to use linear deliveries of radiofrequency energy to connect the scar to either anatomic boundaries or to myocardium which demonstrates normal electrogram characteristics and which is located approximately 2 centimeters away from the scar area.

Infiltrative Myopathies: Sarcoidosis and Chagas' Disease

Sarcoidosis

Epidemiological and Pathological Considerations

Sarcoidosis, a multisystemic granulomatous disease of unknown origin, most frequently presents with mediastinal, pulmonary, and skin or eye involvement. The incidence of clinically apparent cardiac abnormalities in sarcoid patients is relatively low (5–13%).[112,113] Pathological cardiac involvement at autopsy has been demonstrated in 27–60% of patients with systemic sarcoidosis.[113,114] Clinical cardiac manifestations of sarcoidosis include conduction disturbances, paroxysmal arrhythmias, and far less frequently, heart failure. Sudden death due to bradyarrhythmias and tachyarrhythmias were noted in as many as two-thirds of the patients with documented cardiac sarcoidosis.[112,114]

The pathology of cardiac sarcoidosis was first described by Bernstein and colleagues in 1923.[115] Cardiac sarcoid lesions are usually microscopic, consisting of either focal granulomata or discrete areas of fibrosis.[113,114] Because of the patchy nature of involvement, cardiac sarcoid may be missed by endomyocardial biopsy.[116] Data suggests [201]thallium or [67]gallium scintigraphy and MRI may be more useful for monitoring disease activity.[117–119] Patients with widespread granuloma and myocardial fibrosis generally have arrhythmias and often die suddenly,[113,120] but even asymptomatic patients with previously electrically "silent" lesions may experience ventricular tachyarrhythmias.[112,113,121] Rarely, sustained VT and congestive cardiomyopathy may be the only signs of systemic sarcoidosis with cardiac involvement.[122] There are no studies that specifically address the electrophysiological risk stratification of asymptomatic cardiac sarcoid patients.

Electrophysiological Considerations

There is little data describing the electrophysiological characteristics of ventricular arrhythmias associated with cardiac sarcoidosis. It is speculated that ventriuclar myocardial scarring produced by sarcoid granulomas provides the substrate for reentrant arrhythmias.[120,121] Inducibility of monomorphic VT with programmed stimulation in at least some of these patients also supports a reentrant mechanism.[120,123,124]

The surface electrocardiogram morphology of inducible VT in cardiac sarcoid varies. Investigators have reported right and left bundle configuration ventricular tachycardias, ranging in cycle length from 220–400 milliseconds.[121,123,124] Both superiorly and inferiorly directed frontal plane axes have been described.[121,123,124] One case report described a RBBB right inferior axis QRS morphology tachycardia with positive R waves in the precordial leads, suggesting a lateral inferobasal left ventricular site of origin.[124] We have seen recurrent VT in cardiac sarcoid patients with minimal ventricular dysfunction. In these patients, multiple morphologies of tachycardia were inducible, all arising from the basal setpum or the posterolateral left ventricle with corresponding ^{201}T1 defects (unrelated to coronary artery disease) in these anatomic distributions (Figure 6). Unfortunately, there is no data describing radiofrequency ablation methods, acute success, and/or long term success in cardiac sarcoid patients. Given the diffuse and often progressive nature of the disease process, one might speculate that tachyarrhythmia recurrence would prove the rule. Further investigation needs to be performed to determine which, if any, patients with cardiac sarcoidosis and VT might benefit from radiofrequency ablation.

Chagas' Disease

Epidemiological and Pathological Considerations

Chagas' disease is a major cause of cardiac dysfunction in Latin American populations. The causative parasite, *Trypanosoma cruzi,* is spread to humans via the insect vector reduviid bug. Recent data suggest that 16 million people, or more than 4%, are infected in Latin American countries. In certain areas, seropositivity as assayed by blood donors exceeds 60%.[125] In North America, the incidence of Chagas' disease has been increasing, owing perhaps to increasing immigrant populations. For example, in Los Angeles, California, Chagas' seropositivity occurs in 1.1% of all voluntary blood donors.[126]

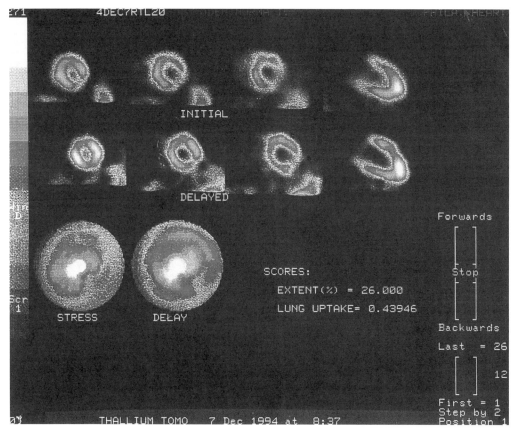

Figure 6. Top: Short axis and polar plot[201] T1 images obtained from a patient with biopsy-proven cardiac sarcoid. Note inferobasal thallium uptake defects corresponding to myocardium supplied by the left circumflex artery distribution. This patient did not have epicardial coronary disease. Bottom: Surface ECG demonstrating clinical VT from the same patient. This right bundle right superior axis VT was mapped to the endocardial surface corresponding to the thallium defect. See color plate.

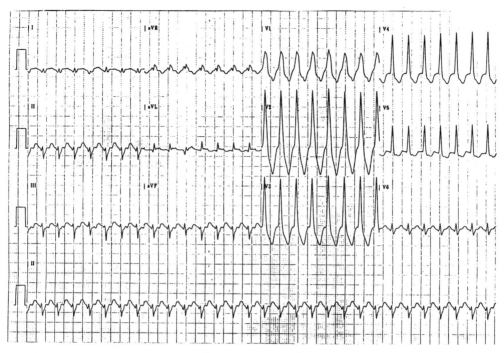

Figure 6. (*continued*)

Following acute infection, most patients are essentially asymptomatic. After a latent period that can last decades, approximately 10–40% of patients with Chagas' seropositivity develop chronic heart disease. This cardiomyopathy is manifested by both congestive heart failure as well as bradyarrhythmias and tachyarrhythmias, syncope, and sudden death.[127,128]

The latter may account for up to 30% of chagasic deaths. Interestingly, patients with Chagas' disease who present with hemodynamically-tolerated monomorphic ventricular tachycardia usually do not have severe myocardial disease and appear to have a relatively good prognosis.[129] In contrast, patients who present with recurrent syncope ascribed to VT on the basis of electrophysiological study generally have a poorer prognosis.[127]

The causative role of the parasite in chronic chagasic cardiomyopathy is not fully clarified. Most investigators have found active parasitemia is not a prominent feature, leading to the speculation that autoimmune, neurogenic, and microvascular etiologies are involved in the development of chagasic cardiomyopathy. However, Belloti et al have demonstrated that detection of *T. cruzi* antigen correlates with the presence of moderate or severe myocarditis in both autopsy specimens as well as in patients undergoing MRI-guided endomyocardial biopsy.[130] Furthermore, using a Langendorff-perfused rabbit heart model, de Carvalho and colleagues have shown that exposure of adult rabbit hearts to sera from chronic chagasic rabbits results in acute abnormalities of sinus node automaticity and conduction.[131] Whether these latter findings are applicable to humans is unknown.

Electrophysiological Considerations

Patients with Chagas' disease who present with hemodynamically tolerated VT usually have baseline ventricular premature depolarizations, STT wave abnormalities, and left axis deviation. Unlike "classic" patients with chronic chagasic cardiomyopathy, right bundle branch block is often not present at baseline, and left ventricular function is usually not severely depressed.[129] In the majority of patients, the clinical arrhythmia can be reproducibly initiated with programmed stimulation, implying a reentrant mechanism. The surface ECG QRS morphology during VT may vary from patient to patient.[132,133] In at least some patients, tachycardias arise near apicoseptal or apicoinferior aneurysmal segments as defined by left ventriculography, although left lateral as well as right ventricular sites of origin have been described.[134]

There is extremely limited data regarding catheter ablation of VT associated with Chagas' disease. In a very small group, electrical fulguration has been successful in controlling the clinical arrhythmia in approximately 50% of patients.[134–136] One case report describes use of intracoronary ethanol to successfully ablate a VT.[137] With regard to radiofrequency ablation targeting the endocardial surface, one case series describes results in 11 consecutive chagasic patients with 14 clinical tachycardias.[138] In this small group, mean tachycardia cycle length was 353 ± 50 milliseconds and tachycardia site of origin was septal, anterior, and inferoposterior or lateral in 2, 2, and 7 patients respectively. Sites of radiofrequency energy delivery via an ablation catheter with an 8-millimeter tip were classified as "successful" or "unsuccessful" depending upon whether tachycardia terminated during radiofrequency energy delivery. When compared to unsuccessful sites (n = 99), successful sites (n = 38) were more likely to show 1) entrainment or concealed entrainment (74% vs 48%, respectively, < 0.05); 2) a postpacing interval-tachycardia cycle length difference of <20 milliseconds (32% versus 21%, respectively); and 3) smaller amplitude local ventricular electrograms (0.44 ± 0.35 mV versus 0.54 ± 0.52 mV, respectively). Neither local ventricular electrogram duration nor presystolic activity was predictive of successful versus unsuccessful sites, although all successful sites had at least 30 milliseconds of presystolic activity. In the overall group of 11 patients with 14 clinical tachycardias, 9 tachycardias were rendered noninducible (64% acute success rate); one of these recurred in 12 ± 7 months of follow-up. Ten patients remained on antiarrhythmic therapy.

Recent preliminary data suggest that acute ablation success rates may be higher if ablation methods targeting epicardial sites of origin are used. Sosa and colleagues have reported on 10 consecutive patients with Chagas' disease and VT in whom percutaneous subxyphoid pericardial puncture was used to access the epicardium for mapping and radiofrequency energy delivery.[139] In all patients, coronary angiography was performed at the time of the study to avoid potential complications arising from radiofrequency energy delivery on or near major epicardial arteries. In 7 patients, epicardial mid-diastolic potentials and/or continuous electrical activity were seen. Radiofrequency energy was delivered to the epicardial surface in 6 patients and to the endocardial surface in 4 patients. In these latter 4 patients, the clinical VT was still inducible at the termination of the procedure. In contrast, in the 6 patients in whom radiofrequency energy was delivered to the epicardial surface, the targeted VT was no longer inducible following ablation. No procedural complications were noted. However, long-term data describing freedom from tachycardia occurrence following epicardial ablation is lacking.

In summary, the limited data suggest radiofrequency ablation of VT associated with chagasic cardiomyopathy may be acutely successful in at least half of patients. If acutely successful, radiofrequency ablation is usually associated with freedom from recurrence of the clinical tachycardia for at least the medium term. However, it is unknown which chagasic patient subsets are most likely to experience acute success. Furthermore, the optimal strategy for targeting sites for radiofrequency energy delivery has not been determined. It appears that, similar to some patients with idiopathic dilated cardiomyopathy, the major brunt of the pathological process and therefore the site of origin of VT in patients with chagasic cardiomyopathy may be epicardial. Exciting new thoracoscopic or intrapericardial mapping and ablative techniques coupled with a detailed identification of the coronary anatomy may prove safe and effective in ablating VTs associated with epicardial origins in selected patients.

Conclusions and Future Directions

Compared to the literature describing radiofrequency ablation of VT associated with coronary artery disease, there has thus far been limited experience and published data in patients with nonischemic structural heart disease. This relative paucity of information underscores the need for international registry for such patients. Such a registry would facilitate identification of common sites of origin of the particular VTs associated with specific disease subsets. In addition, mapping and ablation strategies for the ablation of VT in specific subsets of patients with nonischemic structural heart disease could be compared.

Finally, radiofrequency ablation in patients with nonischemic structural heart disease is overall less likely to be acutely successful than ablation in patients with coronary disease. This appears particularly true for the subsets with dilated cardiomyopathy and Chagas' disease. One possible explanation for this is the presence of intramural or epicardial reentrant circuits that are currently unapproachable using conventional ablative techniques directed at the endocardial surface. Emerging catheter technology (see Chapter 35) may allow for deeper lesion formation with endocardial energy delivery. Furthermore, percutaneous transpericardial or venous epicardial mapping and ablation techniques may increase the likelihood of successful ablative therapy for VT in this patient population.

References

1. Schamroth L. *The Disorders of Cardiac Rhythm.* Oxford, England: Blackwell, 1971.
2. Fontaine G, Guiradon G, Frank R, et al. Stimulation studies and epicardial

mapping in VT: study of mechanisms and selection for surgery. In: HE Kulbertus, ed. *Reentrant Arrhythmias.* Lancaster, PA: MTP Publishers, 1977. p 334–350.

3. Nava A, Thiene G, Canciani B. Familial occurrence of right ventricular dysplasia: a study involving nine families. *J Am Coll Cardiol* 1988;12:1222–1228.

4. Perloff JK. *The Clinical Recognition of Congenital Heart Disease.* Philadelphia, PA: WB Saunders, 1988.

5. Fontaine G, Guiradon G, Frank R, et al. Dysplasie ventriculaire droite arythmogene et maladie de Uhl. *Arch Mal Coeur* 1982;75:361–372.

6. Marcus FI, Fontaine GH, Guiradon G, et al. Right ventricular dysplasia: a report of 24 adult cases. *Circulation* 1982;65(2):384–398.

7. Thiene G, Nava A, Corrado D, et al. Right ventricular cardiomyopathy and sudden death in young people. *N Engl J Med* 1988;318:129–133.

8. Cherrier F, Floquet J, Cuilliere M, et al. Les dysplasies ventriculaires droites: apropos de 7 observations. *Arch Mal Coeur* 1979;72:766–773.

9. Halphen CH, Beaufils PL, Azancot I, et al. Tachycardies ventriculaires recidivantes par dysplasie ventriculaire droite: association a des anomalies du ventricule gauche. *Arch Mal Coeur* 1981;74:1113–1118.

10. Pinamonti B, Salvi A, Silvestri F, et al. Left ventricular involvement in right ventricular cardiomyopathy. *Eur Heart* 1989;10(suppl D):20–21.

11. Manyari DE, Klein GH, Gulamhusein S, et al. Arrhythmogenic right ventricular dysplasia: a generalized cardiomyopathy? *Circulation* 1983;68:251–257.

12. Webb JG, Kerr CR, Huckell VF, et al. Left ventricular abnormalities in arrhythmogenic right ventricular dysplasia. *Am J Cardiol* 1986;58:568–570.

13. Rowland E, McKenna WJ, Sugrue D, et al. Ventricular tachycardia of left bundle branch block configuration in patients with isolated right ventricular dilatation: clinical and electrophysiological features. *Br Heart J* 1984;51:15–24.

14. Ruder MA, Winston SA, Davis JC, et al. Arrhythmogenic right ventricular dysplasia in a family. *Am J Cardiol* 1985;56:799–800.

15. Nava A, Bottero M, Scognamiglio R et al. Arrhythmogenic right ventricular dysplasia: a familial form [astract]. *PACE* 1985;8:A32.

16. Laurent M, Descaves C, Biron Y, et al. Familial form of arrhythmogenic right ventricular dysplasia. *Am Heart J* 1987;113:827–829.

17. Buja GF, Nava A, Martini B, et al. Right ventricular dysplasia: a familial cardiomyopathy? *Eur Heart J* 1989;10(suppl D):13–15.

18. Rakovec P, Rossi L, Fontaine G, et al. Familial arrhythmogenic right ventricular disease. *Am J Cardiol* 1986;58:377–378.

19. Affatato A, Benedini G, Metra M, et al. Arrhythmogenic right ventricular dysplasia: a report of two familial cases. In: Gomez FP, ed. *Cardiac Pacing: Electrophysiology, Tachyarrhythmias.* Madrid, Spain: Grouz, 1985. p 1344–1350.

20. Marcus FI, Fontaine GH, Frank R, et al. Long-term follow-up in patients with arrhythmogenic right ventricular disease. *Eur Heart J* 1989;10(suppl D):68–73.

21. Leclercq JF, Coumel P. Characteristics, prognosis, and treatment of the

ventricular arrhythmias of right ventricular dysplasia. *Eur Heart J* 1989; 10(suppl D):61–67.

22. Lemery R, Brugada P, Janssen J, et al. Nonischemic sustained ventricular tachycardia: clinical outcome in 12 patients with arrhythmogenic right ventricular dysplasia. *J Am Coll Cardiol* 1989;14:96–105.

23. Wichter T, Haverkamp W, Martinez-Rubio A, et al. Long-term prognosis and risk-stratification of arrhythmogenic right ventricular dysplasia/cardiomyopathy [abstract]. *Circulation* 1995;92[4 part 2]:I97.

24. Reiter MI, Smith WM, Gallagher JI. Clinical spectrum of ventricular tachycardia with left bundle branch morphology. *Am J Cardiol* 1983;51:113–1121.

25. Okano Y, Kamkura S, Katayama K, et al. Electrocardiographic features and their significance in arrhythmogenic right ventricular dysplasia [abstract] *Circulation* 1992;86(I):857.

26. Manyari DE, Duff HJ, Kostuk WJ, et al. Usefulness of noninvasive studies for diagnosis of right ventricular dysplasia. *Am J Cardiol* 1986;57:1147–1153.

27. Blomstrom-Lundqvist C, Hirsch I, Olsson SB. Quantitative analysis of the signal-averaged QRS in patients with arrhythmogenic right ventricular dysplasia. *Eur Heart J* 1988;9:301–312.

28. Kinoshita O, Kamakur S, Ohe T, et al. Frequency analysis of signal-averaged electrocardiogram in patients with right ventricular tachycardia. *J Am Coll Cardiol* 1992;20:1230–1237.

29. Robertson JH, Bardy GH, German LD, et al. Comparison of two-dimensional echocardiographic and angiographic findings in arrhythmogenic right ventricular dysplasia. *Am J Cardiol* 1985;55:1506–1508.

30. Kisslo J. Two-dimensional echocardiography in arrhythmogenic right ventricular dysplasia. *Eur Heart J* 1989;10(suppl D):22–26.

31. Wichter T, Hindricks G, Lerch H, et al. Regional myocardial sympathetic dysinnervation in arrhythmogenic right ventricular cardiomyopathy. An analysis using ^{123}I-meta-iobenzylguanidine scintigraphy. *Circulation* 1994; 89:667–683.

32. Casolo GC, Poggese L, Boddi M, et al. ECG-gated magnetic resonance imaging and right ventricular dysplasia. *Am Heart J* 1989;113:1245–1248.

33. Blake LM, Scheinman MM, Higgins CB. MR features of arrhythmogenic right ventricular dysplasia. *Am J Radiol* 1994;162:809–812.

34. Gill JS, Rowland E, De Belder M, et al. Cardiac abnormalities not visualized by echocardiography are detected by magnetic resonance imaging in patients with idiopathic ventricular tachycardia [abstract]. *Eur Heart J* 1993;14:7A.

35. Auffermann W, Wichter T, Breithardt G, et al. Arrhythmogenic right ventricular disease: MR imaging versus angiography. *Am J Radiol* 1993;161: 549–555.

36. Rossi P, Massumi A, Gillette P, et al. Arrhythmogenic right ventricular dysplasia: clinical features, diagnostic techniques, and current management. *Am Heart J* 1982;103:415–420.

37. Furanello F, Bettini R, Bertoldi A, et al. Arrhythmia patterns in athletes with arrhythmogenic right ventricular dysplasia. *Eur Heart J* 1989;10 (suppl D):16–19.

38. Haïssaguerre M, Le Metayer P, D'Ivernois C, et al. Distinctive response of arrhythmogenic right ventricular disease to high dose isoproterenol. *PACE* 1990;13(2):2119–2226.
39. Nimkhedkar K, Hilton CJ, Furniss SS, et al. Surgery for ventricular tachycardia associated with right ventricular dysplasia: disarticulation of right ventricle in 9 of 10 cases. *J Am Coll Cardiol* 1992;19:1079–1084.
40. Wichter T, Martinez-Rubio A, Kottkamp H, et al. Reproducibility of programmed ventricular stimulation in arrhythmogenic right ventricular dysplasia/cardiomyopathy [abstract]. *Circulation* 1996;94(suppl 1):I626.
41. Yamabe H, Okumura K, Tsuchiya T et al. Demonstration of entrainment and presence of slow conduction during ventricular tachycardia in arrhythmogenic right ventricular dysplasia. *PACE* 1994;17:172–178.
42. Aizawa Y, Funizaki T, Takahashi M, et al. Entrainment of ventricular tachycardia in arrhythmogenic right ventricular tachycardia. *PACE* 1991;14:1606–1613.
43. Guiradon G, Klein GJ. Right ventricular disconnection for refractory multiple reentry site ventricular tachycardia in adult arrhythmogenic right ventricular dysplasia. *Med World News* 1981;22:26.
44. Fontaine G, Guiradon G, Frank R. Mechanism of ventricular tachycardia with and without chronic myocardial ischemia: surgical management based on epicardial mapping. In: Narula OS, ed. *Cardiac Arrhythmias: Electrophysiology, Diagnosis and Management.* Baltimore, MD: Williams & Wilkins. p 529.
45. Leclercq JF, Chouty F, Cauchemez B, et al. Results of electrical fulguration in arrhythmogenic right ventricular disease. *Am J Cardiol* 1988;62:220–224.
46. Guiradon G, Fontaine G, Frank R, et al. Surgical treatment of ventricular tachycardia guided by ventricular mapping in 23 patients without coronary artery disease. *Ann Thorac Surg* 1981;32:439–450.
47. Guiradon G, Klein G, Gulamheisen S, et al. Total disconnection of the right ventricular free wall: surgical treatment of right ventricular tachycardia associated with right ventricular dysplasia. *Circulation* 1983;67:463–470.
48. Fontaine G, Guiradon G, Pavie A, et al. Surgical treatment of arrhythmogenic right ventricular dysplasia: long-term follow-up [abstract]. *Eur Heart J* 1984;1:144.
49. Fontaine G, Frank R, Rougier I, et al. Electrode catheter ablation of resistant ventricular tachycardia in arrhythmogenic right ventricular dysplasia: experience of 13 patients with a mean follow-up of 45 months. *Eur Heart J* 1989;10(suppl D):74–81.
50. Shoda M, Kasanuki H, Ohnishi S, et al. Recurrence of new ventricular tachycardia after successful catheter ablation in patients with arrhythmogenic right ventricular dysplasia [abstract]. *Circulation* 1992;86(suppl 1):I580.
51. Asso A, Farre J, Zayas R, et al. Radiofrequency catheter ablation of ventricular tachycardia in patients with arrhythmogenic right ventricular dysplasia [abstract]. *J Am Coll Cardiol* 1995;25(suppl A):315A.
52. Stabile G, Pappone C, De Simone A, et al. Arrhythmogenic myocardiopathy: radiofrequency catheter ablation of ventricular tachycardia [abstract]. *PACE* 1995;18(part 2):1177.

53. Haverkamp W, Borgreffe M, Chen X, et al. Radiofrequency catheter ablation in patients with sustained ventricular tachycardia and arrhythmogenic right ventricular disease [abstract]. *Circulation* 1993;88(suppl 1):I353.

54. Mitchell SC, Korones SB, Berendes HW. Congenital heart disease in 56109 births: incidence and natural history. *Circulation* 1971;43:323.

55. Lillehei CW, Cohen M, Warden HE, et al. Direct vision intracardiac surgical correction of the tetralogy of Fallot, pentalogy of Fallot, and pulmonary atresia defects: report of first 10 cases. *Ann Surg* 1955;142:418.

56. Waien SA, Liu PP, Robb BL, et al. Serial follow-up of adults with repaired tetralogy of Fallot. *J Am Coll Cardiol* 1992;20:295–300.

57. Wolf MD, Landtman B, Neill CA, et al. Total correction of tetralogy of Fallot: follow-up study of 104 cases. *Circulation* 1965;31:385–393.

58. Burton ME, Leon AR. Radiofrequency catheter ablation of right ventricular outflow tract tachycardia late after complete repair of tetralogy of Fallot using the pace mapping technique. *PACE* 1993;16:2319–2325.

59. James FW, Kaplan S, Chou T. Unexpected cardiac arrest in patients after surgical correction of tetralogy of Fallot. *Circulation* 1975;52:691–695.

60. Quattlebaum TG, Varghese PJ, Neill CA, et al. Sudden death among postoperative patients with tetralogy of Fallot. *Circulation* 1976;54:289–293.

61. Gillette PC, Yeoman MA, Mullins CE, et al. Sudden death after repair of tetralogy of Fallot: electrocardiographic and electrophysiologic abnormalities. *Circulation* 1977;56:566–571.

62. Garson A Jr, Nihill MR, McNamara DG, et al. Status of the adult and adolescent after repair of tetralogy of Fallot. *Circulation* 1979;59:1232–1240.

63. Downar E, Harris L, Kimber S, et al. Ventricular tachycardia after surgical repair of tetralogy of Fallot: results of intraoperative mapping studies. *J Am Coll Cardiol* 1992;20:648–655.

64. Harken AH, Horowitz LN, Josephson ME. Surgical correction of recurrent sustained ventricular tachycardia following complete repair of tetralogy of Fallot. *J Thorac Cardiovasc Surg* 1980;80:779–781.

65. Horowitz LN, Vetter VL, Harken AH, et al. Electrophysiologic characteristics of sustained ventricular tachycardia occurring after repair of tetralogy of Fallot. *Am J Cardiol* 1980;46:446–452.

66. Kugler JD, Pinsky WW, Cheatham JP, et al. Sustained ventricular tachycardia after repair of tetralogy of Fallot: new electrophysiologic findings. *Am J Cardiol* 1983;51:1137–1143.

67. Hebe J, Weib C, Siebels, J, et al. Radiofrequency current treatment of sustained monomorphic ventricular tachycardias in patients with surgically corrected tetralogy of Fallot [abstract]. *PACE* 1995;18(part 2):1767.

68. Josephson ME. *Clinical Cardiac Electrophysiology*. Malvern, PA: Lea & Febiger, 1993.

69. Biblo LA, Carlson MD. Transcatheter radiofrequency ablation of ventricular tachycardia following surgical correction of tetralogy of Fallot. *PACE* 1994;17:1556–1560.

70. Chinushi M, Aizawa Y, Kitazawa H, et al. Successful radiofrequency catheter ablation for macroreentrant ventricular tachycardias in a patient with tetralogy of Fallot after corrective surgery. *PACE* 1995;18(part 1):1713–1716.

71. Josephson ME. *Clinical Cardiac Electrophysiology.* Malvern, PA: Lea & Febiger, 1993.

72. Goldner BG, Cooper R, Blau W, et al. Radiofrequency catheter ablation as a primary therapy for treatment of ventricular tachycardia in a patient after repair of tetralogy of Fallot. *PACE* 1994;17:1441–1446.

73. Kremers MS, Wells PJ, Black WH, et al. Entrainment of ventricular tachycardia in postoperative tetralogy of Fallot. *PACE* 1988;11:1310–1314.

74. Oda H, Aizawa Y, Murata M, et al. A successful ablation of recurrent sustained ventricular tachycardia in a postoperative case of tetralogy of Fallot. *Jpn Heart J* 1986;27:421–428.

75. Gonska BD, Cao K, Rab J, et al. Catheter ablation of ventricular tachycardia late after repair of congenital heart defects [abstract]. *PACE* 1995; 18(part 2):1167.

76. Lemery R, Brugada P, Cheriex EC, et al. Reversibility of tachycardia-induced left ventricular dysfunction after closed chest ablation of the atrioventricular junction for intractable atrial fibrillation. *Am J Cardiol* 1987;60:1406–1408.

77. Cruz ES, Cheriex EC, Smeets JM, et al. Reversibility of tachycardia-induced cardiomyopathy after cure of incessant supraventricular tachycardia. *J Am Coll Cardiol* 1990;3:739–744.

78. Giorgi LV, Hartzler GO, Hamaker WR. Incessant focal atrial tachycardia: a surgically remediable cause of cardiomyopathy. *J Thorac Cardiovasc Surg* 1984;87:466–473.

79. Packer DL, Bardy GH, Worley SJ, et al. Tachycardia-induced cardiomyopathy: a reversible form of left ventricular dysfunction. *Am J Cardiol* 1986;57:563–570.

80. Chow E, Woodward JC, Farrar DJ. Rapid ventricular pacing in pigs: an experimental model of congestive heart failure. *Am J Physiol* 1990;258: H1603–1605.

81. Wilson JR, Douglas P, Hickey WF, et al. Experimental congestive heart failure produced by rapid ventricular pacing in the dog: cardiac effects. *Circulation* 1987;75:857–867.

82. Fife DA, Gilette PC, Crawford FA, et al. Resolution of dilated cardiomyopathy after surgical ablation on ventricular tachycardia in a child. *J Am Coll Cardiol* 1987;9:231–234.

83. Rao PS, Hajjar HN. Congestive cardiomyopathy due to chronic tachycardia: resolution of cardiomyopathy with antiarrhythmic drugs. *Int J Cardiol* 1987;17:216–220.

84. Rakovec DL, Lajovic J, Dolenc M. Reversible congestive cardiomyopathy due to chronic ventricular tachycardia. *PACE* 1988;12:542–545.

85. Fishberger SB, Colan SD, Saul JP, et al. Myocardial mechanics before and after ablation of chronic tachycardia. *PACE* 1996;19:42–49.

86. Jaggarao NS, Nanda AS, Daubert JP. Ventricular tachycardia-induced cardiomyopathy: improvement with radiofrequency ablation. *PACE* 1996;19 (part 1)505–8.

87. Kim Y, Goldberger J, Kadish A. Treatment of ventricular tachycardia-induced cardiomyopathy by transcatheter radiofrequency ablation. *Heart* 1996;76:550–552.

88. Singh B, Upendra K, Talwar K, et al. Reversibility of "tachycardia-induced

cardiomyopathy" following the cure of idiopathic left ventricular tachycardia using radiofrequency energy. *PACE* 1996;19:1391–1392.

89. Cacares J, Jazayeri M, McKinnie J, et al. Sustained bundle branch reentry as a mechanism of clinical tachycardia. *Circulation* 1989;79:256–270.

90. Mehdirad AA, Keim S, Rist K. Long-term clinical outcome of right bundle branch radiofrequency catheter ablation for treatment of bundle branch reentrant ventricular tachycardia. *PACE* 1995;18:2135–2143.

91. Blanck Z, Jazayeri M, Sra J, et al. Bundle branch reentry: a mechanism of sustained wide QRS complex tachycardia in patients with no structural heart disease [abstract]. *J Am Coll Cardiol* 1993;21:24A.

92. Wang CW, Sterba R, Tchou P. Bundle branch reentry tachycardia with two distinct left bundle branch block morphologies. *J Cardiovasc Electrophysiol* 1997;8:688–693.

93. Huang SK, Messer JV, Denes P. Significance of ventricular tachycardia in idiomyopathic dilated cardiomyopathy: observations in 35 patients. *Am J Cardiol* 1983;51:507.

94. Meinertz T, Hofmann T, Kasper W, et al. Significance of ventricular arrhythmias in idiopathic dilated cardiomyopathy. *Am J Cardiol* 1984;53:902.

95. Von Olshausen K, Schafer A, Mehmel H. Ventricular arrhythmias in idiopathic dilated cardiomyopathy. *Br Heart J* 1984;51:195.

96. Milner PG, Dimarco JP, Lerman BB. Electrophysiological evaluation of sustained ventricular tachyarrhythmias in idiopathic dilated cardiomyopathy. *PACE* 1988;11:562–568.

97. Poll DS, Marchlinski FE, Buxton AE, et al. Usefulness of programmed stimulation in idiopathic dilated cardiomyopathy. *Am J Cardiol* 1986;58:992–997.

98. Chen X, Shenasa M, Borgreffe M, et al. Role of programmed stimulation in patients with idiopathic dilated cardiomyopathy and documented sustained ventricular tachyarrhythmias: inducibility and prognostic value in 102 patients. *Eur Heart J* 1994;15:76–82.

99. Mancini DM, Wong KL, Simson MB. Prognostic value of an abnormal signal-averaged electrocardiogram in patients with nonischemic congestive cardiomyopathy. *Circulation* 1993;87:1083–1092.

100. Pelliccia F, Critelli G, Cianfrocca C, et al. Interstitial fibrosis as a substrate of spontaneous nonsustained ventricular tachycardia in idiopathic dilated cardiomyopathy [abstract]. *J Am Coll Cardiol* 1994;23:340A.

101. Lo YSA, Billingham M, Rowan RA, et al. Histopathologic and electrophysiologic correlations in idiopathic dilated cardiomyopathy and sustained ventricular tachyarrhythmia. *Am J Cardiol* 1989;64:1063–1066.

102. Roberts WC, Siegel RJ, McManus BM. Idiopathic dilated cardiomyopathy: analysis of 152 necropsy patients. *Am J Cardiol* 1987;60:1340–1355.

103. Cassidy DM, Vassallo JA, Buxton AE, et al. Endocardial catheter mapping in sinus rhythm: relationship to underlying heart disease and ventricular arrhythmias. *Circulation* 1986;73:645.

104. Perlman RL, Miller J, Kindwall KE, et al. Abnormal epicardial and endocardial electrograms in patients with idiopathic dilated cardiomyopathy: relationship to arrhythmias [abstract]. *Circulation* 1990;82(suppl 3):III708.

105. Pogwizd SM. Nonreentrant mechanisms underlie spontaneously occur-

ring ventricular arrhythmias in dilated cardiomyopathy [abstract]. *Circulation* 1993;88(suppl 1):I326.

106. Kottkamp H, Hindricks G, Chen X, et al. Radiofrequency catheter ablation of sustained ventricular tachycardia in idiopathic dilated cardiomyopathy. *Circulation* 1995;92:1159–1168.

107. Wilber DJ, Glascock DN, Kall JG, et al. Radiofrequency catheter ablation of sustained ventricular tachycardia associated with idiopathic dilated cardiomyopathy [abstract]. *Circulation* 1995;92(suppl 1):I684.

108. Constantin L, Martins JB, Kienzle MG, et al. Induced sustained ventricular tachycardia in nonischemic dilated cardiomyopathy: dependence on clinical presentation and response to antiarrhythmic agents. *PACE* 1989;12:776–783.

109. Rae AP, Spielman SR, Kutalek SP, et al. Electrophysiologic assessment of antiarrhythmic drug efficacy for ventricular tachyarrhythmias associated with dilated cardiomyopathy. *Am J Cardiol* 1987;59:291–295.

110. Bing-Liem L, Swerdlow CD. Value of electropharmacologic testing in idiopathic dilated cardiomyopathy and sustained ventricular tachyarrhythmias. *Am J Cardiol* 1988;62:611–666.

111. Trappe HJ, Klein H, Auricchio A, et al. Catheter ablation of ventricular tachycardia: role of the underlying etiology and the site of energy delivery. *PACE* 1992;15(part 1):411–24.

112. Mayock RL, Bertrand P, Morrison CE, et al. Manifestations of sarcoidosis: analysis of 145 patients, with a review of nine series selected from the literature. *Am J Med* 1963;35:67–88.

113. Silverman KJ, Hutchins GM, Bulkley BH. Cardiac sarcoid: a clinicopathologic study of 84 unselected patients with systemic sarcoidosis. *Circulation* 1978;58:1204–1211.

114. Matsui Y, Iwai K, Tachibana T, et al. Clinicopathological study on fatal myocardial sarcoidosis. *Ann NY Acad Sci* 1976;278;455–469.

115. Bernstein MF, Konzelmann W, Sidlick DM. Boeck's sarcoid: report of case with veisceral involvement. *Arch Intern Med* 1929;44:721–734.

116. Fleming HA. Sarcoid heart disease. *Br Heart J* 1980;43:366.

117. Tawahara K, Kurata C, Okayama K, et al. Thallium-201 and gallium-67 single photon emission computed tomographic imaging in cardiac sarcoidosis. *Am Heart J* 1991;124:1383–1384.

118. Alberts C, Schoot JB, Groen AS. [67]Ga scintigraphy index of disease activity in pulmonary sarcoidosis. *Eur J Nucl Med* 1981;6:205–212.

119. Kinney EL, Jackson GL, Reves WC, et al. Thallium-scan myocardial defects and echocardiographic abnormalities in patients with sarcoidosis without clinical cardiac dysfunction: an analysis of 44 patients. *Am J Med* 1980;68:497–503.

120. James TN. Clinicopathologic correlations. De subitaneis mortibus XXV: Sarcoid heart disease. *Circulation* 1977;56:320–326.

121. Paz HL, McCormick DJ, Kutalek SP, et al. The automated implantable cardiac defibrillator: prophylaxis in cardiac sarcoid. *Chest* 1994;106:1603–1607.

122. Lopez JA, Hogan PJ, Capek P, et al. Cardiac sarcoidosis: an unusual form of acute congestive cardiomyopathy. *Tex Heart Inst J* 1995;22:265–267.

123. Winters SL, Cohen M, Greenberg S, et al. Sustained ventricular tachycardia associated with sarcoidosis: assessment of the underlying cardiac anatomy and the prospective utility of programmed ventricular stimulation, drug therapy, and an implantable antiachycardia device. *J Am Coll Cardiol* 1991;18:937–943.

124. Huang PL, Brooks R, Carpenter C, et al. Antiarrhythmic therapy guided by programmed electrical stimulation in cardiac sarcoidosis with ventricular tachycardia. *Am Heart J* 1991;121:599–601.

125. World Health Organization. *TDR News* 1992;40:3–5.

126. Hagar JM, Rahimtoola SH. Chagas' heart disease in the United States. *N Engl J Med* 1991;325:763–768.

127. Filho MM, Sosa E, Nishioka S, et al. Clinical and electrophysiologic features of syncope in chronic heart disease. *J Cardiovasc Electrophys* 1994;5:563–570.

128. Andrade ZA. Mechanisms of myocardial damage in *Trypanosoma cruzi* infection. *Ciba Foundation Symposium 99: Cytopathology of Parasitic Diseases.* London, England: Pitman Books, 1983. p 214–233.

129. Bestetti RB, Santos CRF, Machado-Junion OB, et al. Clinical profile of patients with Chagas' disease before and during sustained ventricular tachycardia. *Int J Cardiol* 1990;29:39–46.

130. Bellotti G, Bocchi EA, de Moreas AV, et al. In vivo detection of *Trypanosoma cruzi* antigens in hearts of patients with chronic Chagas' heart disease. *Am Heart J* 1996;131:301–307.

131. De Carvalho ACC, Masuda MO, Tanowitz HB, et al. Conduction defects and arrhythmias in Chagas' disease: possible role of gap junctions and humoral mechanisms. *J Cardiovasc Electrophysiol* 1994;5:686–698.

132. Mendoza I, Camardo J, Moleiro F, et al. Sustained ventricular tachycardia in chornic chagasic myocarditis: electrophysiologic and pharmacologic characteristics. *Am J Cardiol* 1986;57:423–427.

133. Giniger AG, Retyk EO, Laino RA, et al. Ventricular tachycardia in Chagas' disease. *Am J Cardiol* 1992;70:459–462.

134. Rosas F, Velasco V, Arboleda F, et al. Catheter ablation of ventricular tachycardia in chagasic cardiomyopathy. *Clin Cardiol* 1997;20:169–174.

135. Galvao S, Medeiros J, Santos R, et al. Treatment of recurrent ventricular tachycardia by endocardial catheter fulguration in patients with Chagas' cardiomyopathy [abstract]. *Eur J CPE* 1992;2:153.

136. Sosa E, Scalabrini A, Rati M, et al. Successful catheter ablation of the "origin" of recurrent ventricular tachycardia in chronic chagasic heart disease. *J Electrophysiol* 1987;1:58–61.

137. de Paola AAV, Gomes JA, Miyamoto MH, et al. Transcoronary chemical ablation of ventricular tachycardia in chronic chagasic myocarditis. *J Am Coll Cardiol* 1992;20:480–482.

138. de Paola AAV, Tavora MZP, Silva RMF, et al. Radiofrequency catheter ablation of sustained ventricular tachycardia in patients with chronic chagasic cardiomyopathy [abstract]. *PACE* 1996;19:693.

139. Sosa E, Scanavacca M, D'Avila, A. Non-surgical transthoracic epicardial ablation of recurrent ventricular tachycardia [abstract]. *Circulation* 1997;96:I–318.

Part VII

Miscellaneous Topics

Chapter 34

Complications Associated With Radiofrequency Catheter Ablation

Albert C. Lin, M.D., David Wilber, M.D.

Radiofrequency (RF) current delivered by percutaneous catheters has become the energy source of choice in the safe and effective treatment of a variety of supraventricular and ventricular arrhythmias. RF energy delivered via a catheter produces well-localized areas of coagulative necrosis in the myocardium through resistive heating at the point of contact.[1] However, cardiovascular complications have been reported in a small number of patients undergoing catheter ablation. These can be divided into complications inherent in any cardiac catheterization procedure (perforation, vascular injury, and venous or arterial thrombosis) and more specific complications related to RF energy application such as unintended atrioventricular (AV) block, new arrhythmias, or systemic embolism. In order to minimize the risk of performing catheter ablation, a thorough understanding of the potential complications of the procedure, and a fastidious attention to detail are paramount.

Complications Associated with Specific Procedures

Accessory Atrioventricular Connections

RF ablation is a highly effective and curative treatment for arrhythmias due to accessory AV connections.[1-4] RF current may be applied to right-sided accessory pathways and septal pathways via a superior or inferior venous approach to the tricuspid annulus. Left-sided accessory pathways can be ablated

From Huang SKS, Wilber DJ (eds.): *Radiofrequency Catheter Ablation of Cardiac Arrhythmias: Basic Concepts and Clinical Applications,* 2nd ed. Armonk, NY: Futura Publishing Company, Inc. ©2000.

via a transseptal approach or retrograde aortic approach with comparable efficacy and safety. Several studies have reported a success rate in excess of 90% and a complication rate that ranges from 2% to 7%.[2–7]

Reported complications related to ablation of accessory pathways include death, systemic and pulmonary thromboembolism, vascular injury, pneumothorax, coronary occlusion and spasm,[8–9] cardiac perforation, pericardial effusion, pericardial tamponade,[10] aortic valve perforation,[11,12] entrapment of the ablation catheter in the mitral valve apparatus,[12–14] and inadvertent AV block.[12,15,16]

The 1995 North American Society for Pacing and Electrophysiology (NASPE) Survey reported the results of 5427 patients undergoing RF ablation of accessory AV connections from 175 centers in North America during 1993.[12] Ablation was attempted in 3096 left free wall pathways, 885 right free wall pathways, and 1446 septal pathways. The success rates were 93%, 85%, and 87%, respectively. There were a total of 99 (1.8%) reported significant complications, defined as any complication delaying discharge, including 4 deaths (0.07%). Table 1 delineates some of the significant complications. Other complications noted without reported numbers included deep venous thrombosis, pneumothorax, and pulmonary embolism. The Multicentre European Radiofrequency Survey (MERFS) was conducted by the Working Group on Arrhythmias of the European Society of Cardiology with voluntary and retrospective data collection from 68 centers in Europe from 1987 to 1992.[15] MERFS reported the results of 2222 RF ablations of accessory pathways. The total number of complications was 98 (4.4%). Severe complications (unintended complete AV block, torsades de pointes, cardiac perforation/tamponade, arterial and venous thrombosis, pulmonary embolism, cerebral embolism with persistent neurological disorders, and death) occurred in 2.3% of patients. Of note, there were 3 deaths (0.13%), 16 perforations and tamponade (0.72%), and 12 clinically significant pericardial effusions (0.54%).

Persistent AV block is an uncommon complication of accessory pathway ablation, with a reported range of 0.2–1.0%.[12,15,16] This complication occurs almost exclusively during ablation of septal pathways, particularly midseptal location. The risk of heart block during anteroseptal pathway ablation can be minimized by precise mapping and careful power titration, beginning at very

Table 1
Complications of RF Ablation of Accessory Pathways

Complication	MERFS N = 2222	NASPE Registry N = 5427
Death	3 (0.13%)	4 (0.1%)
Cardiac tamponade	16 (0.72%)	7 (0.1%)
Pericarditis or significant pericardial effusion	12 (0.54%)	10 (0.2%)
Stroke or TIA	11 (0.49%)	8 (0.1%)
Aortic valve perforation	Not reported	4 (0.1%)
Mitral valve damage	Not reported	2 (0.04%)
Coronary artery injury	Not reported	3 (0.06%)
Vascular injury or major bleeding at puncture site	7 (0.32%)	3 (0.06%)
Venous thrombosis	4 (0.18%)	Not reported
Permanent AV block	14 (0.63%)	9 (0.2%)

low energies. The accessory pathways appear to be much more sensitive to thermal injury than the His bundle.[17,18]

Although less frequently described than with AV node modification, inappropriate sinus tachycardia has been reported following accessory pathway ablation.[19,20] This may result from damage to autonomic inputs of the sinus node or more nonspecific parasympathetic denervation. Symptoms due to inappropriate sinus tachycardia usually resolve after several months and rarely require long-term therapy.

Atrioventricular Nodal Modification

The treatment of AV nodal tachycardia by RF catheter ablation is also safe and highly successful.[21,22] The vast majority of the 5423 patients with AV nodal reentrant tachycardia reported in the 1995 NASPE survey underwent slow pathway (posterior) ablation (93%).[12] Although the NASPE survey reported a much lower success rate with an anterior (fast pathway) approach (46%) compared to a posterior approach (97%), a randomized trial comparing the 2 methods reported similar success rates.[23] The occurrence of heart block in the NASPE survey was low (0.11%), and the anatomic approach used in the 6 patients developing this complication was not specified. The risk of heart block is reported to be higher with an anterior approach in several comparative studies.[23–25] The risk of heart block with a posterior approach ranges from 0–3% in single center series.[21–24] A detailed analysis of the risk of heart block was performed in 880 patients undergoing attempted AV nodal modification in MERFS.[15] The incidence of complete AV block with fast pathway ablation (3.3%) is statistically higher than the incidence of complete AV block with slow pathway ablation (2.0%). In addition, centers treating more than 30 patients had lower incidence of complete AV block (2.3%) than those with less experience (6.3%). The lowest incidence of complete AV block, 1.5%, occurred in patients ablated by a posterior approach in experienced centers (≥30 patients).

Complications other than heart block occur infrequently (Table 2). In the 1995 NASPE survey of 5423 patients undergoing attempted AV nodal modification, pericarditis or tamponade was reported in 18 (0.3%), pneumothorax in 5 (0.1%), vascular injury in 3, (0.1%), and deep venous thrombosis in 5 (0.1%).

Table 2
Complications of RF Catheter Modification of the
AV Junction in the NASPE Registry and MERFS

Complication	MERFS N = 815	NASPE Registry N = 5423
Permanent AV block	41 (5.1%)	6 (0.11%)
Tamponade or significant pericardial effusion	5 (0.61%)	18 (0.3%)
Pneumothorax	Not reported	5
Vascular injury or major bleeding at puncture site	2 (0.24%)	3
Venous thrombosis	9 (1.1%)	5 (0.1%)
Pulmonary embolism	2 (0.24%)	Not reported

Similar results were reported in the MERFS registry of 815 patients undergoing attempted AV node modification. Major complications included a 0.24% incidence of perforation and tamponade, a 0.37% incidence of a clinically significant pericardial effusion, and a 1.1% incidence of venous thrombosis. No procedure-related deaths were reported in either study.

In addition to permanent AV block, other new rhythm disturbances have been reported following AV nodal modification. As with ablation of accessory pathways, inappropriate sinus tachycardia may develop.[19] Other investigators have noted the occurrence of atypical AVNRT ("slow/slow" or posterior tachycardia) following an anterior approach.[26] In these cases, it is unclear whether the ablation played a role in the genesis of the tachycardia, or was simply ineffective in eliminating a preexisting posteriorly located circuit. Rare patients with poor or absent baseline antegrade fast pathway conduction may develop marked PR prolongation, and second or third degree AV block following slow pathway ablation. This complication may be avoided in such patients by an anterior approach targeting the retrograde fast pathway.[27]

Atrial Flutter and Atrial Tachycardia

RF ablation of typical isthmus-dependent flutter and atrial tachycardia are well established as effective means of achieving a long-term cure.[28–c31] The 1995 NASPE survey included 570 patients undergoing ablation of atrial flutter and 569 patients undergoing ablation of atrial tachycardia. Overall significant complication rates were 0.7% and 1.7%, respectively.[12] Complete heart block occurred in one patient with flutter and one with atrial tachycardia. One patient had tamponade. In MERFS, 141 patients underwent RF ablation for atrial tachycardia and atrial flutter.[15] There were 7 complications (5%) including 1 perforation/tamponade, 2 clinically significant pericardial effusions, and 1 complete AV block. No deaths were reported in either study.

Atrioventricular Junction

In the 1995 NASPE survey, permanent complete heart block was achieved in 97.3% of patients.[12] There were a total of 2084 AV junction ablation procedures performed with a 3.7% overall complication rate (79 patients) including 4 deaths (0.2%), 1 acute myocardial infarction (0.04%), 2 cerebrovascular accidents associated with left-sided His bundle ablations (0.1%), and 2 patients with pericarditis or tamponade (0.1%). In MERFS , 900 patients underwent RF ablation of the AV junction.[15] The overall incidence of severe complications was 1.8%, including 1 perforation/tamponade (0.11%), 4 clinically significant pericardial effusions (0.44%), 1 tricuspid valve injury (0.11%), and 1 death (0.11%).

A worrisome complication associated with RF ablation of the AV junction is the occurrence of ventricular arrhythmias and sudden death. Randomized trials suggest that the incidence of this complication may be less with RF ablation compared to direct current shock.[32,33] However, a small risk of early sudden death persists with RF techniques.[32,34,35] A majority of these deaths occurred in patients with significant structural heart disease, and mortality risk may not differ from a comparable group of patients with atrial fibrillation and structural heart disease treated medically.[35,36] Retrospective data suggest that the risk of sudden death is greater in patients with slower programmed pacing rates ($\leq$ 70 beats per minute) in the initial weeks following the procedure.[34,35] High pacing rates (90 beats per minute) have been advocated for the initial 1–3 months postablation to reduce this risk.[34] A potential mechanism for these observations is the experimental demonstration of greater than expected prolongation of repolarization following the transition from a rapid rate to a slower paced rate, associated with increased vulnerability to early afterdepolarizations and ventricular arrhythmias.[37]

One issue related to ablation of the AV junction is the risk of damage to previously implanted pacemakers. However, in a majority of patients, RF lesions remote from the electrode tip have little effect on either pacemaker or defibrillator function, and minimal change in pacing and sensing thresholds. Occasionally, decreased electrogram amplitude and increased pacing thresholds may be observed, but generally revert back to normal during follow-up.[38] However, persistent late exit block has been reported.[38a] Device function should be tested routinely before and after all ablation procedures.

Ventricular Tachycardia

RF ablation of ventricular tachycardia in structurally normal hearts in the setting of coronary disease and cardiomyopathies is increasing in numbers and efficacy. The 1995 NASPE survey confirms the safety of RF ablation of ventricular tachycardia in 844 patients. Overall, there was a 2.4% significant complication rate and no deaths.[12] The complications included 6 patients (0.7%) with tamponade, 3 patients (0.4%) with systemic emboli, and 1 patient with unintended heart block (0.1%). Approximately 50% of the patients had no structural heart disease (Table 3).

A higher overall complication incidence was reported in MERFS in 320 patients undergoing RF ablation of ventricular tachycardia.[15] Complications occurred in 24 patients (7.5%). Thromboembolic events were more frequent than

Table 3
Complications of RF Catheter Ablation of Ventricular Tachycardia

Complication	MERFS N = 120	NASPE Registry N = 844
Death	1 (0.31%)	0
Cardiac Tamponade	1 (0.31%)	6
Arterial thrombosis	1 (0.31%)	1
Peripheral and cerebral embolism	6 (1.9%)	3
Permanent AV block	1 (0.31%)	1
Major bleeding at puncture site	2 (0.63%)	Not reported

in other types of ablation with an overall incidence of 2.8%. These included arterial thrombosis (0.31%), pulmonary emboli (0.63%), peripheral arterial emboli (0.63%), and cerebral emboli (1.5%). Other complications included complete heart block (0.3%), and perforation/ tamponade (0.3%). In addition, there was a 0.63% incidence of clinically significant pericardial effusions and a 0.63% incidence of major bleeding at the puncture site.

General Comments

Cardiac Perforation and Tamponade

Cardiac perforation is one of the most serious complications of RF ablation procedures, with an incidence of 0.1% to 0.7%. A high index of clinical suspicion should be maintained, and any period of significant hypotension, irrespective of initial response to fluids or alternative potential cause (such as excessive sedation) should be promptly investigated. Fluoroscopy of the left heart border in the left anterior oblique view is a sensitive and quickly obtained clue to the presence of significant pericardial fluid. Two-dimensional echocardiography should be available either in the electrophysiology suite or in close proximity thereto, and will provide sufficient confirmation of diagnosis and treatment outcome. Pericardiocentesis with placement of a multiple sidehole drainage catheter with fluoroscopic and/or echocardiographic guidance is safe, rapid, and effective therapy for acute pericardial tamponade.[39,40] Perforation due to catheter ablation rarely requires surgical intervention if treated promptly. Routine echocardiography following uncomplicated ablation is not clinically useful.[41] The risk of perforation during RF application, typically related to an impedance rise, can be minimized by monitoring of catheter tip temperature, particularly in areas of low flow. However, diagnostic catheters may also result in mechanical perforation, which can be minimized by continued attention to catheter positioning throughout the procedure, use of "floppy" catheters, and avoidance of prolonged positioning at thin-walled regions such as the apices of both ventricles.

Thromboembolic Events

Vascular complications including deep venous thrombosis and systemic embolization associated with catheter ablation range from 0.06% to 1.3%.[7,12,42,43] The incidence of these events is slightly higher if left-sided procedures are considered alone.[42,43] Thermometry may not eliminate the risk of thromboembolism directly related to RF lesion generation. In a multicenter study of a closed loop temperature controlled RF system, 4 patients had systemic emboli without evidence of impedance or temperature rise, or coagulum formation.[16] The use and intensity of systemic anticoagulation or antiplatelet agents during and after catheter ablation is varied and controversial, particularly for procedures limited to the venous circulation.[43,44] Systemic embolization has occurred despite intraprocedural heparinization and postprocedure platelet inhibitors, leading some investigators to question the utility of anticoagulation protocols.[42] In the absence of data from controlled clinical trials, it is our practice to systemically heparinize all patients undergoing left-sided procedures and selected "high risk" right sided procedures (history of heart failure or prior thromboembolism, prior or anticipated periods of prolonged immobilization, and lengthy or complex procedure). The potential utility of more intense intraprocedural monitoring of anticoagulation through the use of activated clotting times (ACT) is similarly unknown, though it may be prudent for patients with atrial fibrillation undergoing left atrial procedures, and patients with significant left ventricular dysfunction undergoing ablation of ventricular tachycardia.

Pediatric Ablation

Complications of pediatric ablation procedures were recently reported from the voluntary Pediatric Radiofrequency Catheter Ablation Registry.[45] A total of 3653 procedures in 3277 patients aged less than 21 years (median 13.3 years) without structural heart disease were reported. Only ablation of accessory pathways (67%) or AV nodal modification were included. There was an overall 3.2% incidence of procedure-related complications. The most common were unintended heart block (0.7%), cardiac perforation/tamponade (0.7%), and thromboembolic events (0.2%). Procedural mortality was 0.11%. The risk of complications was significantly greater for left free wall pathways, body weight less than or equal to 15 kg, and relative operator inexperience (less than 20 procedures performed). Overall, these data are comparable to those reported in adult series.

Limitations of Reported Data

Most of the available data is subject to the limitations of voluntary reporting in multicenter registries and retrospective review. The true incidence of significant complications may be underestimated. However, procedural complications were similar between 2 retrospective registries[12] and a prospective multicenter clinical trial[16] conducted during approximately the same time period. Currently available data largely reflect the outcome of procedures performed between 1990 and 1995, during the period of explosive growth in the number of procedures performed and while many centers were on the steep portion of the procedural learning curve. Finally, the relatively low incidence of major complications renders identification of high risk patients difficult. However, in patients undergoing ablation of supraventricular arrhythmias, the presence of structural heart disease,[16] multiple ablation targets,[16] and procedural inexperience[25,38] have all been identified as potential risk factors.

References

1. Huang SK, Graham AR, Hoyt RH, et al. Transcatheter dessication of the canine left ventricle using radiofrequency energy: a pilot study. *Am Heart J* 1987;1134:43–48.

2. Jackman WM, Wang X, Friday KJ, et al. Catheter ablation of accessory atrioventricular pathways (Wolff-Parkinson-White syndrome) by radiofrequency current. *N Engl J Med* 1991;324:1605–1611.

3. Kuck KH, Schlüter M, Geiger M, et al. Radiofrequency current catheter ablation of accessory atrioventricular pathways. *Lancet* 1991;337:1557–1561.

4. Calkins H, Langberg JJ, Sousa J, et al. Radiofrequency catheter ablation of accessory atrioventricular connections in 250 patients: abbreviated therapeutic approach to Wolff-Parkinson-White syndrome. *Circulation* 1992; 85:1337–1346.

5. Lesh MD, Van Hare GF, Schamp DJ, et al. Curative percutaneous catheter ablation using radiofrequency energy for accessory pathways in all locations: results in 100 consecutive patients. *J Am Coll Cardiol* 1992;19:1303–1309.

6. Lesh MD, Van Hare GF, Scheinman MM, et al. Comparison of retrograde and transseptal methods for ablation of left free wall accessory pathways. *J Am Coll Cardiol* 1993;22:542–549.

7. Chen SA, Chern-En C, Chiang-Tai T, et al. Complications of diagnostic electrophysiologic studies and radiofrequency catheter ablation in patients with tachyarrhythmias: an eight-year survey of 3,966 consecutive procedures in a tertiary referral center. *Am J Cardiol* 1996;77:41–46.

8. Chatelain P, Zimmerman M, Weber R, et al. Acute coronary occlusion secondary to radiofrequency catheter ablation of a left lateral accessory pathway. *Eur Heart J* 1995;16:859–861.

9. Kosinski DJ, Grubb BP, Burket M, et al. Occlusion of the left main coronary artery during radiofrequency ablation for the Wolff-Parkinson-White syndrome. *Eur J Cardiac Pacing Electrophysiol* 1993;1:63–66.

10. Voci P, Tritapepe L, Critelli G. Iatrogenic pneumohemomediastinum mimicking cardiac tamponade: a complication of catheter ablation procedure. *PACE* 1997;20:138–139.

11. Seifert MJ, Morady F, Calkins H, et al. Aortic leaflet perforation during radiofrequency ablation. *PACE* 1991;14:1582–1585.

12. Scheinman MM. NASPE survey on catheter ablation. *PACE* 1995;18:1474–1478.

13. Conti JB, Geiser E, Curtis AB, et al. Catheter entrapment in the mitral valve apparatus during radiofrequency ablation. *PACE* 1994;17:1681–1685.

14. Mandawat MK, Turitto G, El-Sherif N. Catheter entrapment in the mitral valve apparatus requiring surgical removal: an unusual complication of radiofrequency ablation. *PACE* 1998;21:772–773.

15. Hindricks G. The Multicentre European Radiofrequency Survey (MERFS): complications of radiofrequency catheter ablation of arrhythmias. *Eur Heart J* 1993;14:1644–1653.

16. Calkins H, Yong P, Miller JM, et al. Catheter ablation of accessory pathways, atrioventricular nodal reentrant tachycardia, and the atrioventricular junction: final results of a prospective multicenter clinical trial. *Circulation* 1999;99(2):262–270.

17. Kuck KH, Schlüter M, Gürsoy S, et al. Preservation of atrioventricular nodal conduction during radiofrequency current catheter ablation of midseptal accessory pathways. *Circulation* 1992;86:1743–1752.

18. Schlüter M, Kuck KH. Catheter ablation from the right atrium of anteroseptal accessory pathways using radiofrequency current. *J Am Coll Cardiol* 1992;19:663–670.

19. Friedman PL, Stevenson WG, Kocovic DZ. Autonomic dysfunction after catheter ablation. *J Cardiovasc Electrophysiol* 1996;7:450–459.

20. Pappone C, Stabile G, Oreto G, et al. Inappropriate sinus tachycardia after radiofrequency ablation of para-Hisian accessory pathways. *J Cardiovasc Electrophysiol* 1997;8:1357–1365.

21. Jackman WM, Beckman KJ, McCleland J, et al. Treatment of supraventricular tachycardia due to atrioventricular nodal reentry by radiofrequency catheter ablation of a slow pathway conduction. *N Engl J Med* 1992;327:313.

22. Haïssageurre M, Gaita F, Fischer B, et al. Elimination of atrioventricular nodal reentrant tachycardia using discrete slow potentials to guide application of radiofrequency energy. *Circulation* 1992;85:2162.

23. Langberg JJ, Leon A, Borganelli M, et al. A randomized, prospective comparison of anterior and posterior approaches to radiofrequency catheter ablation of atrioventricular nodal reentry tachycardia. *Circulation* 1993;87: 1551–1556.

24. Mitrani RD, Klein LS, Hackett FK, et al. Radiofrequency ablation for atrioventricular node reentrant tachycardia: comparison between fast (anterior) and slow (posterior) pathway ablation. *J Am Coll Cardiol* 1993;21:432.

25. Hindricks G. Incidence of complete atrioventricular block following attempted radiofrequency catheter modification of the atrioventricular node in 880 patients: results of the Multicenter European Radiofrequency Survey (MERFS), the Working Group on Arrhythmias of the European Society of Cardiology. *Eur Heart J* 1996;17:82–88.

26. Langberg JJ, Kim Y-N, Goyal R, et al. Conversion of typical to "atypical" atrioventricular nodal reentrant tachycardia after radiofrequency catheter modification of the AV junction. *Am J Cardiol* 1992;69:503–508.

27. Verdino RJ, Burke MC, Kall JG, et al. Retrograde fast pathway ablation for atrioventricular nodal reentry associated with markedly prolonged PR intervals. *Am J Cardiol* 1999;83:455–458.

28. Chen S-A, Chiang C-E, Yang C-J, et al. Sustained atrial tachycardia in adults: electrophysiological characteristics, pharmacological response, possible mechanisms, and effects of radiofrequency ablation. *Circulation* 1994;90:1262–1278.

29. Tracy CM, Swartz JF, Fletcher RD, et al. Radiofrequency catheter ablation of ectopic atrial tachycardia using paced activation sequence mapping. *J Am Coll Cardiol* 1993;21:910–917.

30. Nakagawa H, Lazzara R, Khastgir T, et al. Role of the tricuspid annulus and the eustachian valve/ridge on atrial flutter: relevance to catheter ablation of the septal isthmus and a new technique for rapid identification of ablation success. *Circulation* 1996;94:407–424.

31. Fisher B, Jaïs P, Shah D, et al. Radiofrequency catheter ablation of common atrial flutter in 200 patients. *J Cardiovasc Electrophysiol* 1996;7: 1225–1233, 1996

32. Olgin J, Scheinman M. Comparison of high energy direct current and ra-

diofrequency catheter ablation of the atrioventricular junction. *J Am Coll Cardiol* 1993;21:557–564.

33. Morady F, Calkins H, Langberg J, et al. A prospective randomized comparison of direct current and radiofrequency ablation of the atrioventriuclar junction. *J Am Coll Cardiol* 1993;21:102–109.

34. Geelen P, Brugada J, Andries E, et al. Ventricular fibrillation and sudden death after radiofrequency catheter ablation of the atrioventricular junction. *PACE* 1997;20:343–348.

35. Darpo B, Walfridsson H, Aunes M, et al. Incidence of sudden death after radiofrequency ablation of the atrioventricular junction for atrial fibrillation. *Am J Cardiol* 1997;80:1174–1177.

36. Ozin B, Mackall J, Van Hare M, et al. A case control study of mortality after radiofrequency ablation of the AV junction. *J Am Coll Cardiol* 1997;29:199A.

37. Satoh T, Zipes DP. Rapid rates during bradycardia prolong ventricular refractoriness and facilitate tachycardia induction with cesium in dogs. *Circulation* 1996;94:217–227.

38. Newby KH, Zimerman L, Wharton JM, et al. Radiofrequency ablation of atrial flutter and atrial tachycardia in patients with permanent indwelling catheters. *PACE* 1996;19:1612–1617.

38a. Wolfe DA, McCutcheon J, Plumb VJ, et al. Radiofrequency current may induce exit block in chronically implanted ventricular pacing leads [abstract]. *PACE* 1995;18:919.

39. Krikorian JG, Hancock EW. Pericardiocentesis. *Am J Cardiol* 1978;65:808.

40. Callahan JA, Seward JB, Nishimura RA, et al. Two-dimensional echocardiographically guided pericardiocentesis: experience in 117 consecutive patients. *Am J Cardiol* 1985;55:476.

41. Pires LA, Huang SK, Wagshal AB, et al. Clinical utility of routine transthoracic echocardiographic studies after uncomplicated radiofrequency catheter ablation: a prospective multicenter study. *PACE* 1996;19:1502–1507.

42. Thakur RK, Klein GJ, Yee R, et al. Embolic complications after radiofrequency catheter ablation. *Am J Cardiol* 1994;74:278–279.

43. Epstein MR, Knapp LD, Martindill M, et al. Embolic complications associated with radiofrequency catheter ablation. *Am J Cardiol* 1996;77:655–658.

44. Scheinman M. Patterns of catheter ablation practice in the United States: results of the 1992 NASPE survey (editorial). *PACE* 1994;47:873–875.

45. Kugler JD, Danford DA, Houston K, et al. Radiofrequency catheter ablation for paroxysmal supraventricular tachycardia in children and adolescents without structural heart disease. *Am J Cardiol* 1997;80:1438–1443.

Chapter 35

Cooled Radiofrequency Ablation

J. Marcus Wharton, M.D., Carlton Nibley, M.D.,
Larry Nair, M.D.

Introduction

Conventional radiofrequency (RF) ablation has achieved remarkable success for ablation of most supraventricular and some ventricular tachycardias. Given these successes, RF ablation is increasingly being used to treat more difficult arrhythmias, particularly ventricular tachycardias associated with structural heart disease and atrial fibrillation. Although initial results have been promising, overall success rates may be further improved if the lesion size created by RF ablation can be increased. In particular, there is a need to create deeper lesions given the occurrence of critical areas for ventricular tachycardia in mid-myocardial or epicardial ventricular sites and given the need for continuously linear and transmural lesions across trabeculated or thickened atrial myocardium for catheter-based Maze procedures for treatment of atrial fibrillation. Originally described by Wittkampf et al in 1988,[1] an RF ablation approach has evolved which uses saline perfusion or irrigation of the ablation electrode tip during RF current delivery to cool the catheter tip and thereby decrease the probability of impedance rises, allow longer RF current applications, and increase lesion size. This approach is called cooled, chilled, or saline-irrigated RF ablation.

Mechanism of Cooled RF Ablation

With conventional RF ablation, passage of RF current through the tip of the catheter results in a relatively thin shell of resistive heating due to the abrupt change in impedance between the low impedance metallic electrode and

From Huang SKS, Wilber DJ (eds.): *Radiofrequency Catheter Ablation of Cardiac Arrhythmias: Basic Concepts and Clinical Applications,* 2nd ed. Armonk, NY: Futura Publishing Company, Inc. ©2000.

the higher impedance tissues. The relatively thin volume of myocardium surrounding the electrode interface that undergoes resistive heating serves as a radiant heat source for ablation of myocardium several millimeters away from the electrode tip.[2,3] This shell of resistive heating is thought to be thin and to have a diameter only somewhat greater than the diameter of the electrode tip. Maximum tissue temperature is generated at the electrode-myocardial interface and temperature decreases hyperbolically with distance from the electrode tip.[2] Since tissue necrosis occurs with temperatures exceeding approximately 50°C, lesion size will be proportional to the size of the electrode-myocardial interface and the maximum interface temperature. Increasing RF current delivery will increase the amount of resistive heating and the temperature at the electrode-myocardial interface to increase lesion size. However, the maximum lesion size that can be created by increasing RF current is limited by the fact that the maximum temperature that can be achieved at the interface is 100°C, since tissue desiccation, steam, and coagulum formation occur at this temperature. Attempts to increase RF current delivery further will be truncated by the development of abrupt impedance rises that occur when steam and coagulum form around the electrode tip. These impedance rises limit the duration of RF current delivery, thus limiting the total amount of energy delivered and the size of the lesion generated. Electrode tip thermistors or thermocouples have been used to monitor tip temperature and via a servo-system regulated current delivery to prevent temperatures from exceeding a prescribed maximum less than 100°C.[4,5] This allows RF ablation for the desired duration without truncating the duration of RF application because of an impedance rise. Although temperature-controlled RF delivery maximizes lesion size with conventional RF ablation, this occurs at the expense of limiting delivered current or power to maintain tip temperature less than the prescribed value.

With cooled RF ablation, the electrode tip is cooled by saline perfusion within the catheter tip or saline irrigation of the outside of the ablation electrode (Figure 1). These approaches allow cooler saline to internally or externally bathe the ablation electrode to dissipate heat generated during RF ablation. This decreases the electrode-myocardial interface temperature and allows for a larger amount of RF current to be passed before heating of tissue results in the development of impedance rises and "pops." Thus, compared to conventional RF ablation, cooled ablation allows passage of both higher powers and longer durations of RF current with less likelihood of impedance rises.[1,6–11]

As RF current is passed between the electrode and the dispersive element during cooled ablation, resistive heating still occurs at the electrode-myocardial interface. However, unlike standard RF ablation, the area of maximum temperature with cooled ablation is within the myocardium rather than at the electrode-myocardial interface.[10,12] Modeling studies have suggested that the maximum temperature generated by cooled RF ablation will be several millimeters away from the electrode-myocardial interface due to the active electrode or interface cooling. In the study by Jain et al,[12] temperatures greater than 95°C extended from the electrode surface to 1.8 millimeters within the myocardium for conventional RF ablation compared to 1.8–3.8 millimeters within the myocardium for cooled ablation modeled using a catheter cooled by internal perfusion of saline (Figure 2). The temper-

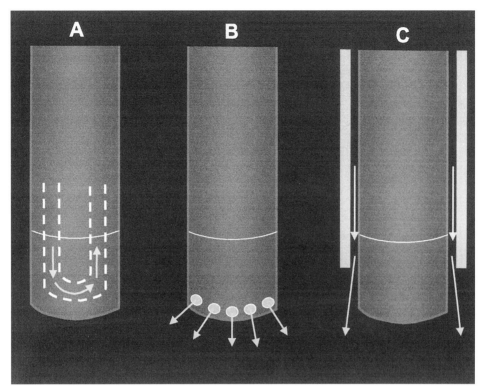

Figure 1. Panels A, B, and C show schematic designs of the 3 major means of cooling an ablation catheter with saline during RF ablation. The 3 methods include (A) internal perfusion of the catheter tip with saline with elimination of saline outside of the body; (B) direct irrigation of the catheter-myocardium interface by forcing saline out small holes in the catheter tip; and (C) direct irrigation of saline through a long sheath slightly larger than the external diameter of the catheter and place up to the myocardial interface.

ature at the electrode-myocardial interface during cooled ablation in this model was 37°C. Thus, tissue temperature generated during cooled RF ablation increased from the electrode tip to a maximum temperature a couple of millimeters within the myocardium, and then gradually decreased beyond 3–4 millimeters from the catheter tip. Estimated power to achieve maximum temperatures at the electrode surface and within the myocardium were 32 watts for conventional and 55 watts for cooled RF ablation, respectively, in this modeling study.[12] Given the greater power that is delivered, the current density and the width of the shell of resistive heating are increased around the electrode-myocardial interface, resulting in a larger effective radiant surface diameter and thus larger lesion depth, width and volume.

Results of modeling studies of cooled ablation have been directly confirmed in the animal model. Nakagawa et al.[10] evaluated cooled ablation in the canine thigh muscle preparation using a saline irrigated catheter. Using thermal probes inserted at the electrode surface and at depths of 3.5 and 7.0 millime-

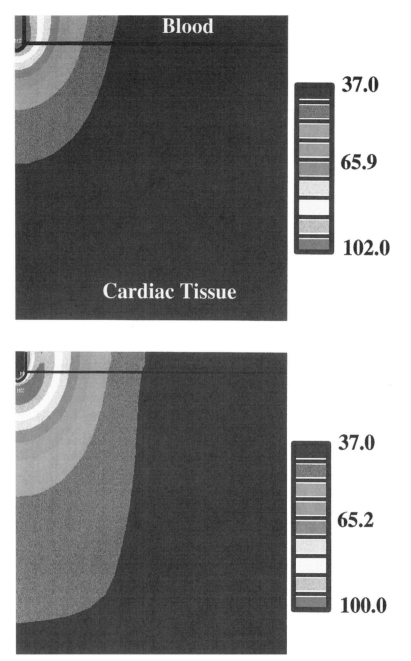

Figure 2. Effect of cooled RF ablation (B) compared to conventional ablation (A) as determined with finite element analysis. Conventional RF ablation (A) has the hottest temperature generated at the electrode-myocardial interface and up to 1.8 millimeters away from the catheter surface. However, during internally cooled ablation (B), the electrode-myocardial interface temperature is lowered, allowing passage of greater RF current, and generation of maximum temperatures 1.8–3.8 millimeters from the catheter surface. See text for further discussion. (Reproduced with permission from Jain MK, Wolf PD, Henriquez C.[5]) See color plate.

ters within the muscle, they demonstrated that the maximum tissue temperature during cooled ablation occurred on the thermal probe that was 3.5 millimeters from the tip of the electrode. This was compared to conventional fixed voltage (66 volts) and temperature-controlled (85°C) RF during which maximum temperatures occurred at the electrode interface and decreased with further distance from the electrode tip. Thus, active cooling during RF ablation generated lesions with greater depth, width, and thus volume than either fixed voltage or temperature controlled RF ablation (Figure 3). Of note, the width of the ablation lesion at the myocardial surface had less diameter than at intramyocardial sites, reflecting that cooling decreases lesion expansion along the myocardial surface.

As with conventional RF ablation, cooled ablation is still limited by the maximum temperature that can be generated within the myocardium and the probability of reaching this maximum temperature will increase with increasing RF power or current. As RF current is increased with cooled RF ablation, heating of intramyocardial tissues to 100°C results potentially in intramyocardial steam formation.[11,13] These pockets of rapidly developing steam can results in abrupt increases in impedance to current flow to limit RF duration. Perhaps more importantly with cooled RF ablation, maximum temperature may now be intramyocardial and surrounded by cooler areas of tissue.[10,12] The development of

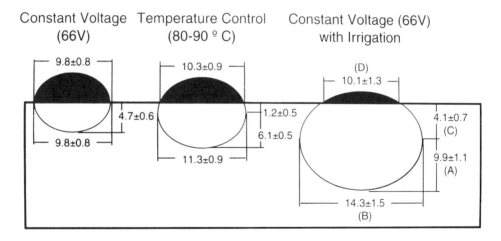

Lesion Volume:
135±33 mm³   275±55 mm³   700 ± 217 mm³

Figure 3. Diagram of average lesion dimensions generated by constant voltage (66 volts) and temperature-controlled (80°C to 90°C) conventional RF ablation versus constant voltage (66 Volts) irrigated tip ablation in the canine thigh muscle preparation. As can be easily seen, lesion size is significantly larger with saline irrigation of the catheter tip during RF ablation, with both greater depth and width of the lesion created. Also note that the maximum width of irrigated tip ablation is not at the surface, as with conventional RF approaches, but several millimeters removed from the surface. The lesser lesion diameter at the surface is presumptively due to direct convective cooling from the saline irrigation from the catheter tip and from cooling from blood flow across the surface. (Reproduced with permission from Nakagawa H, et al.[10]).

intramyocardial steam may result in explosions, typically toward the endocardium, with resultant formation of deep craters, with their potential for dissection, perforation, and thrombus formation.[11,13] Thus, lesion size can be increased with cooled ablation, but the potential for dangerous lesion formation may also be increased. Studies in animal models suggest that powers less than or equal to 50 watts are optimal in terms of avoiding large craters using an internally cooled catheter[13] and less than or equal to 20 watts using an irrigated catheter.[11] Further studies are needed to expand these observations over a range of catheter types and clinical conditions in order to better understand how to limit power of cooled RF ablation in humans to prevent crater formation.

Monitoring tip temperature may not be as helpful in preventing this complication during cooled RF ablation. With conventional RF ablation, maximum tissue temperature occurs at the catheter-myocardial interface and thus a tip-mounted thermistor or thermocouple is a good approximation of this temperature if the catheter tip is directed against the myocardium. Limiting tip temperature to less than 100°C prevents almost all impedance rises with conventional RF ablation.[4,5] However, since maximum tissue temperature is several millimeters from the catheter tip during cooled ablation, the maximum tissue temperature may not be accurately predicted by tip thermometry. If cooling is sufficient, the registered tip temperature will always be less than the maximum, although related to maximum temperature in a complex fashion that is dependent, at least in part, on the rate of convective cooling relative to the rate of resistive and radiant heating at the interface. Thus, the tip temperature predictive of impedance rises due to overheating intramyocardial tissue will be considerably less than 100°C. Studies using internally perfused catheter systems have suggested some utility to using monitored tip temperature for predicting impedance rises, with temperatures of 45°C to 65°C, depending on the clinical model.[14,15] However, optimal parameters and overall utility for tip thermometry have not been well established. In addition, irrigated cooled ablation may be associated with even greater variance in tip temperature, making tip thermometry of little utility with this catheter design.[11]

Technique

Cooling the catheter tip during RF ablation is achieved by circulating saline through or around the tip of the ablation catheter while RF current is being delivered. Saline may be transported to the ablation electrode either within the catheter (see Figure 1, panels A and B) or via a long sheath placed over the catheter (Figure 1, panel C). Catheters transporting saline within the catheter shaft obviously have greater utility for ablation of a larger variety of sites than those relying on sheaths. Two catheter designs for cooled ablation have been designed. With an internally cooled (or closed) system, saline is perfused through the tip of the catheter via a conduit in the catheter shaft (see Figure 1A). After circulating through and cooling the tip of the catheter, the saline is returned back outside the body via a second conduit in the catheter. Thus, no saline is infused into the body and the system is a "closed" loop.[9] The second approach is an externally irrigated (or open) system. With this approach saline is taken to the tip of the catheter via a conduit in the catheter shaft and then extruded through multiple pores at the tip of the catheter. Thus, saline cools the catheter tip both by perfusion through it and by irrigation of the myocardial-electrode tip interface. Since saline is directly infused into the body, the system is an "open" loop.[8,10,11] Another means of irrigating the catheter tip is to infuse saline through a long sheath advanced almost to the tip of the catheter placed within the sheath.[16] A screw-tip needle electrode which allows intramural infusion of saline during RF ablation has also been reported.[17]

Both internally perfused and externally irrigated catheter systems have been shown to increase the size of a lesion compared to conventional RF ablation in investigation models.[1,6–11] Demazunder et al[16] showed in a preliminary study that the openly irrigated cooled ablation system made larger lesions than the closed, internally perfused system. This is probably due to the greater cooling of the electrode-myocardial interface afforded by external irrigation of the catheter tip. However, this finding needs to be confirmed and the safety of the two techniques needs to be compared. It is possible that although the greater cooling may allow for larger lesion formation, the risk of crater formation and complex lesion formation may also be increased (Figure 4).

Larger electrode diameter or length during cooled ablation may generate larger lesions, similar to traditional RF ablation. However, Otomo et al[18] demonstrated that larger electrode length allows passage of increased current to generate larger lesions by increasing the amount of electrode-blood interface to increase convective cooling of the electrode by the blood pool, even without active cooling by saline perfusion or irrigation. Use of saline irrigation may even allow larger lesions to be made with smaller electrodes.[19]

Other factors may also affect the size of a lesion generated with cooled ablation. Saline flow rates can be varied relatively easily within the pressure constraints of the infusion channel of the catheter. Saline flow rate allows modulation of the degree of cooling of the catheter tip, with higher flow rates causing greater cooling to potentially generate larger lesions but with a greater risk of cratering. Lower flow rates will result in lesions sizes approaching conventional RF ablation but will perhaps be associated with greater safety. However, no data is presently available regarding the optimum flow settings for either open or closed cooled RF ablation. Although chilled (rather than room temperature) saline could be infused to further decrease the tip temperature and allow higher RF currents to be used, heating rapidly occurs as the saline passes through the catheter, making this modification of little practical benefit.

For openly irrigated cooled ablation approaches, use of hypertonic saline may also increase lesion size. Hypertonic saline (14.6% NaCl) has 10 times the conductivity of blood, compared to 3 times for normal saline (0.9% NaCl).[20] Therefore, hypertonic saline flowing around the electrode-tissue interface may lower impedance to current flow to allow use of higher currents for generation of larger lesions.[20,21] Application of hypertonic saline for use with electrophysiological cooled ablation catheters has not be performed, and the technique is limited by potential for causing volume overload with intravascular infusion of hypertonic saline.

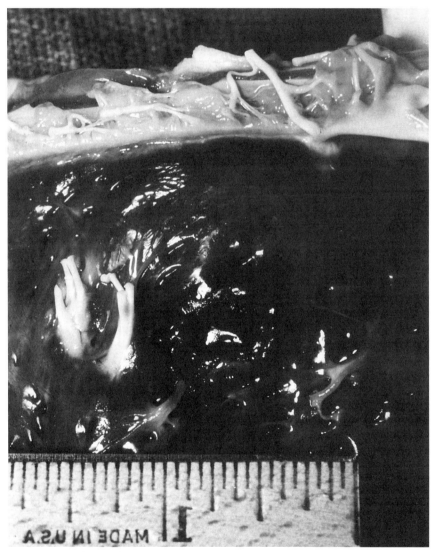

Figure 4. A. Deep ulcerated crater created by an RF application of 70 watts associated with an impedance rise. There is thrombus located in the center of the crater. (*continued*)

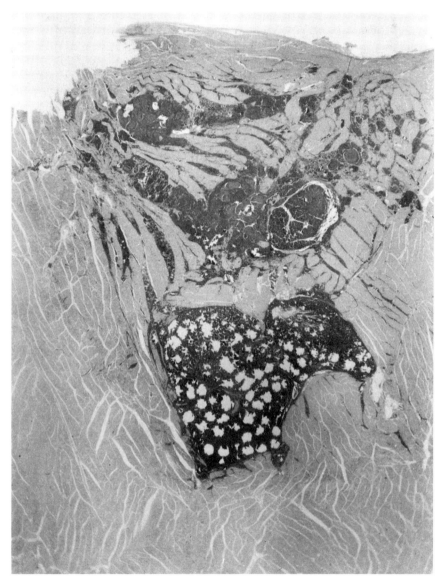

Figure 4. (*continued*) B. Histological section through a nonulcerated lesion demonstrating a hemorrhagic pocket within the mid-myocardium, with mid-myocardial disruption without perforation of the endocardium. The pocket was presumptively formed by intramyocardial steam formation during cooled RF ablation separating the mid-myocardial layers with secondary hemorrhage into the pocket.

Animal Studies

All studies to date comparing cooled to conventional RF ablation have shown that cooled ablation can create larger lesions at some, but not all, power settings. Using a closed catheter system, Sykes et al[6] showed in explanted bovine hearts in a 37°C circulating bath of bovine blood that lesion size increased with increasing power up to a plateau at 15–20 watts delivered power with conventional RF ablation compared with a plateau at 30–35 watts with cooled RF ablation. Thus, cooled RF ablation resulted in larger lesions than conventional RF since higher powers could be used (maximum mean volume was 276 mm^3 at 20 watts conventional versus 481 mm^3 at 30 watts cooled). The plateau curves comparing lesion size generation with increasing powers were due to the fact that impedance rises started occurring with increasing frequency beginning at 15 watts for conventional and 25 watts for cooled ablation, increasingly truncating the duration of RF current delivery from the scheduled 60 seconds. Total energy delivery plateaued at 10–20 watts with conventional

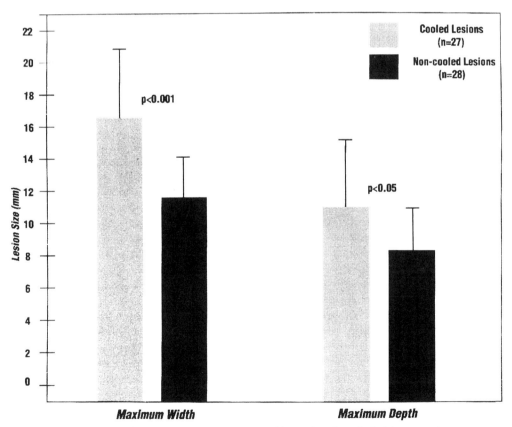

Figure 5. Lesion width and depth using an internally perfused cooled ablation catheter at 30 watts versus conventional temperature-limited ablation (just below 100°C) in the ovine model. As with the irrigated tip catheter design, the internally perfused design results in greater lesion width and depth. (Reproduced with permission from Ruffy R, et al.[9])

RF ablation and then dramatically decreased beyond 20 watts. However, with cooled RF ablation, total energy delivery was only beginning to plateau at the maximum power studied of 35 watts. Ruffy et al[9] demonstrated that lesion depth and width were greater in the ovine model with cooled RF ablation at 30 watts using an internally perfused catheter compared to temperature-controlled standard RF ablation (Figure 5). Nibley et al[7] demonstrated that, compared to conventional RF ablation, lesion size was similar at 20 watts and greater from 30–50 watts with cooled RF ablation. In all of these studies, the benefit of cooling during RF in these conventional power ranges appears to be due to the prevention of impedance rises and longer durations of RF current delivery. At higher powers (greater than 50 watts), although lesion size continues to increase, there is also an increased risk of complex lesion formation with cratering and tissue dissection, suggesting that the optimal power setting in terms of lesion size and safety was 50 watts.[13]

It has been shown that temperature-controlled conventional RF ablation results in larger lesions than fixed-power conventional RF. Thus, it is possible that temperature-controlled conventional RF may generate similar lesion sizes to those seen in cooled RF ablation, since they both optimize the duration of RF current delivery. Nakagawa et al[10] in a canine thigh muscle preparation compared fixed voltage (66 volts), temperature-controlled conventional (80°C to 90°C), and cooled ablation using 66 volts cooled with an open system perfused at 20 cubic centimeters per minute. (Mean lesion dimensions are shown in Figure 3.) As in previous studies, temperature-controlled conventional RF was superior to fixed voltage RF. However, cooled RF was superior in terms of lesion sizes to temperature controlled RF with the irrigated-tip catheter,[10] as was shown for the internally perfused catheter as well.[9]

Human Studies

Limited data exists for the use of cooled ablation in humans. Preliminary studies have shown that the cooled ablation system is effective for ablation of ventricular tachycardia in the setting of heart disease. In the preliminary study comparing cooled tip ablation to medical therapy for treatment of ventricular tachycardia in patients with heart disease, the acute efficacy for ablation of all mappable ventricular tachycardias was 73% with recurrences during long term follow-up in 40%.[22] There was no comparison to conventional RF ablation in this study. Given the high efficacy (ranging from 70–80%) with conventional RF ablation of patients with ischemic disease,[23,24] it is not clear from the available data how much improvement in efficacy, if any, is provided by cooled ablation of ventricular tachycardia. Further studies will be needed to address this issue.

It is not clear what role cooled ablation will have in the treatment of most supraventricular tachycardias. Given the very high efficacy with present technologies for ablation of most of these rhythms, the role of cooled ablation will be limited. However, cooled ablation will potentially have a role in the ablation of supraventricular tachyarrhythmias arising from epicardial or deep posteroseptal accessory pathways or atrial tachycardias arising within thick muscle bundles such as the crista terminalis. In addition, cooled ablation may be useful in the ablation of some isthmus-dependent and independent atrial flutters associated with regions of thickened myocardium (such as a thick eustachian ridge) or surgical scar. Jaïs et al[25] noted that bidirectional isthmus block could not be achieved in 13 (7.6%) of 170 patients who underwent ablation of typical atrial flutter, presumptively due to the inability to transmurally ablate thickened portions of the right atrial isthmus. Using an irrigated tip catheter, bidirectional isthmus block could be achieved in 12 (92%) of these 13 patients, half with a single application of cooled RF, without significant complications. Compared to the mean of 14 ± 6 watts applied with conventional RF ablation, the average power for irrigated tip was 40 ± 6 watts.[25] This is the first human data supporting the clinical application of cooled RF ablation under situations in which conventional RF ablation has failed. Lavergne et al[26] showed that serial linear 50 watts cooled RF applications using an irrigated 4 millimeters tip electrode was relatively safe for making linear lesions, although continuous and transmural lesions could not be made during a single linear series of applications in the right and left atrium. Last, cooled ablation potentially has a major role for the treatment of atrial fibrillation given the potential utility of novel catheter designs utilizing cooled ablation concepts to make linear lesions. Wharton et al[27] demonstrated that a catheter with serial electrode elements surrounded by a saline-filled angioplasty balloon with pores to allow passage of RF current in a uniform fashion and simultaneous extrusion of saline allowed creation of very uniform, non-ulcerated, transmural and continuous linear lesions in the animal model. Similarly, linear electrode element catheters with saline extrusion ports between each metallic electrode to create continuous, nonulcerated lesions may also be useful. Although further development is needed for the improvement of these catheter designs for clinical use, the promise is great that these or similar designs will provide appropriate tools to allow creation of the long, continuous linear lesion needed for atrial fibrillation ablation in an effective, safe, and efficient manner.

References

1. Wittkampf FW, Hauer RN, Robles de Medina EO. Radiofrequency ablation with cooled porous electrode [abstract]. J Am Coll Cardiol 1988;11:17A.
2. Haines DE, Watson DD. Tissue heating during radiofrequency catheter ablation: a thermodynamic model and observations in isolated perfused and superfused canine right ventricular free wall. *PACE* 1989;12:962–976.
3. Haines DE, Watson DD, Verow AF. Electrode radius predicts lesion radius during radiofrequency energy heating: validation of a proposed thermodynamic model. *Circ Res* 1990;67:124–129.
4. Langberg JJ, Calkins H, El-Atassi R, et al. Temperature monitoring during radiofrequency catheter ablation of accessory pathways. *Circulation* 1992; 86:1469–1474.
5. Calkins J, Prystowski E, Carlson M, et al, and the Atakr Multicenter Investigators Group. Temperature monitoring during radiofrequency cathe-

ter ablation procedures using closed loop control. *Circulation* 1994;90: 1279–1286.

6. Sykes C, Riley R, Pomeranz M, et al. Cooled tip ablation results in increased radiofrequency power delivery and lesion size. *PACE* 1994;88:782.

7. Nibley C, Sykes CM, McLaughlin G, et al. Myocardial lesion size during radiofrequency current catheter ablation is increased by intra-electrode tip chilling. *Circulation* 1994;90(Suppl 1):I-485.

8. Mittleman RS, Huang SKS, De Guzman WT, et al. Use of the saline infusion electrode catheter for improved energy delivery and increased lesion size in radiofrequency catheter ablation. *PACE* 1995;18(Part I):1022–1027.

9. Ruffy R, Imran MA, Santel DJ, et al. Radiofrequency delivery through a cooled catheter tip allows the creation of larger endomyocardial lesions in the ovine heart. *J Cardiovasc Electrophysiol* 1995;6:1089–1096.

10. Nakagawa H, Yamanashi WS, Pitha JV, et al. Comparison of in vivo tissue temperature profile and lesion geometry for radiofrequency ablation with a saline-irrigated electrode versus temperature control in a canine thigh muscle preparation. *Circulation* 1995;91:2264–2273.

11. Skrumeda LL, Mehra R. Comparison of standard and irrigated radiofrequency ablation in the canine ventricle. *J Cardiovasc Electrophysiol* 1998; 9:1196–1205.

12. Jain MK, Wolf PD, Henriquez C. Chilled-tip electrode radio frequency ablation of the endocardium: A finite element study. Proceedings of the 17th Annual Conference of the IEEE Engineering in Medicine and Biology Society. Montreal, Cannada, September 1995.

13. Wharton JM, Nibley C, Sykes CM, et al. Establishment of a dose-response relationship for high-power chilled-tip radiofrequency current ablation in sheep [abstract]. *J Am Coll Cardiol* 1995;25:239A.

14. Nibley C, Sykes CM, Rowan R, et al. Predictors of abrupt impedance rise during chilled-tip radiofrequency catheter ablation [abstract]. *J Am Coll Cardiol* 1995;25;293A.

15. Wharton JM, Wilber DJ, Calkins J, et al. Utility of tip thermometry during radiofrequency ablation in humans using an internally perfused saline cooled catheter [abstract]. *Circulation* 1997;96(Suppl 1);I–318.

16. Demazunder D, Kallash HL, Schwartzman D. Comparison of different electrodes for radiofrequency ablation of myocardium using saline irrigation [abstract]. *PACE* 1997;20:1076.

17. Hoey MF, Mulier PM. Fluoroscopic visualization of ventricular ablation after radiofrequency energy application with the saline electrode. *Circulation* 1997;96(Supp 1):I–319.

18. Otomo K, Yamanashi WS, Tondo C, et al. Why a large tip electrode makes a deeper radiofrequency lesion: effects of increase in electrode cooling and electrode-tissue interface area. *J Cardiovasc Electrophysiol* 1998;9: 47–54.

19. Nakagawa H, Yamanashi W, Wittkampf F, et al. Comparison of tissue temperature and lesion size in radiofrequency ablation using saline irrigation with a small versus large tip electrode in a canine thigh muscle preparation. *Circulation* 1994;90(Suppl 1);I–271.

20. Leveillee RJ, Hoey MF, Hulbert JC, et al. Enhanced radiofrequency abla-

tion of canine prostate utilizing a liquid conductor: the virtual electrode. *J Endourol* 1996;10:5–11.

21. Neya K, Lee R, Guerrero JL, et al. Experimental ablation of outflow tract muscle with a thermal balloon catheter. *Circulation* 1995;91:2445–2453.

22. Epstein AE, Wilber DJ, Calkins H, et al, Cooled Ablation of VT Investigators. Randomized controlled trial of ventricular tachycardia treatment by cooled tip catheter ablation vs. drug therapy. *J Am Coll Cardiol* 1998;

23. Gonska B, Cao K, Schaumann A, et al. Catheter ablation of ventricular tachycardia in 136 patients with coronary artery disease: results and long-term follow-up. *J Am Coll Cardiol* 1994;24:1506–1514.

24. Stevenson WG, Khan H, Sager P, et al. Identification of reentry circuit sites during catheter mapping and radiofrequency ablation of ventricular tachycardia late after myocardial infarction. *Circulation* 1993;88:1647–1670.

25. Jaïs P, Haïssaguerre M, Shah DC, et al. Successful irrigated-tip ablation of atrial flutter resistant to conventional radiofrequency ablation. *Circulation* 1998;98:835–838.

26. Lavergne T, Jaïs P, Haïssaguerre M, et al. Evaluation of a single passage RF ablation line in animal atria using an irrigated tip electrode [abstract]. *Circulation* 1997;96(Suppl 1);I-259.

27. Wharton JM, Tomassoni G, Pomeranz M, et al. Saline-perfused, balloon radiofrequency ablation catheter for creation of linear transmural atrial lesions. *Circulation* 1995;94(Suppl):I-492.

Chapter 36

Electroanatomic Imaging as a Guide for Catheter Ablation

David J. Wilber, M.D., Philip A. Cooke, M.B.B.S., and John G. Kall, M.D.

Highly accurate and reproducible electroanatomic correlation has assumed increasing importance in the mapping and ablation of cardiac arrhythmias. The structural basis of several arrhythmias has been extensively documented. Specific macroscopic structures, including venous ostia,[1–3] muscular ridges such as the crista terminalis and eustachian ridge,[4,5] and valve annuli[6] appear to be preferential sites for focal atrial tachycardia. These "normal" structural features, as well as acquired structural abnormalities, may act as conduction barriers, facilitating the maintenance and determining the location of macroreentrant circuits such as typical atrial flutter[7,8] and incisional tachycardias.[9,10] While the precise structural underpinnings of atrioventricular (AV) nodal reentry remain controversial, critical regions for maintenance of this tachycardia appear localized to relatively discrete anatomic sites with specific spatial relationships to the compact AV node and the coronary sinus os.[11,12] Focal ventricular tachycardia also arises from characteristic anatomic sites.[13,14] Finally, the relationship of large reentrant circuits associated with prior myocardial infarction to the structural characteristics of the scar border,[15,16] and adjacent natural barriers such the mitral annulus,[17,18] has received increasing attention.

In consequence, catheter ablation has become increasingly an anatomically-based procedure. This anatomic orientation poses additional demands on mapping systems: 1) realistic and spatially accurate three-dimensional representation of the endocardial surface, permitting simple and reliable recognition of common macroscopic structures, 2) reproducible catheter positioning at specific sites, 3) rapid and continuously updated integration of spatial location with

From Huang SKS, Wilber DJ (eds.): *Radiofrequency Catheter Ablation of Cardiac Arrhythmias: Basic Concepts and Clinical Applications,* 2nd ed. Armonk, NY: Futura Publishing Company, Inc. ©2000.

functional data (electrogram timing and characteristics, response to pacing), and 4) an accurate spatial record of ablation sites. This latter feature is particularly important to guide placement of additional applications (particularly linear lesions connecting anatomic barriers) and to minimize unnecessary energy delivery.

Until recently, attempts to correlate electrophysiological data to anatomic features were predominantly made by documenting the position of the recording electrode in a small number of radiographic planes. The precision and reproducibility of visual estimates of fluoroscopic position remain limited. This qualitative technique is also poorly suited for tracking and display of large amounts of mapping data, and in localizing the position of the mapping electrode within a geometrically and spatially accurate representation of the endocardial surface. Recently, percutaneous devices have been introduced which permit simultaneous acquisition of data from a large number of endocardial sites, either by direct endocardial recording ("basket" catheters)[19,20] or by reconstruction of endocardial electrograms from intracavitary potentials ("noncontact" arrays).[21,22] These techniques permit improved estimates of the spatial relationships and timing between large numbers of recording sites; however precise correlation of this spatial data to a realistic representation of chamber geometry and specific anatomic structures remains problematic.

Overview of Electroanatomic Imaging

An imaging system based on magnetic catheter tracking has been developed recently which addresses several of the requirements for anatomically based mapping and ablation (Carto, Biosense-Webster, Baldwin Park, CA).[23] The method uses a miniature passive magnetic field sensor embedded in the tip of the mapping catheter. A locator pad, placed underneath the patient's thorax, consists of 3 equidistant coils that generate ultralow magnetic fields, which decay as a function of distance from each coil. The sensor measures the strength of each field, enabling determination of the distance from each coil, and thus the position of the catheter tip in three-dimensional space (Figure 1). The third component of the system is a processing unit which displays the catheter tip in real time, permitting nonfluoroscopic navigation. As the catheter is manipulated over the endocardial surface, data points are acquired either manually or by automated acceptance criteria; they are then assigned a color-coded activation time and a three-dimensional spatial location on the computer display. Both location and electrogram timing are gated to a user-defined fiducial point in the cardiac cycle. In addition, these data are recorded relative to a fixed reference catheter, compensating for changes in patient position.

As each point is added, a three-dimensional surface demonstrating the spread of activation is continuously updated. Activation of the surface between acquired points is interpolated within user-defined distances. Individual points can be reviewed and manually edited when appropriate at any time during the mapping procedure. The fidelity with which the reconstruction reflects actual endocardial geometry is to some extent determined by the density of points obtained and the degree of complexity of the surface being imaged. De-

Chapter 36

Color figures.

The illustrations appearing in this chapter have been grouped together for the convenience of the reader. Text resumes on page 781.

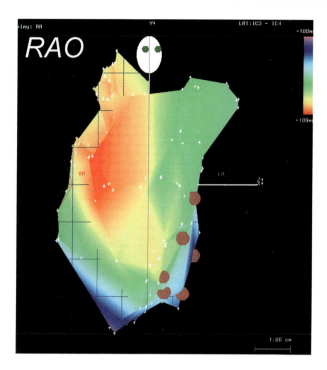

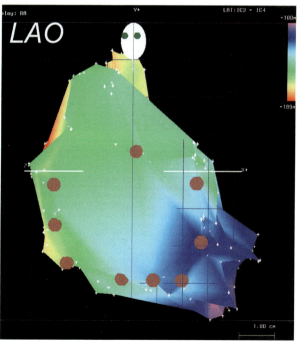

Figure 2. Endocardial reconstruction demonstrating right atrial activation during sinus rhythm. In this and subsequent figures, the earliest activation is in red, and latest activation in purple. In this and subsequent figures, the white disc represents the head of the patient, with "eyes" pointed toward the front (anterior chest wall). The brown tags represent the approximate position of the tricuspid annulus (see text for details).

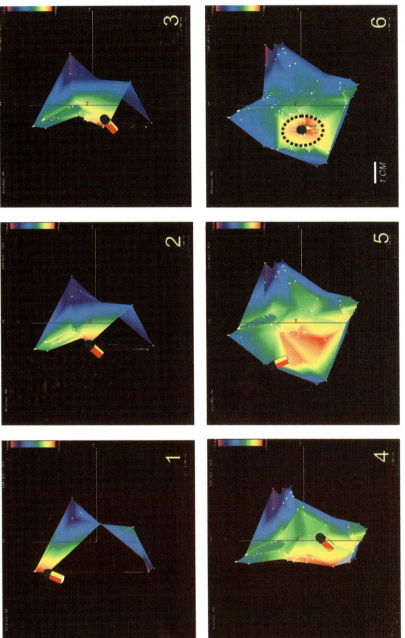

Figure 3. Sequential acquisition of points during mapping of a right atrial focal tachycardia, imaged in the right lateral projection. The icon in the center of the field represents the catheter. The distal tip is a solid green hemisphere. The orientation of the catheter tip in three-dimensional space is accurately represented as an additional guide to navigation. Following delineation of the boundary points of the chamber (panel 1), addition of subsequent points fills in the intervening endocardial surface. Note that subsequent data points are acquired with greatest density in the direction of earliest activation during each successive iteration of the map. While the general region of the site of origin is identified by panel 4, additional data points are required to identify the boundaries of the early activation zone (panel 5), and to completely characterize activation near the site of origin (panel 6). In the final panel, the dotted ellipse (12 × 18 millimeters) defines all points within 10 milliseconds of the site of earliest activation. The catheter tip was positioned in the center of this zone, and a single RF application at that site eliminated the tachycardia.

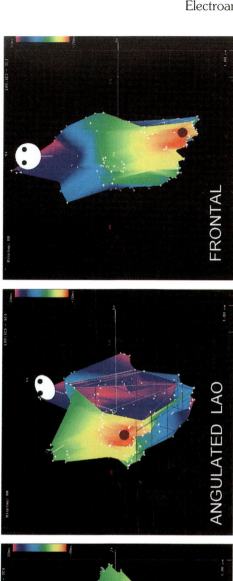

Figure 4. Focal atrial tachycardia arising adjacent to the inferolateral tricuspid annulus viewed in multiple projections. The red and orange colors represent the approximate size of the early activation zone, and the brown tag signifies the site of successful ablation at the center of this zone.

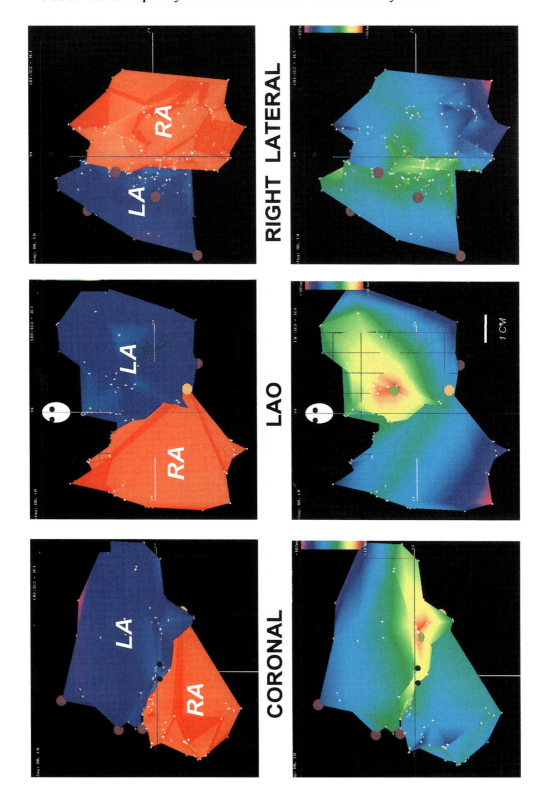

Figure 5. Focal atrial tachycardia arising from the anterior mitral valve annulus near the interatrial septum. Reconstructions of both right and left atria are demonstrated in multiple projections. The top series of panels depicts all points within each atrium as a single solid color, left atrium as blue and right atrium as red. The anterior location of the right atrium in the chest cavity is readily appreciated in the coronal and right lateral views. The bottom series of panels represents the color-coded activation sequence of the tachycardia through both chambers. Note the relatively rapid spread of activation posteriorly along the interatrial septum. If adequate mapping of the anterior left atrium had not been undertaken, the operator might be left with the impression of early activation along the posteriomedial right atrium or the right pulmonary veins. The orange tag represents the region adjacent to the His bundle. The brown tags are adjacent to the ostia of the pulmonary veins.

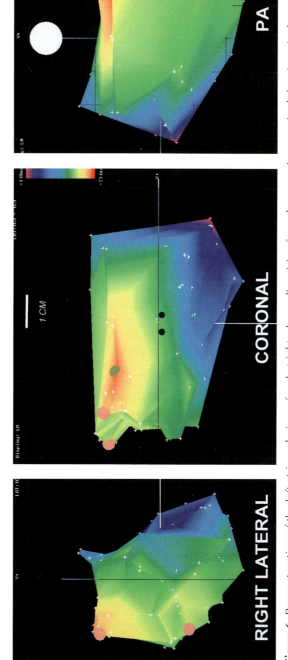

RIGHT LATERAL **CORONAL** **PA**

1 CM

Figure 6. Reconstruction of the left atrium during a focal atrial tachycardia arising from the posterior superior left atrium, in the region of Bachman's bundle. Note the markedly anisotropic conduction, with rapid spread medially and laterally along the bundle from the tachycardia focus. The site of successful ablation is denoted by the green tag. The ostia of the pulmonary veins are signified by the pink tags. The patient had previously undergone unsuccessful ablation of a presumed right superior pulmonary vein focus. Despite the marked anisotropy, note that the successful ablation site remains at the center of the early activation zone; discrimination of this site from the pulmonary vein orifice would have been difficult without high density simultaneous display of activation times and anatomic orientation.

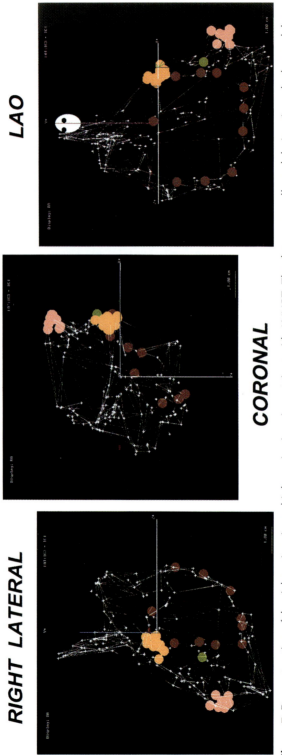

Figure 7. Reconstruction of the right atrium in multiple projections in a patient with AVNRT. The data were collected during sinus rhythm and the reconstruction is displayed as a geometric mesh without activation times. Relevant anatomy of Koch's triangle has been tagged including the tricuspid annulus (brown), coronary sinus os (pink) and region of recordable His potentials (orange). The green tag marks the successful ablation site. This example illustrates the typical "vertical" orientation of Koch's triangle in standard radiographic imaging planes, seen in more than 90% of patients (see text for details).

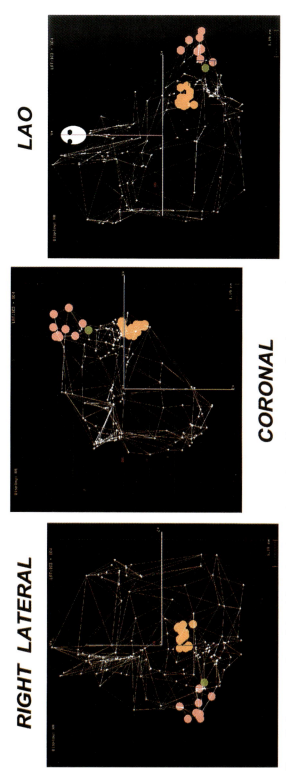

RIGHT LATERAL

CORONAL

LAO

Figure 8. Reconstruction of the right atrium in another patient with AVNRT, with a format similar to that shown in Figure 7. In contrast to the previous patient, note the marked change in orientation of Koch's triangle in the right lateral and LAO projections, with a nearly horizontal axis between the recordable His region and the coronary sinus os. However, the typical relationship between these structures is preserved in the coronal view. This uncommon orientation of Koch's triangle poses a particular challenge for ablation if inadvertent AV block is to be avoided. The successful ablation site is denoted by the green tag. In these patients energy is applied more posteriorly, and closely opposed to the coronary sinus os (compare the coronal views of both patients).

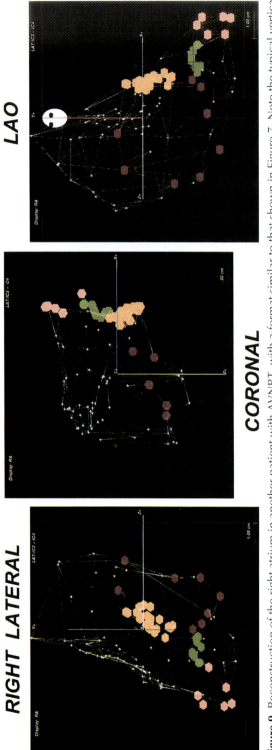

Figure 9. Reconstruction of the right atrium in another patient with AVNRT, with a format similar to that shown in Figure 7. Note the typical vertical axis of Koch's triangle. In this patient, initial applications close to the tricuspid annulus did r ot eliminate tachycardia. Sequential linear applications of RF energy were given during a pullback toward the superior aspect of the coronary sinus os (approximately 14 millimeters). Prolonged junctional rhythm was obtained during each of 7 RF energy applications. Repetitive slow pathway conduction was not eliminated until the final application at the coronary sinus ostium.

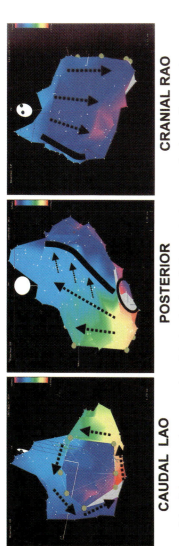

CAUDAL LAO **POSTERIOR** **CRANIAL RAO**

Figure 10. Reconstruction of the right atrium demonstrating global activation during typical counterclockwise flutter in three projections. The arrows indicate the general direction of activation. The heavy black line indicates the area where electrograms demonstrate double potentials in the approximate region of the crista terminalis. The green tags signify points adjacent to the tricuspid annulus. Activation spans the entire flutter cycle length, and the grey region is a software annotation that the earliest and latest activation during the mapped rhythm occur adjacent to one another (see text for details).

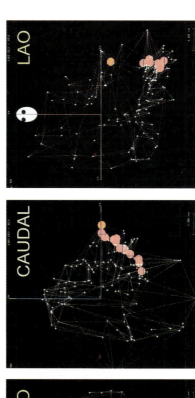

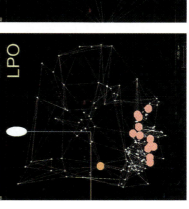

Figure 11. Reconstruction of the right atrium in another patient with typical atrial flutter in three views. The reconstruction is displayed as a geometric mesh to facilitate identification and tracking of the catheter tip and visualization of the ablation line. The pink tags indicate the sequential course of the catheter tip as RF energy is applied during a linear drag across the annular-eustachian ridge isthmus. The orange tag identifies the location of the His bundle. The caudal and LPO (or RAO) views are optimal projections for tracking the catheter tip along the subeustachian isthmus (see text for details).

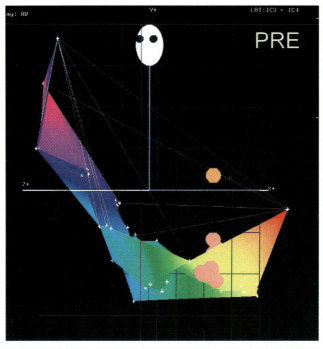

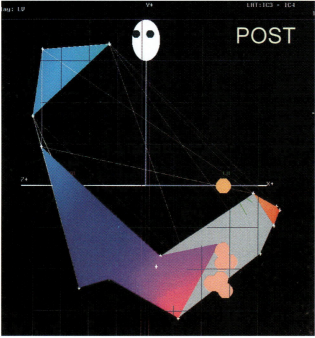

Figure 12. Reconstructions of a limited portion of the right atrium, including the annular-eustachian ridge isthmus, acquired during proximal coronary sinus pacing (cycle length 600 milliseconds) in the same patient as in Figure 6. Both reconstructions are viewed in the LAO projection. The left panel illustrates activation prior to ablation (PRE) and demonstrates rapid clockwise conduction through the isthmus. The right panel illustrates an activation following completion of the ablation line (POST) and demonstrates clockwise activation block, with the latest activation just lateral to the ablation line. The pink tags illustrate the sites of RF energy applications, and the orange tag, the location of the His bundle (see text for details).

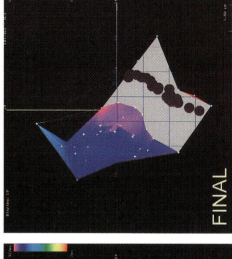
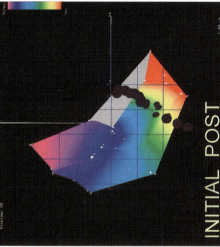
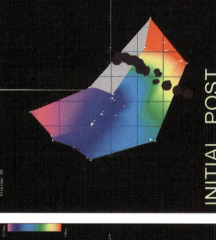

PREABLATION

INITIAL POST

FINAL

Figure 13. Reconstructions of the annular-eustachian isthmus viewed from below (caudal projection) acquired during proximal coronary sinus pacing (cycle length 600 milliseconds) in a different patient. Prior to ablation (far left panel), there is rapid clockwise activation through the isthmus. After placement of the initial ablation line (middle panel), a second acquisition demonstrates delayed activation of the lateral isthmus. However, there is an area of early breakthrough in the posterior portion of the isthmus. Following additional RF applications to the posterior 1 cm of the ablation line, a final acquisition (far right panel) confirms complete clockwise conduction block. The grey tags indicate the sites of ablation. A software feature permits superimposition of tags from previous or subsequent maps provided that the location reference is unchanged, facilitating comparisons of activation following interventions (see text for details).

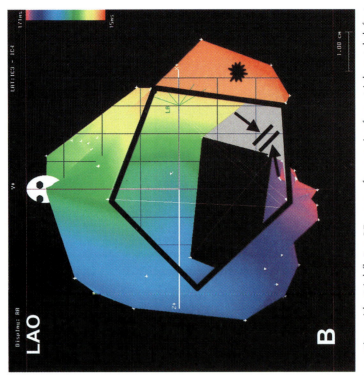

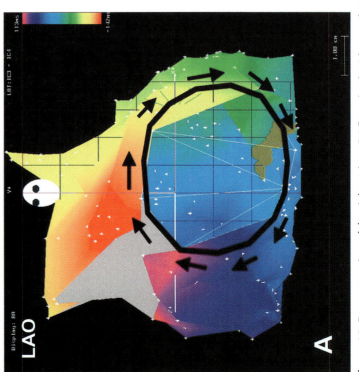

Figure 14. Reconstruction of the right atrium (LAO projection) in a patient presenting with atrial flutter 25 years after repair of an atrial septal defect. The F waves were predominantly positive in the inferior leads. The left panel demonstrates activation characteristic of typical clockwise atrial flutter; the diagnosis of isthmus-dependent flutter was confirmed by pacing maneuvers. The green tags depict the line of ablation in the subeustachian isthmus. The right panel illustrates the results of pacing from the coronary sinus os a cycle length of 600 milliseconds (star). Note that the latest activation is immediately lateral to the ablation line, confirming the presence of clockwise conduction block.

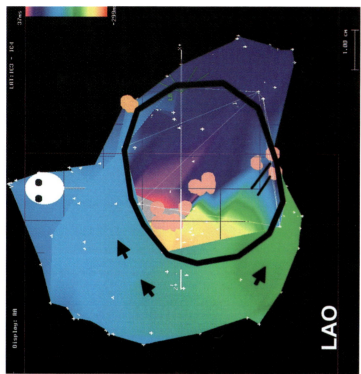

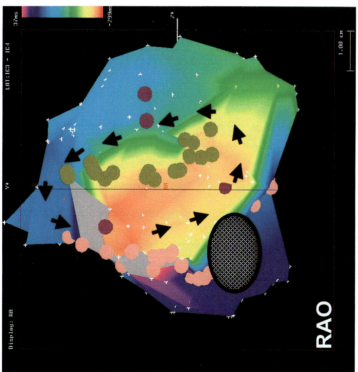

Figure 15. Reconstruction of the right atrium during incisional tachycardia induced in the same patient as in Figure 13, following ablation of the isthmus dependent flutter. Note the markedly different activation of the tricuspid annulus compared to typical flutter, and the persistence of block lateral to medial across the subeustachian isthmus. A complete circuit, accounting for the entire flutter cycle length is confined to the right atrial free wall, with counterclockwise activation around a line of double potentials (olive tags). These double potentials are in the same area as the atriotomy scar (see Figure 16). The circuit is bounded posteriorly by another line of double potentials (pink tags) corresponding to the location of the crista terminalis. The brown tags represent sites where pacing during tachycardia was performed. Each of these sites had short postpacing intervals, confirming their participation in the tachycardia circuit. The electroanatomic map facilitates selection and precise cataloging of pacing sites. The heavy black line outlines the tricuspid annulus. The stippled oval identifies an orifice of the inferior vena cava.

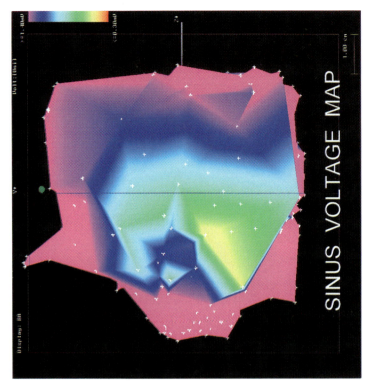

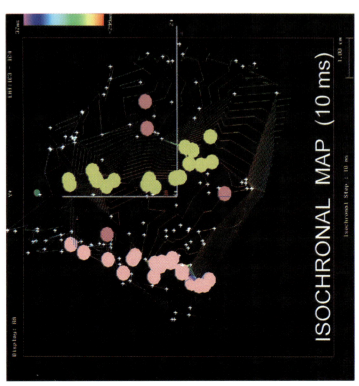

Figure 16. Two additional imaging modalities in the same patient as illustrated in Figure 14, both shown in the right lateral projection. The left panel illustrates an isochronal activation map during incisional tachycardia. This view may be helpful in clarifying regions of slow conduction within a macroreentrant circuit. The right panel illustrates a unipolar voltage map acquired during sinus rhythm. In this map, high voltage ($\geq$1.5 mV) is depicted in pink, while the lowest voltage is depicted in red. Regions of low voltage typically correspond to scar. In this example, the region of low voltage is the same as that containing the central core of double potentials during the tachycardia (green tags, Figure 14). Voltage mapping in sinus rhythm may be useful in identifying regions of scar which play a role in the genesis of tachycardias.

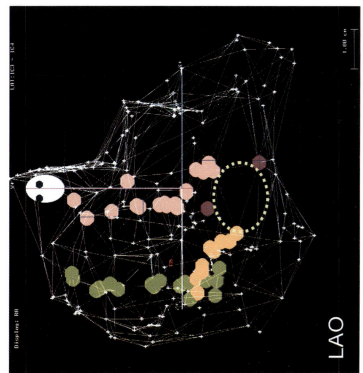

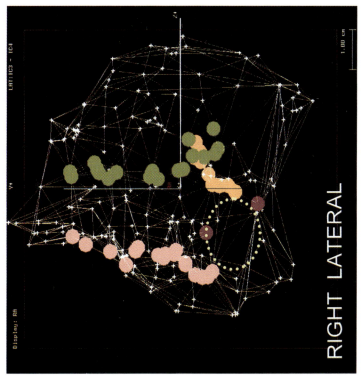

Figure 17. Reconstruction of the right atrium identical to Figure 14, now depicted as a mesh figure to facilitate planning and execution of the ablation strategy. The yellow oval outlines the orifice of the inferior vena cava. The shortest potentially effective ablation line appeared to connect to the lower pole of the atriotomy scar (green tags) to the inferior vena cava. During linear sequential application of RF energy along this line (orange tags), the tachycardia terminated. Following completion of the line, incisional tachycardia could not be reinduced.

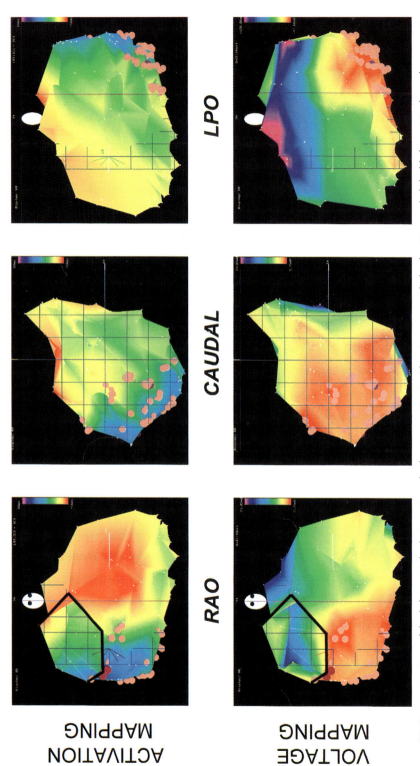

Figure 18. Reconstruction of the left ventricle during sinus rhythm in a patient with prior myocardial infarction and global left ventricular enlargement. The top panels demonstrate activation maps, with earliest activation in red along the intraventricular septum, and latest activation at the base of the heart beneath the mitral annulus. The bottom panels demonstrate bipolar voltage maps with lowest voltage (< 2.5 mV) in red. The extensive low voltage in the inferoseptal, inferior and lateral walls defines a large inferior myocardial infarction. There is extensive fractionation of local electrograms (double potentials or electrogram duration > 100 milliseconds) over a wide area, as indicated by the pink tags. The patient had ventricular tachycardia which was successfully ablated by RF energy application beneath the mitral annulus at the site indicated by the brown tags (see text for details).

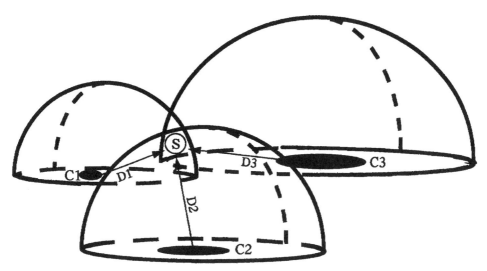

Figure 1. Schematic of the process for location determination. A locator pad consists of three equally spaced magnetic coils (C1, C2, C3), each of which generates a slightly different magnetic field that decays as a function of distance from the coil. The sensor (S) embedded in the mapping catheter tip measures the strength of the magnetic field from each coil, and hence measures the distances from each coil. The location of the catheter in three-dimensional space can be determined as the point of intersection between the three hemispheres whose radii are the distances (D1, D2, D3) measured by the sensor. (From reference 15, with permission).

pending on the specific needs of the operator, the density of data points and the proportion of the chamber that is reconstructed can be varied. The reconstructed surface can be viewed in "traditional" radiographic projections, as well as in any degree of rotation around the X, Y, and Z axes. In vivo assessment of location accuracy compared to known distances averages 0.7 millimeters, and reproducibility of repeated positioning at the same site averages 0.5 millimeters.[23,24] Since the spatial coordinates of each point in three-dimensional space are stored, the precise distance between any two points can be automatically calculated by the mapping software. In the following sections, some of the potential applications of this imaging technique to catheter ablation are examined in detail.

Sinus Rhythm and Inappropriate Sinus Tachycardia

An isochronal reconstruction of the right atrial endocardium during sinus rhythm is displayed in Figure 2. Atrial activation begins in the mid-high posterolateral right atrium, and is most rapid in the cranial-caudal direction. Activation subsequently spreads anteriorly and posteriorly, with the inferoseptal region near the coronary sinus activating last. The total right atrial activation time is 89 milliseconds. The "tagged points" in this map represent sites adjacent to the tricuspid annulus identifed by an AV ratio of less than 1. Annular dimensions measured by this technique correlate closely with those obtained by three-dimensional echo reconstruction of the tricuspid annulus. Electroanatomic imaging appears to be useful in identifying pacemaker foci in patients with inappropriate sinus tachycardia, and in documenting progressive shifts in the focus during the ablation procedure.[25]

Focal Atrial Tachycardia

While catheter ablation of atrial tachycardia guided by standard radiographic imaging has provided effective therapy for atrial tachycardia,[1-3] several features of the magnetic catheter tracking system are well suited to mapping and ablation of this arrhythmia. Simultaneous display of location and activation time facilitates concentration of data acquisition in the region of early activation (Figure 3). In most focal tachycardias, early atrial activation preceding the P wave can be recorded over a relatively large area due to rapid conduction in normal myocardium.[26] This characteristic often confounds attempts to quickly identify and eliminate the tachycardia focus with a minimum number of radiofrequency (RF) applications once the general region of early activation is identified. This point is demonstrated in the focal right atrial tachycardia depicted in Figure 3, panel 6. Sites activating within the first 10 milliseconds of each beat form an ellipse with dimensions of 12 × 18 millimeters (tagged points, dashed line). Given the potential inaccuracies of assigning activation time, any one of these sites may have been designated earliest by isolated sampling of individual points. Viewing the region of early activation as a whole helps to smooth over minor inaccuracies in assigning activation time at individual sites. Placement of the initial RF lesion at the center of the "early activation zone" irrespective of the specific activation time at that site resulted in prompt termination of tachycardia. The location of this focus (mid to slightly posterior in the right lateral view) is typical for tachycardias arising from the crista terminalis, although confirmation of the precise location on the crista requires direct visualization by intracardiac echocardiography. The total time to generate and edit the map, and eliminate the tachycardia was less than 30 minutes.

Foci in both atria are readily identified by this technique (Figures 4–6). Collectively, these figures also illustrate another property of atrial activation during focal tachycardia that may complicate identification of optimal target sites with traditional mapping techniques. The spread of global activation from the site of origin is not uniform, but is often markedly anisotropic, depending on specific anatomic features and fiber orientation in the region.[26] In Figure 3, the tachycardia spreads more rapidly in the superior-inferior axis, parallel to the fibers of the crista terminalis. In Figure 4, activation spreads more rapidly parallel to the annulus than perpendicular to it. In Figure 5, there is marked anisotropic activation away from the focus in the superior left atrium, parallel to the fiber orientation in Bachman's bundle. In this latter example, anisotropic conduction led to early activation of nearby orifice of the right superior pulmonary vein, resulting in inappropriate targeting of this structure for ablation directed by traditional mapping techniques. A more complex example is illustrated in Figure 6. In this case, the tachycardia originated from the anteroseptal left atrium near the mitral annulus. However, there was rapid activation posteriorly along the interatrial septum toward the fossa ovalis, consistent with fiber orientation in this region,[27] resulting in the appearance of relatively early activation in the posteromedial right atrium and right pulmonary veins. The system has the ability to simultaneously display maps from four different chambers.

Preliminary experience has indicated that ablation directed by electroanatomic mapping is highly effective for treatment of focal atrial tachycardias, and is associated with short procedure times and a small number of RF applications.[26,28,29]

AV Nodal Reentry

Ablation of the posterior atrial approaches to the AV node adjacent to the coronary sinus has become the most commonly used approach for elimination of AV nodal reentrant tachycardia (AVNRT).[11,12] Techniques to identify the appropriate site for ablation include both identification of specific electrogram features, and radiographic position relative to coronary sinus and His bundle recording catheters. Electroanatomic imaging with the magnetic catheter tracking system may be useful to identify the spatial relationships between major structures within Koch's triangle.[30] Following generation of a global right atrial or limited atrial septal reconstruction, sites of interest can be tagged. For this purpose, the surface interpolation feature is disabled, and the map is displayed a meshwork of connected points (Figure 7). The right lateral view is generally the most helpful in delineating anatomic relationships, although simultaneous display of additional views are also useful. Sites where a His potential is present on the intracardiac electrogram are tagged with a specific color. The resultant "His cluster" marks the region of the proximal His bundle and adjacent compact AV node and its anterior fast pathway inputs. The practical application of this maneuver is to highlight the area to be avoided during ablation in order to minimize the risk of AV block. Points are then sampled from the CS ostium. Care is taken to delineate the most superior and "septal" aspects of the ostium during catheter withdrawal from the coronary sinus. Finally, the annular border of Koch's triangle is defined by serial acquisition of points recording a low amplitude atrial electrogram and a large amplitude ventricular electrogram.

As illustrated in figure 7, Koch's triangle is usually oriented vertically in the left anterior oblique projection. However, a nearly horizontal variant is occasionally observed (Figure 8), which may be difficult to identify radiographically and may be associated with a greater risk of unintentional heart block if unrecognized.[30] The spatial relationships and dimensions of Koch's triangle as assessed by this method correlate well with published dimensions measured at autopsy.[31]

Creation of a "tagged" endocardial map of Koch's triangle allows rapid selection of the ablation site. In patients with normal anatomic relationships, the tip of the ablation catheter is placed anteriorly at the level of the superior border of the coronary sinus os in the right lateral projection. The initial site is a few millimeters from the annular border of the triangle. Other than using the AV ratio as a guide to the proximity of the catheter tip to the tricuspid annulus, no specific electrogram characteristics are sought. If junctional rhythm and elimination of inducible AVNRT are not produced by the initial RF energy application, the catheter is withdrawn toward the coronary sinus an additional few millimeters and energy again applied. The site of RF application is generally kept at least 10 millimeters from the most inferior "His" location. In our initial experience with this technique in 23 patients, AVNRT was eliminated with a median of 2 RF applications and with no complications or recurrences.[30] Occasionally, initial applications do not eliminate AVNRT or repetitive slow pathway conduction despite the production of junctional rhythm during RF application. In this instance, extension of a linear sequence of applications to the superior aspect of the coronary sinus os has proven effective (Figure 9).

Typical Atrial Flutter

High density electroanatomic maps during typical counterclockwise atrial flutter are useful in delineating the specific features of the flutter circuit and global right atrial activation during flutter (Figure 10). Activation exits the isthmus between the eustachian ridge and the tricuspid valve annulus as a broad wavefront, spreading anterosuperiorly around the tricuspid annulus, and posterosuperiorly. Lateral spread of the posterior wavefront is blocked along a vertical line in the posterolateral right atrium, a region marked by double potentials and demonstrated by intracardiac echocardiography to coincide with the location of the crista terminalis. The posterior wavefront proceeds cranially around the superior vena cava to merge with the activation wavefront circulating around the tricuspid annulus. The anterolateral wall of the right atrium is the last to activate as the wavefront reenters the lateral aspect subeustachian isthmus.

Estimates of regional conduction velocity in the flutter circuit remain controversial. The spatial precision of electroanatomic mapping offers some advantages over radiographically localized measurements. Data from high density electroanatomic reconstructions indicate that conduction velocity through the subeustachian isthmus is somewhat slower (50–70 cm/sec) than the posterior free wall or the superior surface of the right atrium (110–120 cm/sec).[32,33] However, conduction velocity measured parallel and immediately adjacent to the annulus is uniform around the entire annular circumference, approximately 50–60 cm/sec.[33] The flutter cycle length is highly correlated to the circumference of the tricuspid annulus as measured from electroanatomic maps and three-dimensional echocardiographic annular reconstructions, suggesting that the annulus represents the minimal path length for the typical flutter circuit.[34] These observations confirm earlier reports that the tricuspid annulus is the anterior "barrier" for the flutter circuit based on entrainment data during pacing at annular sites.[8]

Delineation of isthmus geometry by electroanatomic mapping may facilitate flutter ablation. Figure 11 illustrates a typical ablation line produced during flutter ablation in the septal portion of the isthmus. As the catheter is dragged across the isthmus, each point is acquired and tagged. The mesh display is used to allow easier visualization of tagged sites. The isthmus region forms a relatively flat rectangular surface in a caudal projection, and a "side-on" view is provided by right anterior or left posterior oblique projections. The ablation line can be planned by a trial run. Typically, the most anterior and posterior points in the isthmus are tagged; during application of RF energy, the line is placed to connect the tags. Each tag is approximately 4 millimeters in diameter, permitting visual estimation of the density of applications needed to produce a linear lesion during the drag. This "bookkeeping" function of the mapping system is particularly useful to avoid redundant lesion application, and to identify potential gaps in the line. In this patient, the width of the isthmus was 3 cm. Data from animal studies indicates a close correlation (r=0.96) between the length of an ablation line measured by the mapping system to that measured by direct inspection at autopsy.[35] The superior indentation of the line as it extends posteriorly is commonly observed (best viewed in the left posterior oblique projection), and is consistent with a prominent eustachian ridge.

The mapping system can be used to verify conduction block following the placement of linear lesions. Figure 12 illustrates the technique used for verification. The left panel illustrates activation during coronary sinus pacing (cycle length 600 milliseconds) prior to ablation in the same patient illustrated in Figure 11. Activation progresses rapidly through the isthmus with the anterolateral wall activated last. The system allows superimposition of data from the ablation on previously or subsequently generated reconstructions acquired during the same setting. The panel on the right illustrates the postablation results. Pacing from the coronary sinus now results in earlier activation of the lateral wall relative to the isthmus, with the latest activation in the septal isthmus immediately lateral to the ablation line, consistent with complete conduction block of clockwise activation through the isthmus. Similar maps can be generated during pacing from the low lateral right atrium to confirm counterclockwise activation block.

The initial ablation line may not always result in complete conduction block. Figure 13 illustrates data from another patient during ablation of typical clockwise flutter. Following the initial ablation line, counterclockwise conduction through the isthmus is modified, but there is persistent early activation of the posterior septal isthmus across the ablation line (middle panel). Since initial RF energy was applied with a 4 millimeters tip catheter, we hypothesized that lesion depth may not have been sufficient to produce transmural ablation of the relatively thick eustachian ridge. Additional RF energy applications were given with an 8 millimeter tip electrode. The subsequent reconstruction during proximal coronary sinus pacing confirmed the attainment of complete counterclockwise conduction block.

Spatially precise tagging of the ablation line also facilitates a second, more precise and rapid technique for identifying gaps in the ablation line. Local electrogram configuration can be easily inspected as the catheter tip "retracks" the ablation line during coronary sinus pacing. Areas of conduction block generally have either no double potentials or widely split double potentials while areas of persistent conduction manifest a single potential, usually of relatively high amplitude. Similar techniques have been advocated by others.[36]

The clockwise variant of typical (subeustachian isthmus-dependent) flutter can be mapped and ablated in a fashion similar to that described above (Figure 14).

Incisional tachycardias

A variety of supraventricular arrhythmias may complicate the long-term clinical course of patients following surgical repair of congenital heart disease. These include typical atrial flutter and focal atrial tachycardia. In addition, macroreentrant circuits may develop around the healed incisions of the surgical procedure, including atriotomy incisions and prosthetic or pericardial patches.[9,10] Electroanatomic mapping often clarifies the complex sequence of activation in these tachycardias,[37] and permits identification of the central line of block, as well as additional conduction barriers that influence global activation during these tachycardias (Figure 15). These circuits usually display the hallmarks of macroreentrant arrhythmias, including electrograms recorded spanning the entire tachycardia cycle length, and close proximity of the earliest and latest activation sites. Lines of conduction block are usually manifest as double potentials, which may be either functional or fixed in nature. These sites can be tagged for easy identification, and may serve as the boundaries for subsequent design of ablation strategies. The activation map can also be used to catalog sites at which pacing maneuvers are performed during assessment of the tachycardia.

In addition to providing spatial information with respect to activation, the mapping system also permits a similar electroanatomic reconstruction of the voltage distribution (either unipolar or bipolar) over the endocardial surface. Preliminary data suggest that low voltage is well correlated to myocardial scarring. Voltage maps obtained in sinus rhythm may thus provide an indirect means of visualizing regions of myocardial scar, and identifying sites of prior atriotomy (see the right-hand panel in Figure 16). Finally, the maps may be used to design and execute the ablation strategy for these arrhythmias, as illustrated in Figure 17. The line of orange tags in this figure identify the sites of RF energy application during stepwise pullback from the lower border of the atriotomy scar to the inferior vena cava. The tachycardia was eliminated following completion of this line.

Ventricular Tachycardia

The approach to electroanatomic mapping and ablation of focal ventricular tachycardias is similar to that for focal atrial tachycardia. Also similar to these latter arrhythmias, activation during focal ventricular tachycardia spreads rapidly away from the site of origin, resulting in a broad zone of early activation. Successful ablation sites are found in the center of this zone. The electroanatomic map may also be used to provide a spatial record of the outcome of pacemapping at various sites in the area of early activation. A more detailed discussion of the electroanatomic imaging of focal ventricular tachycardia may be found in Chapter 36.

The role of electroanatomic mapping for treatment of ventricular tachycardia associated with prior myocardial infarction is evolving. While activation mapping during tachycardia can identify the general region of exit from a slow conduction zone, the system may be more useful for cataloging sites of diastolic activation and associated responses to pacing maneuvers. However, the greatest potential for this system may be in characterization of the anatomic substrate for tachycardia: voltage maps outlining regions of dense scar, spatially detailed maps of late activation and fragmented activity, and spatial maps indicating sites of pacing induced conduction delay (Figure 18). These properties may help direct placement of linear lesions during sinus rhythm which will subsequently serve as conduction barriers, inhibiting the formation of macroreentrant ventricular circuits. Such approaches are the only means of targeting the large number of patients in whom some or all clinical tachycardias are hemodynamically unstable, and thus cannot be approached by traditional mapping techniques. Complete encirclement of the scar may prove impractical, and the precise number, direction, and relationship of linear lesions both to the center of the scar and to natural anatomic barriers such as the mitral annulus are matters of current investigation. Preliminary data suggest that scar-related sinus rhythm ablation is feasible and may reduce the frequency of spontaneous unstable ventricular tachycardia recurrences.[38]

Summary

The electroanatomic imaging system has several additional features useful for catheter ablation. The magnetic technology can be incorporated into any type of ablation catheter. Currently, only a standard 4 mm-tip catheter without temperature monitoring is commercially available. However, a 4 mm-tip thermocouple catheter, as well as an irrigated 3.5 millimeter tip, and an 8 millimeter dual thermocouple tip electrode catheter are undergoing clinical investigation at the present time. Both unipolar and bipolar data can be acquired and stored simultaneously, and either can be displayed on the three-dimensional image. Finally, the ability to display the position and orientation of the catheter tip in real-time permits nonfluoroscopic navigation, reducing fluoroscopy time and radiation exposure.

A few practical issues merit further discussion. As a point-by-point mapping technique, the system requires a stable activation sequence for the duration of the map. Mapping of nonsustained arrhythmias can be performed, provided the rhythm recurs with sufficient frequency and has a similar activation sequence between episodes. To accurately depict chamber geometry and dimensions, a minimum number of well-spaced points need to be obtained (approximately 50 to 100 points in the normal right atrium), and care must be taken to assure that data from all portions of the endocardial surface have been recorded. Finally, it must be emphasized that specific anatomic structures are often not directly visualized, but rather inferred from a combination of spatial information and electrogram characteristics. Intracardiac echocardiography may provide important additional and complementary anatomic information for specific applications.[39]

Electroanatomic imaging with magnetic catheter tracking has enhanced the three-dimensional visualization of endocardial geometry and activation during a variety of cardiac arrhythmias. By providing geometrically accurate and spatially precise localization of the recording electrode, it allows correlation of activation and electrophysiological observations with underlying structure and anatomy. The rapid diagnosis and successful ablation of atrial arrhythmias, such as AV nodal reentry or tachycardias related to an accessory atrioventricular connection, may be accomplished with a variety of imaging techniques. However, magnetic catheter tracking can often provide useful insights in patients with complex or unusual anatomy. For focal atrial and ventricular tachycardias, the system has unique advantages which permit rapid and accurate identification of target sites. Most maps can be acquired and edited where necessary in less than 30 minutes with results immediately available online to guide ablation. In patients with complex atrial arrhythmias, the imaging system permits rapid visualization of potential macroreentrant circuits and critical boundaries. More importantly, the operator can then use this spatial template to identify sites where the response to pacing will clarify the nature of the circuit, and to plan and execute the appropriate ablation strategy. Finally, the maps can serve as a purely spatial template for cataloging and directing placement of a large number of linear lesions, such as recently reported for treatment of atrial fibrillation.

References

1. Triedman JK, Jenkins KJ, Colan SD, et al. Multipolar mapping of the right heart using a basket catheter: acute and chronic animal studies. *PACE* 1997;20:51–59.
1a. Kay GN, Chong F, Epstein AE, et al. Radiofrequency ablation for treatment of primary atrial tachycardias. *J Am Coll Cardiol* 1993;21:901–909.
2. Lesh MD, Van Hare GF, Epstein LM, et al. Radiofrequency catheter ablation of atrial arrhythmias: results and mechanisms. *Circulation* 1994;89: 1074–1089.
3. Poty H, Saoudi N, Haïssaguerre M, et al. Radiofrequency catheter ablation of atrial tachycardias. *Am Heart J* 1996;131:481–489.

4. Shenasa H, Merrill JJ, Hamer ME, et al. Distribution of ectopic atrial tachycardias along the crista terminalis: an atrial ring of fire? [abstract] *Circulation* 1993;88:I–29.

5. Kalman JM, Olgin JE, Karch MR, et al. "Cristal tachycardias": origin of right atrial tachycardias from the crista terminalis identified by intracardiac echocardiography. *J Am Coll Cardiol* 1998;31:451–459.

6. Marchlinski FE, Gottlieb CD, Callans DJ, et al. Tricuspid and mitral annuli: common origin of atrial tachycardias [abstract]. *PACE* 1997;20(part II):1182.

7. Olgin JE, Kalman JM, Fitzpatrick AP, et al. Role of right atrial endocardial structures as barriers to conduction during human type I atrial flutter: activation and entrainment mapping guided by intracardiac echocardiography. *Circulation* 1995;92:1839–1848.

8. Kalman JM, Olgin JE, Saxon LA, et al. Activation and entrainment mapping defines the tricuspid annulus as the anterior barrier in typical atrial flutter. *Circulation* 1996;94:3989–4006.

9. Kalman JM, Van Hare GF, Olgin JE, et al. Ablation of incisional reentrant atrial tachycardia complicating surgery for congenital heart disease: use of entrainment to define a critical isthmus of conduction. *Circulation* 1996; 93:502–512.

10. Triedman JK, Bergau DM, Saul JP, et al. Efficacy of radiofrequency ablation for control of intraatrial reentrant tachycardia in patients with congenital heart disease. *J Am Coll Cardiol* 1997;30:1032–1038.

11. Jackman WM, Beckman K, McClelland JH, et al. Treatment of supraventricular tachycardia due to atrioventricular nodal reentry by radiofrequency catheter ablation of slow-pathway conduction. *N Engl J Med* 1992;327:313–318.

12. Jazayeri MR, Hempe SL, Sra JS, et al. Selective transcatheter ablation of the fast and slow pathways using radiofrequency energy in patients with atrioventricular nodal reentrant tachycardia. *Circulation* 1992;85:1318–1328.

13. Wilber DJ, Baerman J, Olshansky B, et al. Adenosine-sensitive ventricular tachycardia: clinical characteristics and response to catheter ablation. *Circulation* 1993;87:126–134.

14. Coggins DL, Lee RJ, Sweeney J, et al. Radiofrequency catheter ablation as a cure for idiopathic ventricular tachycardia of both right and left ventricular origin. *J Am Coll Cardiol* 1994;1333–1341.

15. DeBakker JMT, van Capelle FJL, Janse MJ, et al. Reentry as a cause of ventricular tachycardia in patients with chronic ischemic heart disease: electrophysiologic and anatomic correlation. *Circulation* 1988;77:589–606.

16. De Bakker JMT, Coronel R, Tasseron S, et al. Ventricular tachycardia in the infarcted, Langendorff-perfused human heart: role of the arrangement of surviving cardiac fibers. *J Am Coll Cardiol* 1990;15:1594–1607.

17. Wilber DJ, Kopp DE, Glascock DN, et al. Catheter ablation of the mitral isthmus for ventricular tachycardia associated with inferior infarction. *Circulation* 1995;92:3481–3489.

18. Hadjis TA, Stevenson WG, Harada T, et al. Preferential locations for critical reentry circuit sites causing myocardial infarction. *J Cardiovasc Electrophysiol* 1997;8:363–370.

19. Schalij MJ, van Rugge FP, Siezenga M, et al. Endocardial activation mapping of ventricular tachycardia in patients: first application of a 32-site bipolar mapping electrode catheter. *Circulation* 1998;98:2168–2179.

20. Triedman JK, Jenkins KJ, Colan SD, et al. Intra-atrial reentrant tachycardia after palliation of congenital heart disease: characterization of multiple macroreentrant circuits using fluoroscopically based three-dimensional endocardial mapping. *J Cardiovasc Electrophysiol* 1997;8: 259–270.

21. Liu ZW, Jia P, Ershler PR, et al. Noncontact endocardial mapping: reconstruction of electrograms and isochrones from intracavitary probe potentials. *J Cardiovasc Electrophysiol* 1997;8:415–431.

22. Schilling RJ, Peters NS, Davies DW. Simultaneous endocardial mapping in human left ventricle using a noncontact catheter: comparison of contact and reconstructed electrograms during sinus rhythm. *Circulation* 1998;98: 887–898.

23. Gepstein L, Hayam G, Ben-Haim SA. A novel method for nonfluoroscopic electroanatomical mapping of the heart: in vitro and in vivo accuracy results. *Circulation* 1997;95:1611–1622.

24. Smeets JL, Ben-Haim SA, Rodriguez LM, et al. New method for nonfluoroscopic endocardial mapping in human. *Circulation* 1998;97:2426–2432.

25. Arruda M, Kall JG, Burke MC, et al. Differences in endocardial activation adjacent to the crista terminalis in patients with inappropriate sinus tachycardia compared to normal subjects. *PACE* 1999; in press.

26. Kall JG, Burke MC, Verdino R, et al. Electroanatomic mapping and ablation of focal atrial tachycardia [abstract]. *PACE* 1998;21:II-984.

28. Kottkamp H, Hindricks G, Breithardt G, et al. Three-dimensional catheter technology: electroanatomic mapping of the right atrium and ablation of ectopic atrial tachycardia. *J Cardiovasc Electrophysiol* 1997;8:1332–1337.

29. Marchlinski F, Callans D, Gottlieb C, et al. Magnetic electroanatomic mapping for ablation of focal atrial tachycardias. *PACE* 1998;21:1621–1635.

30. Cooke PA, Wilber DJ. Radiofrequency catheter ablation of atrioventricular nodal reentry tachycardia utilizing nonfluoroscopic electroanatomic mapping. *PACE* 1998;21(9):1802–1809.

31. Cooke PA, Johnson CT, Lin AC, et al. Mapping of Koch's triangle and slow pathway ablation guided by nonfluoroscopic electroanatomic imaging [abstract]. *J Am Coll Cardiol* 1998;31:255A.

32. Shas DC, Jaïs P, Haïssaguerre M, et al. Three-dimensional mapping of the common flutter circuit in the right atrium. *Circulation* 1997;96:3904–3912.

33. Wilber DJ, Rubenstein D, Burke MC, et al. Global activation patterns during high density electroanatomic mapping of atrial flutter [abstract]. *J Am Coll Cardiol* 1997;29:331A.

34. Wang ZG, Kall JG, Kopp DE, et al. Do tricuspid annular dimensions influence the cycle length of typical atrial flutter? [abstract] *J Am Coll Cardiol* 1998;31:367A.

35. Shpun S, Gepstein L, Hayam G, et al. Guidance of radiofrequency endocardial ablation with real-time three-dimensional magnetic navigation system. *Circulation* 1997;96:2016–2021.

36. Nakagawa H, Jackman WM. Use of three-dimensional nonfluoroscopic mapping system for catheter ablation of typical atrial flutter. *PACE* 1998; 21:1279–1286.
37. Dorostkar PC, Cheng J, Scheinman MM. Electroanatomic mapping and ablation of the substrate supporting intra-atrial reentrant tachycardia after palliation for complex congenital heart disease. *PACE* 1998;21:1810–1819.
38. Lesh MD, Kalman JM, Karch MR. Use of intracardiac echocardiography during electrophysiologic evaluation and therapy of atrial arrhythmias. *J Cardiovasc Electrophysiol* 1998;9:S40–47.

Chapter 37

Radiation Exposure During Radiofrequency Catheter Ablation Procedures

Hugh Calkins, M.D., Lawrence Rosenthal, M.D., and Mahadevappa Mahesh, Ph.D.

Introduction

Since it was first introduced for clinical use in the early 1990s, radiofrequency (RF) catheter ablation has gained widespread acceptance as an effective and safe approach for treatment of many types of cardiac arrhythmias.[1–6] Although electrophysiologists are keenly aware of the acute risks associated with the ablation procedure itself, the long-term risks that result from radiation exposure received by patients and electrophysiologists are less well recognized.[1–12] Recently, several case reports of serious X ray-induced skin injuries during fluoroscopy-guided interventional procedures have been published.[13–15] Because radiation can be neither felt nor seen, and its detrimental effects may not appear until decades later, these hidden risks of catheter ablation are easily ignored. As the number, complexity, and duration of catheter ablation procedures increase, the radiation-related risks of these procedures increase in importance. Determination of the proper role of catheter ablation in treating arrhythmias today and in the years ahead depends both on the efficacy of the procedure but also on the short- and long-term risks of the procedure. The purpose of this chapter is to review the risks of radiation exposure during catheter ablation procedures and to recommend techniques and equipment that may be used to reduce these risks.

From Huang SKS, Wilber DJ (eds.): *Radiofrequency Catheter Ablation of Cardiac Arrhythmias: Basic Concepts and Clinical Applications,* 2nd ed. Armonk, NY: Futura Publishing Company, Inc. ©2000.

Determinants of Fluoroscopy Time during Catheter Ablation Procedures

During catheter ablation procedures, fluoroscopy is needed to position diagnostic electrode catheters, guide manipulation of the ablation catheter, and monitor catheter stability during delivery of RF energy. Several studies have evaluated fluoroscopy time during catheter ablation procedures.[9–12] Calkins et al reported a mean fluoroscopy time of 44 ± 40 minutes during catheter ablation of APs.[9] Lindsay et al reported a mean fluoroscopy time of 50 ± 31 minutes during catheter ablation of atrioventricular nodal reentrant tachycardia (AVNRT) or accessory pathways (APs),[11] and Park et al reported a mean fluoroscopy time of 47 ± 31 minutes during catheter ablation of a wide variety of ablation targets.[10] More recent studies have identified increasing patient age and unsuccessful ablation procedures as predictors of increased fluoroscopy time.[16–18] In the Cardiorhythm (Medtronic, Minneapolis, MN) multicenter clinical trial, the fluoroscopy duration increased with age from 32 ± 12 minutes for patients less than 10 years old, to 45 ± 36 minutes for patients 10 to 20 years old, and to 59 ± 56 minutes for patients greater than 20 years old.[17] This increase in fluoroscopy duration with patient age was observed regardless of the ablation target. In this trial, the cumulative success of catheter ablation rose rapidly during the first 90 minutes of fluoroscopy exposure and then plateaued.[16] Patients undergoing a failed attempt at catheter ablation received more than 50% greater fluoroscopy exposure, compared to those patients in whom the ablation was successful. The fluoroscopy times associated with catheter ablation are considerably longer than has been reported during diagnostic angiography (<10 minutes) and angioplasty (<20 minutes) procedures.[19–21]

Patient Radiation Exposure

Fluoroscopy uses X radiation generated with kilovoltages typically between 65 and 100 kilovolt peak (kV(p)) to image the heart and guide the placement of intracardiac electrode catheters. These X rays have relatively low penetrating power resulting in the delivery of the maximum dose of radiation at the skin surface where the X ray beam enters. For low-energy radiation, 1 rem=1 rad=0.01 sievert (Sv). To date, a number of studies have been published that have evaluated the radiation exposure received by patients during catheter ablation procedures.[9–12] In these studies, somewhat different approaches were used to estimate patient radiation exposure. For example, Calkins et al used lithium fluoride thermoluminescent dosimeter sensors positioned at various sites on patients' bodies to estimate radiation exposure during catheter ablation of accessory pathways.[9] Radiation sensors were placed over the thyroid, over the xiphoid process, on the patients back at the level of the ninth thoracic vertebral body posteriorly, in the right and left midaxillary lines, and on the patient's back in the midline at the level of the iliac crests to assess gonadal radiation exposure. In contrast, Lindsay, Park, and colleagues estimated radiation exposure based on fluoroscopy times and radiation exposure rates which were obtained using an ion chamber dosimeter placed at various sites in a anthropomorphic radiation model of the human chest.[10,11] Yet another approach was used to analyze data from the Medtronic Cardiorhythm Clinical Trial.[18] In this report, radiation exposure was determined based on fluoroscopy times as well as the dose rate, which was estimated based on the kVp and mA settings used during the ablation procedure together with dose rate information obtained from typical fluoroscopy units. Despite the varying approaches used for quantifying radiation exposure, the radiation exposure estimates in these studies are remarkably consistent.

The amount of radiation exposure and radiation exposure rate reported by Calkins et al is shown in Table 1. The site receiving the largest amount of radiation was the ninth thoracic vertebral body posteriorly with a median exposure of 7.26 rem. The radiation exposure at all other sites was less than 2.5 rem. Lindsay and colleagues reported that the entrance radiation exposure rate was greatest using the left anterior oblique projection (2.2 Roentgens per minute, or R/min), intermediate using the right anterior oblique projection (2.0 R/min), and lowest using in the posterior anterior projection (1.6 R/min). The mean entrance radiation dose received by the skin on the back in the Medtronic Cardiorhythm Clinical Trial was 1.3 ± 1.3 Sv,[18] which is similar to the mean entrance radiation dose of 0.9 ± 0.6 Sv reported by Park.[10] The threshold dose of radiation needed to cause the earliest signs of radiation skin injury (2 Sv) was exceeded by 5% of patients in the study by Park and in 19% of patients in the Cardiorhythm study. The absence of any clinical reports of skin erythema by patients in these studies may reflect a lack of awareness of this complication and absence of a formal follow-up to ascertain the effects of radiation which may not appear for 2 to 3 weeks,[14] or the fact that the estimates of radiation exposure in these studies represent an upper limit of radiation dose as it was assumed that the patient's position relative to the fluoroscopy tube remained fixed.

Independent predictors of radiation exposure during catheter ablation procedures include patient age, sex, the target arrhythmia, success or failure, and the hospital center at which the ablation was performed.[18] Children receive less radiation exposure than adults, women received less radiation exposure than men, patients undergoing a successful ablation procedure receive less radiation

Table 1
Patient Radiation Exposure

Sensor Location	Median Exposure (rem)	Exposure Range (rem)	Exposure Rate (millirem/min)
Thyroid	0.46	0.06–7.26	36
Xyphoid process	1.28	0.16–11.58	58
Thoracic ninth vertebra	7.26	0.31–135.7	447
Right axillary line	0.93	0.06–9.99	45
Left axillary line	0.95	0.005–16.8	50
Posterior iliac crest	2.43	0.005–8.3	64

Sievert = 0.01 rem.
From Calkins et al.[9]

than those in whom catheter ablation failed, and patients undergoing ablation of APs receive more radiation than patients undergoing ablation of the atrioventricular node or AVNRT. The greater radiation exposure in men versus women and in adults versus children likely reflect differences in body thickness as well as differences in the difficulty of catheter ablation in these patient groups.

The amount of radiation exposure received by patients during RF catheter ablation is greater than has previously been reported during diagnostic catheterization procedures but is similar to prior reports of radiation exposure during percutaneous transluminal coronary angioplasty (PTCA) procedures.[21–23]

Patient Radiation Risks

An estimate of cancer or genetic risks resulting from radiation received during RF catheter ablation requires knowledge of radiation doses to individual organs as well the organ's specific sensitivity to radiation exposure. These risks can be estimated based on studies of atomic bomb survivors, patients radiated for treatment of spondylitis, and other similar groups, assuming that radiation risk is linear, nonthreshold, and dose rate independent.[24–26] The BEIR V Committee estimated the risk of a fatal malignancy or a genetic defect per rem of exposure to specific organs as a function of age at exposure and sex.[26] The International Commission on Radiological Protection (ICRP, 1977) also has estimated the risk of a fatal malignancy or genetic defect based on radiation exposure.

The estimated absorbed dose of radiation to various organs in the body result from radiation received during catheter ablation procedures is summarized in Table 2. The 3 organs receiving the largest dose of radiation are the lungs, breast, and bone marrow. The estimated risk of a fatal malignancy in both studies was approximately 1 per thousand patients per 1 hour of fluoroscopy. The significance of this risk must be considered in terms of the baseline 20% lifetime risk of a fatal malignancy in the general population. Because the risk of a fatal malignancy resulting from radiation exposure is age dependent (greater in children than adults) the risk of a fatal malignancy in a child less

Table 2
Estimated Absorbed Radiation Dose During RF Catheter Ablation Procedures

Organ	Dose Equivalent (rem)	
	Calkins	Lindsay
Lungs	7.5	6.9
Breast	2.5	2.0
Bone Marrow	2.0	1.1
Thyroid		0.4
Ovaries	0.4	0.4
Testes	0.1	<0.8

Data are compiled from studies by Calkins et al[9] and Lindsay et al.[11]

than 14 years of age would be approximately twice that of a 35-year-old patient. The risk of a genetic disorder resulting from 1 hour of fluoroscopy was estimated by Calkins et al to be 5 per 1 million births for men and 20 per 1 million live births for women and by Lindsay et al to be 12 per 1 million live births.

These risk estimates are higher than in studies that have estimated the radiation risks during cardiac catheterization and PTCA procedures.[23] Faulkner et al estimated a risk of a fatal malignancy of 0.13 per 1000 during cardiac catheterization and 0.08 per 1000 during PTCA procedures. The genetic risks of cardiac catheterization or PTCA were estimated to be 0.001 per 1000 for men and 0.002 to 0.005 per 1000 for women.

Physician Radiation Exposure

The amount of radiation exposure received by physicians manipulating catheters during RF catheter ablation procedures has been studied.[9,11] Calkins et al[9] measured the radiation exposure to physicians manipulating catheters during RF catheter ablation of accessory pathways in 31 consecutive patients. The radiation exposure was measured using 6 lithium fluoride thermoluminescent dosimeter sensors that were taped to the physician before the procedure. Sensors were placed on the physician's left hand, at the waist level outside the lead apron, at the waist level inside the lead apron, on the physician's left axillary process, immediately below the left eye and outside the thyroid collar. The amount of radiation exposure to physicians reported in this study is summarized in Table 3. Radiation exposure was highest at the operator's left hand. The sensors located beneath the lead apron and under the thyroid shield did not exceed the threshold level of the sensor (10 millirem).

Lindsay et al[11] also recently estimated the radiation exposure to physicians who manipulate catheters and to other staff in the electrophysiology laboratory during RF catheter ablation of AVNRT or during catheter ablation of an AP. The radiation exposure rate was measured in the region occupied by physicians

Table 3
Physician Radiation Exposure

Sensor Location	Mean Exposure Per Badge* (millirem)	Mean Exposure per Case (millirem)	Exposure Rate (millirem/min)
Left hand	513±263	99.3	2.25
Waist	275±229	53.2	1.21
Outside lead			
Under lead	<10	<2	—
Left maxilla	146±95	28.1	0.53
Thyroid	81±57	15.6	
Outside lead			
Under lead	<10	<2	—

Values given as mean ± standard deviation.
*Each badge was used in 5 or 6 consecutive cases.
From Calkins, et al.[9]

manipulating catheters using either the femoral or subclavian approach, in the region of the electrophysiology station approximately 8 feet from the patient, and in the region occupied by the nursing staff, also approximately 8 feet from the patient. As expected, this study reported that the exposure rate was related to the distance from the fluoroscopy source being greatest to the physician manipulating catheters and markedly less at the electrophysiology station or in the position occupied by the nursing staff (Table 4). The radiation exposure rate was also related to the imaging projection being highest using the left anterior oblique projection, intermediate using the posterior anterior projection, and lowest using the right anterior oblique projection. The authors estimated that the calculated effective dose equivalent to physicians who manipulate catheters from the femoral area and wear standard leaded collars and aprons rated at 0.5 lead equivalence is 1.8 millirem per case, assuming 55 minutes of fluoroscopy time. If thyroid collars are not worn, the calculated effective dose equivalent was 2.8 rems per case.

The techniques used to measure radiation exposure during catheter ablation procedures by Calkins et al[9] are similar to those used in prior studies of radiation exposure during cardiac catheterization and angioplasty procedures.[22,27] The levels of radiation exposure recorded during catheter ablation of APs are somewhat greater than that reported during diagnostic catheterizations and PTCA procedures. Reuter et al[22] reported a mean physician radiation exposure during diagnostic catheterization at the eye level of 20 ± 16 millirem, mean radiation exposure to the thyroid of 10 ± 4 rem, and the mean exposure to the left hand of 13 ± 11 millirem. In comparison, the mean radiation exposure during catheter ablation procedures reported by Calkins et al[9] was 28 millirem at the left maxilla, 16 millirem at the thyroid, and 99 millirem at the left hand. At least in part, these exposure rates reflect longer fluoroscopy times. The much greater radiation exposure to the left hand of physicians performing the procedure reflects the almost constant placement of the catheter by the operator's left hand at the groin region.

Table 4
Radiation Exposure Rate to Physicians and Staff

Subject	PA	RAO
Cardiologist		
Femoral position	47	21
Beam open: no shield		
Cardiologist		
Subclavian position		
Beam open: no shield	70	30
Beam collimated: no shield	36	11
Beam open: shield used	2	7
Monitoring personnel		
Beam open: no shield	15	9
Nurse		
Beam open: no shield	8	5

PA = posteroanterior; RAO = right anterior oblique; LAO = left anterior oblique.
From Lindsay, et al.[11]

Physician Radiation Risks

The amount of radiation exposure received by the catheter operator during RF catheter ablation procedures is small and well below the occupational radiation exposure limits which have been established by the National Council on Radiation Protection (NCRP).[28] The current guidelines limit the annual whole body dose to 5 rem, the dose to the lens of the eye to 15 rem, and the dose to other organs including the skin, extremities, breast, thyroid, and gonads to 50 rem. Based on the total body calculated effective dose equivalent estimated by Lindsay et al,[11] a physician who wears a lead apron and collar can perform 200 cases per month (mean fluoroscopy duration of 55 minutes) and remain below the 5 rem annual whole body radiation exposure limit for people whose jobs require radiation exposure. However, when the radiation exposure limits to individual organs are considered, more restrictive guidelines can be established.[9] Assuming that the radiation exposure measured at left mandible approximates eye exposure, a single operator should be limited to 52 ablation procedures each month assuming an average fluoroscopy time of 44 minutes. Based on the radiation measured on the left hand, current NCRP guidelines would limit the number of ablation procedures performed by a single operator to 42 ablation procedures each month. If the average fluoroscopy time was significantly greater than the 44 minutes reported by Calkins, et al[9] these limits should be reduced accordingly.

Clinical Implications

Catheter ablation procedures require substantial amounts of fluoroscopy that result in radiation exposure to patients and physicians similar to that received during diagnostic cardiac catheterizations and PTCA procedures. This amount of radiation poses a negligible risk to physicians but poses a measurable risk to the patient of malignancy and genetic defects. Although these risks must be recognized, they appear to be small relative to the risk associated with alternative treatment strategies. Furthermore, the increased risk of a fatal malignancy resulting from radiation received during catheter ablation procedures (approximately 1 per thousand per 1 hour of fluoroscopy) is small relative to the spontaneous fatal cancer risk in the United States which is approximately 20%.[29] Thus, radiation exposure resulting from fluoroscopy received during catheter ablation procedures results in less than a 1% increased risk of a fatal malignancy, as compared with the base line risk.

The significance of the risk resulting from radiation received during catheter ablation procedures must be considered relative to the potential benefits of catheter ablation. In patients with symptomatic proximal supraventricular tachycardia or Wolff-Parkinson-White syndrome, the risk resulting from radiation exposure appears to be small relative to the risk associated with other therapeutic approaches. The risk/benefit ratio must be reassessed for asymptomatic patients demonstrated to have the Wolff-Parkinson-White pattern on an electrocardiogram.[30]

Methods to Reduce Radiation Exposure

Although the risks associated with radiation exposure during catheter ablation procedures appear to be acceptable relative to the risk of alternative therapeutic modalities, these risks are significant and therefore every attempt should be made to minimize radiation exposure. The amount of radiation exposure received by patients during catheter ablation procedures can be reduced either by decreasing the duration of fluoroscopy exposure or by reducing the dose rate of radiation exposure which is delivered to the patient. Factors that have been identified as important determinants of fluoroscopy exposure include the patient age and the success or failure of the procedure. Although patient age cannot be modified, the shorter fluoroscopy times in children suggest that radiation risk is not a reason to delay performing ablation procedures in children. It is important to be aware of the relationship between radiation risk and patient age. A prolonged procedure in a child without a life-threatening arrhythmia may not be appropriate. An increased awareness of the relationship which exists between fluoroscopy duration, the incremental success of the procedure, and the ultimate success or failure of the procedure may also result in a reduction of fluoroscopy duration. Catheter ablation can be accomplished, in most patients, with less than 90 minutes of fluoroscopic imaging. Although further increases in success can be achieved with more prolonged attempts, this small increase is associated with a continuous (0.2% per hour of fluoroscopy) increase in the risk of a fatal malignancy. It is also important for the electrophysiologist to recognize that even in the most skilled hands catheter ablation cannot be successfully performed in all patients.

The radiation entrance dose rate is also an important determinant of a patient's radiation exposure. The dose rate can be influenced by the type and settings of the fluoroscopy unit. It has recently been demonstrated that very low-frame-rate pulsed fluoroscopy may reduce radiation exposure by 50% while achieving a nearly equivalent image quality.[31] This technique involves delivering short X ray pulses which are acquired at a lower frame rate (7.5 or 15 acquisitions per second). A standard 30 frames per second display is achieved by using gap filling techniques whereby a single image is repeatedly displayed. The result is a clear but slightly "choppy" display. This type of system is now being used routinely at many institutions. The avoidance of cinefluorography, electronic magnification modes, and high dose fluoroscopy can also help minimize radiation exposure. Geometric and patient factors including the patient thickness and the distance from the source to the patient also influence the radiation dose rate. The great majority of fluoroscopic systems which are in use today employ an automatic brightness system (ABS) which automatically compensates for variations in patient size and density by automatically adjusting the output on the X ray generator so that an approximately constant intensity emerges from the beam exit surface. The ABS thus ensures that thin patients receive a lower skin dose than thick or dense patients and compensates for variations in absorption by different body tissues. Special attention has to be given for proper adjustment of ABS and it should be checked on a regular basis through regular quality control activities.

It is essential that the physicians who perform catheter ablation procedures are trained in radiation safety and have an awareness of the techniques that are available to reduce radiation exposure to the patient as well as the staff performing the procedure.[32] For example, it is important to collimate the field of the image. It is also important to avoid magnification or the use of high dose cine imaging because the entrance radiation dose nearly doubles for 3:2 magnification. Physicians should also monitor and record the duration of fluoroscopy exposure received by each patient and, when possible, estimate the amount of radiation exposure received by the patient. Patients who require either markedly prolonged fluoroscopy exposure as well as those with an estimated exposure of >2 Sv should be reexamined at selected intervals to monitor for development of the late manifestations of radiation-induced skin injury. The wide variability of dose rate among different machines configurations and body sizes, underlines the need for some means for dynamic monitoring of the patient dose during the procedure. A prototype device has been designed that dynamically records and displays to the clinician the cumulative skin dose estimate as well as the instantaneous dose rate during the procedure.[33] These types of monitoring devices may in the future aid in the avoidance of significant skin injury to patients from prolonged fluoroscopic procedures such as RF catheter ablation.

The above techniques will also reduce the radiation exposure to the physician performing the study. It is also important that the operator wear a thyroid shield and be located behind a suspended lead shield.

References

1. Scheinman MM, Morady F, Hess DS, et al. Catheter-induced ablation of the atrioventricular junction to control supraventricular arrhythmias. *JAMA* 1982;851–855.
2. Gallagher JJ, Svenson RH, Kasell JH, et al. Catheter technique for closed-chest ablation of the atrioventricular conduction system: a therapeutic alternative for the treatment of refractory supraventricular tachycardia. *N Engl J Med* 1982;306:194–200.
3. Weber H, Schmidt L. Catheter technique for closed-chest ablation of an accessory pathway. *N Engl J Med* 1983;308:653–654.
4. Calkins H, Langberg J, Sousa J, et al. Radiofrequency catheter ablation of accessory atrioventricular connections in 250 patients. *Circulation* 1992; 85:1337–1346.
5. Jackman WM, Xunzhang W, Friday KJ, et al. Catheter ablation of accessory atrioventricular pathways (Wolff-Parkinson-White syndrome) by radiofrequency current. *N Engl J Med* 1991;324:1605–1611.
6. Kay GN, Epstein AE, Dailey SM, et al. Role of radiofrequency ablation in the management of supraventricular arrhythmias: experience in 760 consecutive patients. *J Cardiovasc Electrophysiol* 1993;4:371–389.
7. Hindricks G, on behalf of the Multicentre European Radiofrequency Survey (MERFS) Investigators of the working group on arrhythmias of the Euro-

pean Society of Cardiology. The Multicentre European Radiofrequency Survey (MERFS): Complications of radiofrequency catheter ablation of arrhythmias. *Eur Heart J* 1993;14:1644–1653.

8. American College of Cardiology Cardiovascular Technology Assessment Committee. Catheter ablation for cardiac arrhythmias: clinical applications, personnel and facilities. ACC Position Statement. *J Am Coll Cardiol* 1994;24(3):828–833.

9. Calkins H, Niklason L, Sousa J, et al. Radiation exposure during radiofrequency catheter ablation of accessory atrioventricular connections. *Circulation* 1991;84:2376–2382.

10. Park TH, Eichling JO, Schechtman KB, et al. Risk of radiation-induced skin injuries from arrhythmia ablation procedures. *PACE* 1996;19:1363–1369.

11. Lindsay B, Eichling J, Ambos H, et al. Radiation exposure to patients and medical personnel during radiofrequency catheter ablation for supraventricular tachycardia. *Am J Cardiol* 1992;70:218–223.

12. Geise RA, Peters NE, Dunnigan A, et al. Radiation doses during pediatric radiofrequency catheter ablation procedures. *PACE* 1996;19(1):1605–1611.

13. U.S. Food and Drug Administration. Avoidance of serious X ray induced skin injuries to patients during fluoroscopically-guided procedures. September 30, 1994.

14. Wagner LK, Eifel PJ, Geise RA. Potential biological effects following high X ray dose interventional procedures. *J Vasc Interv Radiol* 1994;5:71–84.

15. Rosenthal LS, Beck TJ, Williams JR, et al. Acute radiation dermatitis following radiofrequency catheter ablation of atrioventricular nodal reentrant tachycardia. *PACE* 1997;20:1834–1839.

16. Calkins H, Berger R, Tomaselli G, et al, Atakr Investigators. Relationship between fluoroscopy duration, ablation target, and success during catheter ablation procedures [abstract]. *J Am Coll Cardiol* 1995;Feb:294A.

17. Rosenthal LS, Klein LS, Prystowsky E, et al. The relationship between age, fluoroscopy duration, and arrhythmia target: a multicenter study [abstract]. *PACE* 1997;20:1088.

18. Rosenthal LS, Mahesh M, Beck TJ, et al. Predictors and risk of radiation exposure during catheter ablation procedures: results of a multicenter study. (AHA 1997 abstract)

19. Finci L, Meier B, Steffenino G, et al. Radiation exposure during diagnostic catheterization and single- and double-vessel percutaneous transluminal coronary angioplasty. *Am J Cardiol* 1987;60:1401–1403.

20. Pattee PL, Johns PC, Chambers RJ. Radiation risk to patients from percutaneous transluminal coronary angioplasty. *J Am Coll Cardiol* 1993;22:1044–1051.

21. Cascade PN, Peterson LE, Wajszczuk WJ, et al. Radiation exposure to patients undergoing percutaneous transluminal coronary angioplasty. *Am J Cardiol* 1987;59:996–997.

22. Rueter FG. Physician and patient exposure during cardiac catherization. *Circulation* 1978;58:134–139.

23. Faulkner K, Love HG, Sweeney JK, et al. Radiation doses and somatic risk to patients during cardiac radiological procedures. *Br J Radiol* 1986;59:359–363.

24. Shapiro J. Radiation protection: a guide for scientists and physicians. Cambridge, MA: Harvard University Press, 1981.
25. International Commission on Radiological Protection. Problems involved in developing an index of harm. 1977;26:1–17.
26. National Research Council. Health effects of exposure to low levels of ionizing radiation, BEIR V. Washington, DC: National Academy Press, 1990.
27. Dash H, Leaman DM. Operator radiation exposure during percutaneous transluminal coronary angioplasty. *J Am Coll Cardiol* 1984;4:725–728.
28. National Council on Radiation Protection and Measurements. Limitation of Exposure to Ionizing Radiation: NCRP Report No. 116. Bethesda, MD: NCRP, 1993.
29. Boring CC, Squires TS, Tony T. Cancer statistics, 1991. In: Murphy GP, ed. *Cancer J Clinicians* 1991;41:19–35.
30. Klein GJ, Prystowsky EN, Yee R, et al. Asymptomatic Wolff-Parkinson-White: should we intervene? *Circulation* 1989;80:1902–1905.
31. Aufrichtig R, Xue P. Perceptual comparison of pulsed and continuous fluoroscopy. *Med Phys* 1994;21(2):245–256.
32. Brinker JA, American College of Cardiology Cardiac Catheterization Committee. Use of radiographic devices by cardiologists. *J Am Coll Cardiol* 1995;25:1738–1739.
33. Mahesh M, Beck TJ, Azar N. Radiation bode monitor for fluoroscopic procedures. *Med Phys* 1997;24(6):991.

Chapter 38

Follow-up Evaluation for Patients after Radiofrequency Catheter Ablation

Alan B. Wagshal, M.D.,
Shoei K. Stephen Huang, M.D.

Introduction

Previous chapters of this book have dealt primarily with the mapping and ablation procedure itself, but in this chapter we will deal with the care of the patient following the ablation procedure, particularly in regards to 3 issues:

1) Recurrence of arrhythmias and late perturbations of the arrhythmia substrate;
2) Late appearance of side effects;
3) Utility of routine ancillary testing after ablation.

Fortunately a significant amount of data exists to help us address these questions, from prospective and retrospective studies to formal follow-up evaluation of patients undergoing radiofrequency (RF) ablation as part of studies for the purpose of obtaining regulatory agency approval of specific catheters or ablation systems. These studies often included postablation studies such as Holter monitoring, echocardiography, and postablation electrophysiological testing as a means of assessing side effects and long-term procedural efficacy. These studies served not only to validate the specific ablation catheter or system but also to evaluate the technique of catheter ablation itself, and incidentally they also provide data on the utility of routinely performing these studies in everyday clinical practice.

From Huang SKS, Wilber DJ (eds.): *Radiofrequency Catheter Ablation of Cardiac Arrhythmias: Basic Concepts and Clinical Applications,* 2nd ed. Armonk, NY: Futura Publishing Company, Inc. ©2000.

Section 1: Recurrence of Arrhythmias and Late Perturbations of the Arrhythmia Substrate

Accessory Pathway Ablations

Following apparently successful ablation of an accessory pathway or slow atrioventricular (AV) nodal pathway, a fairly significant recurrence rate of between 8% and 20% for accessory pathways,[1-8] and up to 14% for AV nodal modification has been reported.[9-16]

Several studies have specifically addressed the problem of recurrence using follow-up electrophysiological studies, usually performed between 1 and 3 months after the initially successful ablation, to help define the recurrence rate (Table 1).[6,8-10] In the study by Twidale et al,[6] there was a recurrence of accessory pathway conduction in 17 (8%) of 212 patients after a mean follow-up of 8.55±5.4 months, with 90% of the recurrences already discovered within 2 months. Four factors were identified that were associated with a higher incidence or accessory pathway recurrence:

1) concealed accessory pathway conduction (16% recurrence rate compared with a 5% rate for manifest accessory pathways);
2) absence of an accessory pathway potential in the electrogram at the successful ablation site;
3) pathway location (right free wall and posteroseptal locations being associated with a 13% recurrence rate compared with a 5% rate for left-sided pathways);
4) and a longer time interval of the energy delivery ablation pulse until pathway block during ablation.

In a series of 130 patients reported by Langberg et al there was an overall recurrence rate of 12% (16 out of 130 patients), again with a significantly higher

Table 1
Recurrences after accessory pathway ablation

Reference	Date	# of patients	Overall recurrence rate (%)	Left sided accessory pathway recurrence rate (%)	Right sided and posteroseptal accessory pathway recurrence rate (%)
Schlüter[17]	1991	92	4	1	12
Chen[18]	1992	53	9	9	(left sided pathways only)
Twidale[6]	1991	204	8	5	13
Langberg[8]	1992	130	12	6	24
Swartz[3]	1993	114	8	7	25
Wagshal[63]	1993	53	9	7	18
Wagshal (Atakr Registry)[111]	1995	176	9	4	14
Lesh[4]	1992	100	9	5	11

incidence of recurrence in right sided or posteroseptal pathways (24%) compared with left-sided pathways (6%).[8] Other series describing ablation attempts in large series of patients have also reported similar incidences of pathway recurrence with an approximately twofold greater incidence of recurrence for right sided or posteroseptal pathways than left sided pathways (see Table 1).[3,4,17,18] We will later in this chapter discuss the issue of recurrences with regard to the need for performance of routine follow-up electrophysiological testing after successful ablation. Suffice it to say here, however, that most recurrences of accessory pathway function, whether detected clinically or by follow-up electrophysiological testing, will occur within the first few months of ablation. Thereafter, with only rare exceptions, patients can be considered as having been permanently cured of their arrhythmia. From a practical point of view it is also worth noting that patients exhibiting a successful ablation and then a recurrence have a very high long-term success rate if a repeat ablation session is performed.[6,8]

The higher recurrence rate for right sided or posteroseptal pathways has been suggested to result from the lower electrode-tissue interface temperature associated with ablation in these locations.[19] Unlike left sided lesions where ablation is usually performed by wedging the catheter in the space between the mitral annulus and the left ventricular wall, right sided lesions are usually performed with the catheter in the body of the right atrium against the tricuspid valve annulus. RF catheter ablation operates by causing resistive heating of the tissues surrounding the catheter, which constitute the region of the circuit having the highest impedance. The efficiency of tissue heating is dependent upon strong catheter-tissue contact, which allows optimal resistive heating. Signs of good tissue contact and tissue heating include (in addition to high catheter tip temperatures in catheters equipped with temperature monitoring) a high baseline impedance[20,21] and a rapid early fall in impedance at the start of energy delivery, reflecting heat-induced alterations in electrical properties of the tissue at the tissue-catheter interface.[22,23] Right sided lesions often have suboptimal heating because of both the decreased contact pressure and relative instability of the catheter against the tissue as well as convective heat loss through the greater exposure to the circulating blood pool. Accordingly, particular attention should be paid to factors such as either the baseline impedance or impedance changes, or temperatures achieved when ablating these pathways in an effort to minimize recurrences.

Studies using temperature monitoring have confirmed that ablation lesions applied on the right side of the heart are associated with lower peak temperatures than left sided lesions.[19,24] Langberg et al, using a thermistor-tipped electrode, achieved a mean temperature of $49 \pm 7°C$ for right sided accessory pathways and $60 \pm 16°C$ for left sided pathways,[19] while the corresponding temperatures by Calkins et al using a catheter fitted with a thermocouple positioned just within the distal catheter tip and closed-loop temperature control (usually with a target temperature of 70°C) were $58 \pm 10°C$ and $66 \pm 10°C$, respectively.[24] It is important to realize that temperatures recorded by thermistors or thermocouples represent the heat that is reflected back from the tissue-tip interface to the catheter tip. They are thus dependent upon factors such as tissue contact and stability and particularly catheter tip orientation relative to the tissue and may underestimate the actual tissue temperature when some of these factors are suboptimal.[25,26] In experimental models, better definition of the actual tissue temperature has been achieved by actually inserting probes into tissue slices themselves during experimental ablation procedures.[27–29]

The minimum temperature necessary to achieve complete necrosis of accessory pathways is 50°C,[30,31] so the increased tendency to recurrence of right sided accessory pathway ablations may be explained by the borderline temperature responses achieved, such that the pathway is damaged but true necrosis is not produced.[32–34] In fact, in experimental models, tissue temperatures between 43°C and 50°C were associated with reversible tissue injury.[30] Langberg et al, in the study mentioned above, also showed that transiently effective RF applications (that is, pulses that cause conduction pathway block that recurs within the initial session, often within minutes of the application) were associated with a mean temperature of 50 ±8°C, whereas applications that permanently eliminated accessory pathway function were associated with a temperature of 62±15°C.[19] These transiently effective pulses presumably represent stunning of the pathway rather than complete necrosis and thus are analogous to applications that cause conduction block with recurrence after the ablation session. Similar observations were made by Chen et al.[18]

Using data from the Atakr (Medtronic CardioRhythm, Inc. San Jose, CA) thermocouple-tipped ablation catheter, Calkins et al directly analyzed the relationship between the maximum temperature recorded by the catheter tip during the ultimately successful ablation with the incidence of recurrence.[35] They showed that the electrode temperature achieved at successful sites associated with recurrence of conduction was not different than the electrode temperature achieved at successful sites without recurrence (61.1±8.9°C, range 44°C to 78°C, median 62°C versus 61.6±9.1°C, range 43°C to 105°C, median 61°C; $P = 0.8$). The most reasonable explanation for the lack of a measurable temperature difference is the inability to actually measure the tissue temperature at the actual site of the accessory pathway. Thus, a patient with a more epicardially situated pathway would presumably have a higher incidence of recurrence and might well have a lower peak ablation temperature at the site of the pathway (since ablation temperature drops off rapidly with increasing distance from the catheter tip) even though the temperature recorded at the thermocouple in the distal electrode tip might be high. A similar lack of correlation between peak ablation temperature achieved and the incidence of recurrence was shown by O'Connor et al.[36]

In contrast, Laohaprasitiporn et al, also using the Atakr system with closed-loop temperature control, showed that initially successful lesions that recurred (either during the ablation session itself or later) were associated with a higher temperature at the actual moment of conduction block than lesions that were permanently successful (55.0±7.9°C for transient lesions versus 49.8±7.7°8C for permanently effective lesions).[37] Although at first glance this seems contradictory to what we have written above, one explanation might be that conduction block achieved at a lower temperature may be a reflection of close proximity between the pathway and the electrode tip that allows optimal and rapid heat transference from the catheter to the actual accessory pathway location. Conversely, a high temperature might indicate greater than average separation between the catheter and the accessory pathway, a situation in which the actual temperature at the site of the accessory pathway might be significantly lower than that measured at the electrode tip. This would also explain why the maximal temperature achieved (as opposed to the temperature recorded at the moment of conduction block) might not correlate with success as was true for both this study and the 2 studies mentioned above. Further support for this hypothesis is that in the Laohaprasitiporn study there was also a correlation between the rapidity of the time to pathway disappearance and permanently successful lesions with a breakpoint between successful and only transiently successful ablations of 2.3 seconds. Again, longer time to pathway disappearance would also be an indicator of a greater distance between the ablation catheter and the actual pathway. Nevertheless these values are at variance with the earlier study of Langberg where the actual temperature at the time of either permanent or transient pathway conduction block was also measured and showed a much higher temperature for permanent as opposed to transient lesions. However, Langberg et al used a power-controlled ablation system and many applications were at only 20 or 30 watts of power, whereas the Atakr system used by Laohaprasitiporn used closed-loop power control, which would serve to partially negate any situation of suboptimal catheter-tissue contact by automatically continuing to increase power in an attempt to reach 70°C as well as, hopefully, a therapeutic temperature at the actual pathway site.

Slow Pathway Modification for AV Nodal Reentrant Tachycardia and Complete AV Block

In terms of slow pathway ablation for AV nodal reentrant tachycardia (AVNRT), factors that have been reported to correlate with recurrence include an inferior-posterior ablation site (at or caudal to the coronary sinus orifice) rather than more medial or superior ablation sites;[38] presence of residual slow pathway conduction, and/or a single AV nodal reentrant echo beat after ablation;[13,39] and absence of an accelerated junctional rhythm during the successful ablation pulse.[13] However, other investigators have failed to show any correlation between these factors and the incidence of slow pathway recurrence and the need for completely eliminating residual slow pathway function in patients rendered noninducible (with and without isoproterenol provocation) by ablation remains controversial.[16,38,40,41] Results of some of the larger studies analyzing recurrences in slow pathway ablations are shown in Table 2.

An analogous situation to the case of transient block of an accessory pathway may exist in the case of both slow pathway AV nodal modification and complete AV node ablation where successful ablation sites are usually associated with an accelerated junctional rhythm. Nath et al demonstrated that accelerated junctional rhythm could be produced by lower temperatures than those required to produce at least some degree of AV nodal block (51 ± 4°C versus 58 ± 6°C respectively) and that permanent AV block required temperatures in the range of 60 ± 7°C.[42] Since permanently successful ablations are also preceded by junctional rhythm, this may be a model for the ability of suboptimal

Table 2
Recurrences after AVNRT ablation

Reference	Date	# of patients	Recurrence rate of AVNRT (%)	Comments
Baker[13]	1994	143	7	40% recurrence rate in patients with residual SP function; 5% in patients without
Lindsay[40]	1993	59	2	41% of patients had residual SP function after ablation— 0% recurrences
Hummel[122]	1995	104	7	5% recurrence rate in patients with residual SP function; 8% without
Li[39]	1993	51	14	55% recurrence rate in patients with residual SP function; 3% without
Manolis[38]	1994	55	13	5% recurrence rate in patients with anterior ablation site
Chen[16]	1995	362	2.5	no association between recurrence rate and presence or absence of residual SP function
Jackman[10]	1992	80	0	ablation guided by slow-pathway potentials
Jazayeri[11]	1992	35	0	
Haïssaguerre[12]	1992	64	0	ablation guided by slow-pathway potentials
Wagshal (Atakr Registry)[111]	1995	138	5	

heating to produce electrophysiological effects on a target tissue without causing permanent conduction block. In further analogy to accessory pathway block, it was shown that the median time to onset of junctional rhythm was significantly shorter during successful applications compared with unsuccessful applications (1.8 seconds versus 7.7 seconds respectively).

Atrial Flutter Ablation and Other Ablation Targets

Other ablation targets may have an even higher recurrence rate, such as atrial flutter in which a comparatively large region (the isthmus between the tricuspid valve, coronary sinus, and inferior vena cava), as opposed to a single discrete pathway, must be ablated completely; and ventricular tachycardia associated with coronary artery disease where not only is there a large area but often multiple and/or deep tissue sites requiring ablation.[43,44] A survey of the larger studies of atrial flutter ablation reveals fairly significant recurrence rates for atrial flutter ranging from 9% to 44% (Table 3).[45–54] Saxon et al identified right atrial enlargement (defined as an end-systolic mediolateral dimension exceeding 4.6 centimeters) as an independent risk factor for atrial flutter recurrence.[45] This can be readily understood as increasing the size of the criti-

Table 3
Recurrences after atrial flutter ablation

Reference	Date	# of patients	Recurrence rate of atrial flutter (%)	Comments
Saxon[45]	1996	51	22	
Nath[46]	1995	22	23	
Philipon[47]	1995	59	9	
Poty[57]	1995	12	0	used isthmus conduction block as criterion for ablation success
Steinberg[48]	1995	16	25	
Fischer[49]	1995	80	19	
Kirkorian[50]	1994	22	16	
Chen[123]	1996	60	9	
Cauchemez[56]	1996	20	20	used isthmus conduction block as criterion for ablation success
Schwartzman[55]	1996	35	20	used isthmus conduction block as criterion for ablation success
Lesh[51]	1994	18	29	
Calkins[52]	1994	16	31	
Cosio[53]	1993	9	44	
Feld[54]	1992	16	17	

cal isthmus required for permanent successful atrial flutter ablation. The recurrence rate of atrial flutter can be significantly decreased by using as an end point for ablation success not only non-inducibility of atrial flutter but also conduction block in the isthmus reflecting ablation of the entire isthmus region (see also Chapter 12).[55–57]

In summary, recurrence of pathway conduction is a potential procedure complication for all forms of RF ablation. In most cases part of the difficulty is the inability to distinguish between transient stunning of the pathway with loss of conduction and total irreversible coagulation necrosis of the pathway. Many centers routinely deliver a booster pulse at the successful site in an attempt to assure adequate lesion size. While some investigators have suggested that this is helpful,[58] other studies have not shown any obvious improvement in the incidence of recurrence when using booster pulses.[7] Furthermore, Wittkampf et al demonstrated in an experimental study that repeated RF applications had little effect on lesion size or maximum intramyocardial temperature.[59] Most centers also use isoproterenol infusion and a waiting time of 30 to 60 minutes after the successful ablation pulse to verify that the ablation effect was not transient, although obviously this will not help with recurrences that become manifest only several days later. Adenosine infusions have also been used as an attempt to verify complete pathway ablation. Walker et al administered adenosine to a series of 107 patients after undergoing apparently successful ablation with no evidence of residual accessory pathway function and unmasked latent accessory pathway conduction in 12 patients.[60] These 12 patients underwent continued ablation attempts and 7 achieved adenosine-induced block, while 5 patients continued to demonstrate persistent accessory pathway conduction only with adenosine. All 5 of these patients experienced clinical recurrence of accessory pathway function. In a smaller study, however, Keim et al were unable to identify any patients in whom the use of adenosine brought out any latent antegrade or retrograde accessory pathway function.[61]

"A Late Cure" and Other Late Postablation Phenomena—Accessory Pathways

The opposite effect of pathway recurrence—so-called late cure—has also been described, in which conduction block is only achieved some time after an apparently unsuccessful ablation session, or following an apparently successful ablation session there is a recurrence of conduction followed only later by complete and often permanent conduction block.

Leitch et al observed several patients undergoing seemingly unsuccessful ablation who subsequently exhibited delayed loss of preexcitation 3 to 5 days after ablation.[62] However, the success was not permanent, as all patients regained preexcitation between 3 and 5 months later. It is quite reasonable to hypothesize that these patients' accessory pathways were located not in the area of necrosis but in the surrounding area of inflammation; thus, between 3 and 5 days later, when the inflammatory response would be expected to be at its height there could be loss of accessory pathway function, only to recur later after healing had occurred. Chen et al also reported that 5 of 10 patients undergoing an unsuccessful ablation attempt (out of a total group of 123 patients undergoing attempted accessory pathway ablation) developed late block of accessory pathway conduction after 1 to 3 days.[7] In all cases the original ablation session achieved only transient accessory pathway block. However 4 of these 5 patients subsequently had recurrence of the accessory pathway.

On the other hand, we have presented a group of patients from our laboratory who underwent initially successful RF ablation of accessory pathways (that is, leaving the lab with an apparently successful result, not just transient pathway block) who then developed recurrence of accessory pathway function but later progressed to complete pathway block which was subsequently shown to be a permanent cure based on follow-up electrophysiological testing and long-term clinical observation.[63] An example of such a patient is shown in Figure 1. The best explanation is that these patients' accessory pathways were on the edge of the original necrotic lesion in such a way that complete necrosis did not occur immediately but only several days later. Since these patients demonstrated immediate loss of preexcitation, presumably the accessory pathways of these patients were closer to the central zone of necrosis than those reported by Leitch et al.[62] Reports of similar patients have also been published by other investigators.[64–69] It is known from histological observations after lesion formation that the zone of coagulation necrosis is surrounded by a zone of inflammation and edema, where transient pathway effects could certainly be understood to occur (Figure 2). Furthermore, Nath et al have shown that this zone of tissue injury is characterized by a marked reduction in microvascular blood flow and associated with histological findings of microvascular endothelial injury.[70] Progression or resolution of this area of potential ischemia could account for either the late progression or regression of the RF-induced tissue injury.

The important lesson to be learned from these reports is that there can be considerable evolution of the ablation-induced lesion during the first few days postablation, which can lead to either recurrent accessory pathway conduction or to a long-lasting complete cure. Accordingly, we feel that it is appropriate to observe the patients for several days before making a decision as to whether or not a repeat ablation procedure is required, and then to obtain full electrophysiological evaluation of the residual accessory pathway characteristics before actually undertaking repeat RF energy deliveries.

A variety of other interesting, and so far not well understood, phenomena have been documented after accessory pathway ablation procedures. For example, patients with manifest preexcitation have been reported who developed recurrent accessory pathway conduction after ablation only in the retrograde direction (and who of course are still capable of orthodromic AV reciprocating

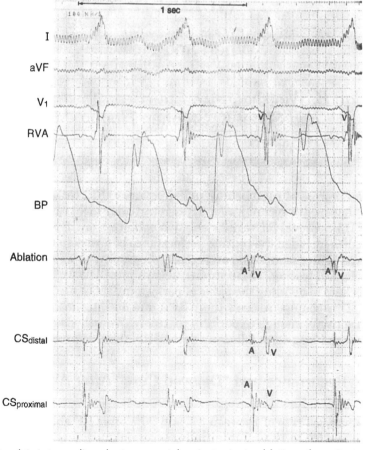

Figure 1. Panel A: Intracardiac electrograms taken just prior to ablation of a patient with a right free wall accessory pathway, demonstrating a short AV interval in the ablation electrogram (20 milliseconds). (*continued*)

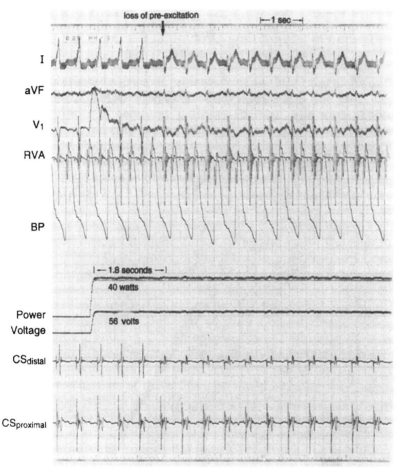

Figure 1. (*continued*) Panel B: After application of RF energy, there is prompt loss of preexcitation (1.8 seconds). (*continued*)

2 HOURS POST ABLATION

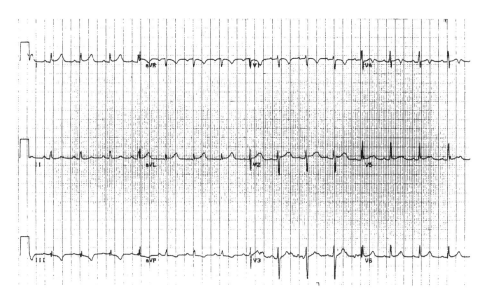

48 HOURS POST ABLATION

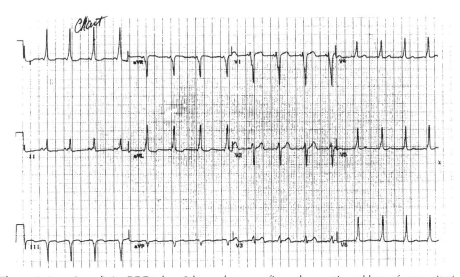

Figure 1. (*continued*) An ECG taken 2 hours later confirms the continued loss of preexcitation (Panel C). However, shortly thereafter the patient developed return of preexcitation (Panel D), (*continued*)

72 HOURS POST ABLATION

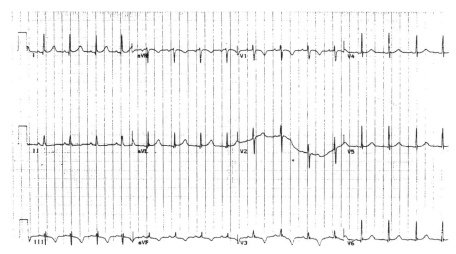

Figure 1. (*continued*) which persisted for more than 48 hours before finally disappearing (Panel E). Preexcitation remained absent and a follow-up electrophysiological study obtained a month later revealed no evidence of accessory pathway function either antegrade or retrograde. The patient has been followed for several years since and has remained free of recurrent preexcitation or supraventricular tachycardia. (Reprinted with permission from The American Journal of Cardiology, Excerpta Medica, Inc.[63])

tachycardia).[8] This would suggest that either the antegrade and retrograde-conducting limbs of the pathway are longitudinally separate pathways or that there is just 1 pathway and that partial damage resulted in loss of ability to conduct antegradely while retaining the ability to conduct retrogradely. Even harder to explain, Willems et al presented a group of patients in whom the converse situation was exhibited: they initially presented with a concealed accessory pathway but following catheter ablation they developed manifest preexcitation, apparently for the first time ever.[71]

Previous work has established that the site of conduction block in the antegrade direction of accessory pathways in patients with concealed accessory pathways is at the accessory pathway-ventricular interface.[72] This would suggest that 1 of the RF lesions had somehow modified the ventricular insertion of the accessory pathway so as to now allow bidirectional conduction. The ability of RF catheter ablation (apparently in a "subtherapeutic" dose) to result in the new appearance of manifest conduction suggests that pathways are intrinsically bidirectional in nature; i.e., not that concealed pathways are missing something that somehow prevents them from conducting bidirectionally, but rather that there is a specific structure that results in antegrade block in concealed pathways and that somehow this structure itself can be "ablated" by RF energy, thereby allowing antegrade pathway conduction.

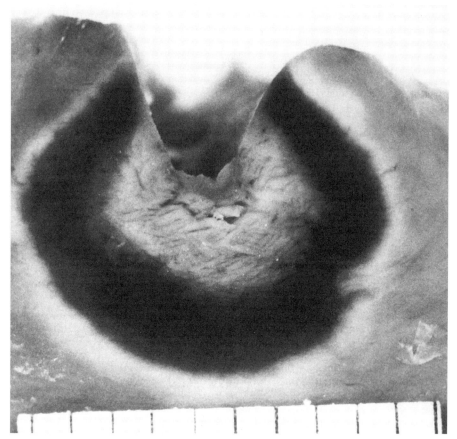

Figure 2. A cross-sectional view of a spherical lesion resulting from RF catheter ablation (15 watts × 30 seconds) of the canine left ventricular myocardium in the subacute stage (4 days following ablation). The sharply circumscribed coagulation necrosis was separated from the normal myocardium by a hemorrhagic zone and a rim of mononuclear cell infiltration. The lesion measured 9 × 8 × 5.5 mm. (The reader should note that this lesion was created under ideal circumstances in a laboratory model. It is certainly known that typical clinical lesions are much smaller and it may well be in such lesions that the ratio of inflammation to the actual area of coagulation necrosis itself might be considerably larger). Reprinted with permission from the C.V. Mosby Company from Huang, SKS. RF catheter ablation of cardiac arrhythmias: appraisal of an evolving therapeutic modality. *Am Heart J* 1989; 118:1317–1323.

AVNRT

A variety of interesting observations have also been noted following modification of dual AV nodal pathways for treatment of AVNRT. One example is the occurrence of new atypical AVNRT following the anterior approach to AV nodal modification, in which a slow pathway is now used for retrograde conduction resulting in "slow-slow" tachycardia.[11,14,73,74] Avoidance of this new tachycardia by the posterior ablation approach which targets the slow pathway is an advantage of the slow pathway approach.

Ehlert et al were the first to describe persistent inappropriate sinus tachycardia following fast pathway AV nodal modification.[75] Chen et al described 8 patients out of a series of 314 undergoing slow pathway AV nodal modification with recurrent palpitations after a mean follow-up of 27 ± 11 months who were found to not have recurrent AVNRT but rather inappropriate sinus tachycardia (2 patients) or atrial flutter/fibrillation (5 patients) documented both by event monitoring and by follow-up electrophysiological testing.[16] Skeberis et al specifically addressed the issue of symptomatic inappropriate sinus tachycardia (i.e., sinus tachycardia not related to activity or other precipitants) and reported an incidence of 12 of 118 patients—all of whom had received fast-pathway AV nodal modification.[76] In all but 3 patients, the inappropriate sinus tachycardia lasted less than 1 week, and a total of 4 patients required β-blocker therapy for between 1 and 3 months after the procedure.

Madrid et al used Holter monitoring with heart rate variability analysis to study inappropriate sinus tachycardia after ablation.[77] They discovered an incidence of inappropriate sinus tachycardia on the day after ablation in 10 of 170 patients associated with altered heart rate variability parameters; the remaining 160 patients had, in addition to normal heart rates, normal postprocedure heart rate variability parameters. These 10 patients included 5 patients with ablations for AVNRT and 4 patients with posteroseptal accessory pathway ablations. All Holter and heart rate variability parameters normalized on Holter monitoring 3 months later.

Kocovic et al reported a significant reduction in heart rate variability and attenuation of the parasympathetic component (high frequency) of heart rate variability immediately after AVNRT or posterosepetal accessory pathway ablation in 58% of their patients.[78] This is in agreement with animal studies on the parasympathetic innervation of the AV and sinus nodes which have shown that postganglionic vagal fibers ultimately destined for the sinus node travel across the inferior inter-atrial septum near the opening of the coronary sinus.[79–81] Thus, these fibers could certainly be easily affected by either posteroseptal accessory pathway or AV nodal ablations. Also of note was that these abnormalities tended to disappear between 1 and 6 months on follow-up Holter recordings, in agreement with the time expected for re-innervation of the parasympathetic nerves (about 6 weeks in animal modes).[82] The authors speculated that this parasympathetic denervation may also play a role in the shortening of the effective refractory period of the fast AV nodal pathway after successful slow pathway ablation described by several investigators.[10–12,83] However, other authors have explained this phenomenon as the result of release of electrotonic inhibition on the fast pathway from the slow pathway after slow pathway ablation, in part based on the lack of effect of parasympathetic inhibition on these changes.[84,85]

Another reported sequelae of AV node modification is the delayed development of complete AV block, presumably analogous to other forms of "late cure," although here, of course, it is unintentional and unwanted. This has been reported to occur as late as 6 to 30 days after the ablation. Late development of AV block has been reported following modification of the AV node using the fast-pathway or anterior approach[9,11,83,86–88] as well as the slow pathway or posterior approach.[67,89] Williamson et al reported 3 late complete AV blocks up to 3 days after posterior AV node modification for rate control of rapid atrial fibrillation.[90] Common to all these reports has been the finding that late complete AV block is always preceded by transient AV block during the procedure itself. This would suggest that patients manifesting transient AV block should be observed carefully for at least several days after the procedure to watch for sudden recurrent symptomatic AV block. Transient ventriculo-atrial block during the junctional rhythm that is often associated with successful ablation sites and/or faster than usual rates for the junctional rhythm during AV node modification may presage either transient or permanent AV block and may be valuable early signs to watch for during ablation to minimize the chances of unwanted late AV block.[89,91]

Section 2: Late Appearance of Side Effects

Most side effects occur during the ablation procedure and are thus outside the subject matter of this chapter. However, other side effects manifest later and are worthy of discussion here, particularly as they have an impact on the follow-up of the patient.

Effects on Nearby Coronary Arteries

Two studies have specifically addressed the issue of possible effects on the nearby coronary artery after RF ablation of accessory pathways located along either the tricuspid or mitral annulus.[92,93] In both studies no effects were seen. In the series of 100 patients undergoing RF ablation of accessory pathways described by Lesh et al,[4] 1 patient developed chest pain and transient ST elevation during application of RF energy. Coronary spasm was suspected, but results of coronary angiography were normal. The demonstration of lack of effect of RF ablation on coronary arteries is not unexpected given the small size of the RF lesion produced during ablation as well as the fact that the rapid blood flow through the coronary arteries would prevent any local heat build-up. However, inadvertent cannulation of the coronary artery resulting in spasm or occlusion and leading to acute myocardial infarction has been reported,[94] and care should therefore certainly be taken to avoid this. Obviously, at the current time, follow-up after ablation procedures is still only short-term and it is possible that there may be some subtle changes in coronary arteries that are not visible after ablation but which might result in accelerated atherosclerosis 10 or 20 years later. It should also be pointed out that T wave abnormalities are common after ablation of manifest accessory pathways but are related to repolarization changes and "T wave memory" and do not represent ischemia.[95–97]

Proarrhythmic Effects of Ablation Lesions

We previously reported the appearance of new inducible atrial tachycardia in 6 of 37 patients following RF catheter ablation of the slow AV nodal pathway on 1 month follow-up study. The tachycardia origin was from the low right atrium and potentially from the site of an ablation attempt or attempts. Correspondingly, this arrhythmia was more frequently demonstrated in patients receiving a larger number of RF applications during the ablation session. However, all of these patients were asymptomatic and none demonstrated any episodes of tachycardia on Holter monitoring. There is also a report of 1 case of an atrial tachycardia caused by DC ablation of a bypass tract more than 10 years ago.[98]

Strickberger et al performed programmed ventricular stimulation after accessory pathway ablation in a small group of patients and found no evidence of ventricular proarrhythmia either by electrophysiological testing (using 3 extrastimuli) or by Holter monitoring both immediately after and several months after the ablation procedure.[92]

An interesting report showed that over time RF lesions delivered to newborn sheep myocardium grew larger as the animal and its heart grew larger.[99] The clinical implications of this finding are unknown, although the authors suggest that because of the paucity of long-term follow-up data available that appropriate caution be advised particularly in infants or children undergoing RF cardiac ablation regarding the possibility of late proarrhythmic or other cardiac effects from the ablation lesions.

Thromboembolism

At least theoretically the creation of a RF ablation lesion in the ventricle could be a nidus for thromboembolism. Experimental ablation procedures in animal models have also shown that occasionally there is a thin layer of thrombus overlying the endocardial surface of the ablation lesion (Figure 3).[21,100] Manolis et al studied the thrombotic tendency for ablation lesions by measuring plasma levels of D-dimer, a product of fibrin degradation, immediately before and after RF ablation procedures and showed a significant increase after ablation that persisted at least 48 hours after the procedure.[101] Similar changes in D-dimer levels were not seen after routine electrophysiological study testing, and thus are presumably from the ablation lesions themselves. These increases in D-dimer levels all occurred in patients despite systemic heparinization. However the clinical relevance of this finding is completely unknown—in particular, it is unknown whether these elevations in D-dimer levels are related to a tendency for clinical embolic events and whether a higher level of D-dimer corresponds to a higher risk of embolic events; also unknown is whether these elevations are irrelevant such that when clinical events do occur they are unassociated with the pathophysiology that raises the D-dimer levels. There is also speculation that ablation pulses associated with an acute impedance rise and coagulum formation on the catheter tip can be a potential nidus of embolic complications. Because of all these concerns about embolic side effects, most investigators use systemic level heparinization during the ablation (particularly for left sided ablations) and approximately 325 mg of aspirin for 1–3 months after ablation.

Although fairly uncommon, some embolic events have been reported following ablation. In 1 of the first reports of the efficacy of RF ablation, 1 case of a postprocedure transient neurological ischemic event was reported.[94] In the Atakr ablation system registry, 1 child suffered a small nonhemorrhagic stroke shortly after an ablation procedure.[102] No embolic complications occurred in a report of complications after over 300 ablations from our laboratory.[103]

Thakur et al specifically addressed the incidence of embolic complications in 153 patients undergoing left sided accessory pathway ablations and reported 3 patients with symptoms of systemic embolization (2 patients with a cerebral emboli and 1 patient with a renal embolus) all of whom, somewhat surprisingly, developed their embolic event only after 1–3.5 months after ablation.[104] In the European catheter ablation registry, there was also a small percentage of patients suffering embolic complications from ablation.[105] The results of this study are described in detail in chapter 34.

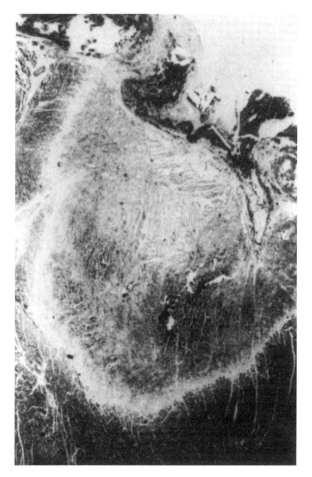

Figure 3. Low power photomicrograph of an acute lesion (7 days old) from an animal model showing a well-circumscribed area of ablated myocardium with a small adherent fibrinous mural thrombus. (Trichrome stain; original magnification × 18.) Reprinted with permission from the C.V. Mosby Company from Ring ME, Huang SKS, Graham AR, et al. Catheter ablation of the ventricular septum with RF energy. *Am Heart J* 117:1233–1240.

Sudden Death Following Complete AV Node Ablation

Perhaps most importantly, there have been several reports of sudden cardiac death, presumably the result of torsades de pointes or polymorphic ventricular tachycardia/ventricular fibrillation after complete AV node ablation. This was first reported after direct current ablation of the AV junction and as it was not reported with RF ablation for many years, sudden death was presumed to be secondary to extension of the lesion from the AV node into the ventricle as a result of the known propensity of high current DC ablation to cause large and/or far field lesions.[106,107] Subsequently, however, reports of sudden cardiac death following RF ablation of the AV node also were reported.[108] We have reported from the Atakr database 3 instances of late sudden cardiac death (2 patients with documented ventricular fibrillation) between 7 and 272 days after complete ablation of the AV node using RF energy.[109] All 3 patients had significant preexisting left ventricular dysfunction, and all were paced at a lower rate limit of between 70 and 90 beats per minute.

Conti et al described 3 patients (out of a pool of 38 patients) after complete AV node ablation with polymorphic ventricular tachycardia after the procedure and showed that in these patients (but not in patients without polymorphic ventricular tachycardia postablation) there was a significant increase in QT dispersion.[110] These patients all had severely depressed left ventricular function. The runs of ventricular tachycardia appeared to be bradycardia dependent and could be suppressed by increasing the ventricular pacing rate to 90 beats per minute. This change in pacing rate also significantly decreased the QT dispersion. This postablation polymorphic VT appeared to be a transient phenomenon because no patient had a recurrent life-threatening arrhythmia after discharge (with 13±3 months of follow-up)—although data on follow-up QT dispersion measurements were not reported.

Section 3: Utility of Ancillary Testing After Ablation

Electrophysiological Testing

Given the recurrence rate following ablation discussed in the first section of this chapter, as well as the occasional appearance of unusual ablation-related electrophysiological effects, the need for routine follow-up studies in patients after apparently successful RF ablation needs to be defined. We have addressed this issue as well as the role of trans-telephonic event monitoring as an alternative modality for follow-up in 310 patients undergoing successful RF catheter ablation (134 undergoing slow pathway ablation for AV nodal reentrant tachycardia, 172 undergoing ablation of accessory pathways, and 4 undergoing both procedures) who participated in the Atakr registry.[111] A routine follow-up electrophysiological study between 1 and 3 months postablation was performed in 247 out of the 310 patients as part of the study protocol, and patients developing palpitations postablation were encouraged to use an event monitor. Of these, 23 patients (7.4%) developed a recurrence of their supraventricular tachycardia (7, or 5.2%, with AVNRT and 16, or 9.3%, with an accessory pathway-related tachycardia) at a mean of 46 ± 47 days (range 1 day to 8 months) postablation. This is comparable to the results of other studies discussed earlier in this chapter. As shown in Figure 4, only 2 of these 23 recurrences were discovered by follow-up electrophysiological testing in asymptomatic patients (both of whom had concealed accessory pathways and 1 of whom was a 4-year-old child); in the remaining 21 patients a positive follow-up electrophysiological study was heralded by either recurrent symptoms (17 patients), recurrent preexcitation on ECG (9 patients), and/or by an episode of recurrent supraventricular tachycardia documented by a rhythm strip (9 patients). In this series, event monitoring was shown to be a valuable complementary technique to follow-up electrophysiological study, in that it not only correctly identified patients with a recurrence who had a symptomatic episode of supraventricular tachycardia while activating the event monitor, but also that event monitoring correctly eliminated recurrent supraventricular tachycardia as the cause of palpitations in all 8 symptomatic patients in whom another rhythm was identified as the cause of the symptoms (nonsustained atrial

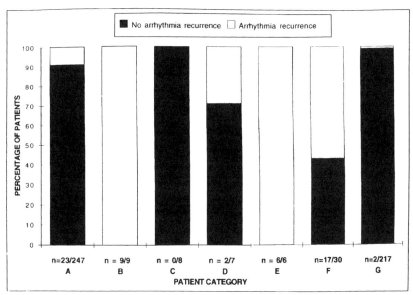

Figure 4. Yield of follow-up electrophysiological studies after ablation by various patient categories. The numbers separated by a slash are the incidence of positive electrophysiological studies/total number of patients in that category. A = all patients; B = electrocardiographic evidence of recurrent preexcitation; C = postablation palpitations with an etiology other than arrhythmia recurrence detected by event monitoring; D = postablation palpitations and normal event monitoring; E = documented arrhythmia recurrence by electrocardiogram or event monitoring; F = all patients with symptoms of postablation palpitations; G = patients without symptoms or electrocardiographic findings. The use of event monitoring and symptoms was sufficient to either rule in or exclude arrhythmia recurrence in all but 2 patients out of the entire sample of 247 patients. (Reprinted with permission from the America Journal of Cardiology, Excerpta Medica, Inc.[111])

tachycardia in 2 patients, atrial premature contractions in 1 patient, atrial flutter in 1 patient, sinus tachycardia in 3 patients, and a slow junctional rhythm in 1 patient).

Based on this study, we conclude that the yield of follow-up electrophysiological study in patients who are either asymptomatic or have palpitations with another etiology shown on event monitor is very low (only 2 of 247 patients, or 0.8% in this series); so that in most cases, routine follow-up electrophysiological study does not appear to be warranted. Furthermore, event monitoring is a useful modality to identify the cause of palpitations after RF catheter ablation and it can further reduce the need for follow-up electrophysiological studies. A study by Mann et al similarly noted that although palpitations occur frequently following RF catheter ablation, many times these palpitations do not represent pathway recurrence, but instead represent other usually benign rhythm disturbances such as sinus tachycardia or isolated premature atrial or ventricular contractions.[112] This study is discussed later in this chapter under the subheading of Holter monitoring. A similar conclusion was reached by Chen et al after performing 326 follow-up studies which provided the first evidence of recurrence in only 4 patients.[113]

It must be kept in mind that most patients undergoing RF catheter ablation for supraventricular arrhythmias are at least moderately symptomatic, thus the absence of recurrent symptoms over a long period following ablation suggests that a recurrence is unlikely. Similarly patients with manifest preexcitation can usually be followed merely by a 12-lead ECG, although it is theoretically possible, as described above, for an occasional patient who presented initially with manifest preexcitation to develop a recurrence of concealed (retrograde-only) pathway function. Possible exceptions might include patients whose initial presentation of supraventricular tachycardia was associated with syncope and/or hemodynamic collapse, or patients in high risk professions such as commercial vehicle drivers, airplane pilots, or professional athletes where even a single recurrence could have grave consequences.

Doppler Echocardiography

Several studies have performed echocardiograms routinely after ablation and noted abnormal findings in a small percentage of patients, such as cavity thrombus, aortic valve leaflet perforation, or aortic regurgitation. These findings, however, might not necessarily have been related to the ablation in that most studies did not include preablation echocardiograms. Minich et al did compare preablation and postablation (within 24 hours after ablation) echocardiograms and noted a 30% incidence of new mild (1+) aortic regurgitation by Doppler echocardiography after retrograde left sided ablation procedures.[114] In all cases, however, the aortic regurgitation was only mild, and without any hemodynamic consequences. An interesting case was recently reported of a patient who developed fever and elevated white count following a retrograde left sided ablation procedure in which an aortic valve mass (presumably a thrombus) was documented by echocardiography on the day following ablation. This mass subsequently disappeared after heparin therapy.[115] The use of transesophageal echocardiogram, which is superior to transthoracic studies in detecting mural thrombus, has identified rare cases of small intraventricular thrombus after catheter ablations of accessory pathways using the ventricular approach. As suggested by the authors, however, in many cases the location of these thrombi suggests that they may have been unrelated to the ablation lesions themselves, although prolonged catheter placement might have played a role. None of these patients suffered an embolic event over a several-month-long period of follow-up.[116] Seifert et al reported a single case of aortic leaflet perforation following left sided ablation.[117]

We previously reported the results of a systematic multicenter trial to assess the utility of echocardiography using pre- and postablation (within 24 hours of ablation) echocardiograms as part of the aforementioned Atakr study.[102] In a series of 355 consecutive patients from 10 participating centers who underwent a total of 373 uncomplicated RF catheter ablations of accessory pathways (n=214), slow pathway of the AV node (n=120), and complete AV junction (n=39), we found that the routine use of postablation 2-dimensional Doppler echocardiography rarely identified clinically unsuspected abnormalities. Intracardiac thrombus was not identified in any patient. New wall motion abnormalities were noted in 6 patients (1.6 %), although for the group as a whole, the overall left ventricular ejection fraction was unchanged. New mild (1+) mitral, aortic, or tricuspid valve regurgitations were noted in a small number of patients: 21 (5.4%), 9 (2.3%), and 20 (5.2%) patients respectively, but there were no cases of significant valvular dysfunction. Furthermore, in many cases these new postablation echocardiographic findings did not appear to correlate with the type or approach to ablation in that they were often anatomically disparate from the site of ablation. For example, several of the cases of mild aortic regurgitation were found in patients who did not have the aortic valve crossed as part of the procedure, and 5 of the 6 patients with new mild wall motion abnormalities had these findings in areas of the heart remote from the ablation. Even when the echo changes occurred in proximity to the ablation catheter, it was unclear if they were related to the RF ablation lesion itself or from catheter manipulation. A small pericardial effusion was identified in 11 patients (5 other patients were excluded from the study because they developed clinically overt cardiac perforation and cardiac tamponade during the procedure). There was a variety of minor findings on the preablation echocardiograms, all of which were either unchanged or improved postablation. With a mean follow-up of 15±6.0 months, there were no clinical sequelae possibly related to any of the echo findings. Because of this and the seeming lack of relationship between the ablation and the echocardiogram findings, most of which were trivial, there did not appear to be any value to routine postablation echocardiography. The 1 patient in this series who had an embolic complication (a 6-year-old girl who had a nonhemorrhagic stroke several hours after ablation of a left sided pathway) had normal pre- and post-ablation echocardiograms. Calkins et al described 1 patient who experienced a transient cerebral ischemic event 5 days after an uncomplicated ablation; again, the echocardiogram was normal.[94] Similar results were reported in the ablation series of Lesh et al, in which routine echocardiography was performed in all patients.[4] They reported that no cases of pericardial effusion (except in clinically overt pericardial tamponade from catheter perforation), intracardiac thrombus, or valve disruption were detected. A study using pre- and post-ablation echocardiography in 74 left sided pediatric ablation procedures using the transseptal approach revealed only 1 1-month-old infant who developed new mitral regurgitation after an ablation.[118] Furthermore, the mitral regurgitation was mild and remained mild after 1 year of follow-up.

Cardiac Enzyme Determinations

Many studies also routinely collected blood specimens for serial cardiac enzyme determinations following RF catheter ablation. All of these studies showed that cardiac enzymes following ablation were always in the normal range and did not reveal any significant myocardial necrosis as a result of the ablation procedures.[1,94] Although important initially to document the safety of this technique, all investigators are in agreement that this is no longer necessary. Furthermore, an interesting report by Haines et al suggested that creatine kinase enzyme determinations are useless for another reason, namely that the local heating at the site of the lesion inhibits enzyme release, so that any small local myocardial damage at the ablation site itself would probably not be detected by enzyme measurements.[119]

Holter Monitoring

Earlier in this section we described our results from the Atakr registry showing the value of Holter or event monitoring in identifying the cause of palpitations after ablation. An even higher incidence of 58% for postablation palpitations (with 61% of these patients reporting palpitations severe enough that they were suspicious of pathway recurrence) was reported by Mann et al using outpatient surveys 1 month after ablation.[111] However, on follow-up electrophysiological testing 3 months after ablation only 8 patients (10%) had tachycardia recurrence and 1 additional patient had inducible atrial tachycardia; the remainder had negative follow-up studies. It is not clear how many of these symptoms were related to anxiety or undue concentration on the heartbeat by these patients, or were organic in nature such as inappropriate sinus tachycardia or premature beats perhaps related to the procedure itself. Similar incidences of symptomatic sinus tachycardia and atrial and ventricular premature beats were reported by Jordaens et al using event monitoring.[120] Johnson et al also performed serial Holter monitoring before, immediately after, and 1–2 months after ablation and found no overall increase in supraventricular or ventricular ectopy in pediatric patients undergoing ablation, although 3 out of 31 patients in the study experienced occasional episodes of nonsustained ventricular tachycardia in the immediate postablation period without symptoms and without recurrence.[121] Similar results of Holter monitoring after ablation, namely infrequent arrhythmias in the immediate postablation period without long-term sequelae, were also shown in a study by Chen et al.[16]

Conclusions

Based on the above observations, we feel that in all cases of uncomplicated RF catheter ablation, no specific follow-up procedures are mandatory. Certainly the development of fever, a new heart murmur, or other evidence of a problem would, of course, require a detailed work-up to elicit the exact cause. Such an approach of avoiding routine follow-up studies would certainly result in considerable saving of costs. Palpitations following ablation may indicate an arrhythmia recurrence but also may indicate a variety of other rhythm disturbances, either related or unrelated the ablation procedure. If possible, these should be investigated with either Holter monitoring or event monitoring prior to a follow-up electrophysiological study, with the possible exception of patients in certain high risk professions as discussed earlier.

Because of the possibility of a late cure, all patients undergoing an initially successful ablation procedure and then developing recurrence of the targeted arrhythmia should undergo a period of at least 1 to 2 weeks of waiting and then, if evidence of recurrence is still present, a comprehensive repeat electrophysiological study before undergoing repeat attempts at catheter ablation or, even more so, surgical ablation.

Finally, this somewhat long chapter must be kept in perspective. Many of the phenomena described here are rare, many based on only a few case reports. However, because of the relative infancy of RF catheter ablation procedures, every reported side effect spurs further research that enhances our knowledge of the effects of RF ablation, as, for example, a few cases of idiopathic sinus tachycardia after AV nodal modification led to research and enhanced understanding of the anatomy and possible effects of RF ablation on the parasympathetic supply to the heart, a few cases of "late cure" led to research on the microvascular pathology of RF lesions, a few cases of pathway recurrence helped promote the use of temperature monitoring, and a few cases of new onset of manifest preexcitation in previously concealed accessory pathways changed our concepts of the nature of conduction block in these pathways, and so on. The vast majority of patients (80% to 90% or more, in fact) will have a successful ablation without recurrence or late side effects, and will be truly cured of their arrhythmia without the need of medications or, at least in the case of supraventricular tachycardia, the need for any long-term follow-up. Furthermore, through greater understanding of the nature of accessory pathways and of the effects of RF energy on the heart, as well as continued improvements in catheter design and ablation techniques, we can expect only continued increases in the percentages of patients undergoing long-term, complication-free cures of their arrhythmias.

References

1. Jackman WM, Xunzhang W, Friday KJ, et al. Catheter ablation of accessory AV pathways (Wolff-Parkinson-White syndrome) by radiofrequency current. *N Engl J Med* 1991;324:1605–1611.

2. Calkins H, Langberg JJ, Sousa J, et al. Radiofrequency catheter ablation of accessory AV connections in 250 patients: abbreviated therapeutic approach to Wolff-Parkinson-White syndrome. *Circulation* 1992;85:1137–1346.

3. Swartz JF, Tracy CM, Fletcher RD. Radiofrequency endocardial catheter ablation of accessory AV pathway atrial insertion sites. *Circulation* 1993; 87:487–499.

4. Lesh MD, Van Hare GF, Schamp DJ, et al. Curative percutaneous catheter ablation using radiofrequency energy for accessory pathways in all locations: results in 100 consecutive patients. *J Am Coll Cardiol* 1992;19:1303–1309.

5. Wang L, Hu D, Ding Y, et al. Predictors of early and late recurrence of AV accessory pathway conduction after apparently successful radiofrequency catheter ablation. *Int J Cardiol* 1994;46:61–65.

6. Twidale N, Wang X, Beckman KJ, et al. Factors associated with recurrence of accessory pathway conduction after radiofrequency catheter ablation. *PACE* 1991;14:2042–2048.

7. Chen X, Kottkamp H, Hindricks G, et al. Recurrence and late block of accessory pathway conduction following radiofrequency catheter ablation. *J Cardiovasc Electrophysiol* 1994;5:650–658.

8. Langberg JJ, Calkins H, Kim Y, et al. Recurrence of conduction in accessory AV connections after initially successful radiofrequency catheter ablation. *J Am Coll Cardiol* 1992;19:1588–1592.

9. Kay GN, Epstein AE, Dailey SM, et al. Selective radiofrequency ablation of the slow pathway for the treatment of AV nodal reentrant tachycardia: evidence for involvement of perinodal myocardium within the reentrant circuit. *Circulation* 1992;85:1675–1688.

10. Jackman WM, Beckman KJ, McClelland JH, et al. Treatment of supraventricular tachycardia due to AV nodal reentry by radiofrequency catheter ablation of slow-pathway conduction. *N Engl J Med* 1992;327:313–318.

11. Jazayeri MR, Hempe SL, Sra JS, et al. Selective transcatheter ablation of the fast and slow pathways using radiofrequency energy in patients with AV nodal reentrant tachycardia. *Circulation* 1992;85:1318–1328.

12. Haïssaguerre M, Gaita F, Fischer B, et al. Elimination of AV nodal reentrant tachycardia using discrete slow potentials to guide application of radiofrequency energy. *Circulation* 1992;85:2162–2175.

13. Baker JH, Plumb VJ, Epstein AE, et al. Predictors of recurrent AV nodal reentry after selective slow pathway ablation. *Am J Cardiol* 1994;73:765–769.

14. Morady F, Calkins H, Langberg JJ, et al. A prospective randomized comparison of direct current and radiofrequency ablation of the AV junction. *J Am Coll Cardiol* 1993;21:102–109.

15. Olgin JE, Scheinman MM. Comparison of high energy direct current and radiofrequency catheter ablation of the AV junction. *J Am Coll Cardiol* 1993;21:557–564.

16. Chen S-A, Wu T-J, Chiang C-E, et al. Recurrent tachycardia after selective ablation of slow pathway in patients with AV nodal reentrant tachycardia. *Am J Cardiol* 1995;76:131–137.

17. Schlüter M, Geiger M, Siebels J, et al. Catheter ablation using radiofrequency current to cure symptomatic patients with tachyarrhythmias related to an accessory AV pathway. *Circulation* 1991;84:1644–1661.

18. Chen X, Borggrefe M, Hindricks G, et al. Radiofrequency ablation of accessory pathways: Characteristics of transiently and permanently effective pulses. *PACE* 1992;15:1122–1130.

19. Langberg JJ, Calkins H, El-Atassi R, et al. Temperature monitoring during radiofrequency catheter ablation of accessory pathways. *Circulation* 1992;86:1469–1474.

20. Wagshal AB, Pires LA, Bonavita GJ, et al. Does the baseline impedance measurement during radiofrequency catheter ablation influence the likelihood of an impedance rise? *Cardiology* 1996;87:42–45.

21. Hoyt RH, Huang SKS, Marcus FI, et al. Factors influencing trans-catheter radiofrequency ablation of the myocardium. *J Appl Cardiol* 1986;1986:469–485.

22. Harvey M, Kim Y-N, Sousa J, et al. Impedance monitoring during radiofrequency catheter ablation in humans. *PACE* 1992;15:22–27.

23. Strickberger SA, Vorperian VR, Man KC, et al. Relation between impedance and endocardial contact during radiofrequency catheter ablation. *Am Heart J* 1994;128:226–229.

24. Calkins H, Prystowsky E, Carlson M, et al. Temperature monitoring during radiofrequency catheter ablation procedures using closed loop control. *Circulation* 1994;90:1279–1286.

25. Blouin LT, Marcus FI, Lampe L. Assessment of effects of a radiofrequency energy field and thermistor location in an electrode catheter on the accuracy of temperature measurement. *PACE* 1991;14:807–813.

26. Haines DE, Whayne JG. Accuracy of a single tip thermistor in the measurement of the peak tissue temperature during radiofrequency ablation [abstract]. *Circulation* 1993;88:I–400.

27. Wittkampf FHM, Simmers TA, Hauer RNW, et al. Myocardial temperature response during radiofrequency catheter ablation. *PACE* 1995;18:307–317.

28. Nakagawa H, Yamanashi WS, Pitha JV, et al. Comparison of in vivo tissue temperature profile and lesion geometry for radiofrequency ablation with a saline-irrigated electrode versus temperature control in a canine thigh muscle preparation. *Circulation* 1995;91:2264–2273.

29. Kottkamp H, Hindricks G, Horst E, et al. Intramural temperature measurements during radiofrequency catheter ablation in chronic myocardial infarction [abstract]. *Eur Heart J* 1995;16(II):318.

30. Nath S, Lynch C, Whayne JG, et al. Cellular electrophysiological effects of hyperthermia on isolated guinea pig papimuscle: implications for catheter ablation. *Circulation* 1993;88:1826–1831.

31. Simmers TA, Wittkampf FHM, de Bakker JMT, et al. Relationship between myocardial temperature gradient and volume of permanently and transiently affected tissue: implications for radiofrequency ablation [abstract]. *Circulation* 1993;88:I–399.

32. Haines DE, Watson DD. Tissue heating during radiofrequency catheter ablation: a thermodynamic model and observations in isolated perfused and superfused canine right ventricular free wall. *PACE* 1989;12:962–976.

33. Haines DE, Verow AF. Observations on electrode-tissue interface tempera-

ture and effect on electrical impedance during radiofrequency ablation of ventricular myocardium. *Circulation* 1990;82:1034–1038.

34. Hindricks G, Haverkamp W, Gulker H. Radiofrequency coagulation of ventricular myocardium: improved prediction of lesion size by monitoring catheter tip temperature. *Eur Heart J* 1989;10:972–984.

35. Calkins H, Prystowsky E, Berger RD, et al. Recurrence of conduction following radiofrequency catheter ablation procedures: relationship to ablation target and electrode temperature. *J Cardiovasc Electrophysiol* 1996; 7:704–712.

36. O'Connor BK, Knick BJ, Taylor SJ, et al. Electrode-tissue interface temperature as a predictor of pathway recurrence after successful radiofrequency ablation during childhood [abstract]. *Circulation* 1994;90:I–99.

37. Laohaprasitiporn D, Walsh EP, Saul JP, et al. Predictors of permanence of successful radiofrequency lesions created with controlled catheter tip temperature. *PACE* 1997;20:1283–1291.

38. Manolis AS, Wang PJ, Estes NA. Radiofrequency ablation of slow pathway in patients with AV nodal reentrant tachycardia: do arrhythmia recurrences correlate with persistent slow pathway conduction or site of successful ablation? *Circulation* 1994;90:2815–2819.

39. Li HG, Klein GJ, Stites HW, et al. Elimination of slow pathway conduction: an accurate indicator of clinical success after radiofrequency AV node modification. *J Am Coll Cardiol* 1993;22:1849–1853.

40. Lindsay BD, Chung MK, Gamache C, et al. Therapeutic end points for the treatment of AV node reentrant tachycardia by catheter-guided radiofrequency current. *J Am Coll Cardiol* 1993;22:733–740.

41. Wang CC, Yeh SJ, Wen MS, et al. Late clinical and electrophysiological outcome of radiofrequency ablation therapy by the inferior approach in AV node reentry tachycardia. *Am Heart J* 1994;128:219–226.

42. Nath S, DiMarco JP, Mounsey JP, et al. Correlation of temperature and pathophysiological effect during radiofrequency catheter ablation of the AV junction. *Circulation* 1995;92:1188–1192.

43. Callans DJ, Schwartzman D, Gottlieb CD, et al. Insights into the electrophysiology of ventricular tachycardia gained by the catheter ablation experience: A learning while burning." *J Cardiovasc Electrophysiol* 1994;5:877–894.

44. Blanchard SM, Walcott GP, Wharton JM, et al. Why is catheter ablation less successful than surgery for treating ventricular tachycardia that results from coronary artery disease? *PACE* 1994;17:2315–2335.

45. Saxon LA, Kalman JM, Olgin JE, et al. Results of radiofrequency catheter ablation for atrial flutter. *Am J Cardiol* 1996;77:1014–1016.

46. Nath S, Mounsey JP, Haines DE, et al. Predictors of acute and long-term success after radiofrequency catheter ablation of type 1 atrial flutter. *Am J Cardiol* 1995;76:604–606.

47. Philipon F, Plumb VJ, Epstein AE, et al. The risk of atrial fibrillation following radiofrequency catheter ablation of atrial flutter. *Circulation* 1995; 92:430–435.

48. Steinberg JS, Prasher S, Zelenkofske S, et al. Radiofrequency catheter ablation of atrial flutter: procedural success and long term outcome. *Am Heart J* 1995;130:85–92.

49. Fischer B, Haïssaguerre M, Garrigues S, et al. Radiofrequency catheter ablation of common atrial flutter in 80 patients. *J Am Coll Cardiol* 1995;25:1365–1372.
50. Kirkorian G, Moncada E, Chevalier P, et al. Radiofrequency ablation of atrial flutter. *Circulation* 1994;90:2804–2814.
51. Lesh MD, Van Hare GF, Epstein L, et al. Radiofrequency catheter ablation of atrial arrhythmias. *Circulation* 1994;89:1074–1089.
52. Calkins H, Leon AR, Deam AG, et al. Catheter ablation of atrial flutter using radiofrequency energy. *Am J Cardiol* 1994;73:353–356.
53. Cosio FG, Lopez-Gil M, Goicolea A, et al. Radiofrequency ablation of the inferior vena cava-tricuspid valve isthmus in common atrial flutter. *Am J Cardiol* 1993;71:705–709.
54. Feld GF, Fleck RP, Chen P-S, et al. Radiofrequency catheter ablation for the treatment of human type I atrial flutter: Identification of a critical zone in the reentrant circuit by endocardial mapping techniques. *Circulation* 1992;86:1233–1240.
55. Schwartzman D, Callans DJ, Gottlieb CD, et al. Conduction block in the inferior vena caval-tricuspid valve isthmus: association with outcome of radiofrequency ablation of type I atrial flutter. *J Am Coll Cardiol* 1996;28:1519–1531.
56. Cauchemez B, Haïssaguerre M, Fischer B, et al. Electrophysiological effects of catheter ablation of inferior vena cava-tricuspid annulus isthmus in common atrial flutter. *Circulation* 1996;93:284–294.
57. Poty H, Abdel Aziz A, et al. Radiofrequency catheter ablation of type I atrial flutter: p0rediction of late success by electrophysiological criteria. *Circulation* 1995;92:1389–1392.
58. Schlüter M, Gursoy S, Kuck KH. Recurrence after radiofrequency current catheter ablation of accessory AV pathways [abstract]. *Eur Heart J* 1992;13:441.
59. Wittkampf FHM, Simmers TA, Hauer RNW. Repeated radiofrequency catheter ablation: Effect of a bonus pulse on myocardial temperature [abstract]. *Eur Heart J* 1993;14:256.
60. Walker KW, Silka MJ, Haupt D, et al. Use of adenosine to identify patients at risk for recurrence of accessory pathway conduction after initially successful radiofrequency catheter ablation. *PACE* 1995;18:441–446.
61. Keim S, Curtis AB, Belardinelli L, et al. Adenosine-induced AV block: a rapid and reliable method to assess surgical and radiofrequency catheter ablation of accessory AV pathways. *J Am Coll Cardiol* 1992;19:1005–1012.
62. Leitch JW, Klein GJ, Yee R, et al. Does delayed loss of preexcitation after unsuccessful radiofrequency catheter ablation of accessory pathways result in permanent cure? *Am J Cardiol* 1992;70:830–832.
63. Wagshal AB, Pires LA, Mittleman RS, et al. Early recurrence of accessory pathways after radiofrequency ablation does not preclude long-term cure. *Am J Cardiol* 1993;72:843–846.
64. Langberg JJ, Borganelli SM, Kalbfleisch SJ, et al. Delayed effects of radiofrequency energy on accessory AV connections. *PACE* 1993;16:1001–1005.

65. Dick M II, Dorostkar PC, Serwer G, et al. Delayed response to radiofrequency ablation of accessory connections. *PACE* 1993;16:2143–2145.

66. Stein KM, Lerman BB. Delayed success following radiofrequency catheter ablation. *PACE* 1993;16:698–701.

67. Fenelon G, Brugada P. Delayed effects of radiofrequency energy: mechanisms and clinical implications. *PACE* 1996;19:484–489.

68. Klein LS, Shih HT, Hackett FK, et al. Radiofrequency catheter ablation of ventricular tachycardia in patients without structural heart disease. *Circulation* 1992;85:1666–1674.

69. Delacey WA, Nath S, Haines DE, et al. Adenosine and verapamil-sensitive ventricular tachycardia originating from the left ventricle: radiofrequency catheter ablation. *PACE* 1992;15:2240–2244.

70. Nath S, Whayne JG, Kaul S, et al. Effects of radiofrequency catheter ablation on regional myocardial blood flow: possible mechanism for late electrophysiological outcome. *Circulation* 1994;89:2667–2672.

71. Willems S, Shenasa M, Borggrefe M, et al. Unexpected emergence of manifest preexcitation following transcatheter ablation of concealed accessory pathways. *J Cardiovasc Electrophysiol* 1993;4:467–472.

72. Kuck K-H, Friday KJ, Kunze K-P, et al. Sites of conduction block in accessory AV pathways: basis for concealed accessory pathways. *Circulation* 1990;82:407–417.

73. Goldberger J, Brooks R, Kadish A. Physiology of atypical AV junctional reentrant tachycardia occurring following radiofrequency catheter modification of the AV node. *PACE* 1992;15:2270–2282.

74. Mitrani RD, Klein LS, Hackett FK, et al. Ablation for AV node tachycardia: comparison between fast (anterior) and slow (posterior) pathway ablation. *J Am Coll Cardiol* 1993;21:432–441.

75. Ehlert FA, Goldberger JJ, Brooks R, et al. Persistent inappropriate sinus tachycardia after radiofrequency current catheter modification of the AV node. *PACE* 1992;16:1645–1649.

76. Skeberis V, Simonis F, Tsakonas K, et al. Inappropriate sinus tachycardia following radiofrequency ablation of AV nodal tachycardia: incidence and clinical significance. *PACE* 1994;17:924–927.

77. Madrid AH, Mestre JL, Moco C, et al. Heart rate variability and inappropriate sinus tachycardia after catheter ablation of supraventricular tachycardia. *Eur Heart J* 1995;16:1637–1640.

78. Kocovic DZ, Harada T, Shea JB, et al. Alterations of heart rate and of heart rate variability after radiofrequency catheter ablation of supraventricular tachycardia: delineation of parasympathetic pathways in the human heart. *Circulation* 1993;88:1671–1681.

79. Randall WC, Ardell JL. Nervous control of the heart: anatomy and pathophysiology. In: Zipes D, Jalife, J, eds. *Cardiac Electrophysiology: From Cell to Bedside.* Philadelphia, PA: WB Saunders Co., 1990. pp 291–300.

80. Lazzara R, Scherlag BJ, Robinson MJ, et al. Selective in situ parasympathetic control of the canine sinoatrial and AV nodes. *Circ Res* 1973; 49:48–57.

81. Ardell JL, Randall WC. Selective vagal innervation of sinoatrial and AV nodes in canine heart. *Am J Physiol* 1986;20:H764–H773.

82. Kaye MP, Hageman GR, Randall WC. Selective parasympathectomy of the heart. *J Appl Physiol* 1975;38:183–186.

83. Lee MA, Morady F, Kadish A, et al. Catheter modification of the AV junction with radiofrequency energy for control of AV nodal reentry tachycardia. *Circulation* 1991;83:827–835.

84. Strickberger SA, Daoud E, Niebauer M, et al. Effects of partial and complete ablation of the slow pathway on fast pathway properties in patients with AV nodal reentrant tachycardia. *J Cardiovasc Electrophysiol* 1994;5: 645–649.

85. Natale A, Klein G, Yee R, et al. Shortening of fast pathway refractoriness after slow pathway ablation: effects of autonomic blockade. *Circulation* 1994;89:1103–1108.

86. Kunze K, Schlüter M, Kuck K. Radiofrequency modulation of AV nodal conduction for treatment of AV nodal tachycardia [abstract]. *Circulation* 1989;880:II–324.

87. Goyal R, Langberg J, Kim Y, et al. Complete atrioventricular (AV) block complicating radiofrequency catheter modification of AV nodal reentrant tachycardia [abstract]. *PACE* 1991;14:658.

88. Fujimura O, Schoen J, Kuo C-S, et al. Delayed recurrence of AV block after radiofrequency ablation of AV node reentry: a word of caution. *Am Heart J* 1993;125:901–904.

89. Jentzer J, Goyal R, Williamson B, et al. Analysis of junctional ectopy during radiofrequency ablation of the slow pathway in patients with AV nodal reentry tachycardia. *Circulation* 1994;90:2820–2826.

90. Williamson B, Man KC, Daoud E, et al. Radiofrequency catheter modification of AV conduction to control the ventricular rate during atrial fibrillation. *N Engl J Med* 1994;331:910–917.

91. Thakur RK, Klein GJ, Yee R, et al. Junctional tachycardia: A useful marker during radiofrequency ablation for AV nodal reentrant tachycardia. *J Am Coll Cardiol* 1993;22:1706–1710.

92. Strickberger SA, Okishige K, Meyerovitz M, et al. Evaluation of possible long-term adverse consequences of radiofrequency ablation of accessory pathways. *Am J Cardiol* 1993;71:473–475.

93. Solomon AJ, Tracy CM, Swartz JF, et al. Effect on coronary artery anatomy of radiofrequency catheter ablation of atrial insertion sites of accessory pathways. *J Am Coll Cardiol* 1993;21:1440–1445.

94. Calkins H, Sousa J, El-Atassi R, et al. Diagnosis and cure of the Wolff-Parkinson-White syndrome or paroxysmal supraventricular tachycardias during a single electrophysiological test. *N Engl J Med* 1991;324:1612–1618.

95. Wood MA, DiMarco JP, Haines DE. Electrocardiographic abnormalities after radiofrequency catheter ablation of accessory bypass tracts in the Wolff-Parkinson-White syndrome. *Am J Cardiol* 1992;70:200–204.

96. Surawicz B. Transient T wave abnormalities after cessation of ventricular preexcitation: memory of what? *J Cardiovasc Electrophysiol* 1996;7: 51–59.

97. Poole JE, Bardy GH. Further evidence supporting the concept of T wave memory: observation in patients having undergone high-energy direct

current catheter ablation of the Wolff-Parkinson-White syndrome. *Eur Heart J* 1992;801–807.

98. Borggrefe M, Breithardt G. Ectopic atrial tachycardia after transvenous catheter ablation of a posteroseptal accessory pathway. *J Am Coll Cardiol* 1986;8:441–445.

99. Saul J, Hulse J, Walsh E. Late enlargement of radiofrequency lesions in infant lambs: implications for ablation procedures in small children. *Circulation* 1994;90:492–499.

100. Ring ME, Huang SKS, Graham AR, et al. Catheter ablation of the ventricular septum with radiofrequency energy. *Am Heart J* 1989;117:1233–1240.

101. Manolis AS, Melita-Manolis H, Vassilikos V, et al. Thrombogenicity of radiofrequency lesions: results with serial D-dimer determinations. *J Am Coll Cardiol* 1996;28:1257–1261.

102. Pires LA, Huang SKS, Wagshal AB, et al. Clinical utility of routine transthoracic echocardiographic studies after uncomplicated radiofrequency catheter ablation: a prospective multicenter study. *PACE* 1996; 19:1502–1507.

103. Greene TO, Huang SKS, Wagshal AB, et al. Cardiovascular complications after radiofrequency catheter ablation of supraventricular tachyarrhythmias. *Am J Cardiol* 1994;74:615–617.

104. Thakur RD, Klein GJ, Yee R, et al. Embolic complications after radiofrequency catheter ablation. *Am J Cardiol* 1994;74:278–279.

105. Hindricks G. The Multicentre European Radiofrequency Survey (MERFS): Complications of radiofrequency catheter ablation of arrhythmias. *Eur Heart J* 1993;14:1644–1653.

106. Scheinman MM, Evans-Bell T. Catheter ablation of the AV junction: a report of the percutaneous mapping and ablation registry. *Circulation* 1984;70:1024.

107. Perry JC, Kearney DL, Friedman RA, et al. Late ventricular arrhythmia and sudden death following direct-current catheter ablation of the AV junction. *Am J Cardiol* 1992;70:765–768.

108. Peters RHJ, Wever EFD, Hauer RNW, et al. Bradycardia dependent QT prolongation and ventricular fibrillation following catheter ablation of the AV junction with radiofrequency energy. *PACE* 1994;17:108–112.

109. Huang SKS, Wagshal AB, Mittleman RS, et al. Sudden cardiac death after complete radiofrequency catheter ablation of the AV junction: a multicenter prospective study [abstract]. *Circulation* 1994;90(II):I–335.

110. Conti JB, Mills RM Jr, Woodward DA, et al. QT dispersion is a marker for life-threatening ventricular arrhythmias after AV nodal ablation using radiofrequency energy. *Am J Cardiol* 1997;79:1412–1414.

111. Wagshal AB, Pires LA, Yong PG, et al. Usefulness of follow-up electrophysiological study and event monitoring after successful radiofrequency catheter ablation of supraventricular tachycardia. *Am J Cardiol* 1995; 75:50–52.

112. Mann DE, Kelly PA, Adler SW, et al. Palpitations occur frequently following radiofrequency catheter ablation for supraventricular tachycardia, but do not predict pathway recurrence. *PACE* 1993;16:1645–1649.

113. Chen S-A, Chiang C-E, Yang C-J, et al. Usefulness of serial follow-up electrophysiological studies in predicting late outcome of radiofrequency ablation for accessory pathways and AV nodal reentrant tachycardia. *Am Heart J* 1993;126:619–625.

114. Minich L, Snider A, Dick M II. Doppler detection of valvular regurgitation after radiofrequency ablation of accessory connections. *Am J Cardiol* 1992;70:116–118.

115. Raitt MH, Schwaegler B, Pearlman AS, et al. Development of an aortic valve mass after radiofrequency catheter ablation. *PACE* 1993;16:2064–2066.

116. Goli V, Prasad R, Hamilton K, et al. Transesophageal echocardiographic evaluation for mural thrombus following radiocatheter ablation of accessory pathways. *PACE* 1991;14:1992–1997.

117. Seifert MJ, Morady F, Calkins HG, et al. Aortic leaflet perforation during radiofrequency ablation. *PACE* 1991;14:1582–1585.

118. Lau YR, Case CL, Gillette PC, et al. Frequency of AV valve dysfunction after radiofrequency catheter ablation via the atrial approach in children. *Am J Cardiol* 1994;74:617–618.

119. Haines DE, Walker J, Whayne JG, et al. Creatine kinase is inactivated by radiofrequency catheter ablation and should not be used to accurately estimate the volume of myocardial injury [abstract]. *Circulation* 1991; 84(2):710.

120. Jordaens L, Vertongen P, Verstraeten T. Prolonged monitoring for detection of symptomatic arrhythmias after slow pathway ablation in AV nodal tachycardia. *Int J Cardiol* 1994;44:57–63.

121. Johnson TB, Varney FL Jr, Gillette PC, et al. Lack of proarrhythmia as assessed by Holter monitoring after atrial radiofrequency ablation of supraventricular tachycardia in children. *Am Heart J* 1996;132:120–124.

122. Hummel JD, Strickberger SA, Williamson BD, et al. Effect of residual slow pathway function on the time course of recurrences of AV nodal reentrant tachycardia after radiofrequency ablation of the slow pathway. *Am J Cardiol* 1995;75:628–630.

123. Chen S-A, Chaing C-E, Wu T, et al. Radiofrequency catheter ablation of common atrial flutter: comparison of electrophysiologically guided focal ablation technique and linear ablation technique. *J Am Coll Cardiol* 1996;27:860–868.

Chapter 39

Future Perspective of Radiofrequency Catheter Ablation: New Electrode Designs and Mapping Techniques

Fernando Mera, M.D., Jonathan Langberg, M.D.

Introduction

Radiofrequency energy application through a conventional catheter with a 4-millimeter distal electrode results in lesion diameters in the range of 3 to 5 millimeters.[1–4] Thee are ideally suited for interruption of atrioventricular (AV) nodal conduction and ablation of the discrete substrates mediating accessory pathway tachycardia and AV node reentry. Preliminary experience with catheter ablation of atrial fibrillation has produced considerable interest in developing new techniques and technologies for definitive treatment of this ubiquitous arrhythmia.[5–7] These efforts have increased our understanding of arrhythmia subtypes and have led to the development of new mapping and ablation tools. The purpose of this chapter is to use these recent developments to make projections regarding future capabilities and challenges of catheter ablation of atrial fibrillation.

New Mapping Technologies

During conventional procedures, mapping is usually performed by recording electrograms from the distal electrodes of the ablation catheter. The time

From Huang SKS, Wilber DJ (eds.): *Radiofrequency Catheter Ablation of Cardiac Arrhythmias: Basic Concepts and Clinical Applications,* 2nd ed. Armonk, NY: Futura Publishing Company, Inc. ©2000.

required to localize an arrhythmia substrate using this point-by-point technique is inadequate in the setting of irregular or hemodynamically unstable rhythms. Catheter-based multi-electrode arrays may speed the mapping process.[8] The ability to simultaneously record from multiple sites may also be beneficial for defining large reentry pathways (e.g., atrial reentry around a surgical scar).[9–10]

Three different multi-electrode arrays are currently in clinical use (Figure 1). These have a similar configuration, with splines arranged radially that are joined at the tip. Withdrawal of a "basket" catheter from a sheath and/or traction on a central pull wire causes the splines to bow outward and assume a spheroidal shape.

These devices can rapidly produce activation maps of the atrium and ventricle. Jenkins and coworkers[11] used a multi-electrode basket in the right atrium during sinus rhythm and induced intra-atrial reentry tachycardia. Adequate signals were observed from more than 95% of electrode pairs. Eldar et al[12] mapped ventricular tachycardia in pigs. Pacing thresholds ≤ 3 mA were found at 78% of sites and presystolic activation representing possible ablation targets was detected during 58% of the tachycardia episodes.

Preliminary clinical use of these devices has also been described. Triedman et al[9] used a 50-electrode basket in the right atrium of 8 patients with recurrent supraventricular tachycardia (SVT) after surgery for congenital heart dis-

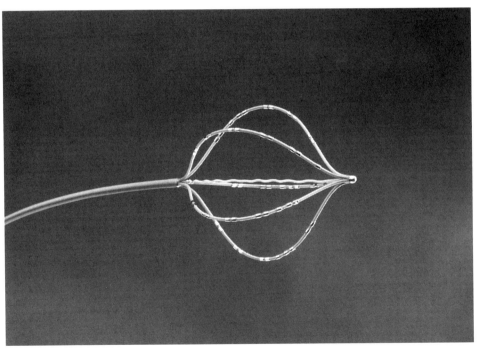

Figure 1. Multi-electrode basket catheter. Five splines are connected distally and can be contained within a sheath. Each spline has 5 pairs of electrodes as well as a marker ring for fluoroscopic identification. Traction on a central pull wire causes the splines to bow outward and assume a spheroidal shape.

ease. Detailed maps were consistently obtained and helped to define the anatomic boundaries of the reentry circuit.

Greenspon et al[13] compared the use of a multi-electrode basket catheter to standard electrode catheters during mapping of patients with atrial flutter, atrial tachycardia, reentrant SVT, and ventricular tachycardia. Comparable electrograms and pacing capture threshold were found were both approaches, and procedure durations were similar.

Although the basket catheters appear useful for rapid generation of multisite activation maps, they have a number of limitations. Variations in chamber size and geometry may impair electrode contact and distort the splines after the basket has been deployed. Manipulation of an ablation catheter within the confines of the basket is challenging and can displace the splines, resulting in a shifting, inaccurate activation map.

A novel non-contact mapping system has been devised that addresses some of the disadvantages of multi-electrode basket catheters. This device consists of a 9F shaft with an 8 millimeter ellipsoidal balloon distally (Figure 2). This is covered by an expansile 64-wire braid which, when inflated, serves as a non-contact electrode array. Virtual endocardial electrograms are reconstructed from these signals using inverse solution mathematics (boundary element method). As many as 3500 virtual electrograms can be used to create isopotential maps. A locator catheter that emits an integrated signal is used to

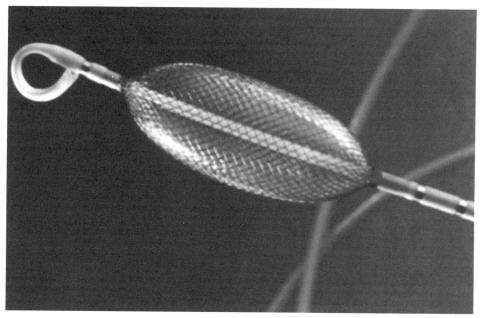

Figure 2. Catheter-mounted electrode array for non-contact mapping. The system consists of a wire braid woven onto an 8 milliliter balloon that is mounted on a 9F catheter shaft. Points of wire overlap serve as sensing electrodes. Recordings from these electrodes floating within the atrium or ventricle are used to reconstruct 2000–3000 virtual electrograms using inverse solution mathematics.

generate an anatomic map of the chamber being studied and to serve as a reference point.

Preliminary reports have described the use of this system in both the experimental and clinical laboratories.[14–16] Another study assessed the resolution of the system by applying the locator signal sequentially to adjacent electrodes with known spacing. The non-contact array measurement error averaged less than 1 millimeter, despite a distance of 3.5 centimeters between the array and the locator.[17] During left ventricular mapping in sinus rhythm,[18] isopotential maps generated from the non-contact array showed a pattern of excitation along the septum from base to apex preceding ventricular activation and consistent with conduction through the left bundle branch (Figure 3). A study in animals showed that the non-contact mapping system was able to localize a left ventricular pacing site within 9 millimeters.[19]

This technology has also been applied to mapping of human atrial flutter and ventricular tachycardia.[20,21] Schilling and coworkers recorded activation wavefronts splitting around the coronary sinus during atrial flutter in 2 of 5 patients and noted activation progressing towards the lateral tricuspid annulus from the surrounding right atrium in 4 of 5 patients.[20] These novel observations would be difficult with a single point mapping technique and suggest that the system may provide useful insights into arrhythmia mechanisms.

Several investigators have used the non-contact array during left ventricular mapping in patients with sustained monomorphic ventricular tachycardia.[21,22] Exits sites were always identifiable, but diastolic activity within the protected isthmus was less consistently seen.

This technology appears useful but is limited by complexity of both the catheter and the signal processing software. In addition, the resolution of the system is degraded by the presence of low amplitude fractionated electrograms, a frequent characteristic of ablation target sites.

A catheter-based "electroanatomic" mapping technology has shown considerable promise. This system consists of a magnetic field sensor incorporated within the tip of an electrode catheter (Figure 4). A location pad containing 3 coil electromagnets is placed beneath the fluoroscopy table. The sensor measures the intensity of each electromagnetic field. Since field strength decays in a predictable way, the distance from each source coil can be calculated, allowing precise localization of the catheter tip through triangulation. During mapping, both a roving catheter and a locatable reference catheter placed in a stable position (e.g., the right ventricular apex or a coronary sinus) are used. The location of the roving catheter is gated to a fixed point in the cardiac cycle and is recorded relative to the position of the reference catheter, thereby compensating for cardiac and respiratory motion. The roving catheter is moved across the endocardium and both electrograms and tip location are continuously displayed. Location and activation timing information from multiple sites can be compiled to form detailed isochronal activation maps (Figure 5).

Studies in animals have confirmed that the technique is accurate, with measurements being reproducible to within less than 1 millimeter.[23] Kollkamp et al used this system to identify the site of earliest ventricular activation in 6 patients with the Wolff-Parkinson-White syndrome and left-sided accessory pathways, resulting in a reduction in fluoroscopy exposure.[24]

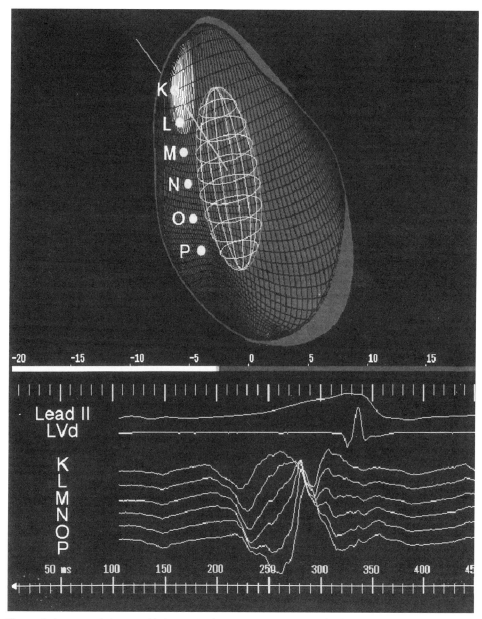

Figure 3. Isopotential map of left ventricular activation in sinus rhythm using a non-contact array. The spheroidal skeleton represents the location of the array within the left ventricle. K-P represent septal sites and their corresponding virtual electrograms. Note the early activation of sites K and L, consistent with the location of the proximal left bundle branch. See color plate.

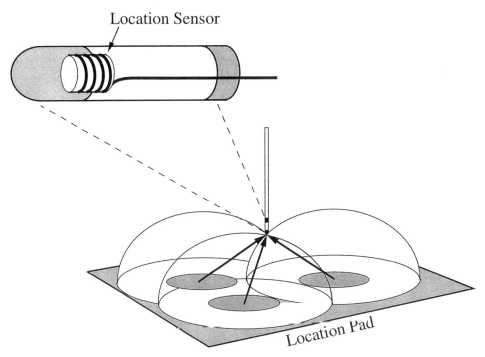

Figure 4. Electroanatomic mapping system. A location pad is placed beneath the patient during the procedure that has 3 electromagnets contained within. By measuring the intensity of each field, the location sensor in the catheter tip can be used to determine a precise position in 3 dimensions.

Preliminary experience with electroanatomic mapping systems in patients with atrial tachycardia has also been described (see Figure 5).[25,26] Right atrial activation patterns could be characterized in an average of 52 minutes. Sites of earliest and latest activity were adjacent in patients with intra-atrial reentry, but were widely separated in those with an automatic mechanism.

The reproducibility of anatomic measurements has also been used to assess the contiguity of linear lesions. Brode and coworkers created lesions between the superior and inferior vena cavae and between the inferior vena cava and the tricuspid annulus in animals.[27] The location and width of gaps in these linear lesions was clearly delineated by the mapping system, as was the presence of residual conduction across the ablation line. These observations suggest that electroanatomic mapping may be a useful adjunct for catheter Maze ablation of atrial fibrillation.

Although the electroanatomic mapping system is accurate and provides spatial information in real time, it is limited in that it is a single-point technique. The time required to generate a map precludes its use during hypotensive arrhythmias. For the same reason, even a small amount of variation in tachycardia cycle length may result in signf. cant inaccuracies of both the anatomic and activation maps.

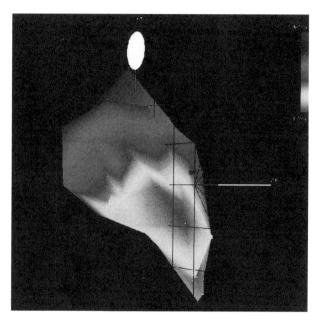

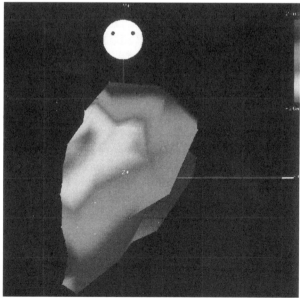

Figure 5. A. Electroanatomic map of the left ventricle during pacing of the right ventricular septum. In this right anterior oblique projection, early activation (red) is seen in the mid-septum, propagating toward the apex and anterior walls, with the lateral and poster-obasal aspects activating last. B. Left anterior oblique isochronal map of the left ventricle during sinus rhythm. As expected, earliest activation is seen in the proximal septum. See color plate.

Challenges Regarding Catheter Ablation of Atrial Fibrillation

The most exciting recent advance in cardiac electrophysiology is the development of catheter techniques to treat selected patients with drug-refractory atrial fibrillation. As described in this text and elsewhere, multiple new technologies are in development in an attempt to make catheter ablation of atrial fibrillation simple, safe, and effective. The initial trials have shown that catheter-based cure of atrial fibrillation is feasible, but have also highlighted challenges that must be addressed.[5,6,28]

Atrial fibrillation is a spectrum of abnormalities. It has been stratified by arrhythmia pattern (paroxysmal persistent or permanent) and by the influence of the autonomic nervous system (adrenergic versus cholinergic dependency). Although these clinical features offer some prognostic information, additional forms of classification will likely be useful for patients being considered for catheter ablation.

Jaïs and colleagues described a cohort of patients with "focal" atrial fibrillation.[29] These patients had little or no structural heart disease and recurrent unifocal atrial premature beats and repeated bouts of atrial tachycardia of the same morphology (Figure 6). Paroxysms of atrial fibrillation were initiated by this atrial tachyarrhythmia. The majority of patients have tachycardia foci located within the upper pulmonary vein ostia. Conventional ablation of these foci result in elimination of atrial fibrillation. These investigators and others have expanded their initial observations. Haïssaguerre et al showed that multiple premature discharges from the pulmonary vein is a common initiating mechanism of atrial fibrillation.[30] Hwang et al studied 14 patients with atrial fibrillation and frequent atrial premature contractions.[31] They, too, found that the arrhythmia originated from the region of the pulmonary veins in all patients and speculated that the automaticity arose from residual atrial tissue from within the ligament of Marshall.

Thus, it seems likely that a significant subset of patients with paroxysmal atrial fibrillation may have a focal source that initiates and maintains the arrhythmia through "fibrillatory conduction" (Figure 7). Identification of this cohort will be important both for patient and ablation target site selection.

The recognition of the importance of the pulmonary veins suggests that ablation of the vein ostia may be a useful strategy. Creation of a circumferential line of block around an ostium would prevent propagation of tachyarrhythmias into the left atrium and obviate the need for detailed mapping within the proximal vein. Swartz and coworkers have described preliminary results using a novel ablation catheter intended to produce electrical isolation of a pulmonary vein.[32] The device consists of a multilumen 8F catheter with 2 balloons. The shaft between the balloons contains a ring electrode and a perfusion lumen as well. The distal balloon is inflated within the pulmonary vein and the proximal balloon at the ostium. Saline is infused through the lumen, purging blood from the space between the 2 balloons. Radiofrequency energy is coupled to the saline via the ring electrode. The saline functions as a virtual electrode, creating a circumferential burn in the region between the 2 balloons. In a preliminary study, complete circumferential lesions were produced in the pulmonary veins in 8 of 9 pigs.

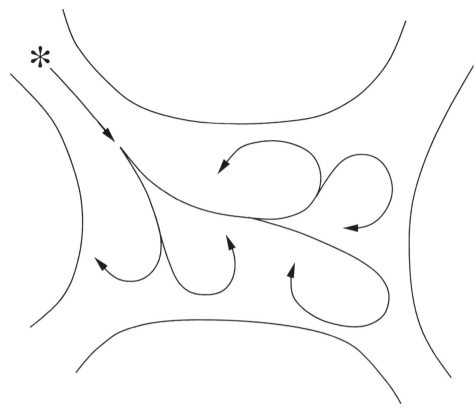

Figure 6. Diagrammatic representation of "fibrillatory conduction." A rapidly firing ectopic focus within the pulmonary vein conducts into the posterior left atrium. There, the uniform activation wavefront encounters inhomogeneously refractory tissue and fragments, resulting in multiple wavelet reentry.

Although the localized nature of this ablation strategy is attractive, it also raises concern regarding a previously unrecognized complication of ablation. Thermal injury within and adjacent to the pulmonary veins using conventional ablation catheters has produced pulmonary venous stenosis and occlusion in patients undergoing Maze ablation of atrial fibrillation.[33] Longer-term animal studies currently in progress will help to characterize this potential problem, as well as the risk for thromboembolism produced by circumferential lesions.

Although some patients with paroxysmal atrial fibrillation in the absence of structural heart disease may be treated with focal ablation, it is clear that linear Maze lesions are required for effective therapy of more severe forms of the arrhythmia. A host of new technologies for the purpose of safely creating continuous, transmural linear lesions are in development, some of which have been described in previous chapters. Determining the optimal lesion set for a given patient is a challenging problem that is just beginning to be addressed.

Initial experience with a simplified surgical Maze procedure suggests that atrial fibrillation in the setting of mitral valve disease may be treated with lesions confined to the left atrium. At the time of mitral valve replacement or re-

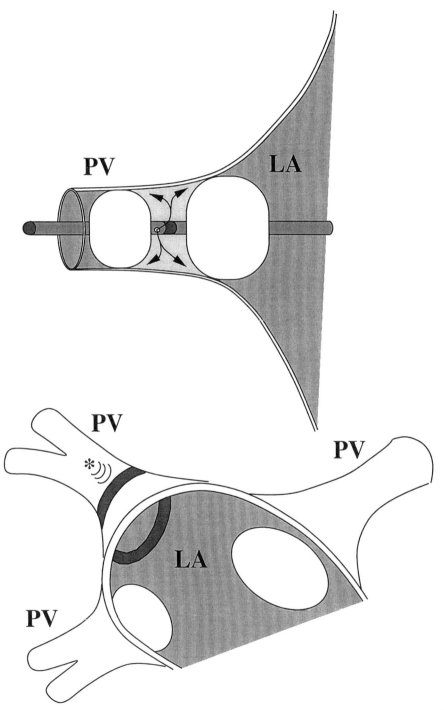

Figure 7. Catheter for creation of circumferential lesions around the pulmonary vein ostia. The catheter is inserted into the pulmonary vein and the balloon inflated. Saline is infused into the space between the balloons, purging it of blood. Radiofrequency energy is applied to the ring electrode and is conducted through the saline, which serves as a virtual electrode. A transmural circumferential burn will electrically isolate the pulmonary vein, preventing a rapidly firing focus (*) from initiating or maintaining atrial fibrillation.

pair, Sueda and coworkers[34] encircled and isolated the pulmonary veins, and connected the suture line to the posterior mitral annulus. Along with the usual left atrial appendectomy, this procedure eliminated atrial fibrillation in 31 of 36 patients (86%). As with the more conventional maze procedure, a majority (71%) of patients with a successful outcome had restoration of left atrial mechanical function.

Results of catheter Maze ablation are also consistent with posterior left atrium acting as the primary "driver" of atrial fibrillation. Haïssaguerre and coworkers[35] noted a success rate (defined as elimination of atrial fibrillation episodes without antiarrhythmic drugs) in only 13% of patients subjected to extensive linear lesions in the right atrium. The patients who went on to receive additional lesions in the left atrium had a 40% success rate. Subsequently, these investigators treated patients exclusively with left atrial lesions—2 lines joining each superior pulmonary vein to the posterior mitral annulus and 1 interconnecting them. This lesion set, which is quite similar to the incisions used by Sueda et al[34] eliminated recurrence of atrial fibrillation in 89% of patients.

The rapid progress in ablative therapy of atrial fibrillation suggests that it will emerge as an important treatment option. An increased understanding of disease subtypes will help identify suitable candidates and predict lesion sets which are likely to be effective in a given patient. Advanced mapping technology may help to identify "hot spots" requiring ablation.[36] It will also be useful for guiding proper placement of lesions and for the identification of gaps in ablation lines. Perhaps the greatest challenge will be the development of the ablation catheters themselves. Creating continuous transmural lesions over several centimeters of irregular atrial endocardium is difficult, especially when widely disparate regions of the atrium are being targeted.[37] Dragging techniques using conventional catheters are inefficient and time-consuming, even when preformed sheaths are used.[38] It is likely that new designs allowing linear lesioning without movement of the catheter will be needed to make Maze ablation practical. The safety of large areas of thermal injury in the left atrium is a critical issue. Preliminary Maze ablation trials have been complicated by embolic strokes. More efficient linear lesioning tools should reduce procedure duration and may decrease unnecessary tissue injury. Ongoing trials of these new devices will determine whether risks can be reduced.

References

1. Hoyt RH, Huang SK, Marcus FI, et al. Factors influencing transcatheter radiofrequency ablation of the myocardium. *J Appl Cardiol* 1986;1:469–486.
2. Langberg J, Lee M, Chin M, et al. Radiofrequency catheter ablation: the effect of electrode size on lesion volume in vitro. *PACE* 1990;13:1242–1248.
3. Huang SKS. New electrode catheter design for improving performance of radiofrequency catheter ablation. In: Huang SKS, ed. *Radiofrequency Catheter Ablation of Cardiac Arrhythmias.* Armonk, New York: Futura Publishing Co., Inc., 1994. pp 569–582.
4. Langberg JJ, Gallagher M, Strickberger SA, et al. Temperature-guided ra-

diofrequency catheter ablation with very large distal electrodes. *Circulation* 1993;88:245–249.

5. Haïssaguerre M, Gencel L, Fischer B, et al. Successful catheter ablation of atrial fibrillation. *J Cardiovasc Electrophysiol* 1994;5:1045–1052.

6. Swartz JF, Pellersels G, Silvers J, et al. A catheter-based curative approach to atrial fibrillation in humans [abstract]. *Circulation* 1994;90:I–335.

7. Nakagawa H, Yamanashi W, Imai S, et al. Long linear atrial lesions by radiofrequency ablation using temperature control: differences of lesion size by ablation during sinus rhythm and atrial fibrillation [abstract]. *PACE* 1997;20:1124.

8. Jenkins KJ, Colan SD, Saul JP, et al. A new catheter for rapid mapping of atrial arrhythmias during percutaneous cardiac catheterization [abstract]. *J Am Coll Cardiol* 1993;21:418A.

9. Triedman JK, Jenkins KJ, Colan SD, et al. Intra-atrial reentrant tachycardia after palliation of congenital heart disease: characterization of multiple macroreentrant circuits using fluoroscopically based-three dimensional endocardial mapping. *J Cardiovasc Electrophysiol* 1997;8:259–270.

10. Davis LM, Cooper M, Johnson DC, et al. Simultaneous 60-electrode mapping of ventricular tachycardia using percutaneous catheters. *J Am Coll Cardiol* 1994;24:709–719.

11. Jenkins KJ, Walsh EP, Colan SD, et al. Multipolar endocardial mapping of the right atrium during cardiac catherization: description of a new technique. *J Am Coll Cardiol* 1993;22:1105–1110.

12. Eldar M, Fitzpatrick AP, Ohad D, et al. Percutaneous multielectrode endocardial mapping during ventricular tachycardia in the swine model. *Circulation* 1996;94:1125–1130.

13. Greenspon AJ, Hsu SS, Haines D, et al. Endocardial mapping and ablation guided by multielectrode "basket" catheter [abstract]. *PACE* 1997;20:II–1076.

14. Schilling RJ, Peters NS, Davies DW. Non-contact mapping of human VT confirms that successful ablation sites activate late during sinus rhythm [abstract]. *J Am Coll Cardiol* 1997;29:202A.

15. Kadish A, Schilling R, Peters N, et al. Endocardial mapping of human atrial fibrillation using a novel non-contact mapping system [abstract]. *PACE* 1997;20:II–1063.

16. Kadish A, Hauck G, Beatty R, et al. Mapping of atrial activation and tachyarrhythmias using a non-contact right atrial catheter [abstract]. *J Am Coll Cardiol* 1979;29:331A.

17. Schilling R, Peters N, Davies DW. Validation of a catheter location system in the human heart [abstract]. *PACE* 1998;21:II–944.

18. Nakagawa H, Beatty G, McClelland JH, et al. New noncontact multielectrode array catheter mathematically reconstructs left bundle branch potential [abstract]. *J Am Coll Cardiol* 1996;27:75A.

19. Adler SW, Pederson BD, Budd JR, et al. Accuracy of endocardial maps using recontructed non-contact unipolar electrograms in locating specific endocardial pacing sites [abstract]. *J Am Coll Cardiol* 1996;27:75A.

20. Schilling R, Peters N, Kakish A, et al. Characterization of human atrial flutter using a novel non-contact mapping system [abstract]. *PACE* 1997;20:1055.

21. Schilling R, Peters N, Jackman W, et al. Mapping and ablation of ventricular tachycardia using a novel non-contact mapping system [abstract]. *PACE* 1997;20:1089.

22. Peters N, Jackman W, Schilling R, et al. Initial experience with mapping human endocardial activation using a novel non-contact catheter mapping system [abstract]. *PACE* 1996;19:600.

23. Gepstein L, Hayam G, Ben-Haim SA. A novel method for nonfluoroscopic catheter-based electroanatomical mapping of the heart. *Circulation* 1997;95:1611–1622.

24. Kottkamp H, Hindricks G, Brunn J, et al. Catheter ablation of left-sided accessory pathways with a new three-dimensional electromagnetic mapping technology [abstract]. *PACE* 1997;20:1121.

25. Hoffmann E, Reithmann C, Nimmermann P, et al. Electroanatomic mapping of atrial activation during atrial tachycardia [abstract]. *PACE* 1997; 20:1146.

26. Kottkamp H, Hindricks G, Brunn J, et al. Initial experience with a new 3-D electromagnetic technology for nonfluoroscopic electro-anatomical mapping and ablation [abstract]. *PACE* 1997;20:1068.

27. Brode SE, Ren J-F, Michele J, et al. Utility of the CARTO™ system for assessing conduction across linear right atrial radiofrequency lesions: correlation with lesion pathology [abstract]. *PACE* 1997;20:1076.

28. Jaïs P, Haïssaguerre M, Shah DC, et al. Efficacy and safety of linear ablation of paroxysmal atrial fibrillation in the left atrium [abstract]. *Circulation* 1997;20:1100.

29. Jaïs P, Haïssaguerre M, Shah DC, et al. A focal source of atrial fibrillation treated by discrete radiofrequency ablation. *Circulation* 1997;95:572–576.

30. Haïssaguerre M, Jaïs P, Shah DC, et al. Predominant origin of atrial panarrhythmic triggers in the pulmonary veins: a distinct electrophysiologic entity [abstract]. *PACE* 1997;20:1065.

31. Hwang C, Chen P-S. Demonstration of ligament of Marshall potential at the orifice of left superior pulmonary vein in humans [abstract]. *PACE* 1998;21:936.

32. Swartz J, Hassett BS, Bednarek M, et al. Single burn pulmonary vein isolation with a virtual circumferential electrode [abstract]. *PACE* 1998;21: 803.

33. Kay GN. Personal communication.

34. Sueda T, Nagata H, Orihashi K, et al. Efficacy of a simple left atrial procedure for chronic atrial fibrillation in mitral valve operations. *Ann Thorac Surg* 1997;63:1070–1075.

35. Haïssaguere M, Jaïs P, Shah DC, et al. Right and left atrial radiofrequency catheter therapy of paroxysmal atrial fibrillation. *J Am Coll Cardiol* 1998;7:1132–1144.

36. Kall JG, Burke MC, Verdfino R, et al. Electroanatomical mapping and ablation of focal atrial tachycardia [abstract]. *PACE* 1998;21:984.

37. Haines DE, Langberg JJ, Lesh MD, et al. Catheter ablation of atrial fibrillation using the multiple electrode catheter ablation (MECA) system: preliminary clinical trial results [abstract]. *PACE* 21:832.

Index

Page numbers in *italics* indicate figures. Page numbers followed by "t" indicate tables.

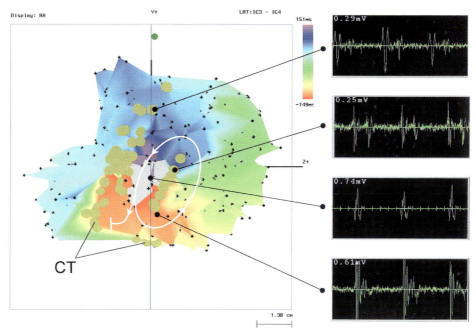

Figure 13-3. A representative electroanatomic right atrial activation map during atypical atrial flutter (410 recording sites; right lateral view). This patient had a history of inferior infarction (right coronary artery occlusion) and no prior cardiothoracic surgery. Activation sequence is color-coded with red indicating relatively early activation and purple indicating late activation (gray indicates a software solution for adjacent sites demonstrating very early and very late activation times, respectively. A line of double potentials (olive pips) was demonstrated along the expected anatomic course of the crista terminalis. An additional discrete line (approximately 1.5 cm in length) of double potentials was identified just anterosuperior to the crista terminalis. Activation was noted to occur in counterclockwise fashion around the discrete line of double potentials. Note block from the reentrant circuit to the inferior interatrial septum at the crista terminalis. The atrium located septal to the crista terminalis is activated passively (see text, Activation and Entrainment Mapping). Electrograms recorded from specific lateral right atrial sites are shown in the panels at the far right (electrogram amplitude in the upper left corner of each panel).

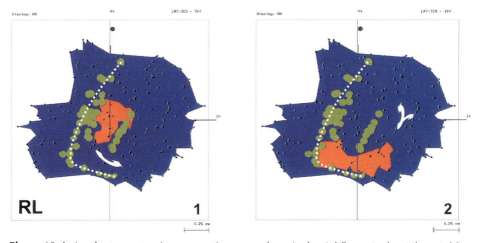

Figure 13-4. An electroanatomic propagation map of atypical atrial flutter in the right atrial free wall (right lateral view). The same tachycardia is depicted in Figure 3. Locations of double potentials are represented by olive pips. The activation wavefront (red) is observed to rotate(arrows) within a midlateral right atrial reentrant circuit in counterlockwise fashion around

(continued)

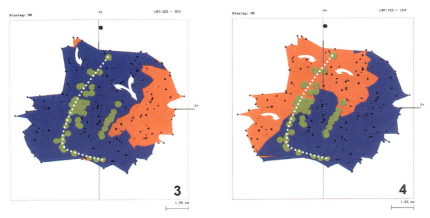

Figure 13-4. (*continued*) a discrete central line of double potentials located approximately 2 cm anterior to the crista terminalis (broken white line). Note late (passive) activation of portions of the right atrium (including the interatrial septum) posterior and septal to the crista terminalis. Clockwise rotation around a central line of double potentials in the midlateral free wall was demonstrated with electroanatomic mapping in 2 additional patients.

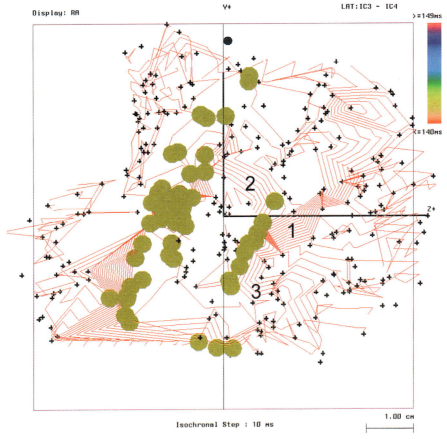

Figure 13-5. An electroanatomic isochronal map of atypical atrial flutter in the right atrial free wall (right lateral view; same patient as in Figure 3). Note crowding of the 10 ms isochrones at several sites (sites 1, 2, and 3) indicating multiple discrete areas of slow conduction (conduction velocities of <0.5 meters per second) within the reentrant circuit. The possible presence of multiple areas of slow conduction within a reentrant circuit should be considered when interpreting activation and entrainment mapping data obtained using conventional mapping techniques.

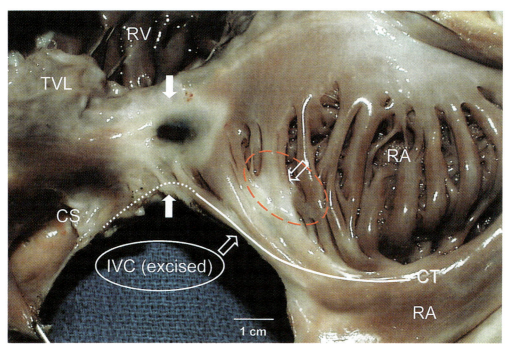

Figure 13-6. Pathological examination of the endocardial surface of the right atrium in a patient after radiofrequency ablation of both typical and right atrial free wall atypical atrial flutter. The heart was obtained following cardiac transplantation. The solid white line indicates the location of the crista terminalis and the adjoining white broken line indicates the eustachian ridge. Note the presence of a typical atrial flutter ablation lesion between the tricuspid valve annulus and the eustachian ridge (solid arrows). An additional lesion (open arrows) is present in the inferior aspect of the right atrial free wall and originates at the the inferior vena cava-right atrial junction, crosses the inferior crista terminalis, and extends into the pectinate musculature. Application of radiofrequency energy was guided using the Biosense electroanatomic mapping and catheter navigation system. Microscopic examination indicated only moderate atrial myocyte hypertrophy and mild interstitial fibrosis. No distinct scar was identified in the right atrium. The putative location of the reentrant circuit based upon analysis of the electroanatomic map superimposed on the right atrial anatomy is indicated by the red broken line. CS = coronary sinus; IVC = inferior vena cava; RA = right atrium; TVL = tricuspid valve leaflet.

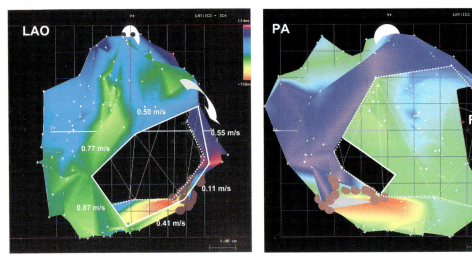

Figure 13-7. Electroanatomic activation maps of left atrial flutter. 7A: Left anterior oblique (LAO) projection. 7B: Posterior-anterior (PA) projection. The results of entrainment mapping indicated that perimitral annular sites were within the reentrant circuit. The electroanatomic map demonstrates clockwise activation around the mitral annulus (visualized best in the LAO view). An extensive electrically silent area was demonstrated in the posterior left atrium (outlined by a broken white line in each view). The electrically silent area was also present during sinus rhythm. Conduction velocities along the mitral annulus are presented in the LAO view. A region of slow conduction (conduction velocity <0.5 meters per second) was identified along the inferolateral aspect of the mitral annulus. Radiofrequency energy application from the electrically silent area to the inferolateral mitral valve annulus resulted in the termination and subsequent inability to reinduce this tachycardia. The ablation line (brown pips) along the inferolateral left atrium was documented using the Biosense mapping system. MVA = mitral valve annulus; FO = fossa ovalis; LAO = left anterior oblique view; PA = posteroanterior view; L LAT = left lateral view.

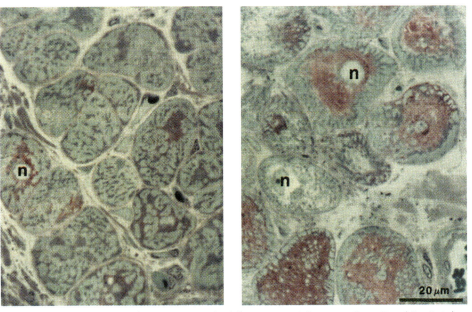

Figure 18-6. Light microscopy of sections 2 μm thick from goat atrial myocardium. Panel 1a: Atrial myocardium sections from goat in sinus rhythm with normally structured cardiomyocytes. PAS staining is almost absent in these cardiomyocytes. Sarcomeres stained with toluidine blue are present throughout cytoplasm of cardiomyocytes. Panel 1b: Section from goat in chronic AF showing severe myolysis. Central part of myocytes is free of sarcomeres and contains abundant glycogen (PAS-positive staining). Magnification × 500. n = nucleus. (From Ausma J, et al. Structural changes of atrial myocardium due to sustained AF in the goat. *Circulation* 1997;96(9):3157–3163.)

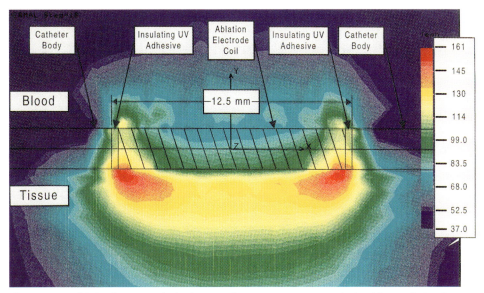

Figure 19-3. This isotherm graph depicts steady-state temperatures derived from a finite element analysis of radiofrequency ablation with a coil electrode 12 mm in length. The legend of temperatures is shown at right; the temperatures range from the physiological normal (violet = 37°C) to maximum tissue temperature (red = 161°C). In this example, the power is adjusted to maintain the temperature at the midpoint of the electrode at 70°C. In this case, tissue temperature may reach 161°C below the electrode edges, resulting in char and coagulum formation. (Reproduced with permission from *Circulation* 1997;96:4057–4064.)

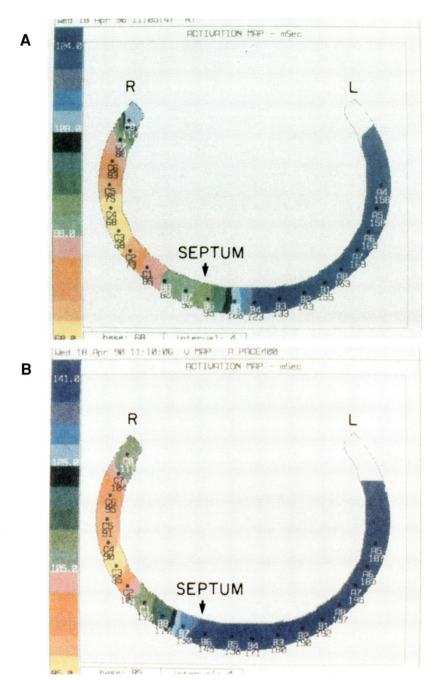

Figure 23-4. Intraoperative maps before (panels A and B) and after (panel C) surgical ablation of a right free wall accessory pathway. Maps are obtained by placing a multielectrode strip on the epicardium along the atrial or ventricular side of the mitral and tricuspid annulus intraoperatively. The strip simultaneously records electrograms extending from the left anterior region (L), the posterior septum and the right anterior region (R). Earliest activation is represented by yellow followed by orange, green, and blue as illustrated in the color scale on the left. In panel A, atrial activation is recorded during orthodromic reciprocating tachycardia. The earliest site of activation is on the right free wall. In panel B, ventricular activation is recorded during atrial pacing, showing earliest anterograde activation in the right free wall region just across the annulus from that in panel A. (*continued*)

C

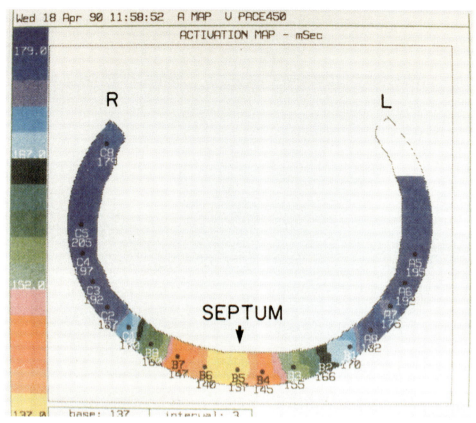

Figure 23-4. (*continued*) In panel C, post ablation, reciprocating tachycardia is no longer inducible. During ventricular pacing, earliest atrial activation is at the posterior septum.

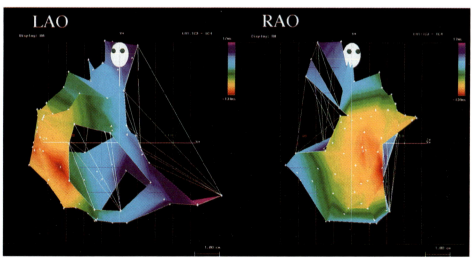

Figure 23-6. Electroanatomic mapping of the right atrium in a patient with a right free wall accessory pathway. Left anterior oblique (LAO) and right anterior oblique (RAO) projections of the right atrium are displayed during ventricular pacing. Earliest atrial activation is indicated by red, followed by yellow, green, blue, and lastly purple. In the LAO view, one can see the entirety of the tricuspid annulus, whereas in the RAO view the annulus is on the right of the image. Note that earliest atrial activation (red) during ventricular pacing is at the lateral aspect of the annulus, consistent with retrograde conduction via a right free wall accessory pathway. (Courtesy of Jeffrey E. Olgin, M.D., Indianapolis, IN.)

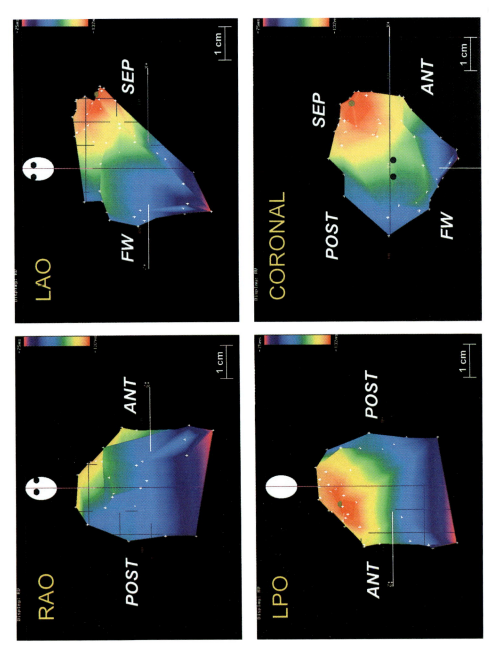

Figure 30-7. Electroanatomic map in multiple projections of the tachycardia illustrated in Figure 6. The color-coded isochrones represent activation times during tachycardia with peak QRS voltage in lead II as the fiducial point. The green dot represents the site of ablation. ANT = anterior; FW = free wall; POST = posterior; LAO = left anterior oblique (45°); LPO = left posterior oblique (45°); RAO = right anterior oblique (45°); SEP = septal.

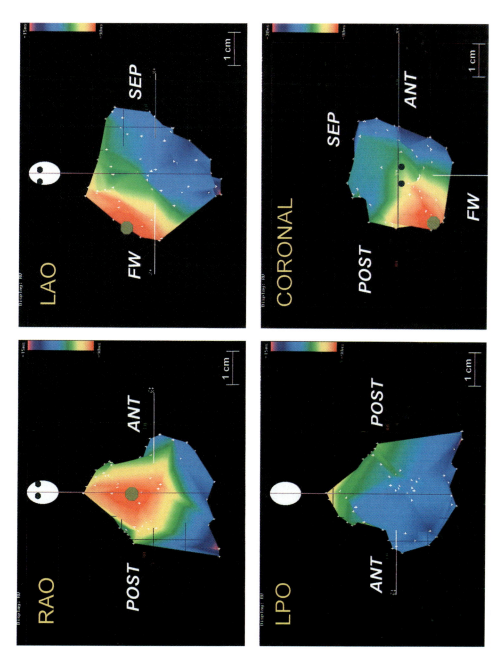

Figure 30-9. Electroanatomic map in multiple projections of the tachycardia illustrated in Figure 8. The format is the same as in Figure 7.

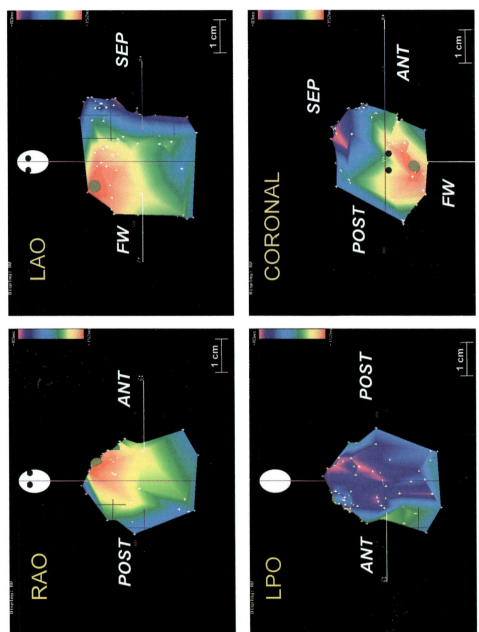

Figure 30-11. Electroanatomic map in multiple projections of the tachycardia illustrated in Figure 10. The format is the same as Figure 7.

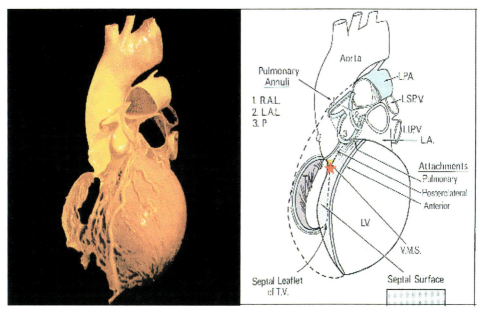

Figure 30-14. Perfusion fixed heart demonstrating the disposition of the right ventricular outflow tract in the 45° LAO imaging plane. The right ventricular free wall has been dissected free, leaving only the attachments to the septum and tricuspid and pulmonary annuli. Note that the entire septal surface of the outflow tract in this projection is to the right of the His bundle region (red star). As the imaging plane moves toward the 60° LAO, the septal surface becomes nearly perpendicular to the imaging plane, but because of the septal curvature as one moves closer to the pulmonary valve, septal points remain to the right or at most vertical to the His bundle region. LA = left atrium; LAL = left anterolateral; LIPV = left inferior pulmonary vein; LPA = left pulmonary artery; LSPV = left superior pulmonary vein; LV = left ventricle; P = posterior; R = right anterolateral; TV = tricuspid valve; VMS = ventricular membranous septum. (Adapted with permission from McAlpine WA. *The Heart and Coronary Arteries.* Berlin, Germany: Springer-Verlag, 1975. p 119.)

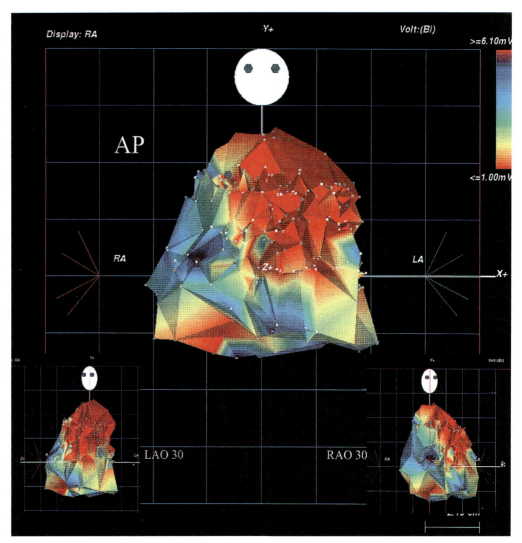

Figure 33-5. Voltage maps of the right ventricular free wall in 2 patients with idiopathic dilated cardiomyopathy. Each map displays a voltage color scale (upper right) and AP, LAO, and RAO views. The interventricular septum is not displayed. Both patients had multiple morphologies of ventricular tachycardia. (*continued*)

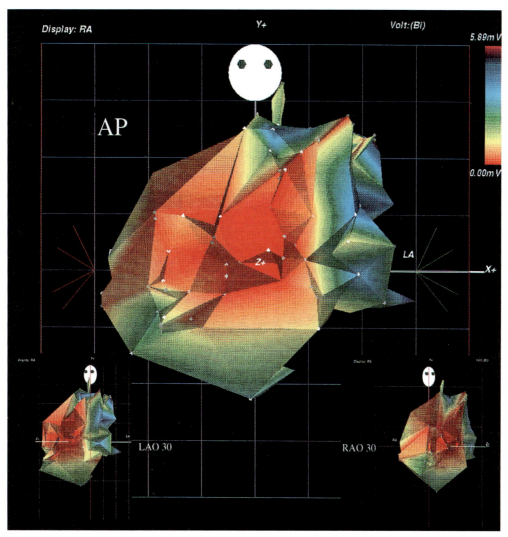

Figure 33-5. (*continued*)

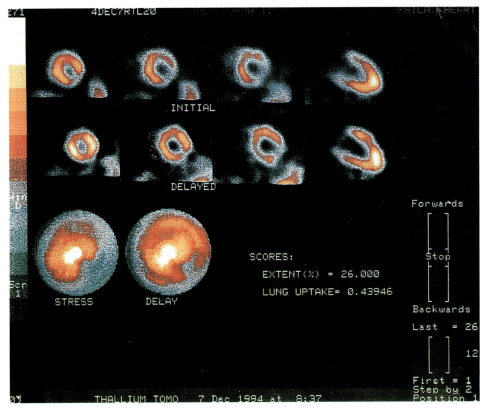

Figure 33-6. Top: Short axis and polar plot ^{201}T1 images obtained from a patient with biopsy-proven cardiac sarcoid. Note inferobasal thallium uptake defects corresponding to myocardium supplied by the left circumflex artery distribution. This patient did not have epicardial coronary disease. Bottom: Surface ECG demonstrating clinical VT from the same patient. This right bundle right superior axis VT was mapped to the endocardial surface corresponding to the thallium defect.

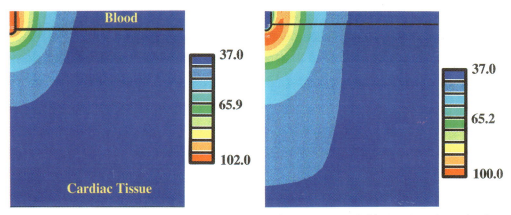

Figure 35-2. Effect of cooled RF ablation (B) compared to conventional ablation (A) as determined with finite element analysis. Conventional RF ablation (A) has the hottest temperature generated at the electrode-myocardial interface and up to 1.8 millimeters away from the catheter surface. However, during internally cooled ablation (B), the electrode-myocardial interface temperature is lowered, allowing passage of greater RF current, and generation of maximum temperatures 1.8–3.8 millimeters from the catheter surface. See text for further discussion. (Reproduced with permission from Jain MK, Wolf PD, Henriquez C.[5])

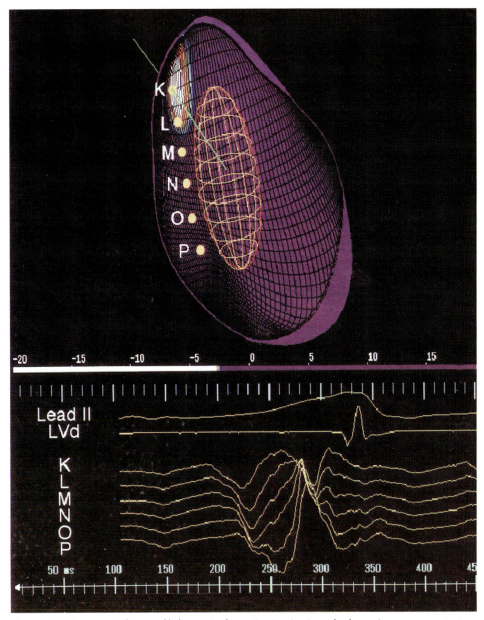

Figure 39-3. Isopotential map of left ventricular activation in sinus rhythm using a non-contact array. The spheroidal skeleton represents the location of the array within the left ventricle. K-P represent septal sites and their corresponding virtual electrograms. Note the early activation of sites K and L, consistent with the location of the proximal left bundle branch.

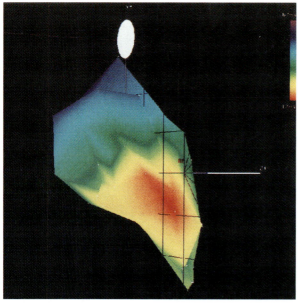

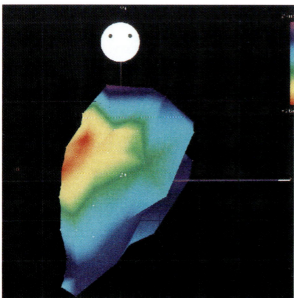

Figure 39-5. A. Electroanatomic map of the left ventricle during pacing of the right ventricular septum. In this right anterior oblique projection, early activation (red) is seen in the mid-septum, propagating toward the apex and anterior walls, with the lateral and poster-obasal aspects activating last. B. Left anterior oblique isochronal map of the left ventricle during sinus rhythm. As expected, earliest activation is seen in the proximal septum.